Computed Tomography

AF729862

Ehsan Samei • Norbert J. Pelc
Editors

Computed Tomography

Approaches, Applications, and Operations

Springer

Editors
Ehsan Samei
Department of Radiology
Duke University
Durham, NC
USA

Norbert J. Pelc
Department of Bioengineering
and Radiology
Stanford University
Stanford, CA
USA

ISBN 978-3-030-26959-3 ISBN 978-3-030-26957-9 (eBook)
https://doi.org/10.1007/978-3-030-26957-9

© Springer Nature Switzerland AG 2020
This work is subject to copyright. All rights are reserved by the Publisher, whether the whole or part of the material is concerned, specifically the rights of translation, reprinting, reuse of illustrations, recitation, broadcasting, reproduction on microfilms or in any other physical way, and transmission or information storage and retrieval, electronic adaptation, computer software, or by similar or dissimilar methodology now known or hereafter developed.
The use of general descriptive names, registered names, trademarks, service marks, etc. in this publication does not imply, even in the absence of a specific statement, that such names are exempt from the relevant protective laws and regulations and therefore free for general use.
The publisher, the authors, and the editors are safe to assume that the advice and information in this book are believed to be true and accurate at the date of publication. Neither the publisher nor the authors or the editors give a warranty, expressed or implied, with respect to the material contained herein or for any errors or omissions that may have been made. The publisher remains neutral with regard to jurisdictional claims in published maps and institutional affiliations.

This Springer imprint is published by the registered company Springer Nature Switzerland AG
The registered company address is: Gewerbestrasse 11, 6330 Cham, Switzerland

To my beautiful spouse, Maija Bell Samei
Who has patiently and admirably supported every step of our ventures
And to my amazing Mani, Mateen, Mitra, and Maryam
Who have perpetually reminded me of the gifts of newness and sheer talent
E.S.

To Lorie Pelc, who has, with love, patience, brilliance, and elegance
Shared this ride with me for 46 years and counting
To our awesome children and grandchildren
And to my parents who taught me the power of learning
N.J.P.

Foreword

The CT scanner is an amazing device, and its continuous development over the past five decades has demonstrated its important role in diagnostic medicine, image-guided intervention, and the assessment of therapeutic and surgical outcomes. To the aficionado, CT technology development has been a case study in the proverb: *necessity is the mother of innovation*. In the early days of CT, innovators sought to overcome inertial limitations of scanner design with the progression through the CT generations. Once the fundamental physics of inertia was overcome with the third-generation slip-ring gantry, the focus of CT vendors was in developing more powerful X-ray sources. With the development of multi-detector array CT (MDCT), the X-ray tube collimators could be opened, making more efficient use of the X-rays that are produced, thereby relaxing X-ray tube power requirements. With the advent of MDCT, spatial resolution and acquisition time were essentially decoupled, making higher-quality CT images and shorter scan times. Cone beam CT (CBCT) systems have taken multi-detector array CT to the extremes, with stationary table sub-second volumetric imaging on whole-body systems and many flat panel-based niche applications of CBCT in dental, orthopedic, angiographic, and others.

As image quality increased and acquisition times decreased, the clinical applications of modern CT have expanded dramatically. In particular, the shorter scan time of modern CT scanners has enabled new clinical opportunities – for example, cardiac imaging is now a routine feature on most high-end CT systems, pediatric scanning can be performed in most settings without anesthesia, and head-to-pelvis imaging can be performed easily within a breath hold. The worldwide demand for CT – approaching 100 million exams each year in the United States alone – is a demonstration of the clinical demand for information that CT images provide to physicians and their patients, and it is also a testimony to the innovation of the scientists, physicians, and engineers who have helped develop CT technology to where it is today. *Necessity was the mother of innovation.*

This new book on computed tomography (CT) represents a much-needed discussion of the many new trends that have occurred over the past decade in CT technology and will be of interest to neophytes and aficionados alike. It is an extension of a very successful categorical course offered at the annual meeting of the Radiological Society of North America, and many of the authors were participants in the course. These authors are elite scientists including several members of the national academies, former AAPM gold and silver medalists, former scientific association presidents, and former department chairs. More importantly, the authors are active research scientists, physicians, and engineers involved in advancing CT technology, applications, and clinical utility; they represent the depth and breadth of experience in the science of computed tomography and include pioneers in whole-body CT technology, early developers of cone beam CT, and international experts on CT reconstruction, perfusion imaging, photon counting detectors, multi-energy CT applications, quantitative CT imaging, radiation dosimetry, image quality assessment, CT practice optimization, and clinical utility.

Progress in CT technology and its applications continues, and this text not only describes recent advances and current research but also lays out a broad vision of where CT technology will go – and the technologies and applications which will continue to drive innovation as we enter the sixth decade of CT research, development, and clinical use – showing once again, *mater artium necessitas.*

Davis, CA, USA John M. Boone

Preface

Computed tomography (CT), as a diagnostic imaging modality, has a 50-year history. Enabled by innovation and investment by EMI from the proceeds of the extraordinary success of the The Beatles, the technology quickly found its place and became an essential tool in the mainstream of medical diagnosis. The impact was so significant that Godfrey Hounsfield and Allan Cormack were awarded the Nobel Prize in Physiology and Medicine in 1979. The success of CT was also a major driver to making radiology the high-technology field that it is today. Major developments since the earlier days of CT include helical acquisition (enabling sub-second acquisition speeds), spectral acquisition (enabling material discrimination), flux modulation (reducing radiation dose), and advanced image reconstruction (enabling notable image quality improvement). As a result, CT has become a leading medical imaging modality, thanks to its superb spatial and temporal resolution and ability to depict anatomical details with low ambiguity. New advances are extending the technology to increasingly depict physiological information. This has enabled a wide and expanding range of clinical applications.

We are most pleased to offer this book as a comprehensive and topical presentation of technological and applicational advances of CT. Penned by leading scientists, developers, and practitioners, the book not only reviews innovations in CT hardware and software but also covers methods to characterize CT performance, techniques for an effective clinical practice with high quality and safety using medical physics technique, as well as exciting and emerging functional, quantitative, and site-specific applications. The authors are leading experts on the topics. We hope the book will serve as a helpful resource for developers and users of CT in medicine, including physicians, engineers, and scientists.

Durham, NC, USA — Ehsan Samei
Palo Alto Stanford, CA, USA — Norbert J. Pelc
May 2019

Contents

Contributors

Andres Abadia, PhD Medical Physics Graduate Program, University of Florida, Gainesville, FL, USA

Samuel G. Armato III, PhD Department of Radiology, The University of Chicago, Chicago, IL, USA

Wesley E. Bolch, PhD Department of Biomedical Engineering, University of Florida, Gainesville, FL, USA

Guang-Hong Chen, PhD Department of Medical Physics and Department of Radiology, School of Medicine and Public Health, University of Wisconsin-Madison, Madison, WI, USA

Aiping Ding, PhD Clinical Imaging Physics Group, Duke University, Durham, NC, USA

André Euler, MD Institute of Diagnostic and Interventional Radiology, University Hospital Zurich, Zurich, Switzerland

Joseph J. Foy, MS Department of Radiology, The University of Chicago, Chicago, IL, USA

Maryellen L. Giger, PhD Department of Radiology, The University of Chicago, Chicago, IL, USA

Fatemeh Homayounieh, MD MGH Webster Center for Quality and Safety, Department of Imaging, Massachusetts General Hospital, Boston, MA, USA

Harvard Medical School, Boston, MA, USA

Jocelyn Hoye, BS Carl E. Ravin Advanced Imaging Laboratories (RAI Labs) and Medical Physics Graduate Program, Department of Radiology, Duke University, Durham, NC, USA

Arya Iranmanesh, MD Duke University School of Medicine, Department of Radiology, Durham, NC, USA

Mannudeep K. Kalra, MD MGH Webster Center for Quality and Safety, Department of Imaging, Massachusetts General Hospital, Boston, MA, USA

Harvard Medical School, Boston, MA, USA

Cameron Kofler, PhD Medical Physics Graduate Program, University of Florida, Gainesville, FL, USA

Nicole Lafata, MS Clinical Imaging Physics Group, Duke University Health System, Durham, NC, USA

Ting-Yim Lee, PhD, FCCPM Imaging Program, Lawson Health Research Institute & Robarts Research Institute, Medical Biophysics, Medical Imaging and Oncology, The University of Western Ontario, London, ON, Canada

Fiona Li, BSc Medical Biophysics, The University of Western Ontario, London, ON, Canada

Ke Li, PhD Department of Medical Physics and Department of Radiology, School of Medicine and Public Health, University of Wisconsin-Madison, Madison, WI, USA

Christopher J. MacLellan, PhD Clinical Imaging Physics Group, Duke University Health System, Durham, NC, USA

Raanan Marants, BSc Medical Biophysics, The University of Western Ontario, London, ON, Canada

Daniele Marin, MD Department of Radiology, Duke University Medical Center, Durham, NC, USA

Cynthia H. McCollough, PhD Department of Radiology, Mayo Clinic, Rochester, MN, USA

Achille Mileto, MD Department of Radiology, Division of Body Imaging, University of Washington, Seattle, WA, USA

Edmond Olguin, PhD Medical Physics Graduate Program, University of Florida, Gainesville, FL, USA

Norbert J. Pelc, ScD Department of Bioengineering and Radiology, Stanford University, Stanford, CA, USA

Jonathan W. Revels, DO Department of Radiology, Division of Body and Thoracic Imaging, University of New Mexico, Albuquerque, NM, USA

Francesco Ria, PhD Clinical Imaging Physics Group, Duke University, Durham, NC, USA

Geoffrey D. Rubin, MD, FACR Duke University School of Medicine, Department of Radiology, Durham, NC, USA

Ehsan Samei, PhD Department of Radiology, Duke University, Durham, NC, USA

Sebastian Schafer, PhD Siemens Healthineers, Advanced Therapies, Madison, WI, USA

Sebastian T. Schindera, MD Institute of Radiology, Cantonal Hospital Aarau, Aarau, Switzerland

Taly Gilat Schmidt, PhD Department of Biomedical Engineering, Marquette University and Medical College of Wisconsin, Milwaukee, WI, USA

Jeffrey H. Siewerdsen, PhD Department of Biomedical Engineering, Johns Hopkins University, Baltimore, MD, USA

Ramandeep Singh, MD MGH Webster Center for Quality and Safety, Department of Imaging, Massachusetts General Hospital, Boston, MA, USA

Harvard Medical School, Boston, MA, USA

Aaron So, PhD Imaging Program, Lawson Health Research Institute, London, ON, Canada

Justin Solomon, PhD Department of Radiology, Duke University Health System, Durham, NC, USA

Charles M. Strother, MD Department of Radiology, University of Wisconsin School of Medicine and Public Health, Madison, WI, USA

Timothy P. Szczykutowicz, PhD, DABR University of Wisconsin Madison, School of Medicine and Pubic Health Department of Radiology, Madison, WI, USA

Federica Vernuccio, MD Department of Radiology, Duke University Medical Center, Durham, NC, USA

Department of Health Promotion, Mother and Child Care, Internal Medicine and Medical Specialties, University of Palermo, Palermo, Italy

Adam Wang, PhD Department of Radiology, Stanford University, Stanford, CA, USA

Dae Myoung Yang, MSc Medical Biophysics, The University of Western Ontario, London, ON, Canada

Lifeng Yu, PhD Department of Radiology, Mayo Clinic, Rochester, MN, USA

Wojciech B. Zbijewski, PhD Department of Biomedical Engineering, Johns Hopkins University, Baltimore, MD, USA

Part I

CT Systems

Fan-Beam CT Systems

1

Norbert J. Pelc

Introduction

Technology continues to advance rapidly for diagnostic computed tomography (CT) systems. One of the biggest drivers for technical improvements in CT is image quality. This includes improving speed for motion blurring and artifact immunity, improving spatial resolution for enhanced image sharpness, and improving low-contrast performance which has been a unique capability in the x-ray imaging field. In addition, development of new clinical applications also drives new technology, as does the desire for improving dose efficiency and ease of use and reducing cost.

While the early development period of clinical CT systems included a number of system architectures ("generations") and research into new measurement geometries continues [1], for many years now, all commercial diagnostic CT systems (as distinct from cone beam systems discussed in the next chapter) have used the so-called "third-generation" fan-beam measurement geometry. These are the systems discussed in this chapter. The x-ray detectors and sources used in CT systems are critical determinants of the system's performance. For this reason, in this chapter we focus on the recent advances and current development directions in x-ray sources and detectors for CT and how they relate to the performance advances discussed above.

Perhaps the strongest long-term trend in CT performance is the increase in scanning speed. Figure 1.1 shows the CT scanning speed characterized in two somewhat different ways as a function of the year the CT system was introduced. One plot shows the number of pixels that can be reconstructed from the data measured by a system divided by the time it took to acquire the data. The second plot is the number of detector samples that are measured per unit time. As can be seen, the speed of CT measured in these ways has increased essentially exponentially since the introduction of CT scanning. The improvement in speed is more than eight orders of magnitude over the past three and a half decades. These speed increases have come about through two pathways: (1) gantries that rotate faster and (2) the acquisition of multiple slices in parallel using multi-detector row CT technology. With earlier single-slice scanners, the detector was segmented in only one direction along the fan beam, whereas in multi-detector row systems, the detector is segmented in the fan-beam direction and also the slice or axial direction, allowing an improvement in speed by a factor comparable to the number of detector rows operating in parallel.

Figure 1.2 shows a plot of the minimum scan time versus the year the system was introduced. While can see a dramatic reduction in the first decade after the introduction of CT scanning, the trend has continued, albeit at a slower pace since

N. J. Pelc (✉)
Department of Bioengineering and Radiology, Stanford University, Stanford, CA, USA
e-mail: pelc@stanford.edu

© Springer Nature Switzerland AG 2020

E. Samei, N. J. Pelc (eds.), *Computed Tomography*, https://doi.org/10.1007/978-3-030-26957-9_1

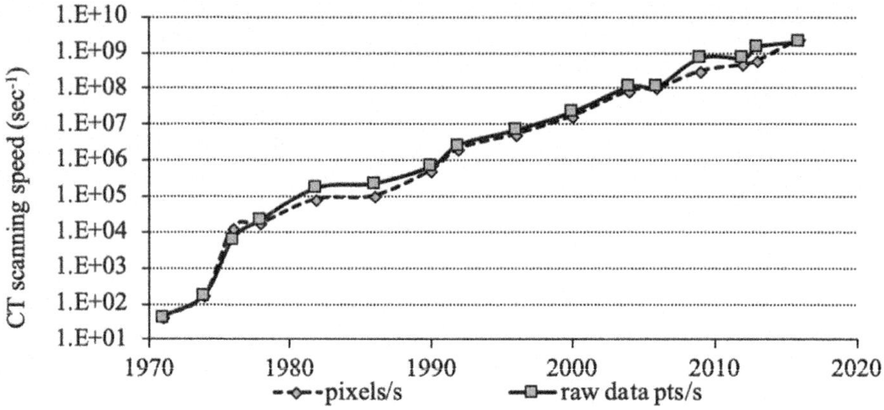

Fig. 1.1 CT scanning speed since CT was commercially introduced. (Updated from [2])

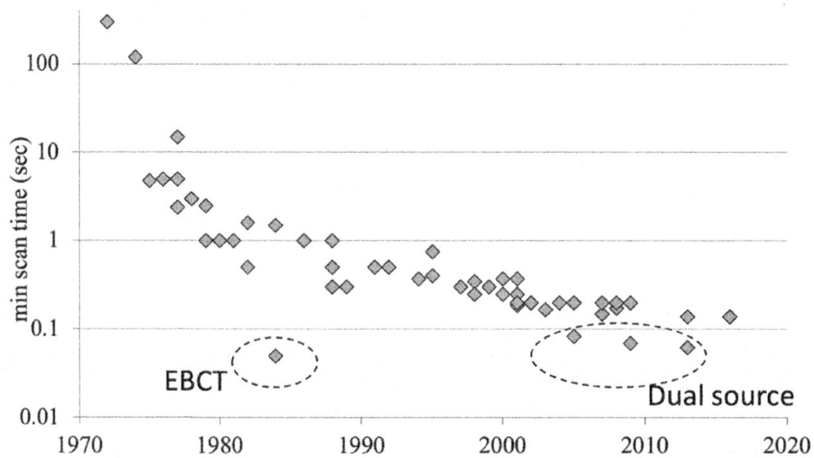

Fig. 1.2 Minimum scan time in seconds vs. year the system was introduced. (Updated from [2])

1980. There are notable outliers to the general trend – systems that are significantly faster than their cohort at the same period in time. One, in the mid-1980s, is the electron beam CT scanner [3], which didn't require any mechanical motion and, as a result, was more than an order of magnitude faster than any other scanner of its time. More recently we see the dual-source scanner configurations [4], which are a factor of two faster than others at the same period in time.

In the following sections, we discuss the impact of these and other trends on CT sources and detectors.

X-Ray Sources

Given the overall trend shown in Fig. 1.2, can we expect gantries to continue to get faster? One main limitation to further increases in gantry rotation speed is the related increase in centrifugal force on the x-ray tube, which depends on the gantry rotation speed and distance of the source from the center of rotation. Figure 1.3 shows the g-force (for Siemens systems only for simplicity of display, other vendors' systems show a similar trend) as a function of the year the system was introduced. We can observe that g-forces on x-ray

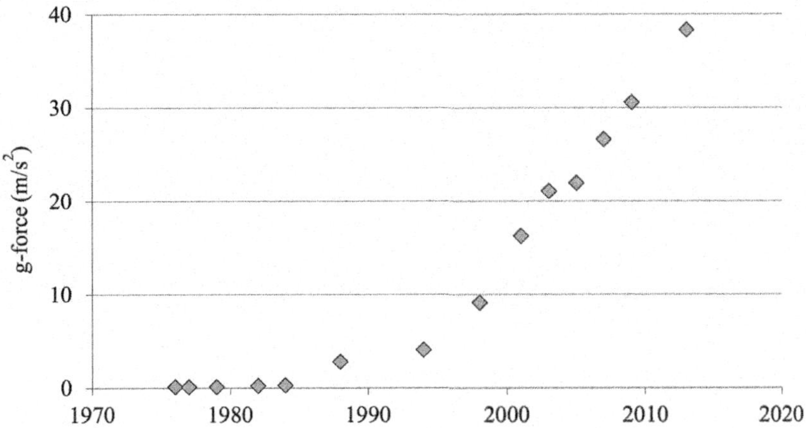

Fig. 1.3 g-force at the position of the x-ray tube since the introduction of CT. (Adapted from [2])

tubes have increased approximately linearly and, interestingly, do not show any trend to stop or slow down; it does not appear that we have reached a physical limit. This impressive increase as a function of time over the historical development of CT has been handled by more robust x-ray tubes that can handle these significant forces and also by using shorter source-to-isocenter distances so as to reduce the centrifugal force.

Another impact on x-ray tubes from the scan time reduction shown in Fig. 1.2 is that, as we shorten the scan time by reducing the gantry rotation time, we need higher tube output to maintain a consistent image noise level. This has been handled by higher-power generators, x-ray tubes that can handle higher instantaneous power, and again by shorter source-to-isocenter distances that increase the x-ray flux at the patient by the inverse-square law. Figure 1.4 shows the maximum x-ray source power since the beginning of the development of CT. We again see an increasing trend, which we expect is due to the desire to keep image noise levels reasonably constant in the face of the reduction in scan time. In fact, also shown in Fig. 1.4 is a plot the maximum x-ray tube fluence (i.e., photons per unit area, a key determinant of image noise), we see that this is essentially flat since the 1980s. From these trends, we can expect continued increase in x-ray source power and mechanical ruggedness to enable further reductions in gantry rotation time while maintaining image noise levels at their current levels.

Other drivers on CT x-ray source technology development have been the desire for lower kV and dual kV scanning, smaller x-ray tube focal spots, wider x-ray beam collimation, and focal spot deflection for aliasing reduction and spatial resolution improvement [2].

With respect to kV reduction, the contrast-to-noise ratio (CNR) at a given dose can be improved in certain cases, especially children and smaller patients, by using lower kV. As shown in Fig. 1.5, for large adults the CNR is essentially independent of the kV over the diagnostic kV range, but for smaller adults and children, the CNR can be improved by using lower kV. One of the technical difficulties with this strategy for improving dose efficiency is that when the kV is reduced, the tube current (mA) has to be increased in order to maintain a high enough dose to obtain the desired CNR, but high mA is difficult to achieve at low kV because of space charge effects in the x-ray tube [5]. Space charge limits cause x-ray tubes to have a lower peak mA at low kV, the opposite of what we need. New x-ray tubes have overcome this and have been able to achieve a much higher mA at a low kV, allowing the clinical use of lower kV. Another difficulty with achieving low kV and high mA is blooming of the x-ray tube focal spot. Generally, x-ray tube focal spots tend to get larger as the x-ray current is increased. This, too,

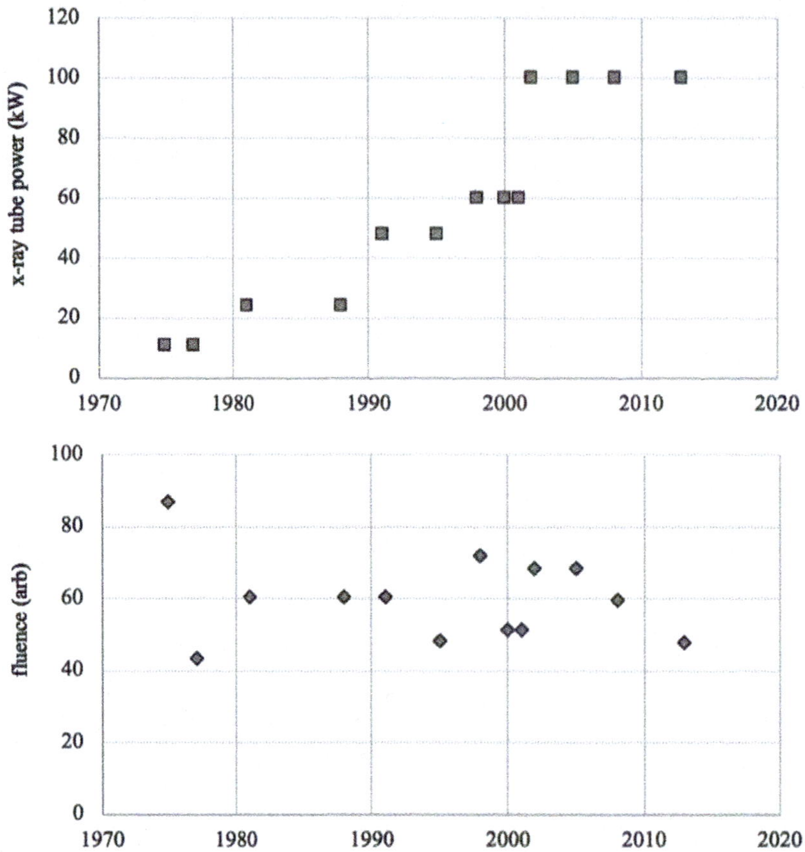

Fig. 1.4 X-ray tube power (left) and fluence at isocenter (right) since the introduction of CT. (Adapted from [2])

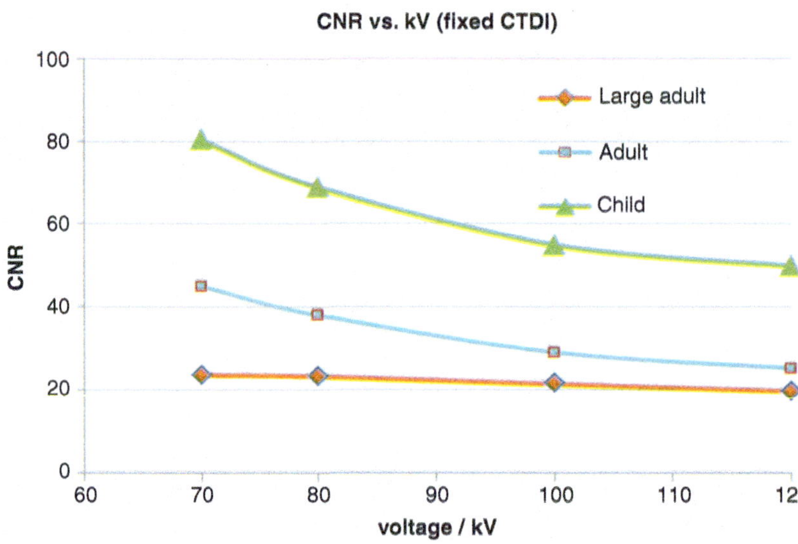

Fig. 1.5 Contrast-to-noise ratio (CNR) vs. kV at constant CTDI, showing the improvement that can be achieved with lower kV for smaller objects. (Courtesy of Thomas Flohr, Siemens Healthineers)

has been overcome by improvements in x-ray tube electron beam focusing.

Optimized filtration has also been used to improve the performance of x-ray tubes and CT systems. One area of application of advanced filtration ideas is dual kV scanning, which can be more dose efficient if the high kV beam is filtered and hardened to decrease the spectral overlap between the two x-ray beams used for spectral imaging [6]. Filtration has also been explored to achieve higher dose efficiency in a single kV imaging as well [7].

Another area of development in x-ray sources is control of the illumination of the patient by the x-ray beam to achieve optimal dose efficiency. The goal is to make sure each ray in the raw data sets has close to the optimal intensity. Two techniques already in use in clinical systems are (1) pre-patient "bowtie" filters [1] that pre-attenuate the edges of the fan beam to account for the fact that patients are more easily penetrated by the x-ray beam in those rays, whereas the center of the fan-beam is less attenuated by the pre-patient filter because that is generally aligned with thicker parts of the body, and (2) mA modulation to control the intensity of the beam at function of gantry angle to account for the fact that, in body imaging, in particular, scanned objects are more oval than round in shape [8]. However, ideally we would like to be able to personalize the intensity distribution of the beam more precisely than is allowed by mA modulation and bowtie filters. Several approaches are under development to customize the fluence illuminating the object. The digital beam attenuator [9] is comprised of wedges that move in the axial direction. The axial position determines the thickness presented to the x-ray beam, so that the ensemble of adjacent wedges produces a piecewise constant attenuation as a function of fan angle that varies continuously as a function of view angle. Another approach is the multiple aperture device [10] comprised of binary attenuators, each of which has a pattern of slits so that ray paths are either open or obstructed at a very small spatial scale. Considering the effect of the finite-sized focal spot, small displacements of each of two or more such apertures can cause a smoothly varying attenuations of the x-ray beam as a function of fan angle. A third approach is the piecewise-linear attenuator [11], which again uses wedges that move in the axial direction, but these wedges have a triangular cross section that varies in height in the axial direction, so that an array of overlapping wedges presents a piecewise-linear (rather than piecewise constant) attenuation as a function in position in the fan beam. Studies have shown that such modulators enable improved dose efficiency by a factor that depends on the object being scanned, but generally up to a factor of two compared to a conventional bowtie filter and mA modulation [11].

X-Ray Detectors

For decades, commercial CT systems have used energy-integrating x-ray detectors based on the scintillator-photodiode architecture. Each detector cell has a small polished scintillator, coated with optical reflector on five sides to prevent cross talk and coupled to a photodiode on the sixth side. The total energy of the photons detected in a sampling interval is converted into electronic charge and digitized. A major driver in technology development has been multi-detector row scanning [12–14]. Figure 1.6 shows the number of slices simultaneously acquired per rotation as a function of time in the development of CT systems. Early during the development of CT, there were several systems, including the first commercial CT scanner that acquired two slices per rotation. Other than those, all commercial CT scanners in the first two decades of clinical CT scanning were single-slice scanners. In the early 1990s, we see the introduction of new multi-detector row systems and then a very rapid increase in the number of detector rows from single digits to now hundreds of detector rows operating simultaneously. Wide-beam scanners enable scanning of an entire organ in a single rotation. This could be useful, for example, for measuring brain perfusion, imaging the entire heart in a single rotation, or pediatric applications.

For this to be useful, the x-ray beam width in the axial direction has to increase substantially. This increases the amount of scatter in the x-ray beam incident on the detectors, so that, in parallel with the development of these wide-beam systems, we have

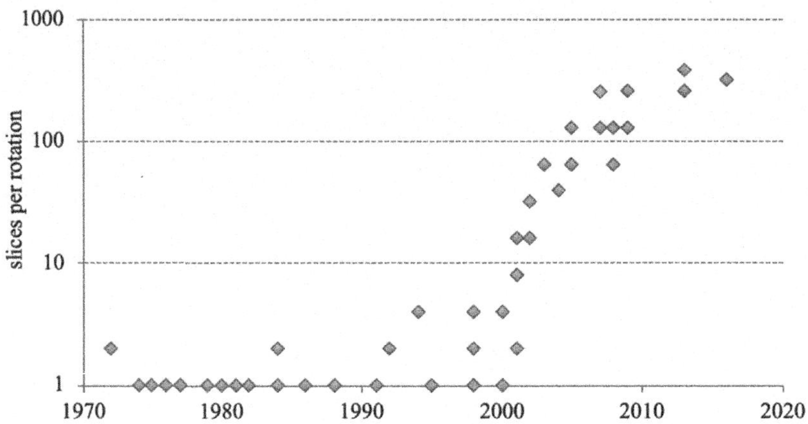

Fig. 1.6 Number of slices acquired per rotation since the introduction of CT. (Updated from [2])

seen the development of improved anti-scatter grids for CT scanners. Most wide-beam scanners have 2D anti-scatter grids with air separating the lamellae so as to not obstruct the primary beam (other than by the lamellae themselves). This significantly improves the detected scatter-to-primary ratio for wide cone beam systems, which is reduced by 50% or more depending on the object size [15].

An additional impact of the increase in gantry speed is that the x-ray detectors require faster scintillators and the sampling speed and electronic bandwidth of the detectors have had increase. Without these changes, azimuthal blurring would result [1]. These changes bring along a potential increase in electronic noise. Further driving the concern about electronic noise are the efforts to reduce radiation dose and to improve image quality when imaging obese patients, as both of these lead to reduced signal amplitude and greater degradation from electronic noise [16]. The increase in the number of detector channels has motivated efforts to improve packaging and manufacturability and to reduce the cost of each electronic channel. Figure 1.7 shows an example of the improvement in the packaging of the CT detectors and electronics. We see a significant increase in the level of circuitry integration, which brings along not only ease of manufacturing and reduced cost but, importantly, also a reduction in electronic noise due to shorter electrical leads and improved circuit designs.

Another detector engineering effort has been the development of dual-layer detectors for spectral imaging. The dual-layer detector separates the broad detected x-ray spectrum into two bands. This detector can achieve dual-energy imaging without requiring two x-ray sources [4] or rapid switching of the kV [16]. Instead, a thin front layer detects primarily low-energy photons and the thicker back layer detects the rest of the spectrum, which, because of the filtration from the front layer, has a higher average energy [17–19]. The signals from the two layers can be combined to produce a conventional CT image, while the two layers can be used separately to deliver spectral information in a single rotation, with the two spectra being perfectly aligned in space and time.

The CT detector is also a major driver of spatial resolution. Figure 1.8 (left), a plot of the detector aperture (mm^2) as a function of time since the introduction of CT, shows a reduction of a factor of about 3 since the mid-1990s, but most of this has been in the slice direction. Shown in Fig. 1.8 (right) is a plot of the in-plane detector width. As can be seen, it has been largely constant for the last 30 years or so. The reason for this lack of progress, at least in the reduction of the detector size/pitch, is the reliance on scintillator-photodiode detector architecture described above. Not only is it difficult to make the scintillators smaller but also the reflectors need to be thick enough to prevent cross talk. The reflectors lead to a reduction in geometric efficiency and make further improvements in spatial resolution more difficult. Interestingly, just in the

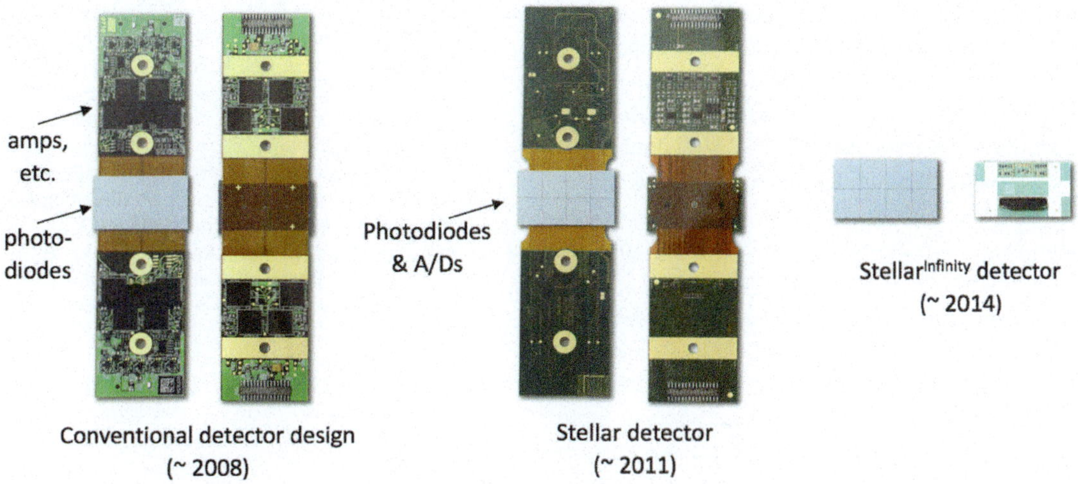

Fig. 1.7 Photographs showing the evolution of CT detector hardware, demonstrating increased integration. The smaller distance between the detector cell and its electronics helps reduce electronic noise. (Courtesy of Thomas Flohr, Siemens Healthineers)

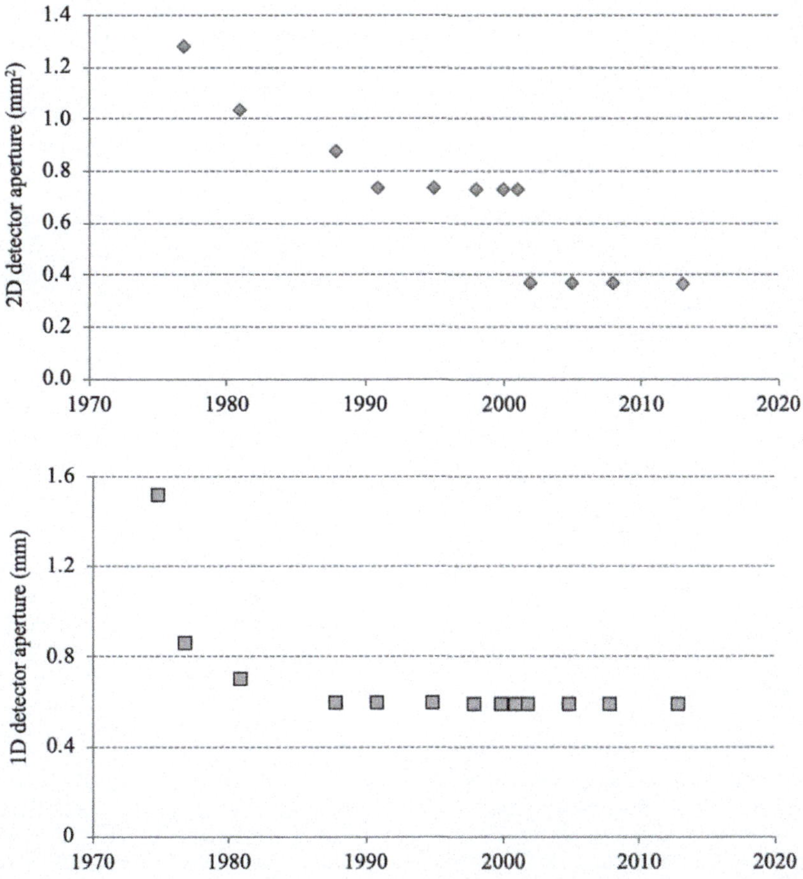

Fig. 1.8 Two-dimensional (left) and one-dimensional (right) detector aperture since the introduction of CT. Plots are for GE systems. (Adapted from [2])

past few years, a scanner has been introduced with a reduction in detector cell size of a factor of 2 in both directions [20]. This reduction in detector size is able to deliver improvement in high-contrast spatial resolution. This was done by a reduction in the scintillator size and also a reduction in the thickness of the reflector material, aiming to keep the geometric efficiency roughly the same as the previous detector.

Another area of active research and development is work toward photon-counting detectors. Instead of measuring the integrated energy in all the photons arriving in a measurement interval, these devices count individual photons and also analyze their energy. Because they count individual photons, they are less susceptible to electronic noise effects at low flux. They also promise improved spatial resolution and geometric efficiency. Photon-counting detectors and their use for spectral imaging are presented in detail in Chap. 14.

Summary

X-ray sources and detectors are key to CT system performance. Even after more than 120 years since Roentgen's discovery of x-rays, x-ray tube technology continues to advance. On the detector side, scintillator-photodiode detectors are very highly refined and continue to be the dominant technology for clinical CT. This is likely to continue for some time to come because this technology is so mature, but there is much investment and research in photon-counting detectors, which offer potential for significant improvements in spatial resolution and dose efficiency, especially at low dose, and no doubt will lead to new applications of CT.

References

1. Hsieh J. Computed tomography principles, design, artifacts, and recent advances. Bellingham: SPIE; 2003.
2. Pelc NJ. Recent and future directions in CT imaging. Ann Biomed Eng. 2014;42:260–8.
3. Lipton MJ, Higgins CB, Boyd DP. Computed tomography of the heart: evaluation of anatomy and function. JACC. 1985;5:55S–69S.
4. Flohr TG, McCollough CH, Bruder H, Petersilka M, Gruber K, Süβ C, Grasruck M, Stierstorfer K, Krauss B, Raupach R, Primak AN, Küttner A, Achenbach S, Becker C, Kopp A, Ohnesorge BM. First performance evaluation of a dual-source CT (DSCT) system. Eur Radiol. 2006;16:256–68.
5. Curry TS, Dowdey JE, Murry RC. Christensen's physics of diagnostic radiology. 4th ed. Philadelphia: Lippincott Williams and Wilkins; 1990. p. 13.
6. Primak AN, Ramirez Giraldo JC, Liu X, Yu L, McCollough CH. Improved dual-energy material discrimination for dual-source CT by means of additional spectral filtration. Med Phys. 2009;36:1359–69.
7. Angel A. Personal Communication.
8. Kalender WA, Wolf H, Suess C. Dose reduction in CT by anatomically adapted tube current modulation. II. Phantom measurements. Med Phys. 1999;26:2248–53.
9. Szczykutowicz TP, Mistretta CA. Design of a digital beam attenuation system for computed tomography: Part I. System design and simulation framework. Med Phys. 2013;40:021905.
10. Stayman JW, Mathews A, Zbijewski W, Gang G, Siewerdsen J, Kawamoto S, Blevis I, Levinson R. Fluence-field modulated x-ray CT using multiple aperture devices. Proc SPIE Int Soc Opt Eng. 2016;9783.
11. Hsieh SS, Pelc NJ. The feasibility of a piecewise-linear dynamic bowtie filter. Med Phys. 2013;40:031910.
12. Taguchi K, Aradate H. Algorithm for image reconstruction in multi-slice helical CT. Med Phys. 1998;25:550–61.
13. Hu H. Multi-slice helical CT: scan and reconstruction. Med Phys. 1999;26:5–18.
14. Klingenbeck-Regn K, Schaller S, Flohr T, Ohnesorge B, Kopp AF, Baum U. Subsecond multi-slice computed tomography: basics and applications. Eur J Radiol. 1999;31:110–24.
15. Vogtmeier G, Dorscheid R, Engel KG, Luhta R, Mattson R, Harwood B, Appleby M, Randolph B, Klinger J. Two-dimensional anti-scatter grids for computed tomography detectors. SPIE Medical Imaging. 2008.
16. Pelc NJ. Statistical aspects of digital x-ray imaging. In Fullerton GD et al., editor. Electronic imaging in medicine. AAPM Monograph 11. New York: American Institute of Physics. 1984;320–31.
17. So A, Lee TY, Imai Y, et al. Quantitative myocardial perfusion imaging using rapid kVp switch dual-energy CT: preliminary experience. J Cardiovasc Comput Tomogr. 2011;5:430–42.
18. Alvarez RE, Macovski A. Energy-selective reconstructions in X-ray computerized tomography. Phys Med Biol. 1976;21:733–44.
19. Carmi, R, Naveh, G, Altman, A. Material separation with dual-layer CT. IEEE Nuclear Sci Symp. 2005;1876–1878.
20. Onishi H, Hori M, Ota T, Nakamoto A, Osuga K, Tatsumi M, Fukui H, Tsukagoshi S, Uranishi A, Saito Y, Taniguchi A, Enchi Y, Sato K, Tomiyama N. Phantom study of In-stent restenosis at high-spatial-resolution CT. Radiology. 2018;289:255–60.

2 Cone-Beam CT Systems

Jeffrey H. Siewerdsen

Basic Principles of Cone-Beam CT

Introduction

Many works have reviewed aspects of cone-beam CT (CBCT). Basic principles are covered in textbooks by Hsieh [1], Buzug [2], Shaw [3], Brock [4], and Zhou [5]. In the following short subsections of the Introduction, we touch on the key principles and considerations of CBCT and provide references to previous sources that treat each topic in depth. The main bulk of this chapter is treated in Sect. 2, which aims to elucidate the distinctions (and commonalities) of CBCT with respect to multi-detector CT (MDCT).

Physical Configurations

The diversity of physical platforms for CBCT and their corresponding clinical applications are described by Siewerdsen and Schafer [5]. These include C-arm [6], U-arm [7], and O-arm [8] gantries and applications ranging from image-guided interventions (e.g., surgery [9], interventional radiology [10], cardiac interventions [11], and radiation therapy [7]) to diagnostic specialties (e.g., dental [12], ENT [13], breast [14], and orthopedics [15]).

J. H. Siewerdsen (✉)
Department of Biomedical Engineering, Johns Hopkins University, Baltimore, MD, USA
e-mail: jeff.siewerdsen@jhu.edu

Image Reconstruction

Methods and algorithms for CBCT image reconstruction are described in the textbooks by Hsieh [1] and Buzug [2]. The first practical, analytical algorithm for CBCT image reconstruction is commonly identified as the Feldkamp-Davis-Kress (FDK) algorithm [16]. Many variations on the FDK algorithm have emerged, but its basic principles – e.g., the cosine weighting associated with the density of rays incident on a 2D flat detector – remain the workhorse underlying algorithm for many CBCT systems. We will retread neither the analytical form nor its common algorithmic implementations here – except perhaps to add one note: CBCT system developers might consider generalization of the (1D) smoothing/apodization filter implemented to counter high-frequency ramp-filtered noise into a more symmetric 2D form (i.e., acting on both rows and columns of the detector) in the interest of more isotropic spatial resolution characteristics in the resulting 3D image reconstruction – as noted in the paper by Uneri et al. [17].

Model-based image reconstruction (MBIR) methods involving iterative optimization represent a major area of research in CBCT – offering potential benefits in image quality and dose reduction compared to FBP. Review of such methods in CBCT can be found in [4] and [18]. As with FBP, will we not retread mathematics or broad range of algorithms associated with MBIR in CBCT – nor the emerging space of deep learning approaches for 3D image reconstruction – except

© Springer Nature Switzerland AG 2020

E. Samei, N. J. Pelc (eds.), *Computed Tomography*, https://doi.org/10.1007/978-3-030-26957-9_2

perhaps to echo the sentiments underlying the work of Stayman et al. [19–21] that CBCT systems with flat-panel detectors (FPDs) and diverse source-detector orbits (e.g., noncircular orbits on a robotic C-arm) may benefit even more from MBIR than their counterparts in MDCT, which tend to feature highly optimized detectors and circular acquisition geometry; therefore, the relative benefits of MBIR may be even greater for FPD-CBCT systems.

Image Quality

The factors affecting CBCT image quality have been described in sources such as [3] and [9]. Among the most important factors are

- Characteristics associated with the detector (e.g., blur, lag, and electronic noise);
- Effects associated with the elevated levels of x-ray scatter in a broad volumetric beam (e.g., reduction of image uniformity and contrast); and
- Susceptibility to patient motion artifacts during the long (5–60 s) scan time for CBCT. Each of these areas presents important challenges motivating ongoing research

Applications

The first clinical applications of CBCT were in two very different areas. By 2000–2001, CBCT began to emerge in a variety of systems for dental imaging, as reviewed by Pauwels et al. [12]. Concurrently, CBCT for image-guided radiotherapy was developed via research led by Jaffray et al. [7]. Development of CBCT capability with fixed-room (floor- or ceiling-mounted) C-arms for 3D angiography [10] progressed rapidly from platforms based on x-ray image intensifiers (XRIIs), with FPD-CBCT C-arms becoming commonplace in interventional radiology by 2010. CBCT on mobile C-arms progressed similarly from XRII systems (e.g., the Siemens Iso-C 3D [22]) to higher-quality systems incorporating a FPD [6] and emerging in image-guided surgery on systems by Medtronic [23], Ziehm [24], and Siemens [25]. In the last decade, a number of specialty diagnostic imaging systems based on CBCT have emerged for applications beyond dental imaging. These include breast CBCT as developed by Boone et al. [14] and Ning et al. [26] and systems for musculoskeletal/orthopedic imaging [15] as evident in the Carestream Onsight 3D, Planmed Verity, and CurveBeam PedCat systems.

Overview of This Chapter

With the very brief overview of CBCT characteristics and systems provided above, the remainder of this chapter attempts to survey and clarify the distinctions and commonalities of CBCT and MDCT. For more in-depth description of algorithms, hardware, and applications, the reader is referred to the various sources mentioned above.

In the following section, we survey numerous important aspects of CBCT compared and contrasted to MDCT – the latter representing the state-of-the-art in CT imaging for diagnostic radiology. Commonalities and distinctions between CBCT and MDCT are delineated, and the considerable gray area between the two is brought somewhat into focus. As we will see, even the name associated with the technology – "cone beam" – is ambiguous and incomplete (and, in fact, incorrect) in distinguishing CBCT from MDCT. With an appreciation of the numerous factors surveyed below, it is hoped that the reader interested in CBCT – be that the physics, algorithms, dosimetry, applications, or even regulatory considerations – will be somewhat clearer, and even if a definitive distinction is not reached, the reader will at least be better able to "know it when she/he sees it" and form an educated perspective on these modalities.

Cone-Beam CT Systems

An accurate assertion: *CBCT is MDCT*. By that, we simply say that a CBCT system employs a detector with multiple rows.

An equally accurate converse: *MDCT is CBCT*. By that, we simply say that a MDCT system involves a volumetric x-ray beam with appreciable extent in the longitudinal direction.

What then – if anything – is the difference? Read on.

Genesis

A variety of CBCT systems began to emerge in the early 2000s for applications ranging from image-guided radiation therapy (IGRT) [27] and 3D angiography [28] to dental/ENT [29] and breast imaging [26]. Such developments were coincident with the independent emergence of MDCT also in the early 2000s [30], igniting the "Slice Wars" among 4-, 8-, 16-, 32-, 64-, 256-, and 320-slice scanners for diagnostic radiology and cardiology. The genesis of these two technologies was simultaneous and independent: CBCT was for the most part born to smaller scale efforts in a diversity of clinical specialty applications via academic research and entrepreneurial startup companies; meanwhile, MDCT was propelled primarily by major industry concerns (e.g., GE, Philips, Siemens, and Toshiba) sparking a revolution in diagnostic CT that advanced the modality beyond its conventional "axial mode" (single-slice) acquisition to enable faster scanning with more isotropic spatial resolution [31].

System Geometry and the (Inaccurately Named) "Cone" Beam

CBCT and MDCT systems share a variety of characteristics in system geometry – e.g., an x-ray beam divergent in and covering an appreciable extent in the longitudinal (z) direction. In this respect, it is difficult to specify a unique definition of what constitutes a "cone-beam" system, since both CBCT and MDCT systems share this aspect of broad-beam geometry. In fact, given the rectangular (vs. circular) format of the detector, "pyramid" beam is a more precise designation than "cone" beam. The basic system geometry for CBCT and MDCT is illustrated in Fig. 2.1, and Table 2.1 lists a number of characteristics of MDCT and CBCT systems, including aspects of the x-ray source, detector, image acquisition, etc. - and considerable areas of overlap between the two.

The X-Ray Source

With some exceptions (e.g., breast CBCT), both CBCT and MDCT systems tend to operate in a similar range of the diagnostic x-ray spectrum – ~80–120 kV. One typical distinction, however, is that CBCT systems tend to be implemented with a pulsed radiographic/fluoroscopic x-ray tube (with fairly limited heat capacity, pulsing at a rate up to ~30 pulses/s consistent with FPD readout rate). MDCT systems, on the other hand, are typified by continuous x-ray exposure (continuous mA) with high-performance x-ray tubes featuring high heat capacity.

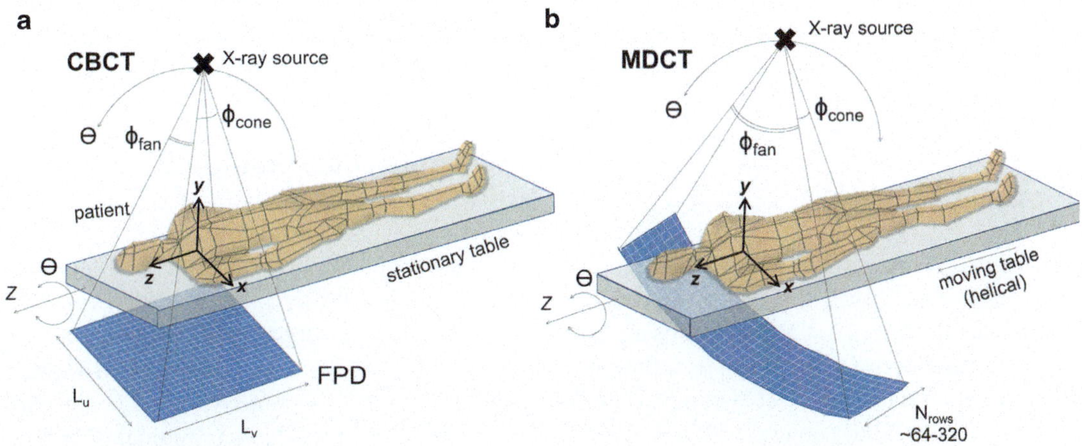

Fig. 2.1 Illustration of cone-beam system geometry. (**a**) CBCT with a flat detector. (**b**) MDCT with a curved detector. (Illustration by Nicole Chernavsky, Johns Hopkins University)

Table 2.1 Characteristics of volumetric x-ray tomography systems, with example (typical) descriptions for MDCT and CBCT systems

	Multi-detector CT (MDCT)	Cone-beam CT (CBCT)
X-ray source	High power (100–240 kW)	Lower power (3–100 kW)
	Continuous mA	Pulsed mA
Detector	64 rows (up to 320 rows)	>1024–2048 rows
	~few cm z coverage (up to 16 cm)	>20 cm z coverage
Acquisition speed	Fast (~3–5 rotations/s)	Slow (~1 rotation in 5–60 s)
	1000s of projections/rotation	100 s of projections/rotation
Orbit	Circular/helical	Circular (semicircular) or
	Fast table feed (>10–50 cm/s)	Noncircular (e.g., dual isocenter)
Image quality	Excellent bone + soft-tissue visualization	Good bone visualization
	Contrast-enhanced scan protocols	Isotropic spatial resolution
	Spectral/dual-energy capability	Modest soft-tissue contrast resolution
		Strong artifacts (scatter and motion)
Applications	Diagnostic radiology (specialty interventional systems)	Image-guided interventions (specialty diagnostic systems)

Each modality is capable of beam modulation (i.e., variation of kV and/or mA), but CBCT systems tend to incorporate such capability only in relation to the automatic exposure control of the detector (to provide a sufficient level of exposure to the detector while avoiding sensor saturation), whereas MDCT systems employ a variety of dedicated modulation schemes designed to reduce dose to the patient.

Multi-source CBCT and MDCT systems present interesting variations within each technology. In CBCT, a distribution of x-ray sources along the z axis has been shown to extend the longitudinal FOVz and reduce cone-beam artifacts [33]. In MDCT, incorporation of two x-ray tubes (and detectors) on the gantry typified the "dual-source" scanner introduced by Siemens primarily to increase temporal resolution, also permitting dual-energy MDCT [34].

The Detector

Among the characteristics that tend to distinguish CBCT and MDCT systems is the x-ray detector. As illustrated in Fig. 2.1, CBCT systems are typified by a flat detector – for example, a flat-panel detector (FPD) formed of CMOS or a-Si:H active matrix readout [25]. By contrast, MDCT systems incorporate a curved detector formed of highly optimized banks of multi-row detector modules, with a diversity of semiconductor and scintillator architectures.

Key differences in detector characteristics and performance include the following:

- For FPDs in CBCT: flat detector format, higher spatial resolution (smaller pixels), multi-mode fluoroscopy/radiography/CBCT imaging, and relatively lower cost
- For MDCT detectors: curved detector format, higher detective quantum efficiency, lower electronic noise, higher frame rate, and deeper bit depth

The distinction in flat or curved detector formats also carries a distinction in weighting factors involved in 3D filtered backprojection (FBP), as described in the textbook by Hsieh [1].

Post-Patient Collimator/Anti-scatter Grid

A broad volumetric beam is associated with high levels of x-ray scatter [35], so scatter rejection (and correction) is an important factor in the uniformity, contrast, noise, and artifact in both CBCT and (esp. 256- or 320-slice) MDCT systems. Post-patient collimation on CBCT systems typically involves a simple anti-scatter grid (usually linear) – if a grid is used at all [36, 37]. The selection of optimal grid (or gridless) configuration is an area of research within CBCT system development, usually concluding that compact CBCT systems with a very short axis-detector distance (small air gap) benefit from the use of a grid, but systems with large air gap may or may not benefit from incorporation of a grid [38]. MDCT systems, on the other hand, employ a highly optimized 2D post-patient collimation grid.

Field of View (FOV)

CBCT systems with a FPD tend to have fairly small lateral FOV, and lateral truncation (of the patient and/or table) is the norm. As illustrated in Fig. 2.1, FPDs have lateral extent (L_u) up to ~41 cm, giving axial FOV (FOV_{xy}) of ~20–25 cm, depending on system magnification. An offset detector geometry (i.e., displacing the detector laterally by up to half its width) and acquisition of projections over a full 360° orbit effectively expands FOV_{xy} to ~(40 × 40) cm^2 at the cost of sampling density and acquisition speed. A sliding or dual-isocenter approach accomplishes an analogous increase in FOV_{xy} for C-arm CBCT systems.

The FOV_{xy} for MDCT is comparatively large and typically avoids lateral truncation of the patient and table (excepting very obese subjects). An MDCT detector has lateral extent sufficient to cover FOV_{xy} ~(50 × 50) cm^2.

Table Motion

CBCT systems typically involve no table motion – i.e., the patient table is fixed, and the source and detector move in an orbit about the patient to acquire a volumetric image. Conversely, MDCT systems typically involve helical motion – i.e., longitudinal motion of the table. In some MDCT implementations (e.g., the Brainlab Airo and BodyTom), helical acquisition is accomplished via longitudinal motion of the gantry [39, 40].

Although algorithms for 3D image reconstruction in "helical CBCT" are tractable (e.g., Katsevich [41]), CBCT systems are not usually implemented for helical scanning (i.e., longitudinal motion of the patient during the scan). Rather, CBCT systems typically operate with the patient stationary on the table, and the source-detector system rotates once to acquire the volumetric image. This is advantageous in requiring only motion of the source-detector gantry (e.g., C-arm, U-arm, or O-arm gantries) and therefore carrying a comparatively simpler system configuration. It is also advantageous in clinical applications involving a complex patient setup and diversity of other systems about the patient – e.g., in surgery.

MDCT, on the other hand, is typified by helical acquisition – with exquisitely engineered tables for longitudinal translation of the patient during the scan. Even 320-slice systems will typically "cone down" to 64-slice coverage plus helical motion to acquire long volumetric scans. The volumetric 320-slice mode is used primarily for whole-organ scanning of the heart, brain, or liver.

Scan Speed

CBCT systems are typically slow. CBCT C-arms rotate up to 45 °/s, with minimum scan time around 5 s. Systems with 15, 30, or 60 s scan time are common. Such long scan times introduce strong susceptibility to artifacts arising from patient motion, as described below. With FPD readout up to ~30 fps, the number of projections acquired in a CBCT scan tends to be fairly low (~200–600 views) compared to MDCT (>1800 views).

MDCT, on the other hand, is typified by fast gantry rotation ~0.2–0.3 s per revolution – more than an order of magnitude increase in speed (per rotation) compared to CBCT. Temporal resolution down to 18–30 ms permits visualization of the beating heart, as discussed below. Susceptibility to patient motion artifacts is correspondingly low, even for helical acquisition covering an extended length of the patient, since motion-related data inconsistencies are mostly limited to the rotation interval (~0.2–0.3 s) rather than the total scan time.

The Imaging Platform and Scan Trajectory

CBCT imaging systems are often implemented in a fairly open geometry, such as a C-arm gantry or mounted on the face of a radiotherapy linac. Accordingly, CBCT systems may enjoy flexibility in scan trajectory – e.g., offset detector geometry to expand the lateral FOV; dual-isocenter (Zeego); noncircular orbit on non-isocentric C-arm (Ziehm); or noncircular orbits designed to improve sampling/image quality (Zeego task-driven orbits).

MDCT systems are typically within a closed ring gantry limited to circular (helical) orbit – the iconic donut that typifies scanners in diagnostic radiology.

Power

The power of the generator is another typical distinction between CBCT and MDCT systems. The former tend to be lower power – e.g., 3–10 kW mobile systems and up to ~200 kW fixed-room C-arm systems. The latter carry the potential for considerably higher power – e.g., up to 240 kW.

Portability

The relative simplicity and flexibility of CBCT systems is reflected in their implementation in numerous mobile systems – e.g., Ziehm, Medtronic, Siemens, Carestream Onsight, etc. That said, many fixed-room implementations exist for CBCT as well – e.g., IGRT and ceiling- or floor-mounted 3D angiography systems.

MDCT systems are typified by dedicated site installation fixed within a shielded room – the backbone of diagnostic CT in radiology. Fixed-room installation is common for MDCT, but not exclusive, and a variety of mobile MDCT systems have also been introduced – e.g., Brainlab Airo, Philips Tomoscan, and Samsung BodyTom and CereTom.

Imaging Modes

Many CBCT systems are capable of acquiring not only 3D volumetric images but also 2D radiographic or fluoroscopic images – or even tomosynthesis imaging (i.e., limited-angle CBCT) [42]. For example, mobile C-arms for image-guided surgery permit "spot-film" or fluoroscopic imaging capability, with 3D images typically acquired infrequently – e.g., at the beginning of the case for purposes of planning, at a milestone during the case to check the integrity of surgical product, or at the end of the case to validate surgical product and/or check for possible complications.

MDCT systems typically do not permit 2D fluoroscopic imaging (i.e., real-time continuous capture of a large-area 2D projection image). Rather, MDCT systems may allow "CT Fluoro" acquisition in which the patient couch is stationary, the source-detector continuously rotates within the slip-ring gantry, and axial slices (covering a relatively narrow longitudinal extent) are acquired in near real-time.

4D Imaging

4D imaging capability (i.e., a time series of 3D volumetric images) is possible in various forms for both CBCT and MDCT systems. The latter are capable of true real-time 4D imaging – i.e., acquisition of fully 3D data at acquisition rates less than 1 s, e.g., 4D MDCT of the heart with volumetric images covering 16 cm longitudinal extent acquired at real-time sampling rates up to ~5 volumes per second.

Other variations of 4D imaging can be found on both CBCT and MDCT systems. Two forms of gated acquisition (prospective and retrospective) work as follows. Prospectively gated acquisition triggers the acquisition of projection data at a particular desired phase of motion (e.g., ECG gating to trigger during diastole), providing 3D imaging of a dynamic scene with reduced motion artifact. Retrospectively gated imaging involves acquisition of projection data throughout all phases of motion and retrospective sorting of the projection data to allow 3D image reconstruction at any particular phase and/or all phases. The latter constitutes a form of 4D imaging, recognizing the difference between true real-time 4D imaging (brute force high-speed real-time volumetric data capture) and retrospectively phase-binned 4D imaging (according to monitoring of some – hopefully periodic – motion signal) to provide a 4D facsimile of (periodic) motion.

Imaging Performance: Spatial Resolution

By virtue of fairly fine pixel spacing of FPDs (typically 0.15–0.4 mm square pixels), CBCT enjoys fairly high spatial resolution in 3D image reconstructions. For FPD readout modes with isotropic pixel binning (1 × 1, 2 × 2, etc.), the spatial resolution in CBCT reconstructions can be similarly isotropic – recognizing that the choice of apodization filter [17] or other post-processing can impose non-isotropic resolution. Depending on the scan protocol and reconstruction method, CBCT images typically provide isotropic spatial resolution with a limiting resolution of ~1–2 lp/mm (minimum feature size ~0.5 mm).

MDCT systems (and certainly conventional single-slice axial CT scanners) conventionally exhibited somewhat coarser spatial resolution than CBCT, but newer detector technologies and scan protocols for MDCT have begun to erase the deficit. Depending on scan protocol and reconstruction method, MDCT systems may provide spatial resolution with limiting resolution ~0.5–1 lp/mm (minimum feature size ~0.65 mm). Emerging MDCT scanner designs push resolution limits further by incorporation of still higher-resolution detectors, for example Canon Precision CT. Higher spatial resolution can be achieved by adjustment of the scan protocol (e.g., fine helical pitch, with a proportional penalty in dose) and application of a sharp apodization filter – e.g., temporal bone scan protocols. The degree to which MDCT reconstructions are isotropic depends on the choice of helical pitch, voxel size (and slice thickness), and reconstruction method.

Imaging Performance: Contrast and Noise

Owing primarily to high levels of x-ray scatter and suboptimal post-patient collimation (anti-scatter grid, or gridless operation), CBCT systems typically exhibit lower subject contrast than MDCT. As a result, soft-tissue imaging capability presents a challenge to CBCT.

Contributing to the challenge are factors of x-ray scatter, lower DQE (quantum detection efficiency ~0.65), a relatively high level of electronic noise, and low digitization bit depth of FPDs for CBCT compared to higher performance detector systems in MDCT. This tends to result in reduced contrast resolution (e.g., contrast-to-noise ratio) for CBCT systems. Many CBCT systems are sufficient only for bone (and metal device) visualization, and soft-tissue contrast resolution is relatively poor.

Improving the soft-tissue contrast resolution of CBCT has presented an important area of ongoing research. For example, the application of MBIR to C-arm and O-arm CBCT systems for image-guided surgery has been shown to enhance soft-tissue visualization in support of soft-tissue surgeries and to provide a check on complications [17, 43]. Similarly, optimal system design was shown to provide reasonable levels of visibility of cartilage, ligament, and tendons in CBCT of the extremities [44]. A particular challenge of contrast resolution was demonstrated in the development of CBCT systems for imaging of acute stage intracranial hemorrhage, where a combination of optimal system design, protocol selection, artifact correction, and MBIR was shown to advance CBCT image quality to a level sufficient for visualization of intracranial hemorrhage [32, 45–48].

MDCT, on the other hand, enjoys a level of contrast resolution suitable to a broad range of low-contrast, soft-tissue anatomy in the brain, abdomen, and pelvis. Such capability has positioned MDCT as the front line for diagnosis for many indications, including detection or rule out of hemorrhage in emergency settings.

Imaging Performance: Artifacts Associated with the X-Ray Beam

As noted above, CBCT and MDCT systems tend to operate in a similar range of diagnostic energies (~80–120 kV) and are therefore susceptible to similar biases associated with the x-ray beam. X-ray scatter and beam hardening are two such effects, leading to shading and streak artifacts in CBCT or MDCT reconstructions.

X-ray scatter increases steeply as the longitudinal extent of the beam is increased above ~1 cm in FOV_z. For CBCT systems, the scatter-to-primary ratio (SPR) incident on the detector is often well in excess of 100% – i.e., the majority of photons incident on the detector are scatter, not primary. MDCT systems up to 64 detector rows (FOV_z ~3.2 cm) have correspondingly lower SPR. MDCT systems with 320 rows, however, experience a similar level of SPR as CBCT and therefore incorporate a highly optimized post-patient collimation (2D focused anti-scatter grid) and scatter correction algorithms to minimize scatter artifacts and maintain soft-tissue contrast resolution.

Imaging Performance: Artifacts Associated with the Detector

CBCT systems based on FPDs contend with a variety of detector characteristics that can introduce artifacts in 3D image reconstructions. Instability (drift) in detector dark current motivates frequent dark/offset correction for FPDs – e.g., collection of dark frames prior to each CBCT scan. Higher levels of image lag (~1–5%) for FPDs can also introduce lag artifacts associated with residual signal from one projection view to the next. A typical example of lag artifact is evident in the "radar artifact" visible as a crescent-shaped non-uniformity in elliptical sites (e.g., head or pelvis) as the FPD signal varies strongly from unattenuated views to heavily attenuated views.

MDCT detectors, on the other hand, tend to exhibit lower levels of image lag and drift in dark current or gain such that they are addressed via regular air calibrations. Highly optimized, modular detector technology combined with low-noise readout electronics with greater digitization bit depth than CBCT tends to minimize such artifacts.

Imaging Performance: Artifacts Associated with the System Geometry

Cone-beam projection data acquisition from a circular source-detector orbit involves incomplete sampling of the 3D object, in accordance with Tuy's condition [49]. Specifically, circular orbit CBCT sampling exhibits a "null cone" about the longitudinal (f_z) Fourier domain axis, with the angular extent of the null cone varying with spatial position in the 3D object – viz., with angular extent equal to the angle subtended between the central axial plane and a particular position within the 3D reconstruction. Therefore, only the central axial plane is fully sampled, and locations "above" or "below" the central plane (i.e., at $z \neq 0$) are subject to undersampling effects that increase with $|z|$. The effect manifests as "cone-beam artifacts" evident as shading and streaks about structures with high f_z spatial-frequency content – e.g., a horizontal edge, as might be found at a joint space oriented parallel to the plane of the source-detector orbit.

In principle, cone-beam artifacts are present for both CBCT systems and MDCT systems with a large cone angle (e.g., MDCT systems with 320 detector rows), since they arise simply as a result of incomplete sampling from a circular geometry. Helical sampling helps to mitigate the effect – as does any orbit that breaks from the axial plane, such as circle-and-line, sinusoid-on-cylinder, or double-semicircle orbits. Such orbits improve f_z sampling, reducing the null cone and mitigating cone-beam artifacts. A helical orbit introduces potential sampling effects of its own, of course, and depending on the choice of helical pitch, undersampling effects and reconstruction errors ("windmill artifacts") may be observed as streaks about high-frequency structures.

Imaging Performance: Artifacts Associated with the Subject

Biases in projection data introduced by the subject include x-ray scatter and beam hardening (as mentioned above – increasing with larger subjects with greater attenuation) as well as photon starvation (strong attenuation resulting in near-zero detector signal). The term "metal artifact" associated with highly attenuating implants, for example, refers to a combination of effects, each of which introduces bias and/or data inconsistency – namely, strong attenuation, strong shift in the transmitted polyenergetic x-ray spectrum, and high-frequency content subject to undersampling effects. Both CBCT and MDCT systems are subject to such effects.

A potentially strong source of image degradation in CBCT is patient motion during the scan – including cardiac motion, respiratory motion, peristalsis, or involuntary drift or jitter. Motion artifacts appear as blur or distortion of anatomical structures and can confound visibility of both low-contrast soft-tissue and high-contrast bone detail. For CBCT systems with long scan times (e.g., >10 s), motion effects can be especially pronounced and present a major source of image degradation.

Such effects are much less severe in MDCT for two reasons. First, the MDCT gantry rotation speed is typically very fast (e.g., ~0.2–0.3 s per rotation) so that the motion within a single rotation is minimal. Secondly, for helical MDCT, the volumetric image is acquired via fast longitudinal motion of the table, and data inconsistencies associated with patient motion tend not to reinforce within angularly sampled, backprojected data in a particular axial plane. That is not to say that MDCT is immune to patient motion artifacts – e.g., "mushroom" artifact sometimes observed in coronal planes at the dome of the diaphragm – but tend to be much less severe than in slow-scan CBCT, which enjoys neither of these two advantages.

Dosimetry

Methods for CBCT dosimetry have been described by Daly et al. [50] and Fahrig et al. [10]. Recognizing that CBCT systems typically operate without table motion, commonly employ short-scan protocols, and have a volumetric beam typically >10 cm in FOV_z, CBCT dosimetry varies somewhat from the methodology established early in the development of axial CT. Specifically, CBCT dosimetry tends to employ a small volume (e.g., 0.6 cc) Farmer ionization chamber to measure the dose (air kerma) at the center and four cardinal peripheral locations in a 16 cm diameter acrylic cylinder. The "point" dose measured at the center (D_o) and periphery (D_p) are combined in 1/3 and 2/3 proportion, respectively, to yield the "weighted" dose (D_w), analogous to $CTDI_w$ or $CTDI_{vol}$ in MDCT. For CBCT scan protocols with orbital extent less than 360° (common for C-arms), the weighted-dose D_w is estimated by 1/3 of D_o plus 2/3 of the *average* D_p measured over the four cardinal peripheral locations.

Clinical Applications

The scope of clinical applications for CBCT and MDCT is vast and is touched upon in numerous instances above. The broad variety in form and function is evident in the diversity of CBCT scanner platforms shown in Fig. 2.2.

There is considerable overlap in application space for these modalities, but a coarse distinction can be stated: CBCT finds primary application in image-guided procedures (e.g., IGRT, image-guided surgery, and interventional radiology) and secondarily in emerging areas of diagnostic specialties (e.g., CBCT of the breast or extremities) – with dental/ENT CBCT being the clear exception; conversely, MDCT is primarily applied in diagnostic radiology and is, in fact, a major frontline workhorse for diagnostic imaging in areas ranging from trauma to cancer and secondarily in image-guided interventions (e.g., portable MDCT systems or CT-on-rails for image-guided procedures). This distinction in primary areas of application is far from absolute, and it is likely to diminish altogether as CBCT systems improve in image quality and, conversely, MDCT systems increase in diversity of form and flexibility.

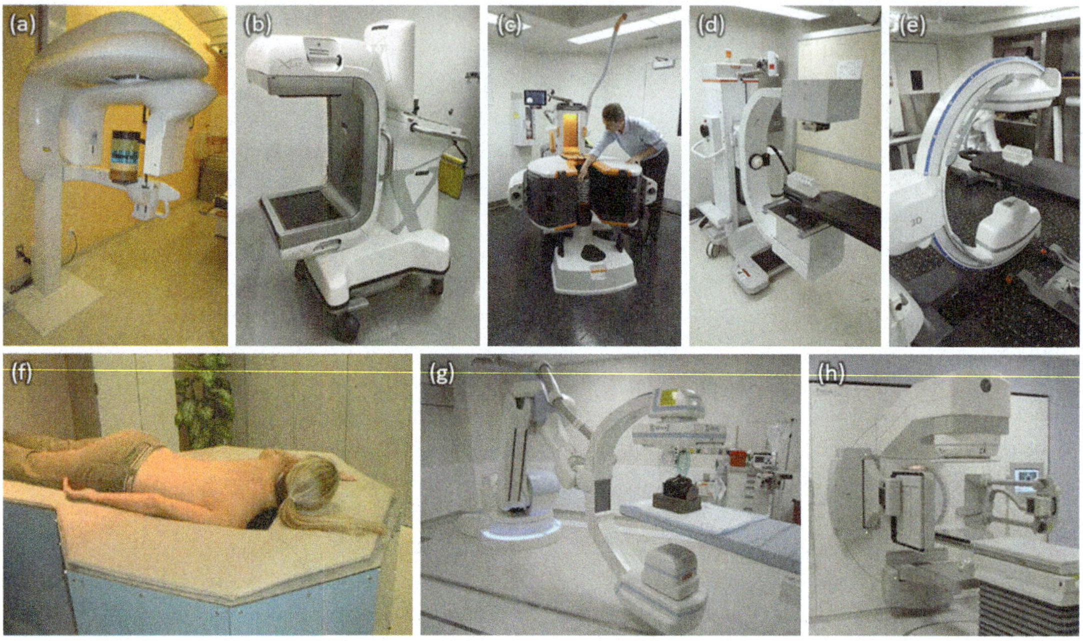

Fig. 2.2 Example CBCT systems. (**a**) CBCT for dental/ENT imaging (Carestream). (**b**) Mobile CBCT for image-guided ENT surgery. (Xoran; photo courtesy of Dr. R. Labadie, Vanderbilt University). (**c**) CBCT for imaging of musculoskeletal/orthopedic extremities (foot, ankle, knee, hand, wrist, or elbow; Carestream). (**d**) Prototype U-arm for CBCT of the head [32]. (**e**) Mobile C-arm CBCT for image-guided surgery (Siemens Healthineers). (**f**) Early prototype CBCT breast scanner. (Photograph courtesy of Dr. J. Boone, University of California – Davis). (**g**) Robotic C-arm for CBCT in interventional radiology (Siemens Healthineers). (**h**) CBCT on a radiotherapy linac for IGRT (Elekta Oncology)

Regulations and Accreditation

MDCT is subject to well-recognized regulatory requirements and accreditation standards established by the American Board of Radiology (ABR). As a result, MDCT systems are subject to well-codified standards of dosimetry, quality assurance (QA), quality control (QC), accreditation, indications for meaningful use, and charge codes.

At the time of this writing, the regulatory requirements, accreditation standards, and charge codes associated with CBCT are nascent by comparison. Recent years have seen emerging effort to establish accreditation standards appropriate to CBCT dental/ENT systems, and one may expect similar efforts in other areas of CBCT clinical application. Example efforts include ongoing Task Group activity by the American Association of Physicists in Medicine (AAPM) – e.g., TG #238 on CBCT-capable C-arms – and IEC MT39 on standards for dental CBCT.

Emerging Topics and Ongoing Research

The areas of ongoing research are as diverse as the topics delineated above, aiming to improve image quality, reduce radiation dose, and extend the application of CBCT (and MDCT) to new applications and capabilities.

Novel X-Ray Sources Research on the development of new x-ray sources for CBCT include multi-source systems. One example is the three-source system incorporated in the Carestream Onsight system for extremity imaging to extend FOV_z and reduce cone-beam sampling effects [33]. Another includes research by Boone et al. to develop breast CBCT systems featuring ~10 x-ray sources [51]. Note that these multi-source systems involve a distribution of sources along the z-axis (cf., sources distributed azimuthally as in dual-source MDCT).

New Scan Protocols Another area of active research involves modulation of the x-ray beam to reduce dose and enable region-of-interest CBCT and MDCT. Modulation of kV and mA is fairly standard. Incorporation of a bowtie filter is standard in MDCT, but less frequent in CBCT [52]. Recent research aims to develop dynamic modulation of the beam during the scan using actuated bowtie filters, multi-leaf partially attenuating collimators, and multi-aperture devices [53].

Novel Detectors and Readout Modes Development of improved x-ray detectors is similarly an active area of research. In CBCT, novel detectors aim to reduce electronic noise, increase dynamic range, and increase spatial resolution. Strategies include development of dynamic gain readout modes and new detector architectures based on CMOS [25] and architectures giving on-pixel amplification [54]. The incorporation of photon-counting detectors (PCDs) has emerged in MDCT, and photon counting with large-area detectors suitable to CBCT is an active area of research [55].

Improved Reconstruction Algorithms Novel algorithms for 3D image reconstruction present a major area of ongoing research and development. By ~2010, MBIR had emerged in mainstream use in MDCT for diagnostic radiology, offering the potential for dose reduction [56]. Parallel activities extended MBIR methods to improve image quality and/or reduce dose in CBCT [43]. Recently, deep learning-based reconstruction methods are emerging to give comparable performance to MBIR with potential advantages of reduced runtime and computational complexity [57]. Such methods, along with adaptive local filtering [58], are likely to contribute to ongoing advances in CBCT and MDCT performance.

New Scanner Platforms and Applications We can anticipate a diversification of the form and application of MDCT systems in the decade ahead not unlike the diverse spectrum of CBCT systems that emerged in their original genesis in dental, C-arm, and IGRT systems. We are already seeing such diversification of MDCT in systems such as the Brainlab Airo. As commented upon below, a diversification of form and function in MDCT with an eye to specialty diagnostic applications, image-guided interventions, and point-of-care imaging signals a vibrant space of MDCT technology development.

Accordingly, one can anticipate adaptation of MDCT to specialty systems specifically designed for diagnostic specialties, adapting to forms beyond the iconic fixed ring gantry that is so iconic of diagnostic radiology. Such specialty areas presented fertile ground for dental CBCT since ~2000 and more recent systems for breast CBCT [59–61], musculoskeletal/orthopedic CBCT [15, 62–64] and even imaging of head trauma [32, 65]. Each of these areas broke new ground in extending certain advantages of CBCT in various diagnostic specialties, but the CBCT systems that emerged carried the challenges of CBCT image quality. We can anticipate the development of specialized MDCT systems to answer the call, evidenced by systems such as MDCT breast scanner [66] and dedicated MDCT head scanner [67].

Similarly, one can anticipate the adaptation of MDCT to forms better suited to image-guided interventional procedures than the conventional fixed ring gantry. Of course, direct translation of a diagnostic CT scanner into the interventional theater has been done, but such direct translation carries a lack of integration with interventional workflow that has presented bottlenecks in patient transfer and operating room (OR) logistics. New MDCT systems specially designed for interventional procedures beckon. Key examples are the BodyTom and Brainlab Airo.

Such diversification in the form and function of CBCT and MDCT systems further emphasizes the need to knowledgeably delineate their distinctions and commonalities as surveyed in the sections above. The ruling factors of cost, workflow, and performance will weigh in what is likely to be an exciting space of technology development – and a challenge to regulatory and accreditation requirements.

Conclusions

The sections above surveyed the distinctions and commonalities among CBCT and MDCT systems, and at each turn, we found areas of overlap.

CBCT is MDCT insofar as it incorporates a detector with multiple rows. On a personal note, I recall the outbreak of the Slice Wars in the early 2000s – marveling at the excitement within the CT community of 4-, 8-, 16-, and 64-slice detectors – and a strange sense as I worked to implement volumetric imaging with a FPD involving 1024 rows. I was not entirely sure if we were onto something big, or if we were beyond the realm of what could be reasonably asked of a large-area detector and 3D image reconstruction algorithm; however, I suspected the former. Moreover, CBCT systems based on XRIIs were already emerging. Many had proven analytically the incompleteness of cone beam sampling: the bumblebee would not fly. It did.

MDCT is CBCT insofar as it employs an x-ray beam that encompasses appreciable extent in the longitudinal (z) direction. On another personal note, I recall first seeing the 256-slice MDCT detector incorporated in the Toshiba Aquilion scanner and its subsequent release as a 320-slice MDCT scanner in diagnostic radiology – and marveling at what I perceived as a quantum leap beyond the performance of FPDs that I knew well in the development of CBCT systems. I thought the technologies of MDCT and CBCT may soon completely converge – and in accordance with the distinctions and commonalities traced in the preceding sections, they had indeed converged at least in principle. Interestingly, as described above, the technological embodiments and clinical applications of MDCT and CBCT remained fairly distinct in the following decades.

The sections above quickly surveyed these distinctions and commonalities in terms of system geometry, choice of x-ray source and detector, image acquisition and reconstruction techniques, imaging modes, image quality, artifacts, dosimetry, clinical applications, and regulatory considerations. So what did we learn?

Interestingly, we see that the term "cone beam" is not only insufficient in precisely distinguishing the modalities, it is somewhat of a misnomer to begin with. Perhaps the distinction between flat and curved detectors is a salient distinction for the time being at least, suggesting a meaningful dichotomy between "flat-detector CT" (FDCT) and "curved detector CT" (CDCT). While that dichotomy may be important with respect to the weighting term in the filtered backprojection algorithm and the design of post-patient collimator, it is not likely to be a durable distinction, and we can anticipate "curved" FPDs on flexible substrates [68]. Neither is the distinction between open-geometry (e.g., C-arms) and closed-bore (e.g., donut) systems meaningful – as FPD-CBCT systems abound in closed geometries as well (e.g., Medtronic O-arm and Varian Halcyon), and we might even envision open-geometry MDCT systems in the future for interventional procedures.

There is, therefore, no absolute distinction according to the survey provided above. Nonetheless, the survey hopefully provides sufficient perspective for the reader interested in these modalities to "know it when she/he sees it" – at least within the current state of the art: CBCT systems with FPDs in open-geometry platforms widespread in image-guidance (and filling specialty niche in diagnostics) and MDCT systems with curved detectors in closed geometry scanners as the backbone of diagnostic radiology (and filling specialty niche applications in image-guided interventions). Alternatively, this chapter may at least equip the reader to speak knowledgeably within the context of technologies between which a simple distinction does not exist.

As a final note, one might anticipate that any remaining confusion between these modalities in their form, application, and capabilities may be temporary and the need to differentiate between the two may melt away. The distinctions in form and application may diminish altogether in years ahead. Advances in x-ray sources, detector technologies, and 3D image reconstruction will advance the performance of volumetric tomography systems (or more generally, "volumetric imaging" systems, since the "tomo" prefix itself is somewhat of a misnomer) and enable application across the spectrum of diagnostic and image-guided procedures described above.

The distinction may be lost from a technological standpoint, leaving the question of whether regulatory administration of volumetric imaging systems will keep up in a manner that properly reflects the spectrum of technologies.

References

1. Hsieh J. Computed tomography: principles, design, artifacts, and recent advances. Computed tomography: principles, design, artifacts, and recent advances. 2nd ed. Bellingham: SPIE; 2015.
2. Buzug TM. Computed tomography: from photon statistics to modern cone-beam CT. Berlin: Springer; 2008.
3. Shaw C, editor. Cone beam computed tomography imaging in medical diagnosis and therapy. Boca Raton: CRC; 2014.
4. Brock KK, editor. Image processing in radiation therapy imaging in medical diagnosis and therapy. Boca Raton: CRC; 2016.
5. Zhou SK, editor. Handbook of medical image computing and computer assisted intervention. Boca Raton: CRC; 2019.
6. Siewerdsen JH, Moseley DJ, Burch S, Bisland SK, Bogaards A, Wilson BC, et al. Volume CT with a flat-panel detector on a mobile, isocentric C-arm: preclinical investigation in guidance of minimally invasive surgery. Med Phys [Internet]. 2005 [cited 2014 May 27];32(1):241–254. Available from: http://www.ncbi.nlm.nih.gov/pubmed/15719975.
7. Jaffray DA, Siewerdsen JH, Wong JW, Martinez AA. Flat-panel cone-beam computed tomography for image-guided radiation therapy. Int J Radiat Oncol Biol Phys [Internet]. 2002 [cited 2014 May 27];53(5):1337–1349. Available from: http://www.ncbi.nlm.nih.gov/pubmed/12128137.
8. Uneri A, Zhang X, Stayman JW, Helm P, Osgood GM, Theodore N, et al. Advanced image registration and reconstruction using the O-arm system: dose reduction, image quality, and guidance using known-component models. In: Webster RJ, Fei B, editors. SPIE medical imaging. Houston: SPIE; 2018. p. 43.
9. Siewerdsen JH. Cone-beam CT with a flat-panel detector: from image science to image-guided surgery. Nucl Instrum Methods Phys Res A [Internet]. 2011 [cited 2014 May 27];648(S1):S241–S250. Available from: http://www.pubmedcentral.nih.gov/articlerender.fcgi?artid=3429946&tool=pmcentrez&rendertype=abstract.
10. Fahrig R, Dixon R, Payne T, Morin RL, Ganguly A, Strobel N. Dose and image quality for a cone-beam C-arm CT system. Med Phys [Internet]. 2006;33(12):4541–50. Available from: http://www.ncbi.nlm.nih.gov/pubmed/17278805.
11. Lauzier PT, Tang J, Chen G-H. Time-resolved cardiac interventional cone-beam CT reconstruction from fully truncated projections using the prior image constrained compressed sensing (PICCS) algorithm. Phys Med Biol [Internet]. 2012;57(9):2461–76. Available from: http://stacks.iop.org/0031-9155/57/i=9/a=2461?key=crossref.9bc9545e6024e4a480c719410b4ec593.
12. Pauwels R, Araki K, Siewerdsen JH, Thongvigitmanee SS. Technical aspects of dental CBCT: state of the art. Dentomaxillofacial Radiol [Internet]. 2015;44(1):20140224. Available from: http://www.birpublications.org/doi/10.1259/dmfr.20140224.
13. Xu J, Reh DD, Carey JP, Mahesh M, Siewerdsen JH. Technical assessment of a cone-beam CT scanner for otolaryngology imaging: image quality, dose, and technique protocols. Med Phys [Internet]. 2012 [cited 2014 May 27];39(8):4932–4942. Available from: http://www.ncbi.nlm.nih.gov/pubmed/22894419.
14. Boone JM, Kwan ALC, Yang K, Burkett GW, Lindfors KK, Nelson TR. Computed tomography for imaging the Breast. J Mammary Gland Biol Neoplasia [Internet]. 2006;11(2):103–11. Available from: http://link.springer.com/10.1007/s10911-006-9017-1.
15. Carrino JA, Al Muhit A, Zbijewski W, Thawait GK, Stayman JW, Packard N, et al. Dedicated cone-beam CT system for extremity imaging. Radiology [Internet]. 2014 Mar [cited 2014 May 27];270(3):816–824. Available from: http://www.ncbi.nlm.nih.gov/pubmed/24475803.
16. Feldkamp LA, Davis LC, Kress JW. Practical cone-beam algorithm. J Opt Soc Am A [Internet]. 1984;1(6):612. Available from: https://www.osapublishing.org/abstract.cfm?URI=josaa-1-6-612.
17. Uneri A, Zhang X, Yi T, Stayman JW, Helm PA, Theodore N, et al. Image quality and dose characteristics for an O-arm intraoperative imaging system with model-based image reconstruction. Med Phys [Internet]. 2018;45(11):4857–68. Available from: https://onlinelibrary.wiley.com/doi/abs/10.1002/mp.13167.
18. Liang JZ, La Riviere PJ, El Fakhri G, Glick SJ, Siewerdsen J. Guest editorial low-dose CT: what has been done, and what challenges remain? IEEE Trans Med Imaging [Internet]. 2017;36(12):2409–16. Available from: http://ieeexplore.ieee.org/document/8125482/.
19. Stayman JW, Dang H, Ding Y, Siewerdsen JH. PIRPLE: a penalized-likelihood framework for incorporation of prior images in CT reconstruction. Phys Med Biol [Internet]. 2013 [cited 2014 Nov 18];58(21):7563–7582. Available from: http://www.pubmedcentral.nih.gov/articlerender.fcgi?artid=3868341&tool=pmcentrez&rendertype=abstract.
20. Gang GJ, Stayman JW, Ehtiati T, Siewerdsen JH. Task-driven image acquisition and reconstruction in cone-beam CT. Phys Med Biol [Internet]. 2015;60(8):3129–50. Available from: http://stacks.iop.org/0031-9155/60/i=8/a=3129?key=crossref.408e80cb449d4c28561d7a6c7f5688c8.

21. Tilley S, Siewerdsen JH, Stayman JW. Model-based iterative reconstruction for flat-panel cone-beam CT with focal spot blur, detector blur, and correlated noise. Phys Med Biol [Internet]. 2016;61(1):296–319. Available from: http://stacks.iop.org/0031-9155/61/i=1/a=296?key=crossref.4796deaf6827d354399470d1f41a47dc.
22. Heiland M, Schulze D, Adam G, Schmelzle R. 3D-imaging of the facial skeleton with an isocentric mobile C-arm system (Siremobil Iso-C 3D). Dentomaxillofacial Radiol [Internet]. 2003;32(1):21–5. Available from: http://www.birpublications.org/doi/10.1259/dmfr/80391180.
23. Zhang J, Weir V, Fajardo L, Lin J, Hsiung H, Ritenour ER. Dosimetric characterization of a cone-beam O-arm imaging system. J Xray Sci Technol [Internet]. 2009;17(4):305–17. Available from: http://www.ncbi.nlm.nih.gov/pubmed/19923687.
24. Ritschl L, Kuntz J, Fleischmann C, Kachelrieß M. The rotate-plus-shift C-arm trajectory. Part I. complete data with less than 180° rotation. Med Phys [Internet]. 2016 12;43(5):2295–2302. Available from: http://doi.wiley.com/10.1118/1.4944785.
25. Sheth NM, Zbijewski W, Jacobson MW, Abiola G, Kleinszig G, Vogt S, et al. Mobile C-arm with a CMOS detector: technical assessment of fluoroscopy and cone-beam CT imaging performance. Med Phys [Internet]. 2018;45(12):5420–36. Available from: https://onlinelibrary.wiley.com/doi/abs/10.1002/mp.13244.
26. Chen B, Ning R. Cone-beam volume CT breast imaging: feasibility study. Med Phys [Internet]. 2002;29(5):755–70. Available from: http://doi.wiley.com/10.1118/1.1461843.
27. Jaffray DA, Siewerdsen JH. Cone-beam computed tomography with a flat-panel imager: initial performance characterization. Med Phys [Internet]. 2000 [cited 2014 May 27];27(6):1311–1323. Available from: http://www.ncbi.nlm.nih.gov/pubmed/10902561.
28. Fahrig R, Holdsworth DW. Three-dimensional computed tomographic reconstruction using a C-arm mounted XRII: image-based correction of gantry motion nonidealities. Med Phys [Internet]. 2000;27(1):30–8. Available from: http://doi.wiley.com/10.1118/1.598854.
29. Arai Y, Honda K, Iwai K, Shinoda K. Practical model "3DX" of limited cone-beam X-ray CT for dental use. Int Congr Ser [Internet]. 2001;1230:713–8. Available from: http://linkinghub.elsevier.com/retrieve/pii/S0531513101001194.
30. Hu H, He HD, Foley WD, Fox SH. Four multidetector-row helical CT: image quality and volume coverage speed. Radiology [Internet]. 2000;215(1):55–62. Available from: http://pubs.rsna.org/doi/10.1148/radiology.215.1.r00ap3755.
31. Pan X, Siewerdsen J, La Riviere PJ, Kalender WA. Anniversary paper: development of x-ray computed tomography: the role of medical physics and AAPM from the 1970s to present. Med Phys [Internet]. 2008;35(8):3728–39. Available from: http://doi.wiley.com/10.1118/1.2952653.
32. Xu J, Sisniega A, Zbijewski W, Dang H, Stayman JW, Mow M, et al. Technical assessment of a prototype cone-beam CT system for imaging of acute intracranial hemorrhage. Med Phys. 2016;43(10):5745.
33. Gang GJ, Zbijewski W, Mahesh M, Thawait G, Packard N, Yorkston J, et al. Image quality and dose for a multisource cone-beam CT extremity scanner. Med Phys [Internet]. 2018;45(1):144–55. Available from: http://www.ncbi.nlm.nih.gov/pubmed/29121409.
34. Flohr TG, McCollough CH, Bruder H, Petersilka M, Gruber K, Süβ C, et al. First performance evaluation of a dual-source CT (DSCT) system. Eur Radiol [Internet]. 2006;16(2):256–68. Available from: http://link.springer.com/10.1007/s00330-005-2919-2.
35. Siewerdsen JH, Jaffray DA. Cone-beam computed tomography with a flat-panel imager: magnitude and effects of x-ray scatter. Med Phys [Internet]. 2001;28(2):220–31. Available from: http://doi.wiley.com/10.1118/1.1339879.
36. Schafer S, Stayman JW, Zbijewski W, Schmidgunst C, Kleinszig G, Siewerdsen JH. Antiscatter grids in mobile C-arm cone-beam CT: effect on image quality and dose. Med Phys [Internet]. 2012 [cited 2014 May 27];39(1):153–159. Available from: http://www.pubmedcentral.nih.gov/articlerender.fcgi?artid=3261054&tool=pmcentrez&rendertype=abstract.
37. Siewerdsen JH, Moseley DJ, Bakhtiar B, Richard S, Jaffray DA. The influence of antiscatter grids on soft-tissue detectability in cone-beam computed tomography with flat-panel detectors. Med Phys [Internet]. 2004. [cited 2014 May 27];31;(12):3506–20.. Available from: http://www.ncbi.nlm.nih.gov/pubmed/15651634
38. Sisniega A, Zbijewski W, Badal A, Kyprianou IS, Stayman JW, Vaquero JJ, et al. Monte Carlo study of the effects of system geometry and antiscatter grids on cone-beam CT scatter distributions. Med Phys [Internet]. 2013 [cited 2014 May 27];40(5):051915. Available from: http://www.pubmedcentral.nih.gov/articlerender.fcgi?artid=3651212&tool=pmcentrez&rendertype=abstract.
39. Weir VJ, Zhang J, Bruner AP. Dosimetric characterization and image quality evaluation of the AIRO mobile CT scanner. J Xray Sci Technol [Internet]. 2015;23(3):373–81. Available from: http://www.medra.org/servlet/aliasResolver?alias=iospress&doi=10.3233/XST-150496.
40. Barsa P, Frőhlich R, Beneš V, Suchomel P. Intraoperative portable CT-scanner based spinal navigation – a feasibility and safety study. Acta Neurochir (Wien) [Internet]. 2014;156(9):1807–12. Available from: http://link.springer.com/10.1007/s00701-014-2184-8.
41. Katsevich A. Analysis of an exact inversion algorithm for spiral cone-beam CT. Phys Med Biol [Internet]. 2002;47(15):302. Available from: http://stacks.iop.org/0031-9155/47/i=15/a=302?key=crossref.a6eb76dffee2c2ce17372b064074320b.

42. Siewerdsen JH, Daly MJ, Bachar G, Moseley DJ, Bootsma G, Brock KK, et al. Multimode C-arm fluoroscopy, tomosynthesis, and cone-beam CT for image-guided interventions: from proof of principle to patient protocols. In: Hsieh J, Flynn MJ, editors. Proc SPIE [Internet]. 2007 [cited 2014 Jul 17];6510:65101A–65101A–11. Available from: http://proceedings.spiedigitallibrary.org/proceeding.aspx?articleid=1299299.
43. Wang AS, Stayman JW, Otake Y, Kleinszig G, Vogt S, Gallia GL, et al. Soft-tissue imaging with C-arm cone-beam CT using statistical reconstruction. Phys Med Biol [Internet]. 2014 [cited 2014 May 27];59(4):1005–1026. Available from: http://www.pubmedcentral.nih.gov/articlerender.fcgi?artid=4046706&tool=pmcentrez&rendertype=abstract.
44. Prakash P, Zbijewski W, Gang GJ, Ding Y, Stayman JW, Yorkston J, et al. Task-based modeling and optimization of a cone-beam CT scanner for musculoskeletal imaging. Med Phys [Internet]. 2011 [cited 2014 May 27];38(10):5612–5629. Available from: http://www.pubmedcentral.nih.gov/articlerender.fcgi?artid=3208412&tool=pmcentrez&rendertype=abstract.
45. Dang H, Stayman JW, Sisniega A, Xu J, Zbijewski W, Wang X, et al. Statistical reconstruction for cone-beam CT with a post-artifact-correction noise model: application to high-quality head imaging. Phys Med Biol [Internet]. 2015 [cited 2015 Aug 18];60(16):6153–6175. Available from: http://www.ncbi.nlm.nih.gov/pubmed/26225912.
46. Dang H, Stayman JW, Xu J, Zbijewski W, Sisniega A, Mow M, et al. Task-based statistical image reconstruction for high-quality cone-beam CT. Phys Med Biol. 2017;62(22):8693–719.
47. Dang H, Stayman JW, Sisniega A, Zbijewski W, Xu J, Wang X, et al. Multi-resolution statistical image reconstruction for mitigation of truncation effects: application to cone-beam CT of the head. Phys Med Biol. 2017;62(2):539–59.
48. Sisniega A, Zbijewski W, Xu J, Dang H, Stayman JW, Yorkston J, et al. High-fidelity artifact correction for cone-beam CT imaging of the brain. Phys Med Biol [Internet]. 2015 [cited 2015 Jan 29];60(4):1415–1439. Available from: http://www.ncbi.nlm.nih.gov/pubmed/25611041.
49. Defrise M, Clack R. A cone-beam reconstruction algorithm using shift-variant filtering and cone-beam backprojection. IEEE Trans Med Imaging [Internet]. 1994;13(1):186–95.. Available from: http://ieeexplore.ieee.org/document/276157/
50. Daly MJ, Siewerdsen JH, Moseley DJ, Jaffray DA, Irish JC. Intraoperative cone-beam CT for guidance of head and neck surgery: assessment of dose and image quality using a C-arm prototype. Med Phys [Internet]. 2006 [cited 2014 May 27];33(10):3767–3780. Available from: http://www.ncbi.nlm.nih.gov/pubmed/17089842.
51. Hernandez AM, Schwoebel P, Boone JM, Becker A. Multisource x-ray system for artifact reduction in dedicated breast CT. In: Krupinski EA, editor. 14th International Workshop on Breast Imaging (IWBI 2018) [Internet]. SPIE; 2018. p. 19. Available from: https://www.spiedigitallibrary.org/conference-proceedings-of-spie/10718/2317846/Multisource-x-ray-system-for-artifact-reduction-in-dedicated-breast/10.1117/12.2317846.full.
52. Xu J. Evaluation of detector readout gain mode and bowtie filters for cone-beam CT imaging of the head. Phys Med Biol [Internet]. 2016;61(16):5973–5992(20). Available from: http://www.ncbi.nlm.nih.gov/pubmed/?term=Evaluation+of+detector+readout+gain+mode+and+bowtie+filters+for+cone-beam+CT+imaging+of+the+head.
53. Stayman JW. Fluence-field modulated x-ray CT using multiple aperture devices. Proc Soc Photo Opt Instrum Eng [Internet]. 2016. Available from: http://proceedings.spiedigitallibrary.org/proceeding.aspx?articleid=2506547.
54. El-Mohri Y, Antonuk LE, Koniczek M, Zhao Q, Li Y, Street RA, et al. Active pixel imagers incorporating pixel-level amplifiers based on polycrystalline-silicon thin-film transistors. Med Phys [Internet]. 2009;36(7):3340–55. Available from: http://doi.wiley.com/10.1118/1.3116364.
55. Stavro J, Goldan AH, Zhao W. SWAD: inherent photon counting performance of amorphous selenium multi-well avalanche detector. In: Kontos D, Flohr TG, Lo JY, editors. 2016. p. 97833Q. Available from: http://proceedings.spiedigitallibrary.org/proceeding.aspx?doi=10.1117/12.2217248.
56. Pickhardt PJ, Lubner MG, Kim DH, Tang J, Ruma JA, del Rio AM, et al. Abdominal CT with model-based iterative reconstruction (MBIR): initial results of a prospective trial comparing ultralow-dose with standard-dose imaging. Am J Roentgenol [Internet]. 2012;199(6):1266–74. Available from: http://www.ajronline.org/doi/10.2214/AJR.12.9382.
57. Chen H, Zhang Y, Kalra MK, Lin F, Chen Y, Liao P, et al. Low-dose CT with a residual encoder-decoder convolutional neural network. IEEE Trans Med Imaging [Internet]. 2017;36(12):2524–35. Available from: https://ieeexplore.ieee.org/document/7947200/.
58. Li Z, Yu L, Trzasko JD, Lake DS, Blezek DJ, Fletcher JG, et al. Adaptive nonlocal means filtering based on local noise level for CT denoising. Med Phys [Internet]. 2013 Dec 31;41(1):011908. Available from: http://doi.wiley.com/10.1118/1.4851635.
59. Lindfors KK, Boone JM, Nelson TR, Yang K, Kwan ALC, Miller DF. Dedicated breast CT: Initial clinical experience. Radiology [Internet]. 2008;246(3):725–33. Available from: http://pubs.rsna.org/doi/10.1148/radiol.2463070410.
60. Kwan ALC, Boone JM, Yang K, Huang S-Y. Evaluation of the spatial resolution characteristics of a cone-beam breast CT scanner. Med Phys [Internet]. 2006;34(1):275–81. Available from: http://doi.wiley.com/10.1118/1.2400830.
61. Zhao B, Zhang X, Cai W, Conover D, Ning R. Cone beam breast CT with multiplanar and three dimensional visualization in differentiating

breast masses compared with mammography. Eur J Radiol [Internet]. 2015;84(1):48–53. Available from: https://linkinghub.elsevier.com/retrieve/pii/S0720048X14002903.

62. Thawait GK, Demehri S, AlMuhit A, Zbijweski W, Yorkston J, Del Grande F, et al. Extremity cone-beam CT for evaluation of medial tibiofemoral osteoarthritis: initial experience in imaging of the weight-bearing and non-weight-bearing knee. Eur J Radiol [Internet]. 2015 [cited 2015 Nov 19]; Available from: http://www.ncbi.nlm.nih.gov/pubmed/26388464.
63. Demehri S, Muhit A, Zbijewski W, Stayman JW, Yorkston J, Packard N, et al. Assessment of image quality in soft tissue and bone visualization tasks for a dedicated extremity cone-beam CT system. Eur Radiol [Internet]. 2015 25(6):1742–1751 [cited 2015 Apr 17]; Available from: http://www.ncbi.nlm.nih.gov/pubmed/25599933.
64. de Cesar NC, Schon LC, Thawait GK, da Fonseca LF, Chinanuvathana A, Zbijewski WB, et al. Flexible adult acquired flatfoot deformity. J Bone Jt Surg [Internet]. 2017;99(18):e98. Available from: http://insights.ovid.com/crossref?an=00004623-201709200-00015.
65. Sisniega A, Xu J, Dang H, Zbijewski W, Stayman JW, Mow M, et al. In: Flohr TG, Lo JY, Gilat Schmidt T, editors. Development and clinical translation of a cone-beam CT scanner for high-quality imaging of intracranial hemorrhage. Orlando: SPIE; 2017. p. 101320K.
66. Kalender WA, Kolditz D, Steiding C, Ruth V, Lück F, Rößler A-C, et al. Technical feasibility proof for high-resolution low-dose photon-counting CT of the breast. Eur Radiol [Internet]. 2017;27(3):1081–6. Available from: http://link.springer.com/10.1007/s00330-016-4459-3.
67. John S, Stock S, Cerejo R, Uchino K, Winners S, Russman A, et al. Brain imaging using Mobile CT: current status and future prospects. J Neuroimaging [Internet]. 2016;26(1):5–15. Available from: http://doi.wiley.com/10.1111/jon.12319.
68. Siewerdsen JH, Sisniega A, Zbijewski W, Wu P, Stayman JW, Koliatsos VE, et al. Image quality, scatter, and dose in compact CBCT systems with flat and curved detectors. In: Chen G-H, Lo JY, Gilat Schmidt T, editors. Medical imaging 2018: physics of medical imaging [internet]. Orlando: SPIE; 2018. p. 163. Available from: https://www.spiedigitallibrary.org/conference-proceedings-of-spie/10573/2293872/Image-quality-scatter-and-dose-in-compact-CBCT-systems-with/10.1117/12.2293872.full.

3 Novel CT Acquisition

Lifeng Yu

Introduction

CT data acquisition geometry went through multiple generations in early days. Currently, almost all commercial scanners employ the third generation geometry, where both the x-ray tube and the detector rotate around the patient to acquire thousands of projection data [24]. After acquisition, raw projection data are transferred to the image reconstruction system (IRS) for reconstruction. To facilitate fast volume coverage speed, the detector width on multi-detector row CT (MDCT) has increased to up to 16 cm (at isocenter), and the gantry rotation time has decreased to as low as 0.25 s. Meanwhile, in order to accommodate large patients and fast scanning speed, the power of the x-ray generator has increased to up to 120 kW. High and isotropic spatial resolution is enabled by small detector pixel size (0.25–0.6 mm at isocenter) and small focal spot size (0.3–0.5 mm). All these advances in hardware have led to a large number of exciting applications in different clinical areas, including thoracic, abdominal, musculoskeletal, neuro, pediatric, cardiovascular, and interventional procedures.

This chapter aims to introduce various CT acquisition techniques, focusing on some of the advanced techniques, including axial scan with large area detector, dynamic or perfusion scan with shuttle mode, helical fast pitch scan on dual-source scanners, helical scan with variable pitch, automatic selection of tube potential, organ-based tube current modulation, electrocardiogram (ECG)-gated cardiac scan, dual-energy and multi-energy CT, and dynamic bowtie filter.

L. Yu (✉)
Department of Radiology, Mayo Clinic, Rochester, MN, USA
e-mail: yu.lifeng@mayo.edu

Basic CT Acquisition Modes

Basic scan modes on clinical MDCT include axial step-and-shoot scan mode with table motion, axial scan without table motion, and helical scans. The axial step-and-shoot mode (Fig. 3.1a) has become almost obsolete since the introduction of the helical scan mode due to its inefficient volume coverage speed. However, it is still being used in several special areas. For example, some radiologists still prefer this mode in brain CT in order to reduce helical artifacts. It is also routinely used in lung scans with a large interval to save radiation dose. Prospectively ECG-triggered cardiac scans also use the axial step-and-shoot mode, which will be described later. Axial scan without table motion (Fig. 3.1b) is typically used for scans monitoring contrast bolus enhancement, perfusion scans, and image guidance for interventional procedures.

Helical scan (Fig. 3.1c) is the most commonly used CT acquisition mode in the majority of exams, thanks to its fast and continuous volume coverage. In combination with a wide detector

© Springer Nature Switzerland AG 2020
E. Samei, N. J. Pelc (eds.), *Computed Tomography*, https://doi.org/10.1007/978-3-030-26957-9_3

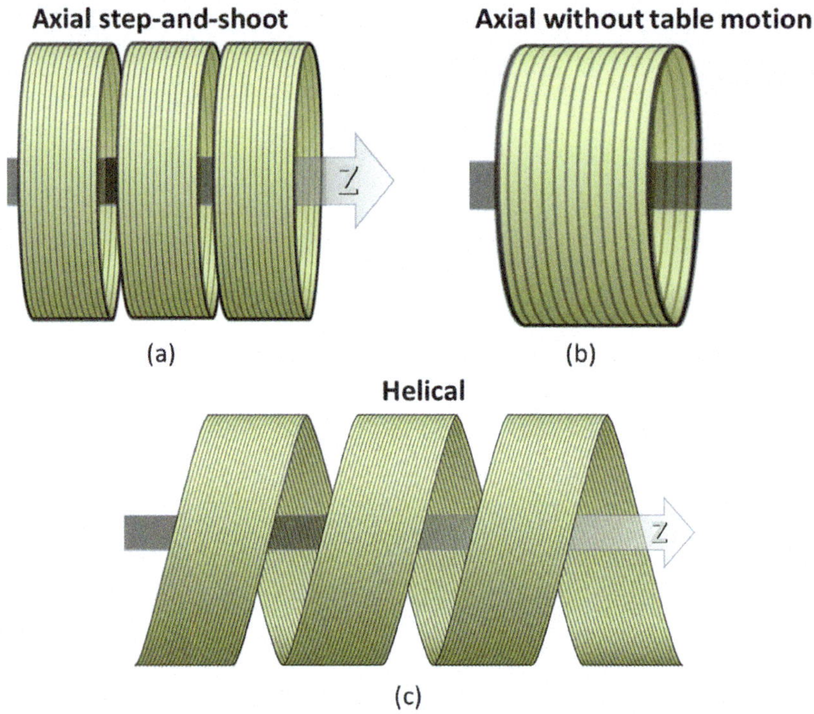

Fig. 3.1 Basic scan modes on clinical MDCT: (**a**) axial step-and-shoot scan with table motion, (**b**) axial scan without table motion, and (**c**) helical scan

and fast gantry rotation time, helical scanning is able to cover the whole body within a few seconds and less than 1 s for many routine exams while providing submillimeter isotropic spatial resolution.

Advanced CT Acquisition Modes

Besides the basic CT acquisition modes, various more advanced data acquisition techniques have been introduced in recent years.

Axial Scan with a Large Area Detector

Some of the major CT manufacturers have large area detectors on their latest scanners, with a longitudinal coverage of up to 16 cm [6, 19, 55]. The benefit of a large area detector is that it can cover many of the major organs in one single axial scan, which facilitates fast volume coverage, provides uniform timing of contrast enhancement within the organ, and enables acquisition of the whole-organ dynamic information without table motion. Another benefit of this scan mode is that it does not require over-ranging scan, which can save radiation dose compared to a helical scan, especially for a short scan range. The over-ranging scan is required in a helical scan to provide sufficient data for reconstructing the volume of interest at both ends of the scan range [9, 66].

Axial scanning with a large area detector also has its limitations. The scattering-to-primary ratio is higher than with a narrow detector. To reduce scatter detection, a two-dimensional anti-scatter grid that is aligned to the focal spot is typically placed in front of the detector. As a result of the large cone-angle, cone-beam artifacts may be more severe, which may lead to distorted geometry and inaccurate CT numbers.

Axial scans with a large area detector may be used for many clinical applications. In pediatric CT, it can facilitate fast scans and reduce motion artifacts [56]. In CT angiography, it can acquire time-series scans to obtain dynamic contrast enhancement information. It can also be used for whole-organ perfusion, such as brain perfusion, which involves repeated volume scans over the brain to generate quantitative blood flow and volume information [55]. Another important application is cardiac CT. This scan mode allows the cardiac images to be acquired within one single heart cycle, as will be described later in this chapter [6, 51].

Dynamic or Perfusion Scan with Shuttle Mode

For most CT scanners, the longitudinal detector coverage is from 2 to 8 cm, which is not wide enough to cover a majority of the organs in one single axial scan. In order to perform dynamic or perfusion scans on these scanners, a so-called "shuttle" mode was introduced (Fig. 3.2).

The shuttle mode can either be axial or helical shuttle [32]. In an axial shuttle, axial scans are performed back and forth between two locations so that the volume coverage can be doubled [71]. In a helical shuttle (or adaptive 4D spiral), the patient is moved smoothly in and out of the gantry over the desired scan range [42, 50]. The longitudinal coverage can be as long as 20–70 cm, well beyond the detector coverage in a single axial scan.

Figure 3.3 shows a clinical example of whole brain perfusion cerebral blood flow (CBF) map acquired on a 128-slice scanner (detector coverage 3.84 cm) with the helical shuttle mode. The longitudinal coverage of the shuttle mode was 10 cm with a scan cycle of 1.5 s. The shuttle mode has also been used to acquire 4D dynamic CT angiography of the lower and upper extremities. The longitudinal coverage was over 70 cm, with each scan cycle taking about 4 s.

Helical Fast Pitch Scan on Dual-Source Scanners

One interesting acquisition technique that is available on a dual-source CT scanner is the fast pitch scan mode [15]. In this mode, the two x-ray sources operate together at the same tube potential. The helical pitch can be as high as 3.4. The scanning speed can be 47 cm/second on the Flash scanner or 70 cm/second on the Force scanner (Siemens Healthcare).

The reason why the fast pitch scan mode cannot be used on a single-source scanner is because there are missing data in longitudinal sampling when the pitch is greater than 1.5 (Fig. 3.4a), which will lead to distortion in reconstructed images (Fig. 3.4b). With two x-ray sources, the gap of missing data from one detector can be compensated with data from the other detector (Fig. 3.4b).

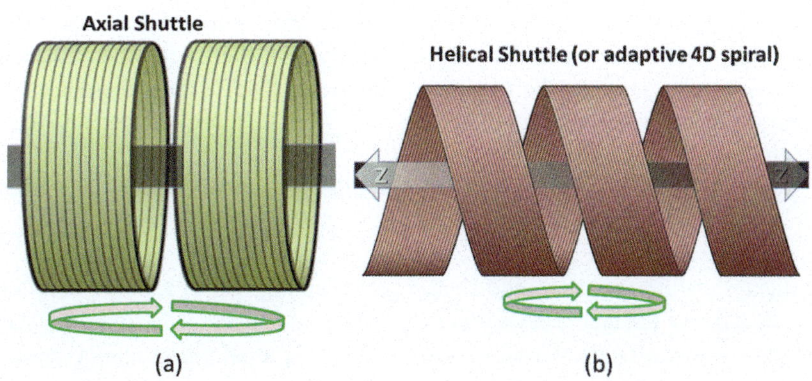

Fig. 3.2 Shuttle scan mode to increase the longitudinal coverage for dynamic or perfusion scans: (**a**) Axial shuttle and (**b**) helical shuttle (or adaptive 4D spiral)

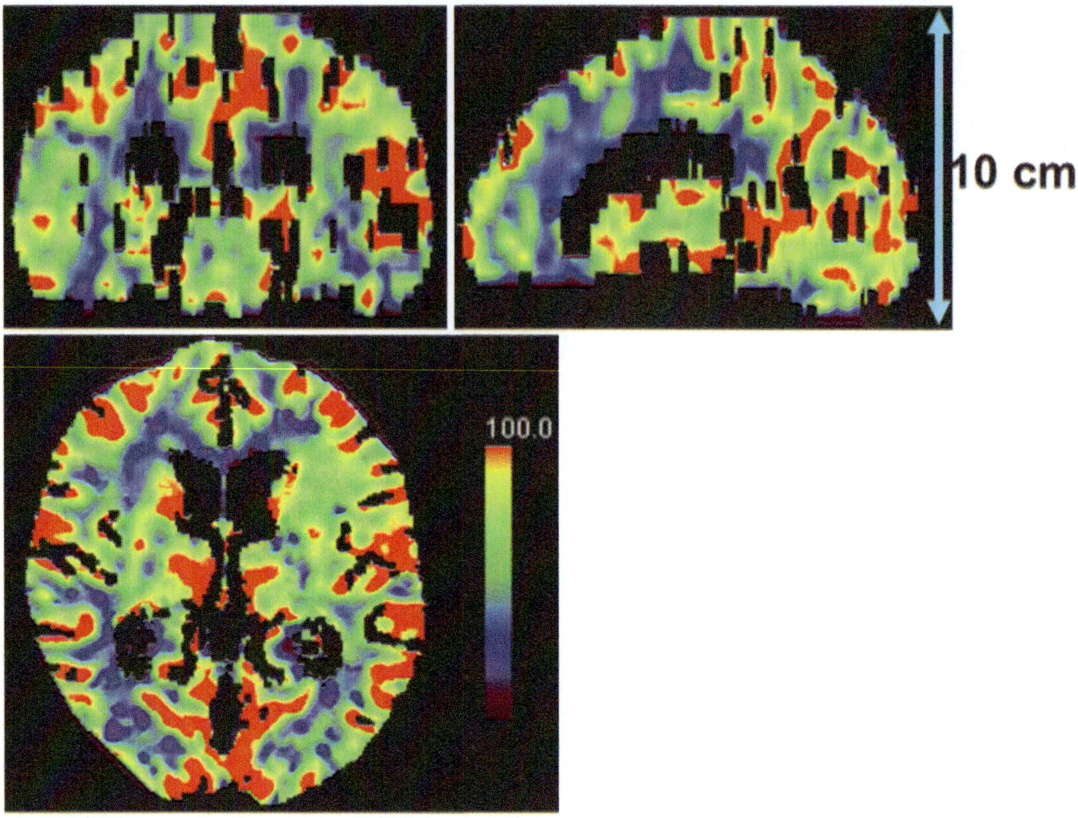

Fig. 3.3 An example of cerebral blood flow (CBF) map acquired from a whole brain perfusion exam with the helical shuttle mode

The fast pitch mode has many important clinical applications. In pediatric CT, it is very useful to suppress motion artifacts from noncooperative patients [33]. In CT angiography of pulmonary embolism, since the scan time is less than 1 s, there is no need for patients to hold their breath, which can significantly improve the stability of contrast enhancement [5]. In cardiac CT angiography, one phase of the heart can be acquired within one heart cycle [15].

The fast pitch mode also has some limitations. First, it has a limited dose output capacity, which limits its use in large patients. Second, helical artifacts are more severe because of the high pitch. The artifacts show up as streaks and shadows (Fig. 3.5). Because of the increased artifacts, the fast pitch mode is generally not recommended for some routine exams, such as the abdomen/pelvis, liver/pancreas, brain, etc. But when reducing motion artifacts outweighs increased artifacts, the fast pitch mode is still appropriate. Finally, one important consideration in the fast pitch scan mode is the safety warning [27]. Since the table needs to travel more than 30 cm before and after the scan range to accelerate and decelerate the table (Fig. 3.6), technologists and nurses need to test the lines and wires connected to the patient before the scan so that they will not be removed during the scan. Otherwise, it could cause unexpected complications.

Helical Scan with Variable Pitch

Another interesting acquisition technique is helical scanning with variable pitch, which involves changing table speed within the same scan [77]. This scan mode has a unique application in cardiovascular exams [37]. When scanning the heart, the pitch is slow to allow for retrospective ECG-gating. After passing through the heart, the pitch becomes regular for a non-ECG-gated scan

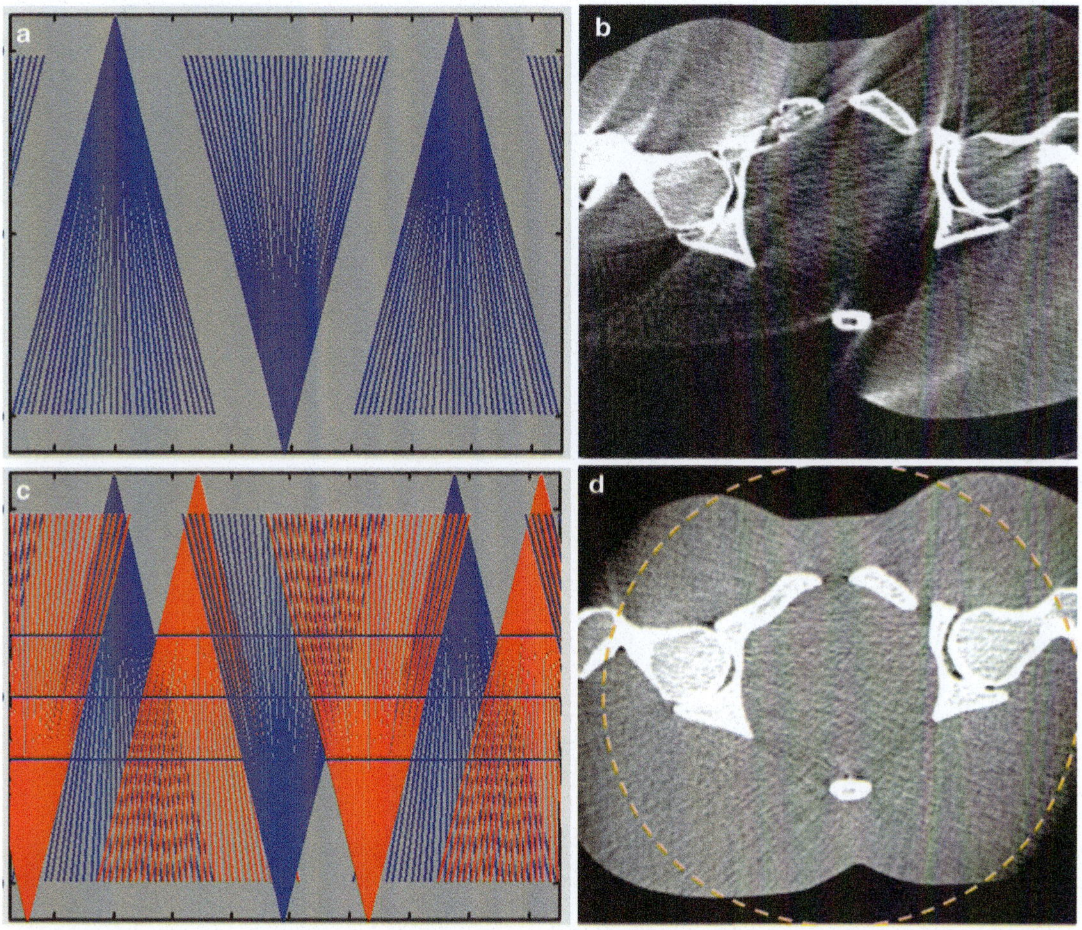

Fig. 3.4 When a fast helical pitch (>1.5) is used on a single-source scanner, missing data in longitudinal sampling (**a**) will lead to distortion in reconstructed images (**b**). The gap of missing data can be compensated with data from the second x-ray source-detector system (**c**), which will remove the distortion in reconstructed images (**d**). Courtesy Drs. Thomas Flohr and Bernhard Schmidt, Siemens Healthcare

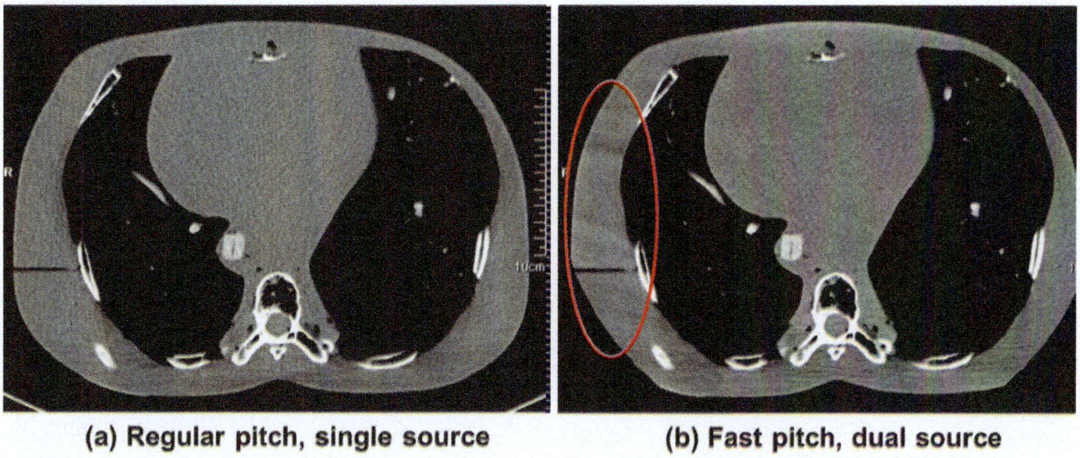

Fig. 3.5 Fast pitch scan mode with dual x-ray sources generates more severe helical artifacts than regular pitch mode with a single x-ray source. (Reprinted with permission from Weber et al. [67])

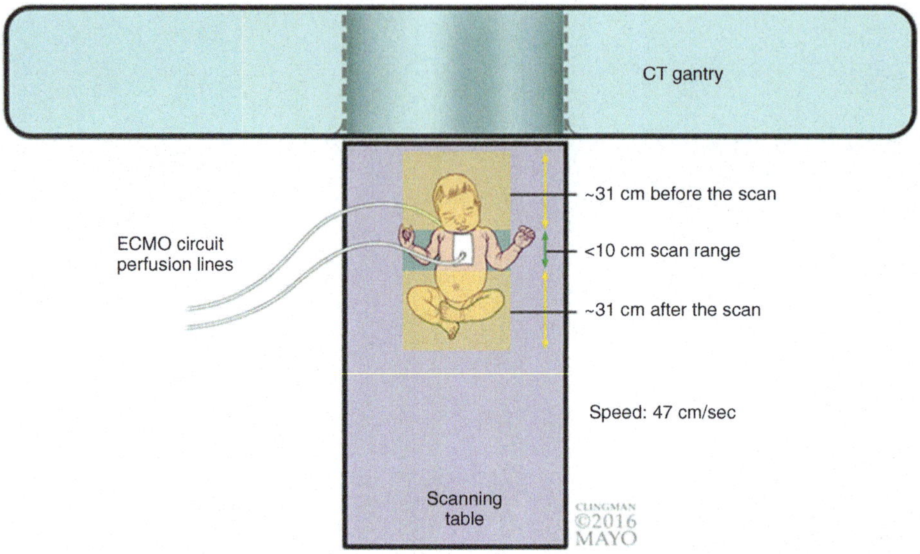

Fig. 3.6 Safety warning when using the fast pitch mode in pediatric CT exams. To accelerate and decelerate the patient table during the scan, the table needs to travel more than 30 cm before and after the scan range. The lines and wires connected to the patient need to be carefully checked before the scan to make sure they will not be accidently removed during the scan. (Reprinted with permission from Hull et al. [27])

portion to save radiation dose. Both radiation dose and contrast dose can be reduced using this mode.

This scan mode also has some applications in imaging trauma, where optimal helical pitch can be used for different parts of the body during one single scan to optimize image quality and scanning speed, for example, slower pitch for head and neck scan, fast pitch for chest scan, and regular pitch for abdomen and pelvis. The helical shuttle (adaptive 4D spiral) also involves a change of helical pitch during the scan.

Organ-Based Tube Current Modulation

Automatic tube current modulation automatically adapts the tube current based on the attenuation level of the patient and has been widely used in clinical CT for radiation dose reduction. The goal of automatic tube current modulation is to produce uniform image quality across different body regions or different patient sizes. However this strategy does not consider the dose distribution to specific organs. It is known that some organs, such as breast or lens of the eye, are more dose sensitive than others. Organ-based tube current modulation was introduced to reduce radiation dose to those specific organs [13, 17]. For example, to reduce radiation dose to the breast, the tube current is reduced substantially when the x-ray source is in front of the patient and increased proportionally along other projection angles. In this way, the dose to the breast can be reduced. For this technique to achieve maximum dose reduction to a specific organ, the angular range for tube current reduction needs to be appropriately defined [64].

Automatic Selection of Optimal Tube Potential

Tube potential is an important scanning parameter that has a major impact on the dose efficiency of the CT exam. Figure 3.7a shows examples of the six x-ray beam spectra used on one CT scanner. How to select the best tube potential for each exam has long been an important clinical question [7]. The main benefit of lower tube potential is that it tends to enhance iodine contrast better than higher tube potentials. However, lower tube potential has its limitation – it tends to increase image noise, especially for relatively larger patients, because of the limited penetration of low energy photons.

To optimize the tube potential, a very common way in practice is to use a manual technique

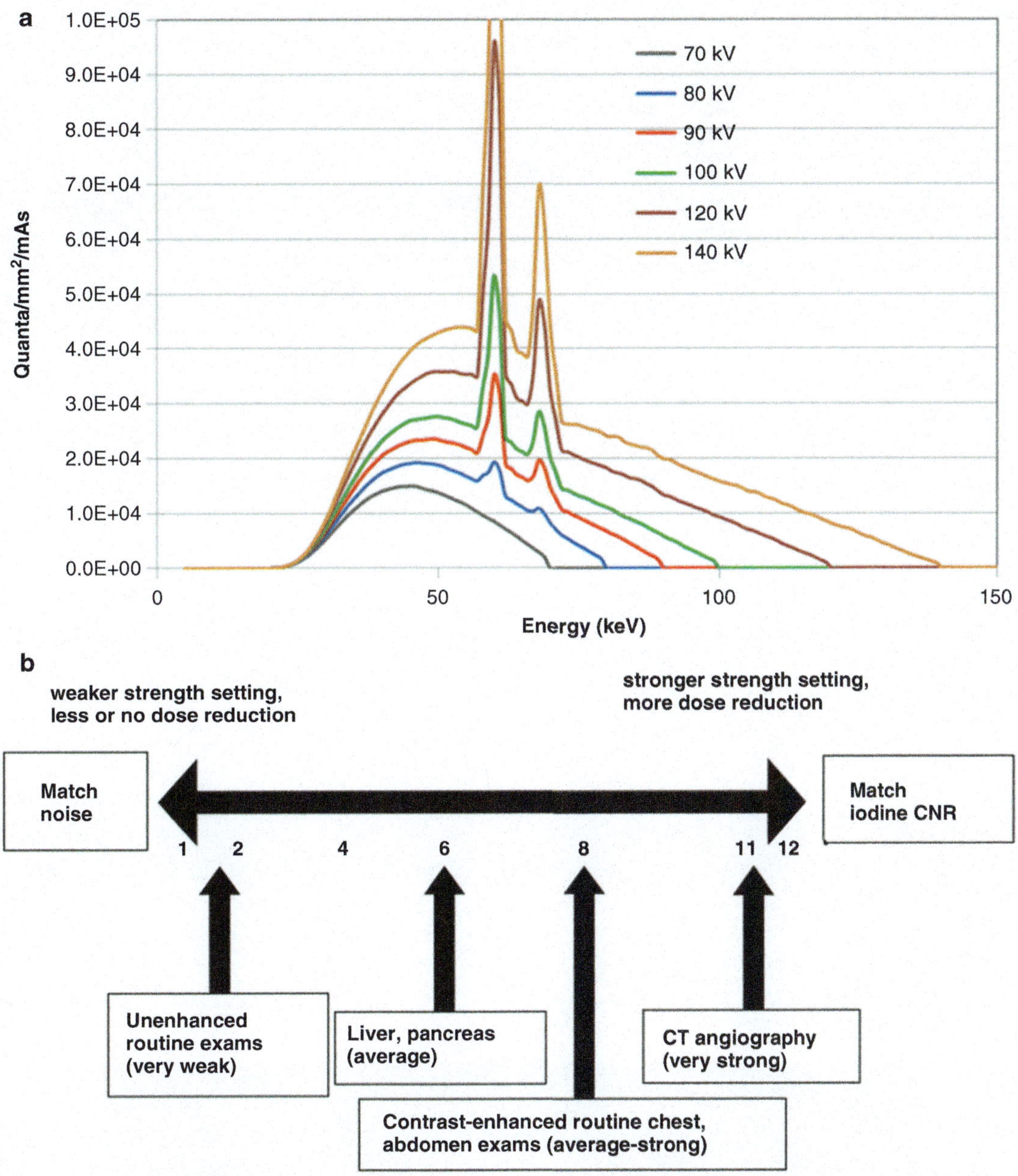

Fig. 3.7 (**a**) Multiple x-ray beam spectra are typically available for selection on CT scanners. (**b**) A software implementation to automatically select the most dose-efficient tube potential based on both patient size and diagnostic task. (Reprinted from Yu et al. [73], with permission from the American Journal of Roentgenology)

chart, i.e., prescribe different kV/mAs combinations for different patient sizes [72]. The chart is empirically determined, and the parameter choice depends on both patient size and diagnostic task. Technologists have to look up the chart for each patient and manually change the technique on the scanner, which is error prone in practice.

A general strategy was proposed to automate this process, which involves determining the most dose-efficient tube potential and the appropriate amount of radiation dose reduction [74]. To predict the most dose-efficient tube potential, an image quality metric has to be defined, which is diagnostic task dependent (Fig. 3.7b). For tasks that would benefit from more iodine contrast enhancement, such as CT angiography, the metric is essential to match the iodine contrast to noise ratio, which allows for more aggressive use of lower tube potential and more dose reduction; for tasks that do not involve iodine, the metric is essential to match the noise, and the dose reduction is minimal, and lower tube potential is typically prohibited. For other tasks, the metric is somewhere in the middle between matching noise and matching iodine contrast to noise ratio.

Based on this strategy, one manufacturer implemented an automatic tool on their scanners. With this tool, there is no need to rely on a manual technique chart. The selection of tube potential and dose reduction becomes automatic and quantitative, which significantly improves the workflow and patient outcome. Many clinical evaluation studies have been performed that demonstrate its effectiveness as a general tool for radiation dose reduction without sacrificing diagnostic image quality [70, 73].

Added Beam Filter to Optimize Beam Quality

Another interesting recent development is to further optimize x-ray beam quality by adding additional beam filtration, such as the tin (Sn) filter [22]. This may improve dose efficiency for some non-contrast exams as low energy photons that do not contribute to image formation are removed by the filter (Fig. 3.8a). Because the added beam filter reduces the x-ray flux, this strategy has only

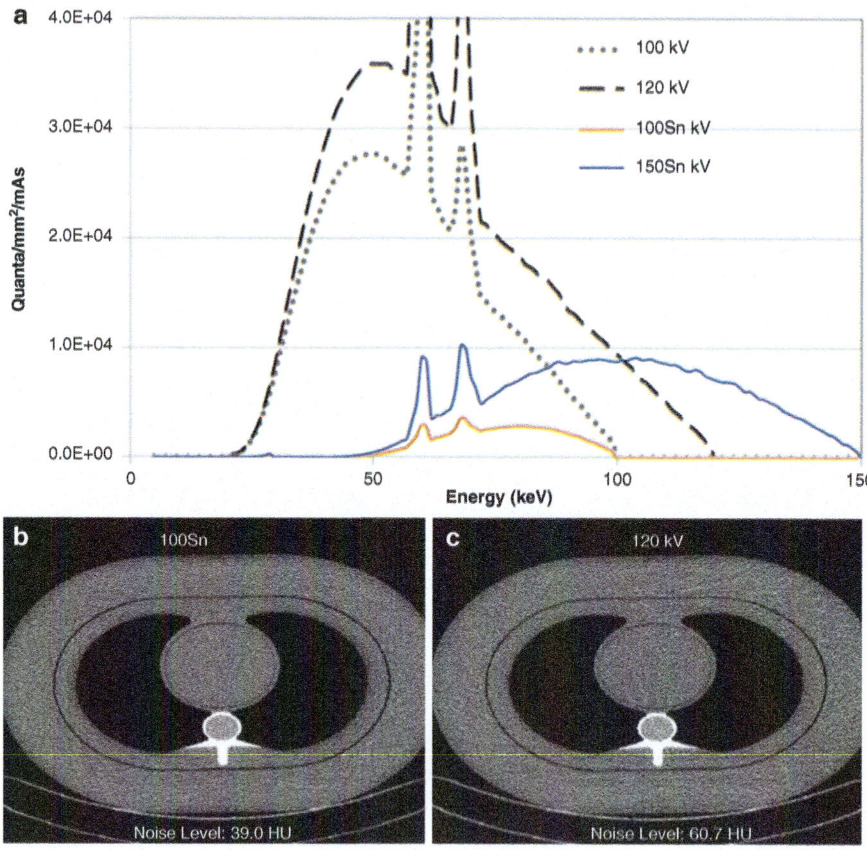

Fig. 3.8 (**a**) X-ray beam spectra of 100 kV, 120 kV, 100 kV with an added tin filter (100Sn), and 150 kV with an added tin filter (150Sn). The added tin filter reduces the radiation output per mAs but absorbs most of the low-energy photons and generates a much harder beam than without the tin filter. (**b**) A phantom image acquired at 100Sn with a volume CT dose index (CTDIvol) of 1.7 mGy. (**c**) A phantom image acquired at 120 kV with a CTDIvol of 1.7 mGy matched to that at 100Sn. Note the much lower noise level at 100Sn than at 120 kV. (Reprinted with permission from Weber et al. [67])

become feasible in recent years after more powerful x-ray tubes become available. Figure 3.8b, c shows two images acquired at the same radiation dose, with Sn and without Sn. Much reduced noise can be observed on image acquired with the Sn filter [67].

Electrocardiogram (ECG)-Gated Cardiac Scan

Cardiac CT requires both a high temporal resolution to "freeze" the heart motion and a high spatial resolution to detect defects in small arteries. Since the temporal resolution is associated with the time duration of the data for image reconstruction, images in cardiac CT are usually reconstructed using half-scan data in order to achieve the highest possible temporal resolution [30]. With half-scan reconstruction, the temporal resolution is roughly half of the rotation time for a single-source CT scanner and quarter of the rotation time for a dual-source CT scanner [16, 39]. In addition, to reconstruct images at specific phases of the cardiac cycle, the ECG signal of the patient is monitored or recorded during the scan. Four different acquisition techniques are currently available for cardiac CT (Fig. 3.9):

1. Retrospectively ECG-gated helical scan

   In this mode, x-rays are continuously on, while data are acquired in helical mode at a very slow pitch (~0.15 to 0.3). The slow helical pitch is to make sure that there is no gap in the data used for image reconstruction in two contiguous cardiac cycles. The helical pitch is determined based on the heart rate to avoid anatomical discontinuities [44]. After data acquisition, images at specific phases are reconstructed. Because of the slow helical pitch and the continuously on x-rays, this scan mode is usually at higher dose than a regular

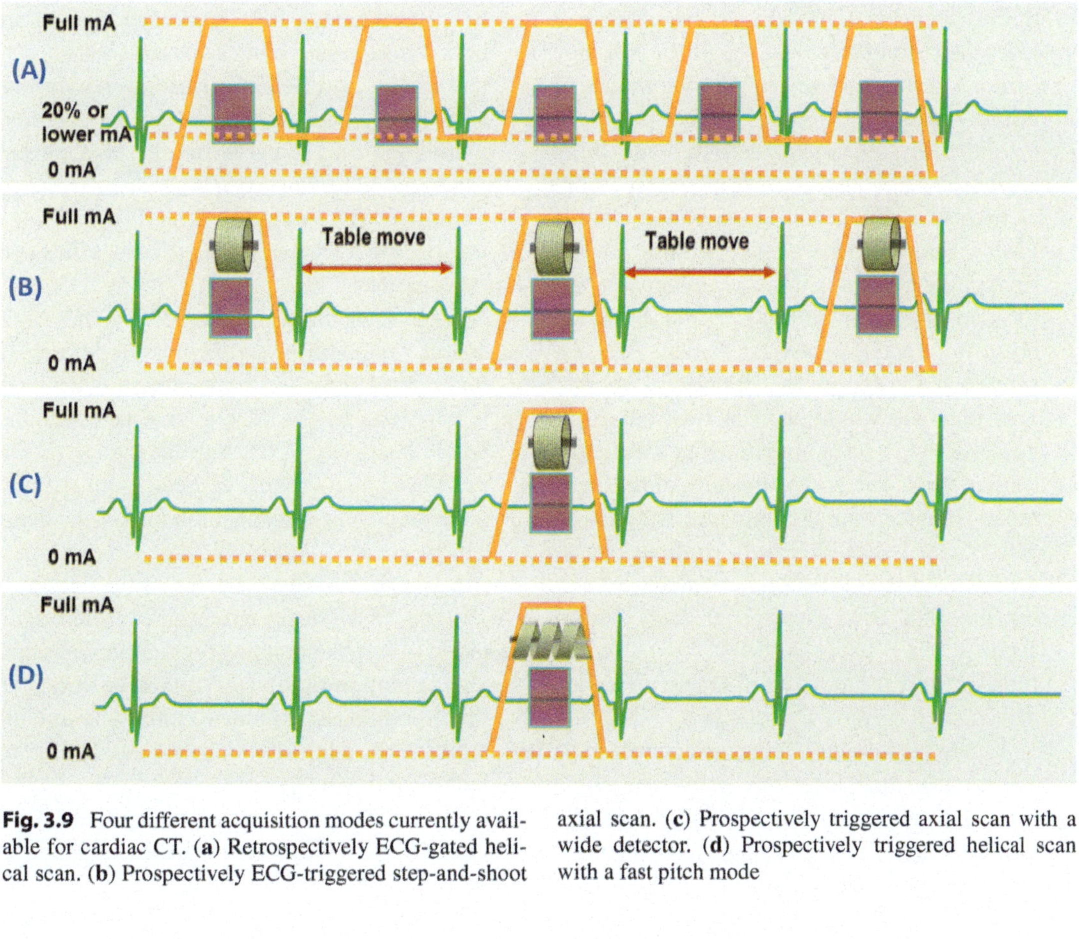

Fig. 3.9 Four different acquisition modes currently available for cardiac CT. (**a**) Retrospectively ECG-gated helical scan. (**b**) Prospectively ECG-triggered step-and-shoot axial scan. (**c**) Prospectively triggered axial scan with a wide detector. (**d**) Prospectively triggered helical scan with a fast pitch mode

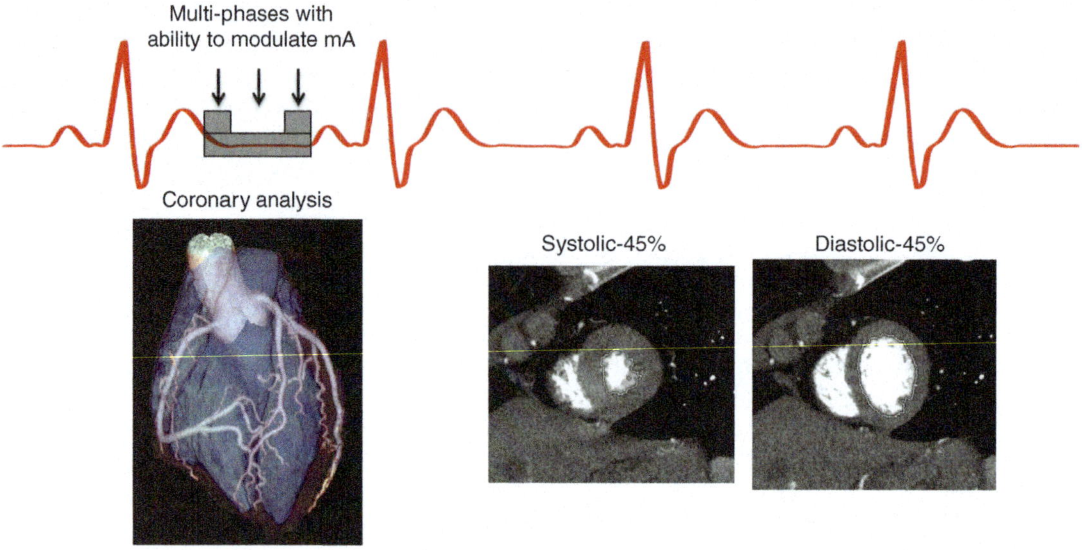

Fig. 3.10 With a wide-detector axial scan, multiple phases of the heart can be acquired within one cardiac cycle, with the tube current modulated at different phases to save radiation dose. (Courtesy Dr. Jiang Hsieh and GE Healthcare)

helical scan. To reduce radiation dose in this mode, ECG-gated tube current modulation or ECG pulsing was introduced, which uses a low tube current (e.g., 4–20% of the full tube current) during cardiac phases that are not of primary interest [28, 68].

2. Prospectively ECG-triggered step-and-shoot axial scan

   In this scan mode, the scanner monitors the ECG signal from the patient, waiting for the right phase to turn on the x-ray beam and perform an axial scan. After each scan, the x-ray beam is turned off, and the patient is translated to the next location to perform another scan until the whole heart is covered. Since x-rays are only on at predefined phases of the cardiac cycle, the dose efficiency of this scan mode is higher than the retrospectively ECG-gated helical scan [53, 58]. Multiple phases can be acquired in this scan mode by extending the axial scan duration at each cardiac cycle.

3. Prospectively triggered axial scan with a wide detector

   When the detector is wide enough (e.g., 16 cm), the whole heart can be covered within one axial scan and one heart cycle [6, 12, 23, 51]. This scan mode provides uniform timing for the whole heart, which resolves an important issue that is commonly seen in the above two scan modes, i.e., gaps and distortions between adjacent volumes caused by inconsistent timing of different cardiac cycles. In this scan mode, multiple phases can be acquired within one cardiac cycle and the tube current can be modulated in between the desired phases to further reduce radiation dose (Fig. 3.10).

4. Prospectively triggered helical scan with a fast pitch mode

   This scan mode is enabled by the dual-source fast pitch mode. In this mode, a very fast helical scan for a pre-determined phase is triggered by the ECG signal to cover the whole heart within one cardiac cycle [1]. On the Flash dual-source scanner, with 3.8 cm detector coverage and a pitch of 3.4, the heart can be covered within 250 ms. On the Force dual-source scanner, the time is reduced to 170 ms. The dose efficiency of this scan mode is just like that in a regular helical scan. One major limitation of this scan mode is that multiphase volumes cannot be reconstructed. In addition, the heart rate needs to be low and regular.

Table 3.1 summarizes the advantages and limitations of the four ECG-gated cardiac scan modes.

Table 3.1 The advantages and limitations of the four ECG-gated cardiac scan modes

Cardiac scan mode	Advantages	Limitations
Retrospectively ECG-gated helical scan	Multiphase reconstruction is built in	Dose higher than regular mode
	Allow ECG editing to identify best phase	Displacement artifacts if pitch is higher than appropriate
	Stable with arrhythmic beat	
Prospectively ECG-triggered axial step-and-shoot scan	Multiphase acquisition is possible	Heart rate needs to be low and regular
	Dose efficiency higher than retrospective helical mode	
Prospectively ECG-triggered axial scan with wide detector	One heart beat	Heart rate needs to be low
	Same phase across heart	More scattering and cone-beam artifacts
	Multiphase acquisition is possible	
	High dose efficiency	
Prospectively ECG-triggered fast-pitch helical scan	One heart beat	Heart rate needs to be low and regular
	Similar phase across heart (from top to bottom between 170 and 250 milliseconds)	No multiphase reconstruction
	High dose efficiency	Limited radiation dose output capacity

Dual-Energy CT

The concept of material decomposition in dual-energy CT (DECT) was originally proposed by Alvarez and Macovski in 1976 [3]. In the diagnostic x-ray energy range, the linear attenuation coefficient of a material can be decomposed into two linearly independent components: photon electric and Compton interactions. By performing material decomposition using DECT, one can obtain material-specific information and virtual monochromatic images. Currently there are five different scanner platforms commercially available to perform DECT (Fig. 3.11a–e). These include slow kV switching, mainly used in low-end scanners; fast kV switching, collecting dual-energy data by quickly switching between low and high kV during one scan [21]; dual-layer detector, collecting low energy data with the upper layer of the detector and higher energy data with the bottom layer of the detector [8, 49];and dual x-ray source, one tube for low kV and the other tube for high kV [16, 45]. Relatively recently, one of the manufacturers also implemented a twin-beam technique, which acquires dual-energy data on a single-source scanner with a split filter in front of the x-ray beam [2, 52]. Many novel applications of DECT have been developed, and some of them have been routinely used in clinical practice, including virtual monochromatic imaging, virtual non-contrast imaging, automatic bone removal, iodine quantification, kidney stone characterization, and gout diagnosis [20, 29, 38, 47, 54, 59, 63].

Multi-energy CT

Recently there have been tremendous efforts to develop techniques that can acquire more than two x-ray spectra and perform multi-energy CT (MECT). MECT has a great potential to enable multi-contrast agent imaging or multi-material decomposition, which may be used to either reduce radiation dose or improve clinical diagnosis. One example is to acquire both the late arterial and portal venous phases of the liver in one single MECT scan by imaging gadolinium and iodine simultaneously, which are reported to potentially reduce radiation dose [43, 60]. Another example is to image iodine and bismuth simultaneously using one single MECT scan to separate the lumen and wall of the bowel so that the diagnosis of tumor in bowel wall and luminal filling defects can be improved [41, 48]. Many other applications of multi-contrast agents or multi-material decomposition have been explored [4, 10, 11, 40].

Energy-resolved photon-counting detector-based CT (PCD-CT) is the most popular platform for MECT [31, 62, 76]. Different from energy integrating detectors, where the x-ray photons are converted to light which is then integrated by photodiodes, PCD counts each photon and resolves its energy using pulse height discriminators. Because of this detection mechanism, PCD has many potential advantages, including improved signal-to-noise ratio and dose efficiency due to optimal energy weighting; improved low-dose performance because of the reduced electronic noise; improved spatial resolution because of small pixel size; and the potential to perform MECT by acquiring multiple energy thresholds. See Chap. 14 for more details on PCD. Currently, there are many ongoing projects trying to develop whole-body PCD-CT systems [38, 69]. Some prototypes have already been tested in patient exams [34, 46] (Fig. 3.11f).

Current PCD-CT systems are not without limitations. The most significant one is spectral distortion caused by non-ideal photon-counting processes, including pulse pileup and many x-ray intensity-independent factors such as charge sharing, K-escape, and Compton scattering [62]. As a result, no obvious advantages have been shown in comparison to traditional energy integrating detector (EID)-based DECT for the same material-decomposition tasks [14]. Much research is ongoing to improve the PCD technology.

Besides PCD-CT, many other techniques have also been proposed to perform MECT based on traditional EID-based CT scanners. One technique is dual-source MECT with split filter [75]. This strategy is based on split-filter DECT technique discussed above [2, 52], which can acquire dual-energy data in a helical scan. When the split filter is applied to one or both x-ray sources on a dual-source scanner, one can acquire three or

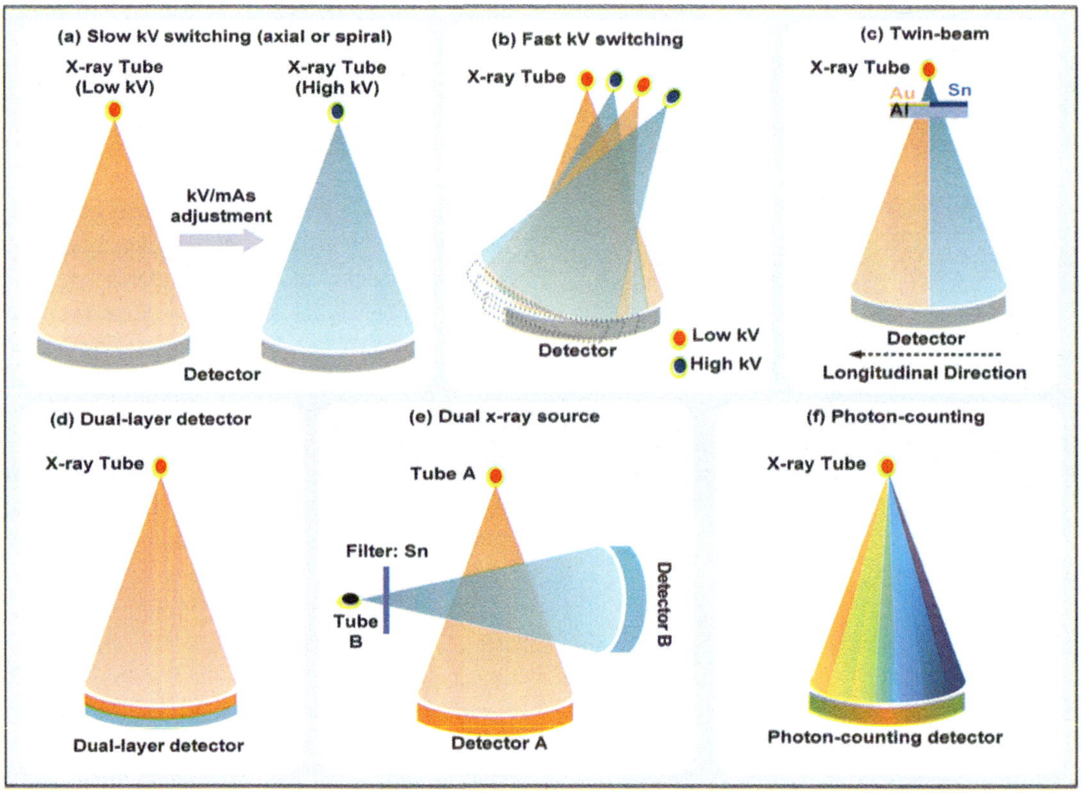

Fig. 3.11 Six different scanner techniques to perform dual-energy and multi-energy CT. (**a**) Slow kV switching at either axial or spiral mode. (**b**) Fast kV switching, collecting dual-energy data by quickly switching between low and high kV. (**c**) Twin-beam configuration, collecting dual-energy data on a single-source CT with an added split filter in front of the x-ray beam. (**d**) Dual-layer detector, collecting low energy data with the upper layer of the detector and higher energy data with the bottom layer of the detector. (**e**) Dual x-ray source, one tube for low energy data and the other tube for high energy data. (**f**) Photon-counting detector, counting each photon and resolving its energy to acquire multi-spectral CT data

four x-ray spectrum measurements nearly simultaneously (Fig. 3.12). Another technique involves spatial modulation of the x-ray beam using a repeating pattern of filter materials, which allows for collection of many different spectral channels within one scan [57, 65] (Fig. 3.13).

Dynamic Bowtie Filter

The goal of a traditional bowtie filter is to adapt x-ray intensity to patient attenuation levels within one projection so that radiation dose can be reduced. The typical bowtie shape is due to

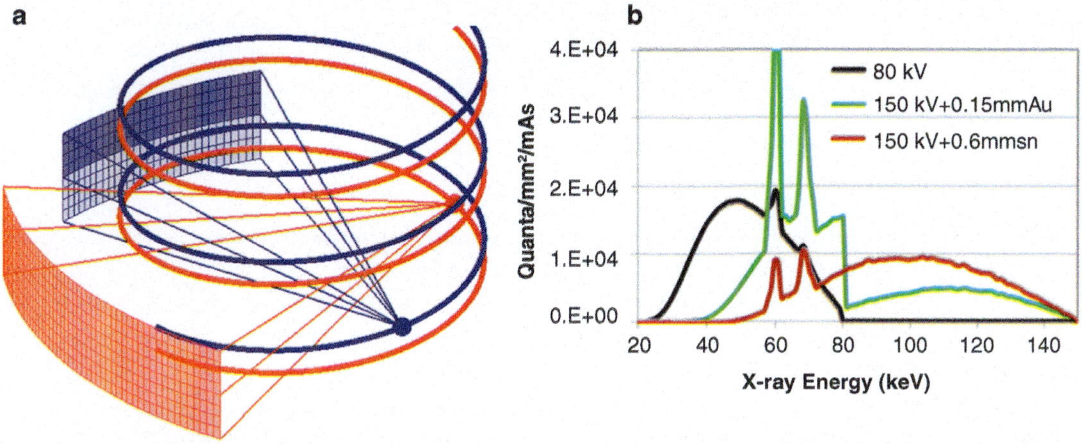

Fig. 3.12 Multi-energy CT using a dual-source CT scanner with added split filters. (**a**) A split filter is added to one of the x-ray sources to acquire three x-ray spectra nearly simultaneously. (**b**) Three x-ray spectra from the triple-beam configuration. (Reprinted with permission from Yu et al. [75])

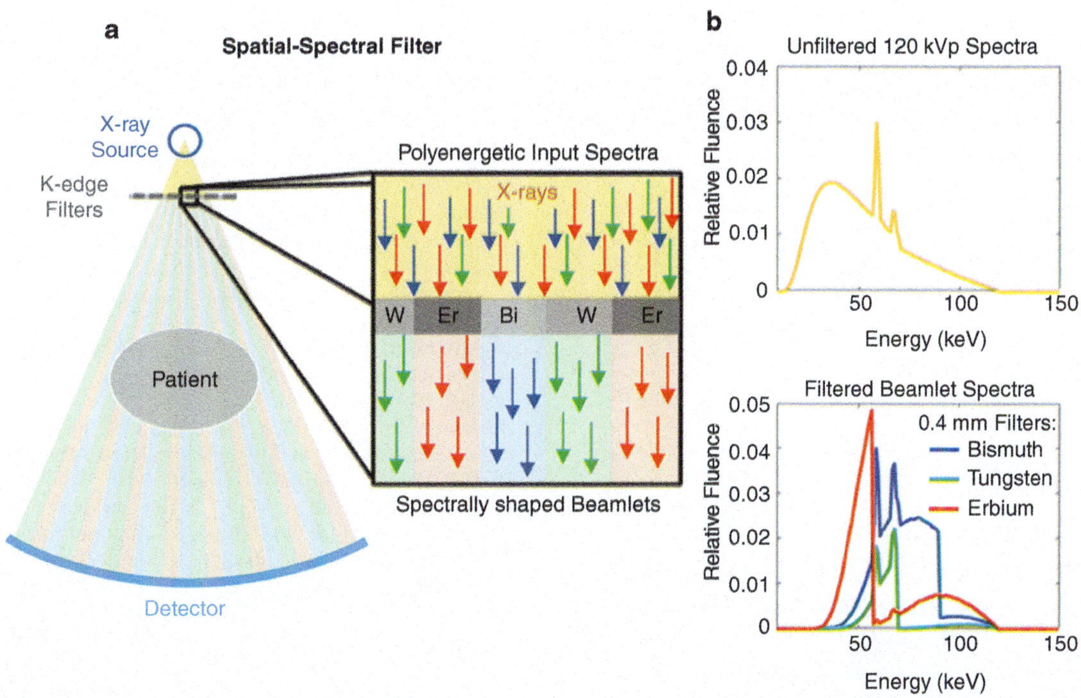

Fig. 3.13 Spatial-spectral filter added to one single x-ray source to enable multi-energy data acquisition on energy-integrating detector CT scanners. (**a**) Illustration of the spatial-spectral K-edge filters to generate spectrally shaped beamlets. (**b**) Spectra before and after the K-edge filters. (Courtesy Dr. J. Webster Stayman, Johns Hopkins University)

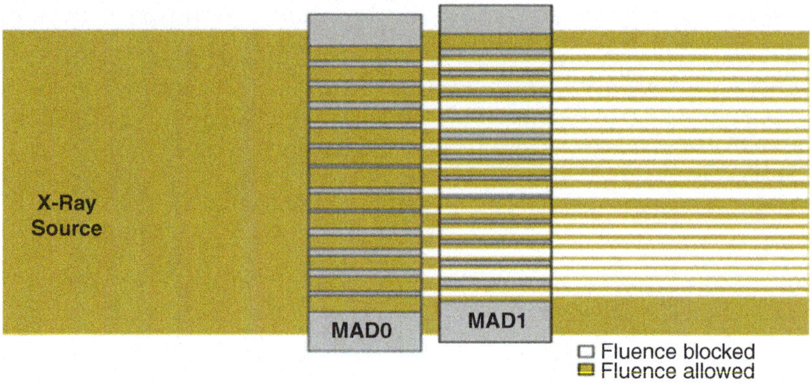

Fig. 3.14 Two sets of multiple aperture device (MAD) are used to modulate the x-ray flux within the beam so that various x-ray intensity profiles can be generated. (Courtesy Dr. J. Webster Stayman, Johns Hopkins University)

the assumption that patient body shape has high attenuation in the center and low attenuation in the peripheral regions. However, patient attenuation varies quite significantly within each projection view, from view to view, and from patient to patient. The fixed shape bowtie filter (or at most a few shapes for different body size and regions) can rarely adapt well for the attenuation variation of the patient. Multiple techniques have been proposed to implement a dynamic bowtie filter so that the x-ray intensity can be fully adapted to patient attenuation for each projection view [25, 26, 36, 61].

One of the designs involves a set of triangular wedges, each wedge independently moved to produce a piecewise-linear attenuation profile based on the specific attenuation level along each ray path [25]. Another design involved the use of two sets of multiple aperture device (MAD) [18, 35, 36]. By shifting the MAD relative to each other, a large variety of fluence profiles can be generated (Fig. 3.14).

Conclusion

The current mainstream clinical MDCT scanners employ the third-generation geometry to acquire CT data. Major advances in x-ray source and detector technology have been made, and many innovative CT acquisition techniques have been developed during the past decades, which dramatically improve volume coverage speed, spatial resolution, temporal resolution, and radiation dose efficiency. As a result of these advances, numerous novel clinical applications have become possible to provide enhanced diagnostic information for CT patients.

Acknowledgments The author would like to thank Drs. James Kofler and Liqiang Ren for helping on some of the figures and Ms. Kris Nunez for preparing the manuscript.

References

1. Achenbach S, Marwan M, Schepis T, Pflederer T, Bruder H, Allmendinger T, Petersilka M, Anders K, Lell M, Kuettner A, Ropers D, Daniel WG, Flohr T. High-pitch spiral acquisition: a new scan mode for coronary CT angiography. J Cardiovasc Comput Tomogr. 2009;3:117–21.
2. Almeida IP, Schyns LE, Ollers MC, van Elmpt W, Parodi K, Landry G, Verhaegen F. Dual-energy CT quantitative imaging: a comparison study between twin-beam and dual-source CT scanners. Med Phys. 2017;44:171–9.
3. Alvarez RE, Macovski A. Energy-selective reconstructions in X-ray computed tomography. Phys Med Biol. 1976;21:733–44.
4. Baturin P, Alivov Y, Molloi S. Spectral CT imaging of vulnerable plaque with two independent biomarkers. Phys Med Biol. 2012;57:4117–38.
5. Bauer RW, Schell B, Beeres M, Wichmann JL, Bodelle B, Vogl TJ, Kerl JM. High-pitch dual-source computed tomography pulmonary angiography in freely breathing patients. J Thorac Imaging. 2012;27:376–81.
6. Benz DC, Grani C, Moch BH, Mikulicic F, Vontobel J, Fuchs TA, Stehli J, Clerc OF, Possner M, Pazhenkottil AP, Gaemperli O, Buechel RR, Kaufmann PA. Minimized radiation and contrast agent exposure for coronary computed tomography angiography: first clinical experience on a latest generation 256-slice scanner. Acad Radiol. 2016;23:1008–14.

7. Boone JM, Geraghty EM, Seibert JA, Wootton-Gorges SL. Dose reduction in pediatric CT: a rational approach. Radiology. 2003;228:352–60.
8. Carmi R, Naveh G, Altman A. Material separation with dual-layer CT. IEEE Nucl Sci Symp Conf Rec. 2005;4:3.
9. Christner JA, Zavaletta VA, Eusemann CD, Walz-Flannigan AI, McCollough CH. Dose reduction in helical CT: dynamically adjustable z-axis x-ray beam collimation. Am J Roentgenol. 2010;194:W49–55.
10. Cormode DP, Roessl E, Thran A, Skajaa T, Gordon RE, Schlomka JP, Fuster V, Fisher EA, Mulder WJ, Proksa R, Fayad ZA. Atherosclerotic plaque composition: analysis with multicolor CT and targeted gold nanoparticles. Radiology. 2010;256:774–82.
11. Dangelmaier J, Bar-Ness D, Daerr H, Muenzel D, Si-Mohamed S, Ehn S, Fingerle AA, Kimm MA, Kopp FK, Boussel L, Roessl E, Pfeiffer F, Rummeny EJ, Proksa R, Douek P, Noel PB. Experimental feasibility of spectral photon-counting computed tomography with two contrast agents for the detection of endoleaks following endovascular aortic repair. Eur Radiol. 2018;28:3318–25.
12. Dewey M, Zimmermann E, Laule M, Rutsch W, Hamm B. Three-vessel coronary artery disease examined with 320-slice computed tomography coronary angiography. Eur Heart J. 2008;29:1669.
13. Duan X, Wang J, Christner JA, Leng S, Grant KL, McCollough CH. Dose reduction to anterior surfaces with organ-based tube-current modulation: evaluation of performance in a phantom study. AJR Am J Roentgenol. 2011;197:689–95.
14. Faby S, Kuchenbecker S, Sawall S, Simons D, Schlemmer HP, Lell M, Kachelriess M. Performance of today's dual energy CT and future multi energy CT in virtual non-contrast imaging and in iodine quantification: a simulation study. Med Phys. 2015;42:4349–66.
15. Flohr TG, Leng SA, Yu LF, Allmendinger T, Bruder H, Petersilka M, Eusemann CD, Stierstorfer K, Schmidt B, McCollough CH. Dual-source spiral CT with pitch up to 3.2 and 75 ms temporal resolution: image reconstruction and assessment of image quality. Med Phys. 2009;36:5641–53.
16. Flohr TG, McCollough CH, Bruder H, Petersilka M, Gruber K, Suss C, Grasruck M, Stierstorfer K, Krauss B, Raupach R, Primak AN, Kuttner A, Achenbach S, Becker C, Kopp A, Ohnesorge BM. First performance evaluation of a dual-source CT (DSCT) system. Eur Radiol. 2006;16:256–68.
17. Gandhi D, Crotty DJ, Stevens GM, Schmidt TG. Technical note: phantom study to evaluate the dose and image quality effects of a computed tomography organ-based tube current modulation technique. Med Phys. 2015;42:6572–8.
18. Gang GJ, Mao A, Wang W, Siewerdsen JH, Mathews A, Kawamoto S, Levinson R, Stayman JW. Dynamic fluence field modulation in computed tomography using multiple aperture devices. Phys Med Biol. 2019;64:105024.
19. Geleijns J, Artells MS, Bruin PW, Matter R, Muramatsu Y, McNitt-Gray MF. Computed tomography dose assessment for a 160 mm wide, 320 detector row, cone beam CT scanner. Phys Med Biol. 2009;54:3141–59.
20. Glazebrook KN, Guimaraes LS, Murthy NS, Black DF, Bongartz T, Manek NJ, Leng S, Fletcher JG, McCollough CH. Identification of intraarticular and periarticular uric acid crystals with dual-energy CT: initial evaluation. Radiology. 2011;261:516–24.
21. Goodsitt MM, Christodoulou EG, Larson SC. Accuracies of the synthesized monochromatic CT numbers and effective atomic numbers obtained with a rapid kVp switching dual energy CT scanner. Med Phys. 2011;38:2222–32.
22. Gordic S, Morsbach F, Schmidt B, Allmendinger T, Flohr T, Husarik D, Baumueller S, Raupach R, Stolzmann P, Leschka S, Frauenfelder T, Alkadhi H. Ultralow-dose chest computed tomography for pulmonary nodule detection: first performance evaluation of single energy scanning with spectral shaping. Investig Radiol. 2014;49:465–73.
23. Hein PA, Romano VC, Lembcke A, May J, Rogalla P. Initial experience with a chest pain protocol using 320-slice volume MDCT. Eur Radiol. 2009;19:1148–55.
24. Hsieh J. Computed tomography: principles, design, artifacts, and recent advances. Bellingham: SPIE Press; 2012.
25. Hsieh SS, Pelc NJ. The feasibility of a piecewise-linear dynamic bowtie filter. Med Phys. 2013;40:031910.
26. Huck SM, Parodi K, Stierstorfer K. First experimental validation of a novel concept for dynamic beam attenuation in CT. In: Fifth computed tomography conference. 2018.
27. Hull NC, Schooler GR, Binkovitz LA, Williamson EE, Araoz PA, Yu L, Young PM. Chest computed tomography angiography in children on extracorporeal membrane oxygenation (ECMO). Pediatr Radiol. 2018;48:1021–30.
28. Jakobs TF, Becker CR, Ohnesorge B, Flohr T, Suess C, Schoepf UJ, Reiser MF. Multislice helical CT of the heart with retrospective ECG gating: reduction of radiation exposure by ECG-controlled tube current modulation. Eur Radiol. 2002;12:1081–6.
29. Johnson TR, Krauss B, Sedlmair M, Grasruck M, Bruder H, Morhard D, Fink C, Weckbach S, Lenhard M, Schmidt B, Flohr T, Reiser MF, Becker CR. Material differentiation by dual energy CT: initial experience. Eur Radiol. 2007;17:1510–7.
30. Kachelriess M, Kalender WA. Electrocardiogram-correlated image reconstruction from subsecond spiral computed tomography scans of the heart. Med Phys. 1998;25:2417–31.
31. Kappler S, Glasser F, Janssen S, Kraft E, Reinwand M. A research prototype system for quantum-counting clinical CT. Proc SPIE. 2010;7622:70.

32. Kim SH, Kamaya A, Willmann JK. CT perfusion of the liver: principles and applications in oncology. Radiology. 2014;272:322–44.
33. Lell MM, May M, Deak P, Alibek S, Kuefner M, Kuettner A, Kohler H, Achenbach S, Uder M, Radkow T. High-pitch spiral computed tomography: effect on image quality and radiation dose in pediatric chest computed tomography. Investig Radiol. 2011;46:116–23.
34. Leng S, Rajendran K, Gong H, Zhou W, Halaweish AF, Henning A, Kappler S, Baer M, Fletcher JG, McCollough CH. 150-mu m spatial resolution using photon-counting detector computed tomography technology technical performance and first patient images. Investig Radiol. 2018;53:655–62.
35. Mao A, Gang GJ, Shyr W, Levinson R, Siewerdsen JH, Kawamoto S, Webster Stayman J. Dynamic fluence field modulation for miscentered patients in computed tomography. J Med imaging. 2018;5:043501.
36. Mathews AJ, Tilley S 2nd, Gang G, Kawamoto S, Zbijewski W, Siewerdsen JH, Levinson R, Webster Stayman J. Design of dual multiple aperture devices for dynamical fluence field modulated CT. Conf Proc Int Conf Image Form Xray Comput Tomogr. 2016;2016:29–32.
37. Matsumoto S, Yamada Y, Hashimoto M, Okamura T, Yamada M, Yashima F, Hayashida K, Fukuda K, Jinzaki M. CT imaging before transcatheter aortic valve implantation (TAVI) using variable helical pitch scanning and its diagnostic performance for coronary artery disease. Eur Radiol. 2017;27:1963–70.
38. McCollough CH, Leng S, Yu L, Fletcher JG. Dual- and multi-energy CT: principles, technical approaches, and clinical applications. Radiology. 2015;276:637–53.
39. McCollough CH, Primak AN, Saba O, Bruder H, Stierstorfer K, Raupach R, Suess C, Schmidt B, Ohnesorge BM, Flohr TG. Dose performance of a 64-channel dual-source CT scanner. Radiology. 2007;243:775–84.
40. Mongan J, Rathnayake S, Fu Y, Gao DW, Yeh BM. Extravasated contrast material in penetrating abdominopelvic trauma: dual-contrast dual-energy CT for improved diagnosis – preliminary results in an animal model. Radiology. 2013;268:738–42.
41. Mongan J, Rathnayake S, Fu Y, Wang R, Jones EF, Gao DW, Yeh BM. In vivo differentiation of complementary contrast media at dual-energy CT. Radiology. 2012;265:267–72.
42. Morhard D, Wirth CD, Fesl G, Schmidt C, Reiser MF, Becker CR, Ertl-Wagner B. Advantages of extended brain perfusion computed tomography: 9.6 cm coverage with time resolved computed tomography-angiography in comparison to standard stroke-computed tomography. Investig Radiol. 2010;45:363–9.
43. Muenzel D, Bar-Ness D, Roessl E, Blevis I, Bartels M, Fingerle AA, Ruschke S, Coulon P, Daerr H, Kopp FK, Brendel B, Thran A, Rokni M, Herzen J, Boussel L, Pfeiffer F, Proksa R, Rummeny EJ, Douek P, Noel PB. Spectral photon-counting CT: initial experience with dual-contrast agent K-edge colonography. Radiology. 2017;283:723–8.
44. Ohnesorge B, Flohr T, Becker C, Kopp AF, Schoepf UJ, Baum U, Knez A, Klingenbeck-Regn K, Reiser MF. Cardiac imaging by means of electrocardiographically gated multisection spiral CT: initial experience. Radiology. 2000;217:564–71.
45. Petersilka M, Bruder H, Krauss B, Stierstorfer K, Flohr TG. Technical principles of dual source CT. Eur J Radiol. 2008;68:362–8.
46. Pourmorteza A, Symons R, Sandfort V, Mallek M, Fuld MK, Henderson G, Jones EC, Malayeri AA, Folio LR, Bluemke DA. Abdominal imaging with contrast-enhanced photon-counting CT: first human experience. Radiology. 2016;279:239–45.
47. Primak AN, Fletcher JG, Vrtiska TJ, Dzyubak OP, Lieske JC, Jackson ME, Williams JC Jr, McCollough CH. Noninvasive differentiation of uric acid versus non-uric acid kidney stones using dual-energy CT. Acad Radiol. 2007;14:1441–7.
48. Qu M, Ehman E, Fletcher JG, Huprich JE, Hara AK, Silva AC, Farrugia G, Limburg P, McCollough CH. Toward biphasic computed tomography (CT) enteric contrast: material classification of luminal bismuth and mural iodine in a small-bowel phantom using dual-energy CT. J Comput Assist Tomogr. 2012;36:554–9.
49. Rassouli N, Etesami M, Dhanantwari A, Rajiah P. Detector-based spectral CT with a novel dual-layer technology: principles and applications. Insights into imaging. 2017;8:589–98.
50. Reiner CS, Goetti R, Eberli D, Klotz E, Boss A, Pfammatter T, Frauenfelder T, Moch H, Sulser T, Alkadhi H. CT perfusion of renal cell carcinoma: impact of volume coverage on quantitative analysis. Investig Radiol. 2012;47:33–40.
51. Rybicki FJ, Otero HJ, Steigner ML, Vorobiof G, Nallamshetty L, Mitsouras D, Ersoy H, Mather RT, Judy PF, Cai T, Coyner K, Schultz K, Whitmore AG, Di Carli MF. Initial evaluation of coronary images from 320-detector row computed tomography. Int J Card Imaging. 2008;24:535–46.
52. Saba L, Porcu M, Schmidt B, Flohr T. Dual energy CT: basic principles. In: De Cecco C, Laghi A, Schoepf U, Meinel F, editors. Dual energy CT in oncology. Switzerland; Springer. 2015.
53. Scheffel H, Alkadhi H, Leschka S, Plass A, Desbiolles L, Guber I, Krauss T, Gruenenfelder J, Genoni M, Luescher TF, Marincek B, Stolzmann P. Low-dose CT coronary angiography in the step-and-shoot mode: diagnostic performance. Heart. 2008;94:1132–7.
54. Scheffel H, Stolzmann P, Frauenfelder T, Schertler T, Desbiolles L, Leschka S, Marincek B, Alkadhi H. Dual-energy contrast-enhanced computed tomography for the detection of urinary stone disease. Investig Radiol. 2007;42:823–9.
55. Siebert E, Bohner G, Dewey M, Masuhr F, Hoffmann KT, Mews J, Engelken F, Bauknecht HC, Diekmann

S, Klingebiel R. 320-slice CT neuroimaging: initial clinical experience and image quality evaluation. Br J Radiol. 2009;82:561–70.

56. Sorantin E, Riccabona M, Stucklschweiger G, Guss H, Fotter R. Experience with volumetric (320 rows) pediatric CT. Eur J Radiol. 2013;82:1091–7.
57. Stayman JW, Tilley II S. Model-based multi-material decomposition using spatial-spectral CT filters. In: International conference on image formation in X-Ray computed tomography. 2018.
58. Stolzmann P, Leschka S, Scheffel H, Krauss T, Desbiolles L, Plass A, Genoni M, Flohr TG, Wildermuth S, Marincek B, Alkadhi H. Dual-source CT in step-and-shoot mode: noninvasive coronary angiography with low radiation dose. Radiology. 2008a;249:71–80.
59. Stolzmann P, Scheffel H, Rentsch K, Schertler T, Frauenfelder T, Leschka S, Sulser T, Marincek B, Alkadhi H. Dual-energy computed tomography for the differentiation of uric acid stones: ex vivo performance evaluation. Urol Res. 2008b;36:133–8.
60. Symons R, Krauss B, Sahbaee P, Cork TE, Lakshmanan MN, Bluemke DA, Pourmorteza A. Photon-counting CT for simultaneous imaging of multiple contrast agents in the abdomen: an in vivo study. Med Phys. 2017;44:5120–7.
61. Szczykutowicz TP, Mistretta CA. Design of a digital beam attenuation system for computed tomography: part I. system design and simulation framework. Med Phys. 2013;40:021905.
62. Taguchi K, Iwanczyk JS. Vision 20/20: single photon counting x-ray detectors in medical imaging. Med Phys. 2013;40:100901.
63. Takahashi N, Hartman RP, Vrtiska TJ, Kawashima A, Primak AN, Dzyubak OP, Mandrekar JN, Fletcher JG, McCollough CH. Dual-energy CT iodine-subtraction virtual unenhanced technique to detect urinary stones in an iodine-filled collecting system: a phantom study. AJR Am J Roentgenol. 2008;190:1169–73.
64. Taylor S, Litmanovich DE, Shahrzad M, Bankier AA, Gevenois PA, Tack D. Organ-based tube current modulation: are women's breasts positioned in the reduced-dose zone? Radiology. 2015;274:260–6.
65. Tivnan M, Tilley S, Stayman JW. Physical modeling and performance of spatial-spectral filters for CT material decomposition. Proc SPIE. 2019;10948:109481A.
66. Tzedakis A, Damilakis J, Perisinakis K, Stratakis J, Gourtsoyiannis N. The effect of z overscanning on patient effective dose from multidetector helical computed tomography examinations. Med Phys. 2005;32:1621–9.
67. Weber NM, Koo CW, Yu L, Bartholmai BJ, Halaweish AF, McCollough CH, Fletcher JG. Breathe new life into your chest CT exams: using advanced acquisition and postprocessing techniques. Curr Probl Diagn Radiol. 2019;48:152–60.
68. Weustink AC, Mollet NR, Pugliese F, Meijboom WB, Nieman K, Heijenbrok-Kal MH, Flohr TG, Neefjes LA, Cademartiri F, de Feyter PJ, Krestin GP. Optimal electrocardiographic pulsing windows and heart rate: effect on image quality and radiation exposure at dual-source coronary CT angiography. Radiology. 2008;248:792–8.
69. Willemink MJ, Persson M, Pourmorteza A, Pelc NJ, Fleischmann D. Photon-counting CT: technical principles and clinical prospects. Radiology. 2018;289:293–312.
70. Winklehner A, Goetti R, Baumueller S, Karlo C, Schmidt B, Raupach R, Flohr T, Frauenfelder T, Alkadhi H. Automated attenuation-based tube potential selection for thoracoabdominal computed tomography angiography: improved dose effectiveness. Investig Radiol. 2011;46:767–73.
71. Youn SW, Kim JH, Weon YC, Kim SH, Han MK, Bae HJ. Perfusion CT of the brain using 40-mm-wide detector and toggling table technique for initial imaging of acute stroke. Am J Roentgenol. 2008;191:W120–W26.
72. Yu L, Bruesewitz MR, Thomas KB, Fletcher JG, Kofler JM, McCollough CH. Optimal tube potential for radiation dose reduction in pediatric CT: principles, clinical implementations, and pitfalls. Radiographics. 2011;31:835–48.
73. Yu L, Fletcher JG, Grant KL, Carter RE, Hough DM, Barlow JM, Vrtiska TJ, Williamson EE, Young PM, Goss BC, Shiung M, Leng S, Raupach R, Schmidt B, Flohr T, McCollough CH. Automatic selection of tube potential for radiation dose reduction in vascular and contrast-enhanced abdominopelvic CT. AJR Am J Roentgenol. 2013;201:W297–306.
74. Yu L, Li H, Fletcher JG, McCollough CH. Automatic selection of tube potential for radiation dose reduction in CT: a general strategy. Med Phys. 2010;37:234–43.
75. Yu L, Ren L, Li Z, Leng S, McCollough CH. Dual-source multienergy CT with triple or quadruple x-ray beams. J Med imaging. 2018;5:033502.
76. Yu Z, Leng S, Jorgensen SM, Li Z, Gutjahr R, Chen B, Halaweish AF, Kappler S, Yu L, Ritman EL, McCollough CH. Evaluation of conventional imaging performance in a research whole-body CT system with a photon-counting detector array. Phys Med Biol. 2016;61:1572–95.
77. Zou Y, Pan X, Xia D, Wang G. PI-line-based image reconstruction in helical cone-beam computed tomography with a variable pitch. Med Phys. 2005;32:2639–48.

CT Statistical and Iterative Reconstructions and Post Processing

4

Norbert J. Pelc and Adam Wang

Introduction

Since the introduction of computed tomography, analytic reconstruction algorithms have been the mainstay for methods used to produce images from the measured projection data. While the original EMI scanner used an iterative algorithm [1] and a great deal of research was conducted on such methods [2], analytical methods, and specifically filtered backprojection [3], were adopted into all commercial systems, largely because of their computational efficiency. In this chapter, we deal with more recent advances in image reconstruction, including iterative reconstruction and methods for noise reduction. These have been helpful in facilitating the reduction of radiation dose in CT.

Mathematical problems include two classes, "forward" and "inverse" problems. With respect to the relationship between the projection data and image (or object) in computed tomography, converting a description of the object to the measured projection data is a forward problem. Suppose we are given full knowledge of the object and are asked what are the ray measurements through that object? We know how x-rays propagate through materials. In principle, we know many things about our system, including the x-ray spectrum, focal spot distribution, and the response of detector. With this information, we can calculate any sample in the raw data. This is an example of a forward problem, often called forward projection in the CT literature. Reconstruction is an inverse problem. We are given raw data (ray measurements) and are asked what is the object that produced these data? As mentioned earlier, for many decades, the mainstay of image reconstruction has been analytic reconstruction methods. In these, we can write down a formula for the relationship between the reconstructed object and the measured data; the best example for this analytic reconstruction approach is filtered backprojection [3].

Analytical reconstruction methods are computationally very efficient because each raw data point is generally touched only once. The amount of computation needed to go from the measured data to the reconstructed image is quite reasonable. An additional property of the analytic reconstruction methods for conventional CT is that they are "exact." This means that when the measured data are perfect and noiseless, the raw data and the resulting image will be perfectly consistent with each other. The problem with analytical reconstruction is that if the measured data are not perfect, as it is often the case, the image may not be ideal; we might be able to obtain a better image with a different approach.

N. J. Pelc (✉)
Department of Bioengineering and Radiology, Stanford University, Stanford, CA, USA
e-mail: pelc@stanford.edu

A. Wang
Department of Radiology, Stanford University, Stanford, CA, USA
e-mail: adamwang@stanford.edu

© Springer Nature Switzerland AG 2020

E. Samei, N. J. Pelc (eds.), *Computed Tomography*, https://doi.org/10.1007/978-3-030-26957-9_4

Iterative Reconstruction

An alternative to analytical reconstruction methods is iterative reconstruction. The process starts with a guess of the object. With this estimate of the object and the forward model, we can generate the projections that would have been measured if the estimate of the object is correct. Example starting guesses are a perfectly transparent object (zero attenuation coefficient throughout) and a round water object. We then compare the projections that would have been measured if the object estimate was correct (our synthetic projections) with the actual projections that were obtained by the scanner. In general, they will not agree, and we update the guess of the object based on the difference between the synthetic and actual projections. This becomes our new estimate of the object, and we apply the forward model to generate a new set of synthetic projections. This process continues until, hopefully, it converges and we obtain an estimate of the object (a reconstructed image) whose synthetic projections agree with the actual projections. This is shown graphically in Fig. 4.1.

The advantage of this approach using a forward model is that it can include as much of the physics of the scanner as desired. Further, the synthetic raw data will contain the effects of the physical processes included in the model, so that when an image is produced using this forward model, it will be intrinsically corrected for those effects. For example, if the real scanner has a polyenergetic x-ray beam but the forward model assumes the source is monoenergetic, the image will have beam-hardening artifacts. On the other hand, if the forward model includes polyenergetic effects with a spectrum that matches that of the scanner, the image will automatically be corrected for beam hardening. Similarly, if the forward model includes scatter in the object, the image will be corrected for this process. The model can be made as realistic and as complicated as we would like. If it includes the focal spot distribution, the real detector cell size and response (e.g., nonlinearity or other imperfections), and finite size voxels, the image will be compensated for blurring or artifacts caused by them. The actual ray paths (e.g., helical scans and divergent beams) and even knowledge that some data are missing can be included in the reconstruction. Indeed, the model can include object motion if it is known. The forward model would then generate synthetic data that reflect what would be measured if in fact all of these assumptions about the system are correct, and because of the way in which the iterative reconstruction method attempts to produce an image consistent with the data (and its imperfections), the image will be corrected for the imperfections included in the model [4].

When the real measured data and the synthetic data generated from the estimated image do not agree, an additional aspect that can be included in iterative reconstruction is any knowledge we have about the precision or reliability of individual measurements. We may know that some measurements may be more reliable than others, for

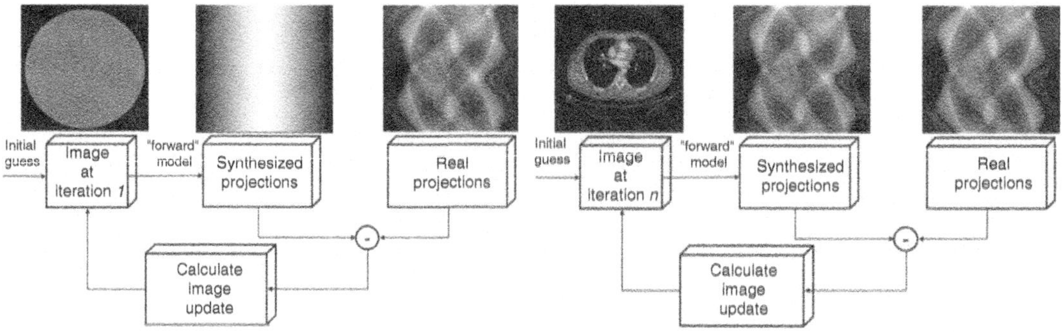

Fig. 4.1 Iterative reconstruction process

example, due to different quantum noise or other stochastic errors. Analytic reconstruction methods do not take measurement error into account, whereas iterative reconstruction methods can incorporate our knowledge of errors in raw data, including uncertainty. In general, the measurement uncertainty is not uniform across the data set, as some measured rays will go through very thin or relatively transparent portions of the object and therefore have excellent statistics and be less noisy, whereas rays that go through bony regions or large soft tissue paths may have far fewer transmitted photons and therefore be much noisier. Analytic reconstruction methods treat all the rays as being equally accurate, but the iterative reconstruction method can incorporate our knowledge of these measurement errors. For example, we can pose the reconstruction problem as finding the object that is "most likely" to have produced the measured data. Of all of the possible objects that might have produced the data, we choose the one that is most likely to have produced it, and in this most likely estimation, we can include measurement errors and physical imperfections that may cause some measurements to be less reliable than others.

The problem with this – even though it is very elegant and convenient – is that if we actually try to use it and generate the object most likely to have produced the data while incorporating our knowledge about our system imperfections, in general it will not converge to a stable answer. The reconstruction process tends to amplify noise, so we have to get this instability under control. We accomplish this with a regularizer that can incorporate prior knowledge or image preference into the reconstruction process. Some aspects we may know about our objects are real physical constraints, e.g., we know density cannot be negative or larger than some value. The reconstruction process can then be constrained to force the map of linear attenuation coefficient be non-negative and less than or equal to the known maximum. In this way, we now try to find the object most likely to have produced the measured data given other things that we may know about our objects. These kinds of prior knowledge constraints can be useful, but in general they are insufficient to stabilize the reconstruction problem. More commonly, we bring other constraints that are sometimes called prior "knowledge" but in reality are preferences. One of them is to promote image smoothness – we prefer images where adjacent pixels have similar attenuation. We can put this constraint into the optimization problem, and this regularizer promotes smoothness. It is important to be realistic about the fact that the regularizer is bringing our own prior bias into the reconstruction problem. The statement that adjacent pixels should have similar values will certainly reduce the noise level, but it may not in fact be true, in which case the image may not accurately represent the object.

One way in which we bring in the regularizer is to minimize a quantity that has two components:

$$\hat{x} = \arg\min_x D(x) + \beta \cdot R(x)$$

We seek to find a reconstruction $\hat{x}$ that minimizes the sum of (1) a data-matching term $D(x)$ which tries to find an object whose forward projections agree with our measured data and can incorporate measurement uncertainty and (2) a second term which is the regularizer. For example, this could be a scalar constant β times the result of an analysis of the difference of adjacent pixels, $R(x)$. As mentioned above, the data-matching term, sometimes called the data-fidelity term, can incorporate our knowledge of statistical uncertainties, such as a log-likelihood model of the Poisson statistics of transmitted photons. A more sophisticated model may also incorporate electronic noise of the detectors or noise from scattered photons [5]. The log-likelihood model is sometimes approximated by a Gaussian model of the line integrals (i.e., after log normalization), simplifying the data-matching term to a weighted least squares approximation, $D(x) = \|y - Ax\|_W^2$, where y is the measured line integral, A is the forward model, x is an estimate of the object, and weights W are inversely related to the statistical uncertainty of the line integrals. Combined with the regularizer, this becomes a penalized weighted least squares (PWLS) problem [6]. While we generally have an accurate forward model A, it is difficult to directly invert the model

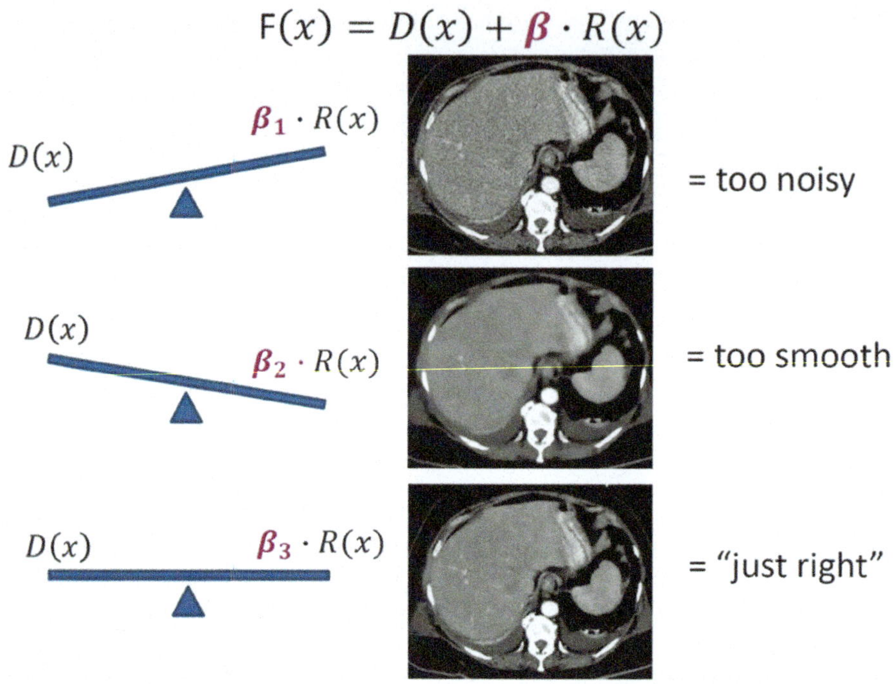

Fig. 4.2 Effect of regularization strength β. (Courtesy of Kevin M. Brown, Philips Healthcare)

due to the size of the inverse matrix, and thus it is difficult to solve the optimization problem directly. Instead, iterative methods are used to progressively improve the reconstruction and get closer to the solution.

The parameter β is very important in the appearance of the image. If β is very small, we are not letting the regularizer affect the image very much, and the image might be quite noisy, as shown in Fig. 4.2. If the regularizer parameter is too large, then the resulting image will be overly smooth. An intermediate parameter may be the one that produces images that we like best, akin to the choice that Goldilocks needed to make.

As shown in Fig. 4.2, the regularizer tends to smooth the image and blur edges. This is much like an analytical reconstruction with a softer reconstruction kernel, but iterative reconstruction can proceed quite a bit differently. It can act differently in different areas of the image. For example, when two nearby pixels are very different, the algorithm could allow it because it could represent a real edge. Thus, if the difference between adjacent pixels is much larger than would be explained by statistical uncertainty, we treat it as being real, whereas if the difference is easily explained by statistical uncertainty, we might treat it as noise and suppress it. This approach is called an edge-preserving regularizer because it will smooth the image and suppress noise except at regions that we have, through our processing, determined are likely to be real edges. We compare local pixel differences to the expected noise level. If the difference between adjacent pixels is low, we suppress that difference by smoothing the image in those regions. If the difference between adjacent pixels is larger and we believe they are true edges, we leave it intact. For intermediate differences, the regularizer will do something intermediate (e.g., lightly smooth).

While this kind of edge-preserving smoothing makes logical sense, it will tend to make images whose texture can be rather strange, an appearance sometimes called "salt-and-pepper" in which isolated black pixels or white pixels that are very much different than adjacent ones are preserved among otherwise gray areas. Another tendency of edge-preserving regularizers is to produce images with noise texture significantly

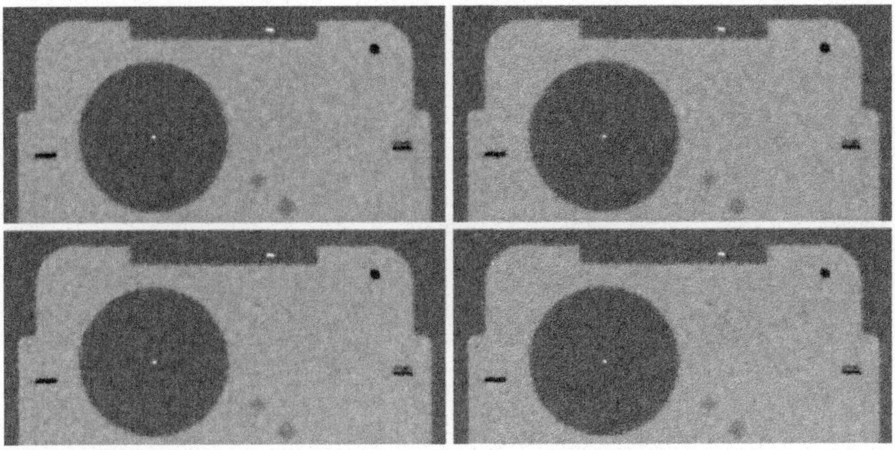

Fig. 4.3 Comparison of images computed with a range of iterative reconstruction parameters [6]. Note the isolated black dots in the lower right panel

different from that of FBP [6]. Often, human observers tend to not like this noise texture, shown in Fig. 4.3. More sophisticated regularizers can avoid this behavior. Many kinds of regularizers can be used, and different iterative reconstruction implementations may use different ones. A complete review of regularizers can be found in [7].

Examples

Edge-preserving smoothing can be quite effective to improve the appearance of clinical images. Figure 4.4 shows a conventional analytic reconstruction of an abdominal section with a particular reconstruction kernel that produced an image with a pixel standard deviation in the liver of 53 HU. This analytical reconstruction image is compared to two other images. One is simply a conventional analytical reconstruction using a softer kernel that reduces the noise level to 21 HU. The other is an iterative reconstruction with five iterations that also has a pixel noise level of 21 HU. While the iterative reconstruction and the image made with the soft kernel both have the same noise level, we see the noise texture is quite different. Difference images between each of the two lower noise images minus the original one show noise in the region of the liver, indicating that each has achieved some noise suppression. However, the difference between the two analytical reconstructions has large values at strong edges in the object (e.g., the skin surface), indicating smoothing of these edges, while the difference between the iterative reconstruction and the original analytical reconstruction has noise, but much lower values at the edges, indicating that the edges were preserved. Thus, the edge-preserving regularizer in the iterative reconstruction changed the noise level in the liver but did not smooth the edges at the skin surface.

Figure 4.5 shows a similar example, comparing a linear filtered backprojection reconstruction of a patient with an aortic stent with an iterative reconstruction of the same data. We see both a reduction in noise level and a sharpening of the high-contrast edges of the stent, demonstrating that we can simultaneously improve the visualization of high-contrast edges while suppressing noise in areas with relatively uniform signal. It is important to keep in mind that these two different effects, noise reduction and edge sharpening, are happening in different areas, as shown in more detail below. Other artifacts, such as blooming and metal artifact, are also often reduced as a result of iterative reconstruction. Although iterative reconstruction is not a dedicated metal artifact reduction algorithm, it does show some robustness to metal artifacts by downweighting the rays that pass through metal and carry little useful information.

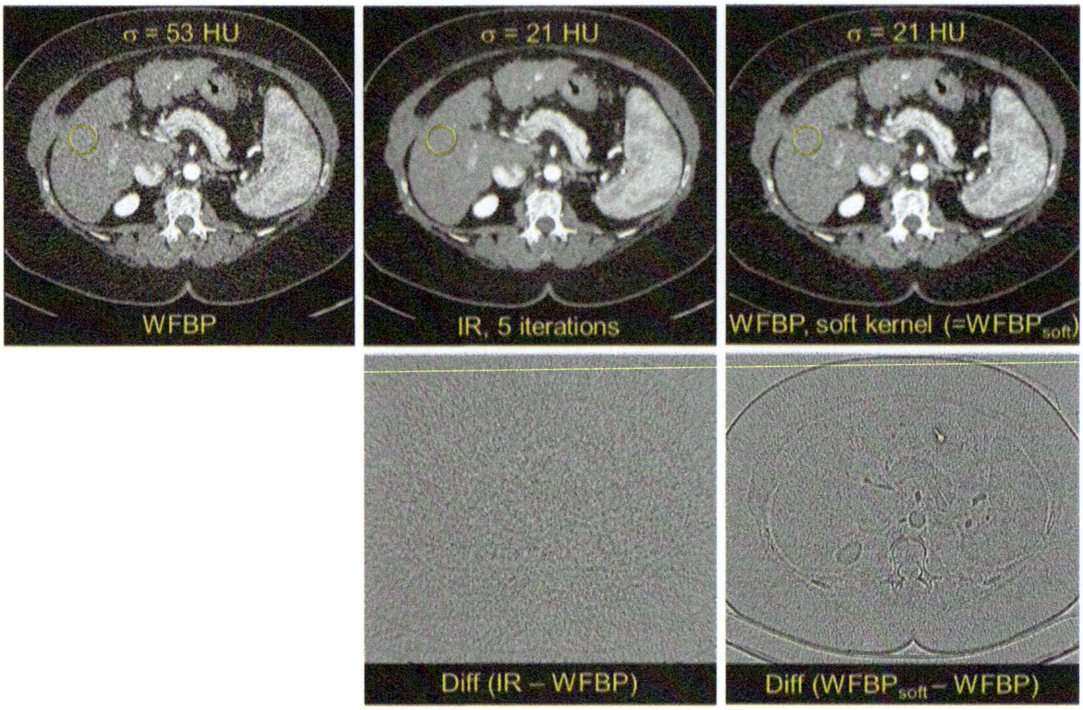

Fig. 4.4 Abdominal scan reconstructed with FBP, IR, and FBP with a soft kernel. (Courtesy of Rainer Raupach, Siemens Healthineers)

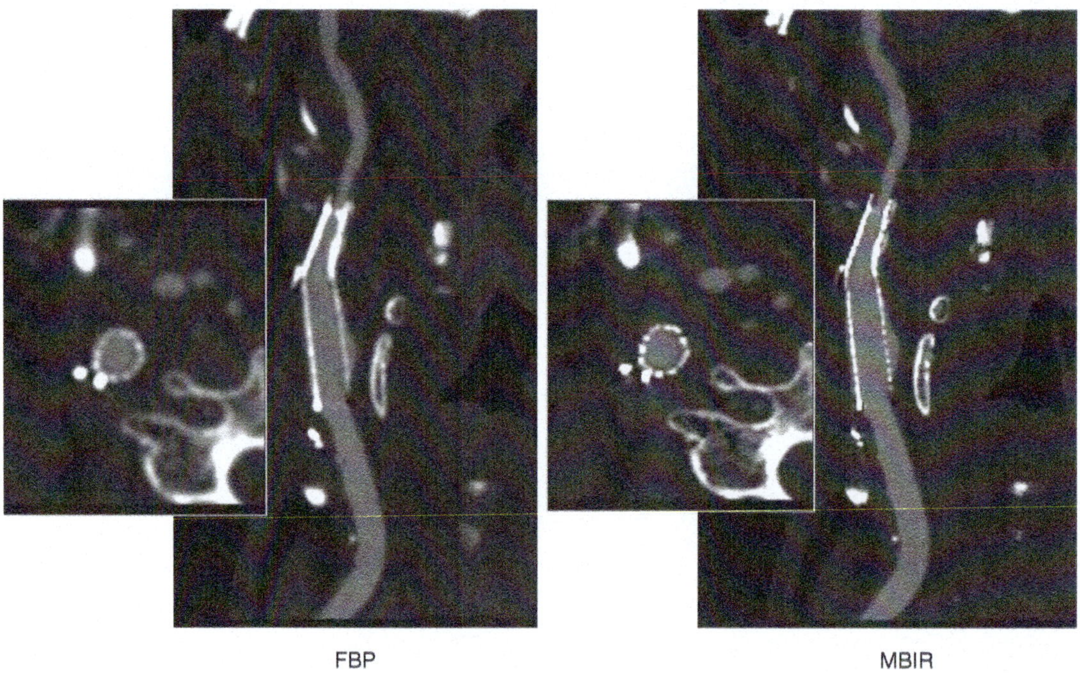

Fig. 4.5 Aortic stent, reconstructed with FBP (left) and model-based iterative reconstruction (right). (Courtesy of Jiang Hsieh, GE Healthcare)

We need to keep in mind that the regularizer can introduce nonlinearities, non-stationarity, and also bias. In a linear system, if we multiply the input by a constant, the output scales by the same constant. A corollary is that spatial resolution (e.g., as reflected by the point spread or modulation transfer functions) does not depend on the local signal difference. By contrast, if the behavior of the algorithm depends on local signal differences, it reflects nonlinearity. The edge-preserving regularizer, which preserves differences between adjacent pixels when they are large but suppresses them when they are small, is a canonical example of nonlinearity. A system is non-stationary if the behavior is different in different areas. The edge-preserving regularizer makes the system non-stationary, with the noise level and the spatial resolution being different in different parts of the image. Lastly, the regularizer can introduce bias if we build into it our own preference for what the image should look like, such as forcing the image to be smooth in areas that do not have strong edges. This property (increased smoothness when there are no strong edges) may not be true, yet the output of the iterative reconstruction may have this behavior. It is merely our preference (or bias), and the image produced will reflect our preference and be in agreement with our prior bias of what the image should look like.

Another example of edge-preserving smoothing is shown in Fig. 4.6, which shows a linear analytical reconstruction (FBP) of a scan of jar of jelly beans. Also shown is the difference between two independent images (two scans) of the same object. The difference shows only noise (which is somewhat higher in the center than at

FBP

MBIR

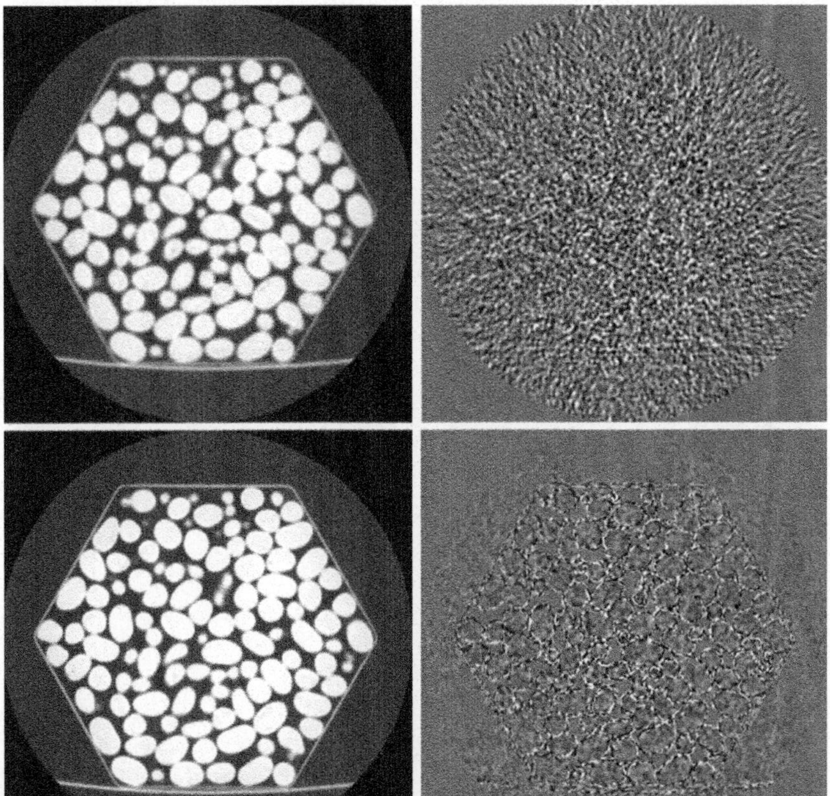

Fig. 4.6 The left column shows reconstructed images of a jelly bean phantom, with filtered backprojection (FBP, top) and model-based iterative reconstruction (MBIR, bottom). The right image shows the difference of two scans, illustrating the noise in the reconstructed images. (Courtesy of Guang-Hong Chen, University of Wisconsin)

the edges due to nonuniform statistics) with no structure from the jar, the jelly beans, or the scanner table. By contrast, when the same data are reconstructed with an iterative algorithm that has edge-preserving smoothing, the difference between two images has much lower noise in all regions with uniform signal (e.g., the interior of the jelly beans) but very high noise in regions corresponding to edges in the original images. The edge-preserving smoothing did not reduce the noise level or the differences between adjacent pixels in these edge regions. It preserves the edges, but it also maintains the high noise level in those local regions, whereas inside the jelly beans or inside uniform parts of the phantom, the noise is suppressed. This is an example of both nonlinearity and non-stationarity.

It is important to keep in mind that the regularizer and these iterative reconstruction methods are operating in three dimensions, i.e., not only the in-plane dimensions that can be appreciated in 2D images but also the slice direction. The noise reduction it can achieve can take advantage of the third dimension, but it will introduce correlations among neighboring pixel values and local smoothing that may be hard to perceive in 2D images. The correlations can be probed by analyzing the noise in volumetric images (stack of slices). Figure 4.7 compares the noise covariance in the slice direction of conventional and iterative reconstructions of a scan of a uniform water phantom. In these displays, the two axes are positions in the slice direction with increasing values to the right and down, and the color portrays the covariance. If the slices are independent, the covariance display would contain non-zero values only along the diagonal, with an amplitude equal to the pixel variance. As can be seen, while the noise in any particular slice (i.e., as represented by the diagonal elements) is lower for iterative reconstruction than filtered backprojection, the correlations in the slice direction (i.e., the off-diagonal elements) are relatively larger in the iterative reconstruction. While the iterative reconstruction has lower absolute covariance, it extends over a wider region, indicating that the method is smoothing in the slice direction. This means that in regions of low contrast (with no strong edges to trigger edge preservation), the slices are effectively thicker than in regions where the reconstruction method has detected edges. This is exactly the same as what we saw earlier with the jelly bean phantom but operating in the slice direction. It is clear that part of the noise reduction in iterative reconstructions comes from (local) smoothing in the slice direction. This approach was used to study iterative reconstruction methods from two different CT system vendors and found that the amount of variance reduction from blurring in the

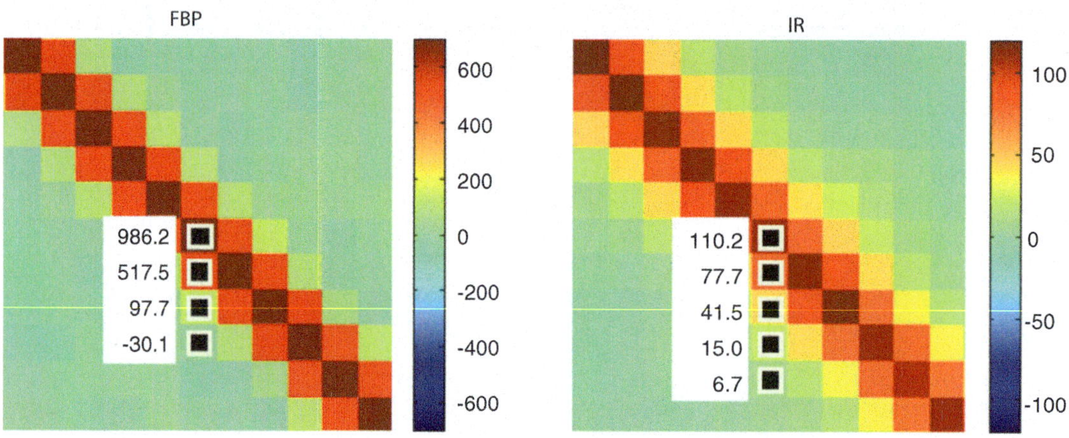

Fig. 4.7 Covariance matrix of noise in the slice direction for a uniform water phantom

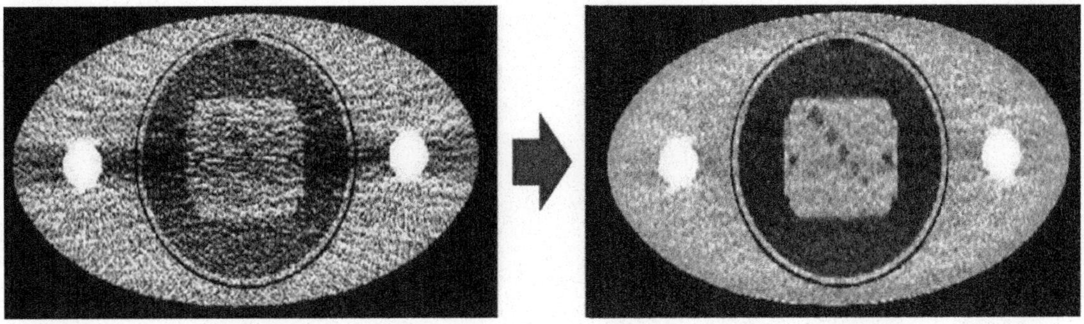

Fig. 4.8 Phantom with dense rods that lead to beam hardening and photon starvation. IR is able to reduce noise and improve visibility of the central object. (Courtesy of Jiang Hsieh, GE Healthcare. Adapted from [9])

slice direction can be quite different among these various methods. It also found that slice-direction smoothing is responsible for a significant amount of the noise reduction from the advanced reconstruction methods [8].

The ability of iterative reconstruction methods to model the physics of the system and to include our knowledge of its imperfections can be very powerful for artifact reduction. Figure 4.8 shows images of a phantom that contains two dense rods and a central region with low-contrast features. Beam hardening and photon starvation can produce artifacts in conventional reconstructions, such as the dark band in the region of the FBP image connecting the two dense rods. Iterative reconstruction can build in knowledge of the data statistics as well as spectral effects, allowing suppression of the artifact and reducing the image noise level to make the low-contrast features to be seen much more easily [9]. While this example is of a phantom, such benefits are readily seen in scans of the shoulder and pelvic regions, which have relatively thick bone cross sections (i.e., beam hardening) and large lateral width (i.e., photon starvation), and traditionally often suffer from streak artifacts in images produced by analytical reconstruction.

Figure 4.9 shows the ability of iterative reconstruction to include cone-beam effects. In this example, the conventional reconstruction of simulated cone-beam CT data has artifacts coming from beam divergence in the slice direction that is not perfectly handled by the analytic reconstruction method. The iterative reconstruction method can include knowledge of the geometry and in some cases generate significant artifact reduction. In this example, only two iterations were needed.

As discussed previously, when data for a 3D volume are available, iterative reconstruction can include the third dimension for purposes of noise reduction. In an extension of this, when the images are dynamic, the time dimension can also be included to further improve image quality [10]. Further, when motion is present and a model of the motion is available, it can be included in the iterative reconstruction model [11]. The method can reduce artifacts and noise at the same time, producing a much more pleasing image, as shown in Fig. 4.10.

Statistical Reconstruction

The iterative reconstruction methods described above that model all the physics can be very powerful. They iterate repeatedly between the raw data and the image domains, and they can include statistical uncertainty, system physics, and prior knowledge and can reduce noise as well as artifacts. The main disadvantage is that

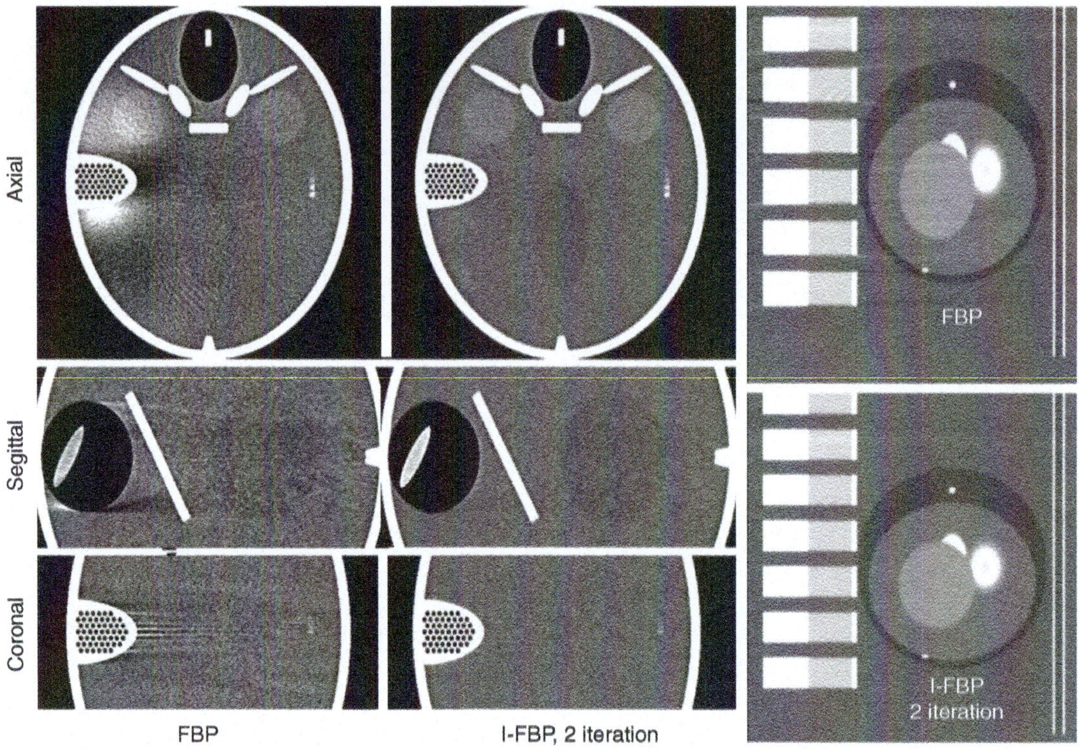

Fig. 4.9 Simulation of a digital phantom. (Courtesy of Karl Stierstorfer, Siemens Healthineers)

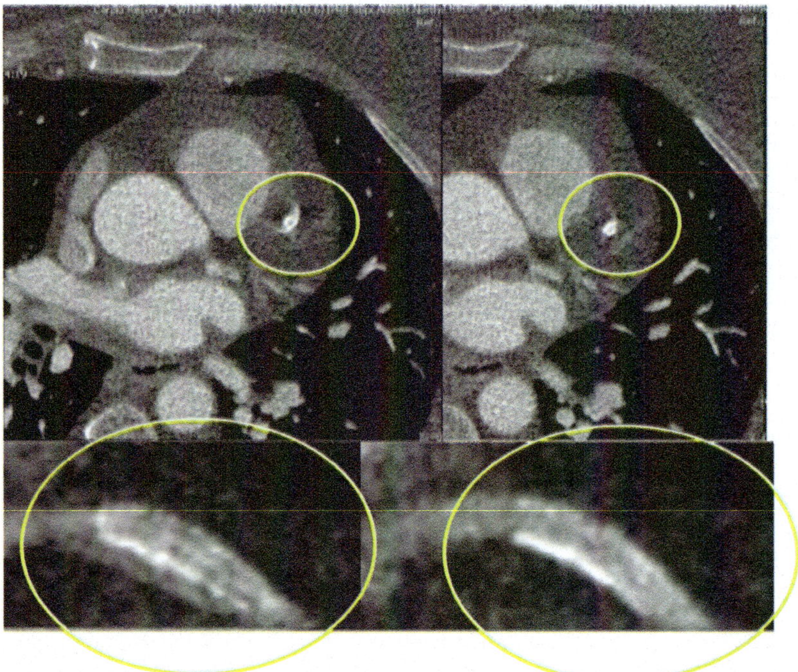

Fig. 4.10 Cardiac CT. Example of iterative reconstruction with built-in motion artifact correction. (Courtesy of Herbert Bruder, Siemens Healthineers)

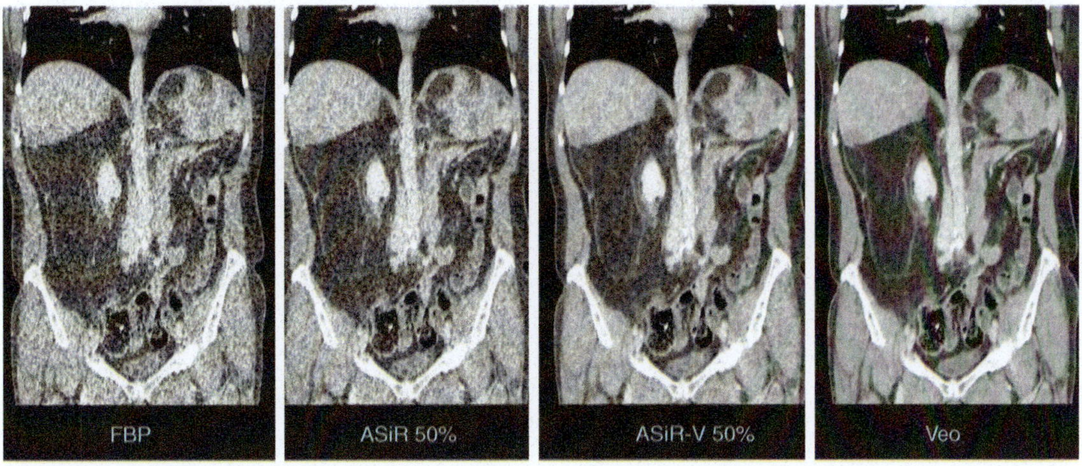

Fig. 4.11 Different reconstruction methods applied to the same acquisition, from left to right, FBP, statistical, and iterative reconstructions ($CTDI_{vol}$ = 1.4 mGy, DLP = 61.8 mGy-cm, effective dose = 0.93 mSv) [13]. (Courtesy of Jiang Hsieh, GE Healthcare)

they are computationally expensive. The amount of computation is much higher than with analytical reconstruction methods; therefore the iterative reconstruction time is much higher. Early releases of iterative reconstruction took upwards of 1 h to reconstruct a scan. While advances in computational hardware, including general-purpose graphics processing units (GPUs), have led to shorter reconstruction times [12], it is still a concern for clinical workflow.

This leads to the question of what other alternatives we might consider. If our need is to correct for artifacts caused by system physics, the iterative reconstruction formalism is often the best solution to that problem, but if one is only trying to reduce image noise caused by statistical uncertainty, it is possible to gain significant benefits with much simpler algorithms. We can choose to apply noise reduction with edge preservation either in the image domain or in the raw data domain or perhaps a mixture of the two. This approach is an example of the third kind of image reconstruction, sometimes called statistical reconstruction. These are algorithms that take into account the known uncertainty in the measured data and in the image domain, but do not necessarily incorporate much or any of the physics of the CT system. Because of the simpler nature of these algorithms, they can be much faster than full iterative reconstruction but usually a bit slower than a simple analytical reconstruction method. We therefore have families of reconstruction methods with filtered backprojection being an example of an analytical reconstruction method, full iterative reconstruction methods that model all of the physics and all of the objects, and statistical reconstruction methods that are intermediate both in their sophistication and also in the reconstruction time. Figure 4.11 shows examples of these various kinds of reconstruction methods and their ability to improve image appearance [13].

Figure 4.12 shows the range of the advanced reconstruction methods available from various vendors and where they fall in the spectrum between iterative reconstruction that models all the physics and rather faster statistical reconstruction methods that operate in one or the other domain in order to improve image appearance.

Image Quality Metrics

The images produced by these advanced nonlinear reconstruction methods have some unusual properties. With standard analytical reconstruction methods, we expect the image noise standard deviation to drop as the inverse of the square root of the dose from the known relationship between noise and the

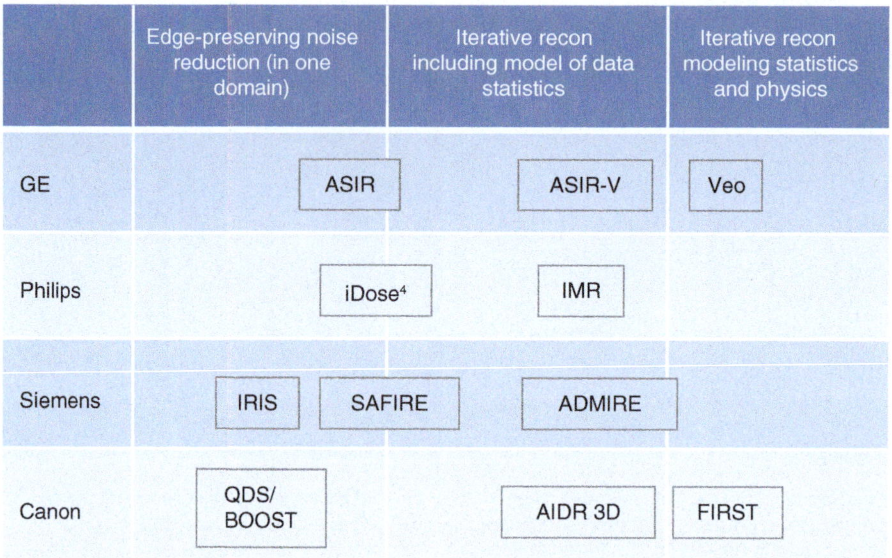

Fig. 4.12 Vendor reconstruction method names and their approaches

number of detected photons. Iterative and statistical reconstruction methods can use the knowledge of the statistics of the measurement to suppress the noise more when the statistics are poor and less when the statistics are quite sufficient, so the relationship between image standard deviation and dose (or the tube current-time product, mAs) of the scan may no longer follow the expected relationship, as shown in Fig. 4.13 (left). Noise was measured in abdominal CT scans. The behavior of the model-based image reconstruction is quite striking, with image noise being almost independent of x-ray tube current. This does not necessarily mean that the image quality (evaluated by radiologists) is also independent of dose or tube current. As shown in Fig. 4.13 (right), image quality rises with increasing tube current for all the methods [14]. When we apply the noise reduction in our iterative reconstruction, the noise standard deviation is reduced, but the image quality does not reflect the lower standard deviation in the way that we are used to in a conventional analytical reconstructions that are linear and (relatively) stationary. The impact of this is that pixel standard deviation is no longer a good predictor of image quality.

With traditional analytical reconstruction, we expect image standard deviation to be predictive of image quality, and we know how to trade off dose and image noise. Users should be careful inferring image quality and the potential for dose reduction from the noise reduction achieved by iterative reconstruction. For example, if iterative reconstruction reduces the noise variance by a factor of 2 compared to FBP, it may not follow that the dose can be reduced by a factor of 2 and that image quality would be comparable to the full-dose FBP. However, to the extent that iterative reconstruction improves subjective image quality, the image quality improvement can be traded off for dose reduction. Typically, the extent to which iterative reconstruction is used for image quality improvement vs dose reduction depends on the clinical application and is generally somewhere in between, where gains in both are achieved. It is also important to use iterative reconstruction in conjunction with other dose reduction methods, such as patient size-specific tube voltage and tube current modulation.

Another unusual property of these advanced reconstruction methods is that the spatial resolution depends on the contrast. The sharpness of the edge of an object will depend on the signal difference across the edge. Again, this is a direct result of the edge-preserving smoothing. When we have a structure with very high contrast, the algorithm will retain a sharp edge in that region. At the opposite extreme, when the contrast or change in attenuation is very low, it may not trigger edge preservation.

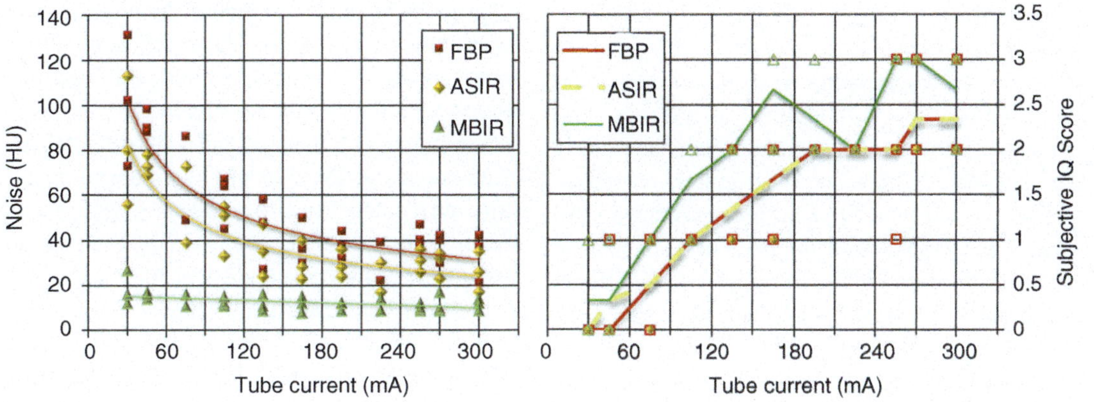

Fig. 4.13 (left) Pixel noise standard deviation in the liver as a function of x-ray tube current. While IR has much lower noise than FBP, especially at lower tube current (i.e., dose), the subjective image quality (right) tells a different story. Image quality for IR is overall higher, but still falls off with tube current. (Adapted from [14]. Courtesy of Dominik Fleischmann, Stanford University)

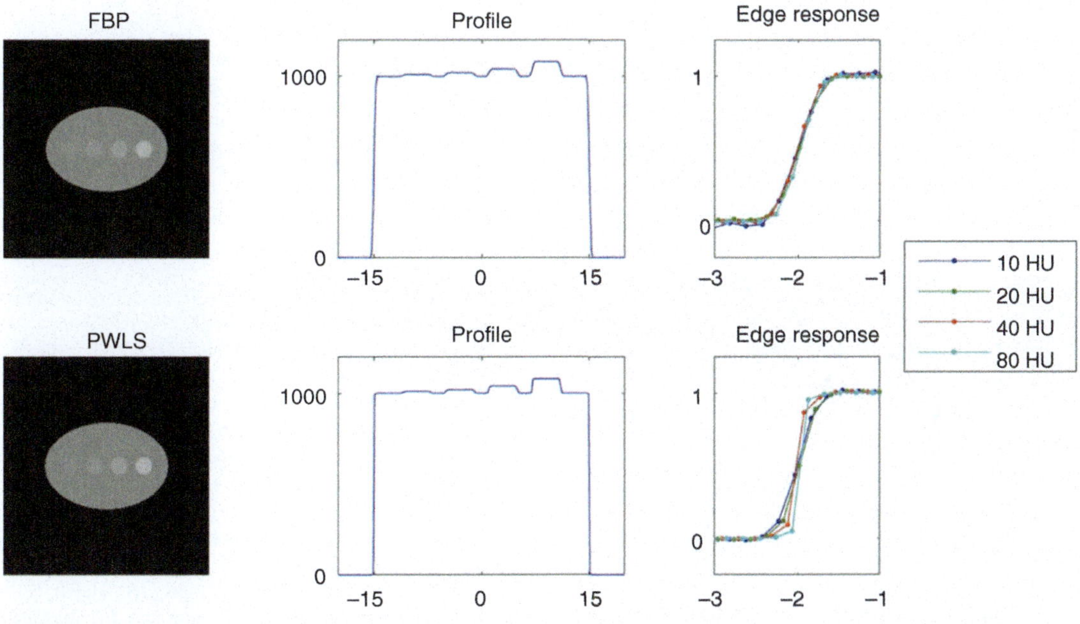

Fig. 4.14 Images from a simulated scan of an elliptical object with round higher density inserts, reconstructed with FBP (left top) and PWLS (left bottom), a form of iterative reconstruction. The middle panels show signal profiles through the round inserts, and the right panels show the edge responses, normalized by the contrast of the insert. The edge response for FBP is independent of contrast level, as we expect, whereas it becomes sharper with increased contrast for PWLS. (Courtesy of Jeff Fessler, University of Michigan)

The real object edge could be quite sharp, but the algorithm may treat this as a region without edges where noise reduction should be applied. This will smooth the edge and cause spatial resolution to depend on image contrast. This effect is shown in Fig. 4.14 [15]. These two properties – that the sharpness of a high-contrast edge does not predict sharpness elsewhere and that the dependence of noise level on dose is different from what we are used to – mean that our usual predictors of image quality, modulation transfer function (MTF) and pixel standard deviations (or even noise texture as measured by the noise power spectrum (NPS)), will have less general applicability and may need to be modified when used in characterizing modern CT systems (see Chap. 7).

Outlook

We expect image quality to continue improving with advances in modeling of physics and statistics. However, a new paradigm is beginning to appear in CT reconstruction, bringing artificial intelligence (AI) to reconstruction [16]. Recently, powerful new methods in AI have been enabled by availability of new software tools (e.g., open-source software such as TensorFlow or PyTorch), computationally efficient methods (deep convolutional neural networks), and hardware (GPUs). Thus far, most methods have incorporated AI as a way to denoise the reconstructed image, much like the regularizer in iterative reconstruction. One approach could be to train an AI model to generate high-dose FBP images from FBP of low-dose data. Another approach could be to produce images like iterative reconstruction images from an FBP reconstruction. One could also incorporate AI into various steps of the reconstruction or even imagine an AI model that directly maps projections to a reconstructed image. Vendors are beginning to announce and introduce AI-driven reconstructions [17, 18], and given the wave of interest in AI, we can expect more to follow. With the nonlinear and even less understood nature of AI, many of the same questions about image quality and behavior at low dose and low contrast will remain.

Conclusions

Analytical reconstruction methods like filtered backprojection are linear, they are fast, and they give us an exact reconstruction when the projection data are perfect. The spatial resolution is independent of contrast, and the standard deviation predicts image quality. We have seen a tremendous advance in statistical and iterative reconstruction methods, and they are being quickly adopted into clinical practice. The trend is certain to continue. The impact of these methods is highest when the data quality is poor, for example, in low-dose scans, thin slices, or obese patients. They can help the image observer be more comfortable with dose reduction because of the ability to reduce the noise level of lower-dose acquisitions. There are large differences among reconstruction methods. Statistical reconstruction methods are nonlinear, have edge-preserving noise reduction, and can help in regions of photon starvation. Model-based iterative reconstruction methods are also nonlinear. They are most effective for noise and artifact reduction but are rather slow. Hybrid methods, which are intermediate between them, are also available. Importantly, these nonlinear methods have contrast-dependent noise and resolution behavior and spatially dependent slice thickness that should be taken into account when the images are interpreted. Their nonlinear behavior challenges the usual image quality metrics. New metrics are needed to allow us to predict image quality.

References

1. Hounsfield GN. Computerized transverse axial scanning (tomography): part 1. Description of system. Brit J Radiol. 1973;46:1016–22.
2. Brooks RA, DiChiro G. Theory of image reconstruction in computed tomography. Radiology. 1975;117:561–72.
3. Kak AC, Slaney M. Principles of computerized tomographic imaging. New York: IEEE Press; 1988.
4. Nuyts J, De Man B, Fessler JA, Zbijewski W, Beekman FJ. Modelling the physics in the iterative reconstruction for transmission computed tomography. Phys Med Biol. 2013;58(12):R63–96.
5. Dang H, Stayman JW, Sisniega A, Xu J, Zbijewski W, Wang X, et al. Statistical reconstruction for cone-beam CT with a post-artifact-correction noise model: application to high-quality head imaging. Phys Med Biol. 2015;60(16):6153–75.
6. Thibault JB, Sauer KD, Bouman CA, Hsieh J. A three-dimensional statistical approach to improved image quality for multislice helical CT. Med Phys. 2007;34(11):4526–44.
7. Zhang H, Zeng D, Zhang H, Wang J, Liang Z, Ma J. Applications of nonlocal means algorithm in low-dose X-ray CT image processing and reconstruction: a review. Med Phys. 2017;44:1168–85.
8. Hsieh SS, Pelc NJ. Limits to dose reduction from iterative reconstruction and the effect of through-slice blurring. Proc SPIE Med Imaging. 2016; 97831C.
9. Chang Z, Zhang R, Thibault JB, Pal D, Fu L, Sauer K, Bouman C. Modeling and pre-treatment of photon-starved CT data for iterative reconstruction. IEEE Trans Med Imaging. 2017;36(1):277–87. https://doi.org/10.1109/TMI.2016.2606338. Epub 2016 Sep 7.

10. Yuki H, Utsunomiya D, Funama Y, Tokuyasu S, Namimoto T, Hirai T, Itatani R, Katahira K, Oshima S, Yamashita Y. Value of knowledge-based iterative model reconstruction in low-kV 256-slice coronary CT angiography. J Cardivasc Comput Tomogr. 2014;4:115–23.
11. Rohkohl C, Bruder H, Stierstorfer K, Flohr T. Improving best-phase image quality in cardiac CT by motion correction with MAM optimization. Med Phys. 2013;40:031901.
12. Després P, Jia X. A review of GPU-based medical image reconstruction. Phys Med. 2017;42:76–92.
13. Hsieh J. Computed tomography: principles, design, artifacts, and recent advances. 3rd ed. SPIE. Bellingham: Washington; 2015.
14. Olcott EW, Shin LK, Sommer G, Chan I, Rosenberg J, Molvin FL, et al. Model-based iterative reconstruction compared to adaptive statistical iterative reconstruction and filtered back-projection in CT of the kidneys and the adjacent retroperitoneum. Acad Radiol. 2014;21(6):774–84.
15. Fessler JA. http://web.eecs.umich.edu/~fessler/irt/irt/example/edge_response_2d.m.
16. Wang G, Ye JC, Mueller K, Fessler JA. Image reconstruction is a new frontier of machine learning. IEEE Trans Med Imag. 2018;37(6):1289–96.
17. Akagi M, Nakamura Y, Higaki T, Narita K, Honda Y, Zhou J, et al. Deep learning reconstruction improves image quality of abdominal ultra-high-resolution CT. Eur Radiol. 2019 (published online).
18. FDA Clears GE's Deep Learning Image Reconstruction Engine. Imaging Technology News. 2019. Retrieved May 24, 2019, from https://www.itnonline.com/content/fda-clears-ges-deep-learning-image-reconstruction-engine.

Part II

CT Performance

Dose and Risk Characterization in CT

5

Cameron Kofler, Edmond Olguin, Andres Abadia, and Wesley E. Bolch

Introduction

It is widely acknowledged that the radiation-absorbed dose received by organs and tissues of the patient undergoing routine CT examination is considered to yield a very low risk of harm [1]. This is particularly the case when (1) the CT exam itself has been medically justified in terms of required diagnostic information and (2) the CT technique factors applied for that exam – including kVp, effective mAs, collimation, and anatomical scan position and length – have been fully optimized for the patient body size and the diagnostic objectives of the image acquisition. Conventional CT dose metrics – such as the volumetric computed tomography dose index ($CTDI_{vol}$) and the dose length product (DLP) – provide information on the x-ray tube output and are thus measures of patient exposure, but not patient organ dose. In order to provide an alternative dose metric that more closely approximates patient organ dose, particularly considering variations in patient size and body morphometry, the AAPM extended the concept of $CTDI_{vol}$ to the size-specific dose estimate or SSDE. Scaling factors applied the $CTDI_{vol}$ to yield the SSDE were first given in AAPM Report No. 204 based upon the concept of *effective diameter* – computed as the square root of the lateral and anterior-posterior dimensions of the patient assessed within the central CT image of the scan range (or possibly averaged across the scan range) [2]. This geometric descriptor of the patient size was further extended in AAPM Report No. 220 to define the *water equivalent diameter* referring to a water cylinder of size giving equivalent x-ray attenuation properties to those of the patient in the CT image [3]. Values of water equivalent diameter require the computation of the mean CT number of the patient region of interest within the CT image, a value that may be computed manually using existing tools available at the CT console or automatically using embedded image processing algorithms.

While the quantities $CTDI_{vol}$, DLP, and SSDE all play central roles in routine CT quality assurance testing and CT scanner commissioning, a full-scale optimization of the CT imaging protocol would entail some estimation of patient risk, however small. Values of radiation risk – including cancer incidence and cancer mortality per organ-absorbed dose – are given by statistical modeling of radiation epidemiology data using subject cohorts exposed to radiation and who have long-term medical follow-up [4–6]. These models thus require as input the absorbed dose to radiosensitive organs and tissues, such as the

C. Kofler · E. Olguin · A. Abadia
Medical Physics Graduate Program,
University of Florida, Gainesville, FL, USA
e-mail: kofler@ufl.edu; eddy64@ufl.edu; pipe86@ufl.edu

W. E. Bolch (✉)
Department of Biomedical Engineering,
University of Florida, Gainesville, FL, USA
e-mail: wbolch@ufl.edu

© Springer Nature Switzerland AG 2020
E. Samei, N. J. Pelc (eds.), *Computed Tomography*, https://doi.org/10.1007/978-3-030-26957-9_5

hematopoietically active bone marrow, thyroid gland, glandular tissues of the breast, and liver. While physical dosimeters embedded in anthropomorphic tissue-equivalent phantoms may yield estimates of these individual organ doses for given CT scanners and imaging protocols [7], Monte Carlo radiation transport techniques are widely considered to provide the closest estimates of ground-truth values of patient organ dose in CT imaging. To perform a radiation transport simulation of a CT imaging session, one must have both (1) a computerized anatomical model of the patient and (2) an experimentally validated source term and geometrical transport model of the imaging system. These are considered briefly in the following sections.

Computational Anatomic Models of Patients

A computational anatomic phantom is a computerized representation of the human body – describing both its external shape and internal organ systems – in a format that is amenable to computing within Monte Carlo radiation transport codes. These codes are computer programs that use random sampling of probability distributions of radiation interaction type (scatter or absorption), energy transfer (full or partial), and scatter/emission angles to follow individual x-ray photons, and potentially their secondary electrons, from a simulated model of the CT x-ray source through the simulated model of patient. Individual computational phantoms have two defining characteristics – their format type and their morphometric category.

Computational Phantom Format Types

Format types of computational phantoms are presently stylized, voxelized, or meshed geometric models of the human body, generally referred to as the first, second, or third generation of phantom technology, respectively (see Fig. 5.1). Stylized (or mathematical) phantoms are composed of 3D geometric surface equations defining both internal organ anatomy and the external body profile. Individual organs are composed of various geometric objects such as spheres, ellipsoids, cones, cylinders, prisms, or toroids either as single entities or as geometric

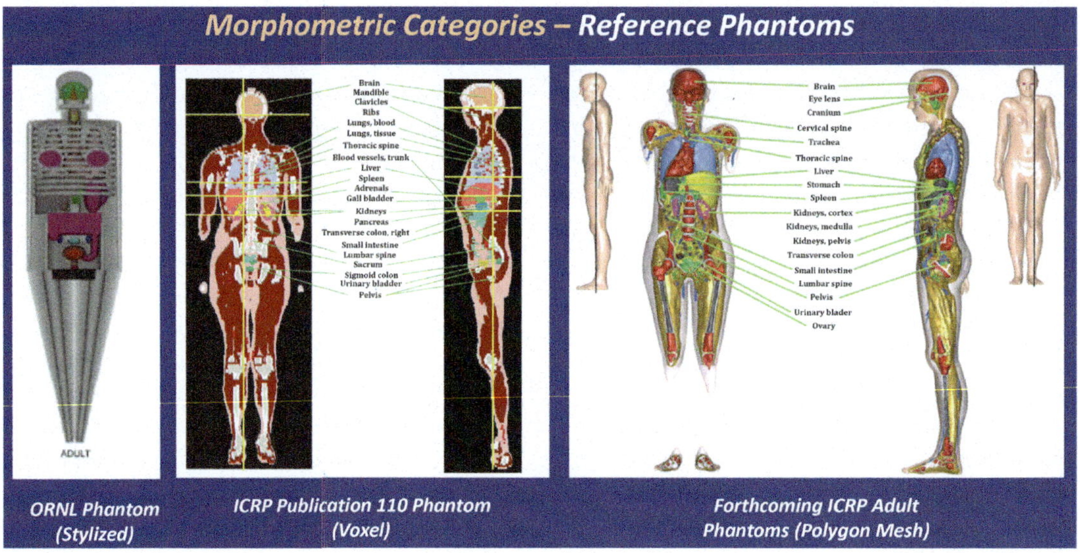

Fig. 5.1 Three generations of ICRP reference computational phantoms

combinations. A targeted organ mass is thus realized in a stylized phantom through assignment of both (1) the object volume (e.g., adjustment of semimajor and semiminor axes of an ellipsoid) and (2) the assigned tissue density. Other anatomic characteristics, however, such as organ shape, depth, and position within the body are only crudely representative of real internal human anatomy. In particular, the limitation on organ shape via geometric modeling of the organ boundary typically results in larger organ-to-organ separation distances than what is seen in true human anatomy. This feature may be far more important in terms of nuclear medicine dosimetry (internal organ cross-fire) than for computed tomography dosimetry (external organ irradiation). Similarly, stylized phantoms typically are limited in their ability to model the exterior body shape of the virtual patient, and most stylized phantoms use at best elliptical cylinders to represent the body torso. The most widely utilized series of stylized computational phantoms are those developed at the Oak Ridge National Laboratory (ORNL) [8, 9].

The second generation of computational phantoms are referred to as voxel (or tomographic) phantoms. These phantoms are based upon the segmentation of computed tomography images of live patients (retrospective image review) or volunteers (prospective image acquisition). Other image sources may include MR images of live patients, CT images of cadavers, or serial color photographs of sectioned cadaveric anatomy. The computational phantom is thus constructed through review of each cross section image whereby pixels belonging to individual tissues or organs are grouped and assigned unique numerical tags. This image segmentation process is performed through combinations of manual contouring, edge-detection, and image intensity thresholding. As each cross-sectional image has a slice thickness (given by the collimation thickness and reconstruction algorithm), the tagged pixels yield corresponding tagged voxels of organ anatomy. The final voxel phantom is thus a 3D array of individual cuboidal elements – a format readily amenable to importation to radiation transport codes [10].

Both stylized and voxel phantoms have important advantages with respect to their application in modeling individual patient anatomy. Stylized phantoms, while lacking in anatomic realism, may be nonuniformly adjusted to alter body region and individual organ size and shape through adjustments in their defining geometric equation parameters. In contrast, voxel phantoms have a high degree of anatomic realism, although this feature is limited to the anatomy of the subject imaged prior to phantom creation. Voxel phantoms can also be rescaled via a redefinition of the voxel dimensions – either uniformly or nonuniformly in the craniocaudal direction or transaxial plane – but the ability to reshape individual organs or body dimensions is more limited than is the case for stylized phantoms.

Hybrid phantoms – the third generation of computational phantom – preserve both the anatomical realism of voxel phantoms and the nonuniform scalability of stylized phantoms [11]. In a hybrid phantom, organ and external body contours are modeled through either NURBS (nonuniform rational B-spline) or polygon mesh surfaces – the same 3D graphical formats used in modern computer animation. NURBS surfaces are composed of an array of individual control points across which a 3D surface is interpolated. Mesh surfaces are arrays of individual triangles or other polygons defined by their vertices in 3D space. Both formats may be used in anatomy modeling within a hybrid phantom, and both provide exquisite flexibility to readjust phantom anatomy to match changes in subcutaneous adipose tissue mass and body distribution; individual organ shape, depth, and position; body height and total mass; and regional body circumference. Only within the past few years have radiation transport codes provided particle tracking algorithms which are compatible with computational phantoms given in a mesh format. Prior to these developments, a mesh-based phantom had to be voxelized – a process by which organ and body surfaces are interiorly filled with voxels of user-defined dimensions – before that phantom could be coupled to the radiation transport code [12].

Computational Phantom Morphometric Categories

Another key feature of a computational phantom – beyond its format type – is the morphometric category of the virtual patient. There are generally four categories to consider: (1) reference, (2) patient-dependent, (3) patient-sculpted, and (4) patient-specific. Each of these four categories (in theory) may be realized by any of the three phantom format types – stylized, voxel, or hybrid.

One of the very first morphometric categories implemented for computational phantoms is that of a *reference* phantom as defined formally by the International Commission on Radiological Protection in ICRP Publications 23 [13] and, more recently, in ICRP Publication 89 [14] for use within the ICRP system of radiological protection. As such, a ICRP reference phantom is defined as the 50th percentile individual in both height and weight at a given age and gender. In ICRP Publication 89, reference phantom characteristics are given in terms of individual organ mass, body height, body weight, and body surface area for the male and female newborn, 1-year-old, 5-year-old, 10-year-old, 15-year-old, and adult (20–30 years of age). Data defining these body characteristics were taken primarily from European and North American populations, and thus many Asian nations have established their own definitions of a reference phantom. Reference phantoms – 12 in total – are ideally applied to assess both internal and external radiation doses from occupational and environmental sources, yet they have been extensively applied in the field of medical patient dosimetry, mostly notable due to a lack of alternative phantom morphometries.

The second morphometric category is that of a patient-dependent phantom [15–17]. In its simplest definition, a patient-dependent phantom is a reference phantom but with the removal of the restriction of 50th percentile height/weight. Patient-dependent phantoms thus allow the creation of a phantom library whereby a specific member from that library may represent, for example, a female patient at 30th height percentile and 65th weight percentile at age 7 years. With increasing trends in both childhood and adult obesity, however, use of height/weight percentiles as the basis for phantom identification can become quickly dated. One solution is to organize the phantom library according a simple array of phantoms at differing combinations of total height and body mass (and hence BMI), yet each constructed to match statistical averages of body region circumferences from a sampled patient population. The advantage of this approach is that the library no longer becomes associated with a given national population. Thus, a given phantom from the patient-dependent library might represent the 45th/70th height/weight individual in one country, but the 55th/85th height/weight individual in another nation.

While ICRP provides definitive values of organ mass for each of its 12 reference phantoms (2 genders/6 ages), no comprehensive database of normal organ masses or volumes exists for which to create a patient-dependent phantom library. One approach is thus to create non-50th percentile members of the library via combinations of 2D and 3D scaling of the head, torso, and legs of a reference phantom for which reference organ masses/volumes are previously modeled. For example, if an adult female phantom with a sitting height larger than the ICRP reference adult female is to be created, a 3D scale of her torso would be performed with a concomitant increase in internal organ mass for all tissues within the torso. Consequently, the process of matching the patient to an individual member of the phantom library would be based upon exterior morphometry such as height/weight/BMI or perhaps body region circumference (such as via the water equivalent diameter of the SSDE). There would remain a degree of uncertainty in internal organ size, shape, and location in the patient-matched phantom.

A third morphometric category of computational phantom is a so-called patient-sculpted phantom [18]. This phantom is generated by first selecting an individual phantom from a patient-dependent phantom library based upon exterior body size (BMI or body circumference) and then reshaping the outer body contour to more closely match the body shape of the individual patient for which CT organ doses are to be assessed. Body contour sculpting is more readily executed using the NURBS and/or polygon mesh surface features of a hybrid phantom. Important features of a patient-sculpted phantom are that no adjustments to phantom height (total or sitting) would be made and that, resultantly, no changes are made to the internal organ anatomy – they remain as is within the phantom selected from the patient-dependent phantom library. Body reshaping will thus only impact the modeling of subcutaneous fat and its body region distribution in the modeled patient. Finally, it is noted that because a patient-sculpted phantom is only created given body size measurements of an individual patient, their use in CT dosimetry would require a radiation transport simulation once created. A pre-CT organ dose library is thus limited to either reference or patient-dependent phantoms.

The final and most accurate computational phantom is a patient-specific phantom whereby both internal organ anatomy and outer body shape are uniquely matched to the patient for which the organ dose estimate is sought. By definition, all voxel phantoms are patient-specific as they are based upon image segmentation of one individual patient, volunteer, or cadaver. However, with sufficient numbers of patient-specific voxel phantoms, a phantom library may be created in a manner analogous to that of a patient-dependent phantom library. Furthermore, modeling software tools now permit the conversion of a voxel phantom into its hybrid equivalent, and thus an array of hybrid phantoms can similarly be used to construct a virtual patient phantom library. This approach, as compared to a rescaling of hybrid reference phantoms, will populate the phantom library perhaps in a more speckled pattern, with variations in individual organ shape, depth, and position inherent in the members of the phantom library. In many dosimetry studies of reference, patient-dependent, and patient-sculpted phantoms, organ doses derived from patient-specific phantoms (CT segmented phantoms) are used as the comparative gold standard.

Organ Dosimetry in CT Imaging

Once a particular patient phantom model is selected for CT organ dose assessment, several steps are needed to complete the computational model of the imaging system [19–24]. These steps are briefly outlined below.

Modeling of the X-Ray Source Term

In a Monte Carlo simulation of a CT imaging examination, one must specify the starting position, emission direction, and energy of each simulated x-ray photon within the virtual imaging beam. Depending upon whether axial or helical scanning is considered, Monte Carlo sampling will be along a simple circle at each slice position on the phantom or along a helical path of a selected pitch. Emission direction will be sampled within an angle defining the fan beam width and should be defined by the beam collimation with additional consideration of the beam penumbra (e.g., over-beaming).

Early attempts at Monte Carlo modeling of CT imaging required explicit knowledge of the material and geometric shape of the bowtie filters to properly model the spatial probability density of emitted x-ray energies. In 2009, Turner et al. published an experimental approach that circumvented the need for this proprietary information [25]. First, the x-ray tube is parked under service mode, and traditional half-value layer measurements are performed as indicated. The method ideally requires measurement of both HVL_1 and HVL_2, although Turner et al. concluded that the former is sufficient for CT imaging simulation. Second, again with a stationary x-ray tube, a series of ion chamber measurements are performed across one-half of the fan beam. These measurements are used to establish a normalized radial beam profile to explicitly model the filtration impact of the bowtie filter on the sampling of x-ray photon emission angles and energies. Finally, a candidate x-ray energy spectrum is generated from standard source term models at the relevant tube potential. This candidate spectrum is then iteratively filtered by a virtual hardening material whose thickness and even material composition is altered – until a simulated HVL measurement is seen to match, within a given tolerance, the HVL measurement. The equivalent energy and filtration method of Turner et al. has been adopted widely in the medical imaging community, not only for CT simulation studies, but in radiography and fluoroscopy studies as well.

Normalization of the Monte Carlo Reported Organ Dose

One additional measurement is generally required for reporting organ doses to patients through Monte Carlo computer simulation. The direct output of the Monte Carlo simulation will yield organ doses per simulated x-ray photon (mGy/photon), while what is required is the organ dose per time-integrated tube current (mGy/100 mAs). As a result, a normalization factor is required to give the number of x-ray photons per 100 mAs for a given irradiation geometry – typically one single axial rotation. This normalization factor is thus acquired as the ratio of measured to simulated free-in-air kerma in a standard CTDI pencil ion chamber:

$$\mathrm{NF}\left(\frac{\text{photons}}{100\,\text{mAs}}\right)=\frac{K_{\text{air, meas}}\left(\frac{\text{mGy}}{100\,\text{mAs}}\right)}{K_{\text{air, MC}}\left(\frac{\text{mGy}}{\text{photon}}\right)}$$

Alternatively, the normalization factor may be expressed as a ratio of CTDI_w values – one measured and one simulated:

$$\mathrm{NF}\left(\frac{\text{photons}}{100\,\text{mAs}}\right)=\frac{\mathrm{CTDI}_{w,\text{ meas}}\left(\frac{\text{mGy}}{100\,\text{mAs}}\right)}{\mathrm{CTDI}_{w,\text{ MC}}\left(\frac{\text{mGy}}{\text{photon}}\right)}$$

The absolute organ dose, normalized to 100 mAs, is then reported as the product of its simulated value and the normalization factor NF:

$$D_{\text{organ}}\left(\frac{\text{mGy}}{100\,\text{mAs}}\right)=\mathrm{NF}\left(\frac{\text{photons}}{100\,\text{mAs}}\right)x\ D_{\text{organ, MC}}\left(\frac{\text{mGy}}{\text{photon}}\right)$$

Generic Axial Dose Libraries Versus Helical Protocol-Specific Dose Libraries

In CT phantom-based dosimetry, two options exist for establishing a pre-CT organ dose library. The first option establishes an organ dose library based upon Monte Carlo simulation of an array of single-rotation axial images at a given collimation beam width, tube potential, and selected computational phantom. This axial slice dose library provides the organ dose, normalized to 100 mAs typically, indexed to each z-position on the computational phantoms, and can in theory extend from across the entire craniocaudal length of the virtual patient. For a given clinical imaging examination, one then linearly sums the slice-specific organ doses over all axial slices that fall within the starting and ending anatomy of the CT examination. For modeling helical protocols, the summed organ doses may then be scaled by the inverse of the exam pitch. This approach thus permits explicit consideration of any combination of starting and ending anatomical landmark. In the second option, when CT imaging studies fall under a specific listing of established clinical protocols, and where the anatomical landmarks of the scan length and the pitch of the exam are well established, the CT organ dose library may be constructed for each imaging protocol through explicit modeling of the helical scan.

Considerations of Starting Angle and Over-Ranging

One significant disadvantage of a protocol-specific organ dose library is that a fixed starting angle is typically assumed during the Monte Carlo simulations of the helical path of the x-ray tube. As has been well documented, variations in CT starting angle can have a significant impact on doses to more superficial organs such as breast, thyroid, and eye lens. One solution is to consider a systematic variation in starting angle for the helical path protocol-specific dose library and populate the organ dose library with the organ dose averaged over all possible starting angles. For axial slice-specific dose libraries, all possible starting angles are implicitly considered, and thus the average value is given directly. In either case, this dose value may differ greatly from the actual organ dose to superficial organs for a given helical scan with an arbitrary starting angle. Over-ranging, which defines additional irradiated anatomy prior to and beyond the edges of the reconstructed image, may be accounted for in the organ dose library through the addition of whole or fractional axial slices in the final dose estimate.

Modeling of Tube Current Modulation: Generic Versus Explicit

One significant challenge to reporting organ doses following CT imaging on a pre-computed basis is how to consider the impact of tube current modulation –in both its angular and axial forms. One solution for prospective application to single axial slice organ dose libraries is to perform a weighted summation of the axial doses in contrast to a straight linear summation. In so doing, a weighting factor should be applied to each axial slice through the computational phantom anatomy in a manner that mimics the TCM algorithm of that particular CT scanner. These slice-specific weighting factors may be developed through computational simulation of central ray x-ray attenuation across several directions of a given axial slice and comparing these values for each z-position along the phantom's anatomy. This approach would, to a first approximation, allow modeling of axial but not angular modulation. The weighted average of the slice-specific organ doses would still be normalized to the entire exam's effective mAs, and thus this value would have to be assumed or extracted to report organ doses in absolute units. In a retrospective assessment of CT organ doses under tube current modulation, one would acquire the effective mA per reconstructed image across the scan length and use this value to weight organ doses from the slice-specific dose library at a fixed mA. This latter approach thus requires extraction of mA information from the entire CT image series.

Risk Modeling in CT Imaging

It is clearly impossible to estimate, with any reasonable degree of certainty, the radiation cancer risk to an individual patient following CT imaging. This is due primarily to four factors. First, there is a significant degree of variation in individual radiation susceptibility to cancer induction owing to different patient generic profiles and DNA repair competencies. Second, our understanding of the dose versus risk relationship is derived from population studies of exposed individuals, and thus by design, these risk models are only valid when applied on a population basis. Third, these dose-response relationships are typically assembled from data on exposed individuals at dose levels that exceed levels seen in individual CT imaging exams. Consequently, methods of extrapolation to lower-dose regions of the dose-response curve must be applied. In a recent review of past and current radiation epidemiological studies, the linear, no-threshold dose-response model is deemed by the National Council of Radiation Protection and Measurements (NCRP) as the most appropriate model presently for use in radiological protection [26]. Still, the exact shape of the dose-response in the lower-dose region, typical of CT imaging, remains uncertain. Fourth, these population-based risk models are typically derived using estimates of life expectancies for the average non-exposed "healthy" population of interest. In most cases, patients undergoing extensive medical imaging should not be considered "healthy" as their underlying disease – which likely triggered the need for the medical imaging exam – will invariably result in a life expectancy perhaps less than that seen in the general "healthy" population.

Nevertheless, population-based risk models may be used to assign nominal values of risk to groups (or populations) of patients for the purpose of CT imaging protocol optimization. It is generally acknowledged that radiation cancer risks are higher for female patients than they are for male patients and these risks are higher for pediatric patients than they are for adult patients. Thus, assignment of a nominal CT imaging risk to a CT imaging study of adult males would necessarily be lower than that assigned to a CT imaging study of pediatric female patients.

Effective Dose and Radiation Detriment

There are two general approaches to modeling patient risk in medical imaging, including computed tomography. The first is the assignment of the radiation protection quantity *effective dose* E in units of sieverts (Sv) as defined in ICRP Publication 103 [27]. The effective dose E is computed as follows:

$$E = \sum_T w_T \sum_R w_R \left[\frac{D_{T,R}^{\text{Male}} + D_{T,R}^{\text{Female}}}{2} \right] \quad (5.1)$$

where w_T is the tissue weighting factor for tissue T, w_R is radiation weighting factor for radiation type R, and $D_{T,R}^{\text{Male}}$ and $D_{T,R}^{\text{Female}}$ are the absorbed doses to tissue T delivered by radiation type R to a male and female reference individual, respectively. Values of w_R are derived from consensus agreement on nominal values of relative biological effectiveness for different forms of ionizing radiation for the induction of stochastic risk (e.g., cancer or hereditary effects). The value of w_R is unity for both photons and electrons, as per ICRP Publication 103, and thus there is no effective radiation weighting under CT imaging of the organ doses. Values of w_T define the relative contribution of radiation detriment to organ T under a hypothetical and uniform whole-body irradiation of the patient. Radiation detriment itself is defined by ICRP as a sex-averaged, age-averaged, and population-averaged cancer incidence risk that is further weighted by a lethality fraction (effectively deriving a cancer mortality risk) and other terms such as the estimated number of years of life lost due to cancer mortality. Because values of w_T are based on sex-averaged cancer risks, Eq. 5.1 clearly denotes that the effective dose itself must be computed using not one but two reference phantoms – one male and one female – for which the organ doses are averaged. Furthermore, the cancer incidence risks are not only sex-averaged, but they are age-averaged as well. In many cases of medical imaging of patients, values of effective dose are computed using Eq. 5.1 but with only a single set of organ-absorbed doses derived from a computational anatomical phantom of the single patient – male or female – at a given age. While termed effective dose, this value is more appropriately a detriment-weighted dose if no sex-averaging is applied to the organ-absorbed doses.

Age- and Sex-Dependent Models of Lifetime Attributable Risk (LAR) of Cancer

As noted above, the effective dose provides only a very broad estimate of radiation detriment that is akin but not exactly equal to a cancer mortality risk. An alternative to the effective dose is the quantity lifetime attributable risk or LAR. Here, the data from radiation epidemiology studies is retained in terms of organ-specific, sex-specific, and age-specific variations in either cancer incidence risk or cancer mortality risk. Thus values of lifetime attributable risk for cancer incidence (CI) might be assessed as follows:

$$\text{LAR}_{T,CI}(s,a) = D_T(s,a) \times \text{RC}_{T,\text{CI}}(s,a) \quad (5.2)$$

where $D_T(s,a)$ is the absorbed dose to organ or tissue T for a patient of sex s and age a and $\text{RC}_{T,\text{CI}}(s,a)$ is the corresponding risk coefficient giving the LAR for cancer incidence per absorbed dose to tissue T and indexed to the same patient sex and age. Values of LAR for cancer mortality (CM) can then be derived as follows:

$$\mathrm{LAR}_{T,CM}\left(s,a\right)=\mathrm{LF}_{T}\left(s,a\right)\times\mathrm{LAR}_{T,\mathrm{CI}}\left(s,a\right) \quad (5.2)$$

where $\mathrm{LF}_T(s, a)$ is the lethality fraction defined as the probability of cancer death following cancer incidence. Data sources for values of LAR include the 2005 National Academy of Sciences BEIR VII report [4], the 2006 UNSCEAR report [5], and EPA Report 402-R-11-001 of the US Environmental Protection Agency [6].

CT imaging protocol optimization, with the goal of maximizing image quality at the lowest patient risk, can be performed using either the effective dose or the lifetime attributable risk as a rough measure of the patient harm to be minimized. The effective dose has been widely used for this purpose across many fields of medical imaging. However, this quantity – as discussed above – has many limitations as it is proportional to a measure of risk (radiation detriment) that does not give explicit consideration of the majority of attributes of many patient subpopulations, particularly in regard to age, gender, and even national population. Lifetime attributable risk can provide these more refined estimates of cancer risk, as shown below in our example problem. Still, they must be applied only in the context of an imaging protocol optimization for patient subpopulations, as they can never be used to assign specific values of cancer risk to individual patients.

Example Dose and Risk Assessment: Pediatric ^{18}FDG PET/CT

As an example of the two methods of patient risk modeling, we now consider the example of pediatric imaging using ^{18}F-fluoro-2-deoxy-D-glucose (FDG) in a series of reference patients under PET/CT hybrid imaging. We consider the organ doses received by the PET imaging portion of the exam, the organ doses received by the CT portion of the exam needed for attenuation corrections of the PET images, and their combined total organ doses. Risks expressed as lifetime excess cancer incidence and mortality are considered, along with estimates of radiation detriment from the effective dose. These doses and risks are further compared to those for a full torso diagnostic CT image of these same reference patients.

Methods of Organ Dose and Risk Modeling in ^{18}FDG PET/CT

Estimates cancer incidence may be determined using the Radiation Risk Assessment Tool (RadRAT), an online calculator that computes the lifetime attributable risk of cancer incidence for members of the USA and other populations of interest in current radiation epidemiological studies. RadRAT was developed and is supported by the Radiation Epidemiology Branch of the National Cancer Institute (NCI).[1] The code includes cancer risk models for 11 organs from the National Academy of Sciences BEIR VII report [4], which are then supplemented by subsequently developed models for 8 additional organs including a remainder tissue category [28]. Given the absorbed dose to an organ, RadRAT will then report the mean, as well as the 90th percentile confidence interval, for the age- and sex-specific cancer incidence rate resulting from that exposure expressed as the excess lifetime risk. Cancer mortality estimates may then be determined using a lethality fraction which itself may be computed as the ratio of cancer mortality risk to cancer incidence risk from other sources such as EPA Report 402-R-11-001 [6].[2] Finally, radiation detriment, a quantity defined in ICRP Publication 103, may be computed as the product of the effective dose to the patient and the ICRP recommended nominal detriment coefficient of 5.5% per Sv [27].

In this example, we consider two types of medical imaging modalities: computed tomography (CT) and positron emission tomography (PET) that are used in combination during ^{18}FDG PET/CT imaging studies. Absorbed doses were computed for individual organs in eight pediatric reference phantoms to include males and females at ages of 1, 5, 10, and 15 years [29] (see Fig. 5.2). Simulations of CT scans were

[1] https://radiationcalculators.cancer.gov/radrat/

[2] https://www.epa.gov/radiation/epa-radiogenic-cancer-risk-models-and-projections-us-population

performed separately from PET dose calculations, and their resulting organ-absorbed doses were summed as needed to estimate the risk of cancer incidence, cancer mortality, and radiation detriment.

CT simulations were performed with the Monte Carlo N-Particle Transport Code (MCNP). The source term modeled had been previously validated against both measurements of $CTDI_{vol}$ and anthropomorphic phantom measurements of organ dose [23]. From these simulations, multiple sets of organ doses were calculated for phantoms in the UF/NCI hybrid phantom library to create an organ dose database that accounts for beam energy, pitch, scan length, $CTDI_{vol}$, and tube current modulation (TCM). The UF/NCI hybrid phantom library consists of 351 hybrid phantoms that vary in height and weight and are comprised of both male and female patient models [16]. The eight reference phantoms were matched to their closest-fitting hybrid phantom based on height, weight, and sex. Each reference phantoms' height, weight, and sex is shown in Table 5.1 along with the height, weight, and sex of their closest matched hybrid

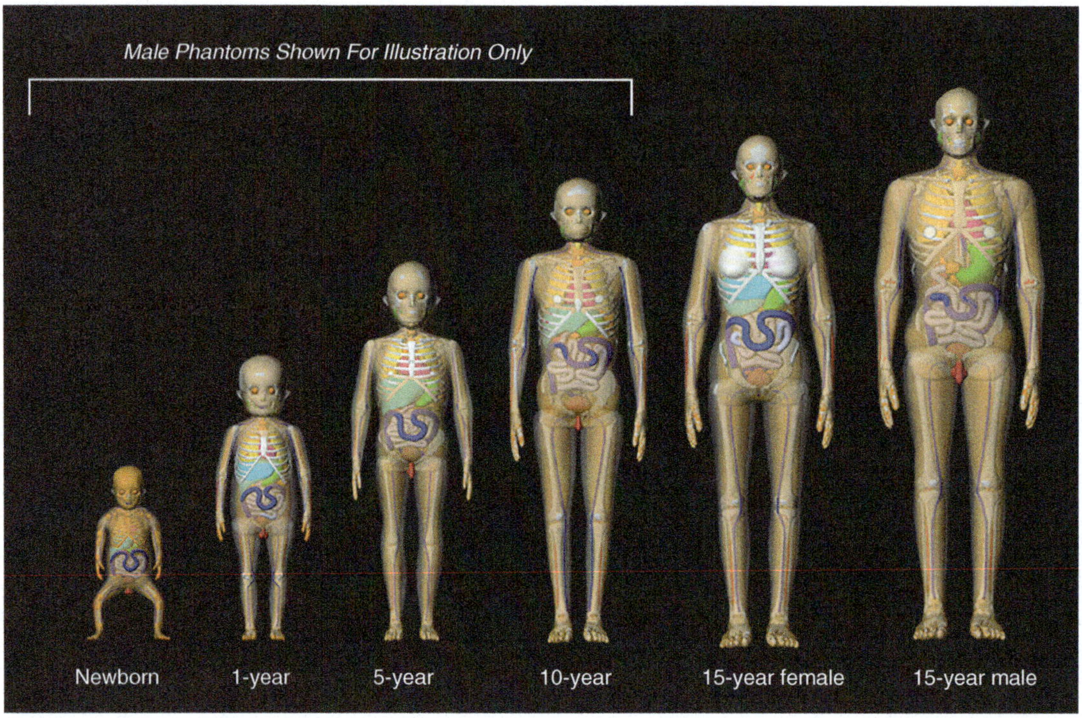

Fig. 5.2 UF/NCI series of pediatric reference hybrid phantoms

Table 5.1 Comparison of reference phantoms to closest matching hybrid phantom

Reference phantom				Hybrid phantom			
Sex	Age [yr]	Height [cm]	Weight [kg]	Sex	Age [yr]	Height [cm]	Weight [kg]
Male	1	76	10	Male	1	85	10
Male	5	109	18	Male	5	105	20
Male	10	138	32	Male	10	135	30
Male	15	167	57	Male	15	165	55
Female	1	76	10	Female	1	85	10
Female	5	109	18	Female	5	105	20
Female	10	138	32	Female	10	135	30
Female	15	161	53	Female	15	165	55

Table 5.2 Input parameters used for all eight hybrid phantoms

Sex	Age [yr]	Beam energy [kVp]	Protocol	Pitch	Scan length [cm]	Vendor $CTDI_{vol}$ [mGy]
Male	1	120	Whole body	1.3	56.0	0.35
Male	5	120	Whole body	1.3	70.4	0.60
Male	10	120	Whole body	1.3	86.4	0.70
Male	15	120	Whole body	1.3	108.8	1.80
Female	1	120	Whole body	1.3	56.0	0.35
Female	5	120	Whole body	1.3	70.4	0.60
Female	10	120	Whole body	1.3	86.4	0.70
Female	15	120	Whole body	1.3	102.4	1.80
Male	1	120	CAP	1.5	41.6	2.80
Male	5	120	CAP	1.5	44.8	3.10
Male	10	120	CAP	1.5	54.4	3.90
Male	15	120	CAP	1.5	73.6	6.10
Female	1	120	CAP	1.5	41.6	2.80
Female	5	120	CAP	1.5	44.8	3.10
Female	10	120	CAP	1.5	57.6	3.90
Female	15	120	CAP	1.5	67.2	6.10

Anatomical landmarks of whole-body scan: base of skull to mid-thigh
Anatomical landmarks of abdomen/pelvis inlet to lesser trochanter

phantom. Once matched to a hybrid phantom, the pre-computed database of organ doses was used to determine organ doses to each hybrid phantom for scan parameters that are commonly used in ^{18}FDG PET/CT imaging studies.

The CT protocols compared in this study were "whole body" (WB) for attenuation correction (AC) and "chest-abdomen-pelvis" (CAP) diagnostic CT scans, respectively. Input parameters were determined from three separate sources. Scan length was defined using the University of Florida Standard Names for Imaging Procedures (SNIPs) using anatomical landmarks for scan start and stop locations.[3] Beam energy, pitch, scan length, and $CTDI_{vol}$ were determined from clinical recommendations from Boston Children's Hospital. TCM was modeled using an algorithm developed at the University of Florida [23]. A complete list of input parameters used for the eight pediatric phantoms is shown in Table 5.2.

For PET organ dose calculations, values of organ-absorbed dose per activity administered [mGy MBq^{-1}] for a reference person at all four ages were obtained from ICRP Publication 128 for ^{18}FDG. These coefficients are listed in Table 5.3 [30]. Once the age-specific absorbed doses per activity administered were known, an injected activity of 5.55 MBq per kg of phantom weight was assumed as utilized at the Boston Children's Hospital to determine the total activity administered. The total activity administered was then multiplied by the age-specific absorbed dose per activity administered to arrive at an absorbed dose to each organ for each phantom. Once phantom-specific organ doses for both PET and CT components were determined, cancer incidence, cancer mortality, and radiation detriment estimates were computed and compared for each of the eight reference phantoms.

In our example study, cancer incidence is only reported but not compared to radiation detriment as a more appropriate comparison should be made to cancer mortality. ICRP Publication 103 considers a lethality fraction when defining radiation detriment along with other factors such as cancer morbidity and years of life lost. Resultantly, radiation detriment is a closer measure to cancer mortality than it is to cancer incidence.

Resulting Organ Doses and Cancer Risks Associated with ^{18}FDG PET/CT

Organ-absorbed doses for each pediatric patient phantom are reported in Tables 5.4, 5.5, 5.6, and 5.7 for the following four imaging exams: (1) a

[3] https://protocols.xray.ufl.edu

Table 5.3 ICRP Publication 128 organ-absorbed dose coefficients for ^{18}FDG

	Absorbed dose per unit activity administered [mGy MBq^{-1}]				
Organ	Adult	15 years	10 years	5 years	1 year
Adrenals	0.012	0.016	0.024	0.039	0.071
Bone surfaces	0.011	0.014	0.022	0.034	0.064
Brain	0.038	0.039	0.041	0.046	0.063
Breast	0.009	0.011	0.018	0.029	0.056
Gallbladder wall	0.013	0.016	0.024	0.037	0.070
Gastrointestinal tract					
Stomach wall	0.011	0.014	0.022	0.035	0.067
Small intestine wall	0.012	0.016	0.025	0.040	0.073
Colon wall	0.013	0.016	0.025	0.039	0.070
Upper large intestine wall	0.012	0.015	0.024	0.038	0.070
Lower large intestine wall	0.014	0.017	0.027	0.041	0.070
Heart wall	0.067	0.087	0.130	0.210	0.380
Kidneys	0.017	0.021	0.029	0.045	0.078
Liver	0.021	0.028	0.042	0.063	0.120
Lungs	0.020	0.029	0.041	0.062	0.120
Muscles	0.010	0.013	0.020	0.033	0.062
Esophagus	0.012	0.015	0.022	0.035	0.066
Ovaries	0.014	0.018	0.027	0.043	0.076
Pancreas	0.013	0.016	0.026	0.040	0.076
Red marrow	0.011	0.014	0.021	0.032	0.059
Skin	0.008	0.010	0.015	0.026	0.050
Spleen	0.011	0.014	0.021	0.035	0.066
Testes	0.011	0.014	0.024	0.037	0.066
Thymus	0.012	0.015	0.022	0.035	0.066
Thyroid	0.010	0.013	0.021	0.034	0.065
Urinary bladder wall	0.130	0.160	0.250	0.340	0.470
Uterus	0.018	0.022	0.036	0.054	0.090
Remaining organs	0.012	0.015	0.024	0.038	0.064
Effective dose [mSv MBq^{-1}]	0.019	0.024	0.037	0.056	0.095

whole-body CT scan for attenuation correction, (2) a^{18}FDG PET scan, (3) a combined PET/CT scan, and (4) a diagnostic chest-abdomen-pelvic (or CAP) CT scan, respectively.

From the organ doses reported estimates of cancer incidence, cancer mortality, and radiation detriment were computed in units of cases per 100,000 individuals exposed. These risk estimates are shown in Tables 5.8, 5.9, 5.10, and 5.11 for (1) an attenuation correction whole-body CT scan, (2) ^{18}FDG PET scan, (3) combined ^{18}FDG PET/CT scan, and (4) a diagnostic chest-abdomen-pelvis CT scan, respectively. Figures 5.3, 5.4, and 5.5 display these data in graphical form.

Figures 5.3 and 5.4 demonstrate graphically the fact that females have a higher estimated risk of cancer incidence and cancer mortality than males when comparing their excess lifetime attributable risk. In contrast, this increased risk is not apparent when comparing radiation detriment among the various male and female reference patients. Table 5.11 shows that, for a diagnostic CAP CT scan, when averaged across all four ages, females have a 129% higher chance of cancer mortality using excess lifetime risk estimates yet only a 2% lower risk when assessed using radiation detriment. This trend is also present in PET scans but not as pronounced with averages of 48% higher and 2% lower for cancer

Table 5.4 Organ dose [mGy] and effective dose [mSv] for all eight phantoms resulting from a typical whole-body, attenuation correction CT scan

	Male				Female			
	1 year	5 years	10 years	15 years	1 year	5 years	10 years	15 years
Adrenals	0.40	0.64	0.70	1.72	0.41	0.64	0.70	1.47
Bladder	0.39	0.71	0.71	1.58	0.39	0.71	0.75	1.91
Bone surface	0.34	0.52	0.53	0.97	0.35	0.52	0.53	1.05
Brain	0.30	0.48	0.51	0.93	0.32	0.48	0.51	0.91
Breasts	0.38	0.59	0.67	1.56	0.44	0.59	0.66	1.26
Colon	0.42	0.71	0.78	1.75	0.42	0.72	0.78	1.65
Extrathoracic region	0.41	0.67	0.72	1.44	0.42	0.66	0.71	1.35
Gall bladder	0.42	0.66	0.74	1.72	0.42	0.66	0.74	1.47
Gonads	0.47	0.79	0.79	1.89	0.36	0.60	0.64	1.76
Heart wall	0.44	0.71	0.80	1.86	0.45	0.71	0.80	1.67
Kidneys	0.42	0.69	0.75	1.69	0.42	0.69	0.75	1.67
Liver	0.42	0.68	0.75	1.73	0.43	0.68	0.75	1.53
Lungs	0.42	0.67	0.77	1.77	0.43	0.67	0.77	1.66
Lymph nodes	0.35	0.57	0.61	1.35	0.36	0.56	0.61	1.32
Muscle	0.29	0.38	0.44	0.96	0.29	0.38	0.44	0.82
Esophagus	0.39	0.65	0.71	1.63	0.40	0.65	0.71	1.51
Oral mucosa	0.33	0.51	0.48	1.02	0.34	0.51	0.48	0.89
Pancreas	0.40	0.70	0.75	1.63	0.40	0.70	0.75	1.53
Prostate/uterus	0.32	0.67	0.76	1.55	0.33	0.59	0.64	1.54
Red bone marrow	0.31	0.40	0.48	1.11	0.28	0.40	0.48	1.12
Salivary glands	0.37	0.60	0.60	1.15	0.37	0.59	0.60	1.13
Skin	0.25	0.33	0.35	0.77	0.25	0.33	0.35	0.77
Small intestine	0.43	0.71	0.79	1.76	0.43	0.71	0.79	1.69
Spleen	0.40	0.68	0.76	1.75	0.41	0.68	0.76	1.65
Stomach	0.42	0.71	0.79	1.79	0.43	0.70	0.78	1.55
Thymus	0.40	0.68	0.73	1.69	0.41	0.68	0.72	1.56
Thyroid	0.51	0.91	0.80	1.82	0.49	0.91	0.80	1.71
Effective dose	0.40	0.65	0.71	1.62	0.40	0.64	0.69	1.50

mortality and radiation detriment, respectively. As noted previously, effective dose, the quantity from which radiation detriment is derived, is a sex-averaged quantity and as such does not adequately account for the larger female cancer incidence rates as are provided in the LAR models of the RadRAT code.

Similarly, larger differences between estimated cancer mortality risk and radiation detriment can be seen at the younger patient ages. For example, Table 5.8 shows that for a whole-body, attenuation correction CT scan, when averaged across both males and females, a 1-year-old has a 172% higher estimated cancer mortality risk as compared to that inferred by radiation detriment. However, a 15-year-old undergoing a whole-body, attenuation correction CT scan has a 54% higher estimated risk of mortality determined by excess lifetime attributable risk as compared to radiation detriment. Radiation detriment is a quantity designed to represent the general population of adults and children. Children, however, are more susceptible to radiation injury owing to their higher rates of cell division, their wider skeletal distribution of active bone marrow, and their longer projected lifespan over which radiation effects may manifest. These factors are not specifically accounted for by radiation detriment, and thus its estimate of cancer mortality is lower than that provided for by the excess lifetime attributable

Table 5.5 Organ doses [mGy] and effective dose [mSv] for all eight phantoms resulting from a typical ^{18}FDG PET scan

	Male				Female			
	1 year	5 years	10 years	15 years	1 year	5 years	10 years	15 years
Adrenals	3.93	3.92	4.31	5.04	3.93	3.92	4.31	4.74
Bladder wall	26.03	34.19	44.87	50.45	26.03	34.21	44.89	47.36
Bone surfaces	3.54	3.42	3.95	4.41	3.54	3.42	3.95	4.14
Brain	3.49	4.63	7.36	12.30	3.49	4.63	7.36	11.54
Breast	3.10	2.92	3.23	3.47	3.10	2.92	3.23	3.26
Colon wall	3.88	3.92	4.49	5.04	3.88	3.92	4.49	4.74
Gallbladder wall	3.88	3.72	4.31	5.04	3.88	3.72	4.31	4.74
Heart wall	21.05	21.12	23.33	27.43	21.05	21.13	23.34	25.75
Kidneys	4.32	4.53	5.21	6.62	4.32	4.53	5.21	6.22
Liver	6.65	6.34	7.54	8.83	6.65	6.34	7.54	8.29
Lower large intestine wall	3.88	4.12	4.85	5.36	3.88	4.13	4.85	5.03
Lungs	6.65	6.24	7.36	9.14	6.65	6.24	7.36	8.58
Muscles	3.43	3.32	3.59	4.10	3.43	3.32	3.59	3.85
Esophagus	3.66	3.52	3.95	4.73	3.66	3.52	3.95	4.44
Ovaries	4.21	4.32	4.85	5.68	4.21	4.33	4.85	5.33
Pancreas	4.21	4.02	4.67	5.04	4.21	4.02	4.67	4.74
Red marrow	3.27	3.22	3.77	4.41	3.27	3.22	3.77	4.14
Remaining organs	3.54	3.82	4.31	4.73	3.54	3.82	4.31	4.44
Skin	2.77	2.61	2.69	3.03	2.77	2.62	2.69	2.84
Small intestine wall	4.04	4.02	4.49	5.04	4.04	4.02	4.49	4.74
Spleen	3.66	3.52	3.77	4.41	3.66	3.52	3.77	4.14
Stomach wall	3.71	3.52	3.95	4.41	3.71	3.52	3.95	4.14
Testes	3.66	3.72	4.31	4.41	3.66	3.72	4.31	4.14
Thymus	3.66	3.52	3.95	4.73	3.66	3.52	3.95	4.44
Thyroid	3.60	3.42	3.77	4.10	3.60	3.42	3.77	3.85
Upper large intestine wall	3.88	3.82	4.31	4.73	3.88	3.82	4.31	4.44
Uterus	4.99	5.43	6.46	6.94	4.99	5.43	6.46	6.51
Effective dose	5.26	5.63	6.64	7.57	5.26	5.63	6.64	7.10

risk of cancer mortality. As the reference patient ages, this effect is not as prevalent as they become less radiosensitive, which is why there is less of a difference between cancer mortality and radiation detriment for a 15-year reference patient as compared to the 1-year reference patient.

When comparing a 1-year reference patient's estimated risk of cancer mortality directly to a 15-year reference patient using the tables and figures presented, this trend of increased radiosensitivity is not immediately evident. The reason is that as the patient ages and increases in body size, so does the average scan parameters applied. For example, in Table 5.8 when comparing a whole-body, attenuation correction CT scan of a 1-year-old averaged across both sexes to a 15-year-old averaged across both sexes, the 15-year-old is imaged with a 414% higher $CTDI_{vol}$ and an 89% longer scan range. With these higher scan parameters, Table 5.8 shows that the 15-year-old has a 131% higher estimated cancer mortality risk than the 1-year reference patient as given by the LAR model and a corresponding 292% higher estimated radiation detriment. These differences are attributed to the higher organ doses received by the 15-year reference patient than received by the 1-year reference patient following changes in scan parameters. At the same time, however, radiation detriment does not account for the lower radiosensitivity of the 15-year reference patient, in comparison to the 1-year patient, and thus its estimated risk is significantly higher than that given by the models of excess lifetime attributable risk.

Table 5.6 Organ doses [mGy] and effective dose [mSv] for all eight phantoms resulting from a typical ^{18}FDG PET/CT scan

	Male				Female			
	1 year	5 years	10 years	15 years	1 year	5 years	10 years	15 years
Adrenals	4.33	4.56	5.00	6.76	4.34	4.56	5.01	6.20
Bladder	26.42	34.90	45.59	52.03	26.42	34.92	45.64	49.27
Bone surfaces	3.88	3.94	4.48	5.38	3.89	3.94	4.48	5.19
Brain	3.79	5.11	7.87	13.23	3.81	5.11	7.87	12.46
Breasts	3.48	3.51	3.90	5.03	3.54	3.51	3.90	4.52
Colon	4.30	4.64	5.27	6.79	4.30	4.64	5.26	6.39
Extrathoracic region	0.41	0.67	0.72	1.44	0.42	0.66	0.71	1.35
Gallbladder	4.30	4.38	5.05	6.77	4.30	4.38	5.05	6.21
Gonads	4.13	4.51	5.10	6.31	4.57	4.93	5.48	7.09
Heart wall	21.49	21.83	24.14	29.30	21.50	21.84	24.14	27.42
Kidneys	4.74	5.21	5.96	8.31	4.74	5.22	5.96	7.89
Liver	7.07	7.02	8.29	10.56	7.07	7.02	8.29	9.82
Lower large intestine wall	3.88	4.12	4.85	5.36	3.88	4.13	4.85	5.03
Lungs	7.07	6.90	8.13	10.92	7.07	6.91	8.13	10.25
Lymph nodes	0.35	0.57	0.61	1.35	0.36	0.56	0.61	1.32
Muscles	3.72	3.70	4.03	5.06	3.72	3.70	4.03	4.67
Esophagus	4.05	4.17	4.65	6.36	4.06	4.17	4.66	5.95
Oral mucosa	0.33	0.51	0.48	1.02	0.34	0.51	0.48	0.89
Pancreas	4.61	4.72	5.41	6.68	4.61	4.72	5.42	6.26
Prostate/uterus	0.32	0.67	0.76	1.55	5.31	6.02	7.10	8.05
Red bone marrow	3.58	3.62	4.25	5.52	3.55	3.62	4.25	5.27
Salivary glands	0.37	0.60	0.60	1.15	0.37	0.59	0.60	1.13
Skin	3.02	2.94	3.04	3.80	3.02	2.94	3.04	3.61
Small intestine	4.47	4.73	5.28	6.80	4.48	4.73	5.28	6.43
Spleen	4.06	4.20	4.53	6.16	4.06	4.20	4.53	5.80
Stomach	4.14	4.22	4.74	6.21	4.14	4.23	4.73	5.69
Thymus	4.06	4.20	4.68	6.42	4.06	4.20	4.67	6.00
Thyroid	4.11	4.33	4.57	5.92	4.09	4.33	4.57	5.56
Upper large intestine wall	3.88	3.82	4.31	4.73	3.88	3.82	4.31	4.44
Effective dose	7.04	6.28	5.97	9.18	7.04	6.27	5.96	8.61

Table 5.7 Organ doses [mGy] and effective dose [mSv] for all eight phantoms resulting from a typical diagnostic chest-abdomen-pelvis (CAP) CT scan

	Male				Female			
	1 year	5 years	10 years	15 years	1 year	5 years	10 years	15 years
Adrenals	2.93	2.93	3.61	5.12	3.26	2.92	3.64	4.32
Bladder	3.16	3.25	3.63	4.59	3.17	3.44	3.77	5.49
Bone surface	2.05	1.89	2.24	2.44	1.63	1.88	2.27	2.68
Brain	0.12	0.08	0.10	0.07	0.10	0.08	0.10	0.06
Breasts	2.71	3.35	3.57	4.70	3.49	3.34	3.55	3.71
Colon	3.35	3.37	3.99	5.26	3.41	3.37	4.00	4.85
Extrathoracic region	1.96	1.18	1.94	2.83	1.52	1.17	1.94	2.19
Gall bladder	3.38	3.23	3.77	5.00	3.34	3.23	3.77	4.34
Gonads	2.99	3.18	4.12	5.63	2.88	3.14	3.35	5.12
Heart wall	3.38	3.40	4.05	5.62	3.54	3.39	4.03	4.88
Kidneys	3.33	3.31	3.85	5.14	3.38	3.31	3.88	4.91
Lens	0.10	0.05	0.07	0.07	0.08	0.05	0.07	0.04
Liver	3.37	3.27	3.89	5.25	3.39	3.27	3.89	4.50
Lungs	3.25	3.17	3.89	5.33	3.33	3.17	3.90	4.85
Lymph nodes	2.67	2.50	2.89	3.84	2.72	2.47	2.91	3.62
Muscle	2.32	1.50	1.64	2.44	2.34	1.49	1.82	1.92
Esophagus	2.97	2.94	3.48	4.88	2.97	2.93	3.49	4.36
Oral mucosa	1.55	0.31	0.36	0.96	0.63	0.31	0.37	0.22
Pancreas	3.52	3.28	3.85	4.94	3.23	3.29	3.86	4.49
Prostate/uterus	3.13	3.03	3.14	4.81	2.68	2.94	3.04	4.43
Red bone marrow	1.71	1.25	2.01	2.94	1.52	1.25	2.04	2.98
Salivary glands	2.06	0.43	0.65	0.51	1.60	0.42	0.65	0.36
Skin	1.74	1.21	1.35	1.85	1.75	1.21	1.43	1.80
Small intestine	3.42	3.42	4.09	5.31	3.48	3.41	4.10	4.97
Spleen	3.17	3.30	3.87	5.29	3.24	3.29	3.88	4.87
Stomach	3.45	3.40	4.01	5.45	3.42	3.39	4.01	4.56
Thymus	3.20	3.13	3.87	5.06	3.10	3.12	3.84	4.47
Thyroid	3.24	3.14	4.43	5.36	3.57	3.13	4.42	4.60
Effective dose	2.90	2.88	3.49	4.70	2.96	2.88	3.44	4.22

Table 5.8 Cancer incidence, cancer mortality, and radiation detriment per 100,000 individuals exposed for a typical whole-body, attenuation correction CT scan

		Incidence per 100,000 people				Mortality per 100,000 people			
Sex	Age [yr]	10% CI	50% CI	90% CI	Mortality fraction	10% CI	50% CI	90% CI	Detriment per 100,000 people
Male	1	4	9	14	0.40	2	4	6	2
Male	5	5	13	21	0.43	2	5	9	4
Male	10	4	11	19	0.45	2	5	8	4
Male	15	8	21	34	0.47	4	10	16	9
Female	1	11	20	34	0.42	4	8	14	2
Female	5	14	25	44	0.44	6	11	19	3
Female	10	11	21	36	0.46	5	9	16	4
Female	15	19	35	60	0.48	9	17	29	8

Table 5.9 Cancer incidence, cancer mortality, and radiation detriment per 100,000 individuals exposed for a typical [18]FDG PET scan

		Incidence per 100,000 people				Mortality per 100,000 people			
Sex	Age [yr]	10% CI	50% CI	90% CI	Mortality fraction	10% CI	50% CI	90% CI	Detriment per 100,000 people
Male	1	82	156	256	0.40	33	63	103	29
Male	5	78	156	276	0.43	34	67	119	31
Male	10	82	169	295	0.45	37	76	133	37
Male	15	83	171	314	0.47	39	80	146	42
Female	1	142	253	413	0.42	60	106	173	29
Female	5	129	228	379	0.44	57	100	166	31
Female	10	128	232	378	0.46	59	107	174	37
Female	15	113	204	338	0.48	54	98	162	39

Table 5.10 Cancer incidence, cancer mortality, and radiation detriment per 100,000 individuals exposed for a typical [18]FDG PET/CT scan

		Incidence per 100,000 people				Mortality per 100,000 people			
Sex	Age [yr]	10% CI	50% CI	90% CI	Mortality fraction	10% CI	50% CI	90% CI	Detriment per 100,000 people
Male	1	86	165	270	0.40	35	67	109	31
Male	5	83	169	297	0.43	36	73	128	35
Male	10	86	180	314	0.45	39	81	141	40
Male	15	91	192	348	0.47	42	89	162	51
Female	1	153	273	447	0.42	64	114	187	31
Female	5	143	253	423	0.44	63	111	186	34
Female	10	139	253	414	0.46	64	116	191	40
Female	15	132	239	398	0.48	63	114	191	47

Table 5.11 Cancer incidence, cancer mortality, and radiation detriment per 100,000 individuals exposed for a typical diagnostic chest-abdomen-pelvis CT scan

		Incidence per 100,000 people				Mortality per 100,000 people			
Sex	Age [yr]	10% CI	50% CI	90% CI	Mortality fraction	10% CI	50% CI	90% CI	Detriment per 100,000 people
Male	1	27	67	121	0.40	11	27	49	16
Male	5	21	54	101	0.43	9	24	44	16
Male	10	22	54	97	0.45	10	24	44	19
Male	15	21	60	100	0.47	10	28	46	26
Female	1	79	149	257	0.42	33	62	108	16
Female	5	63	114	200	0.44	27	50	88	16
Female	10	58	107	185	0.46	27	49	85	19
Female	15	54	98	168	0.48	26	47	81	23

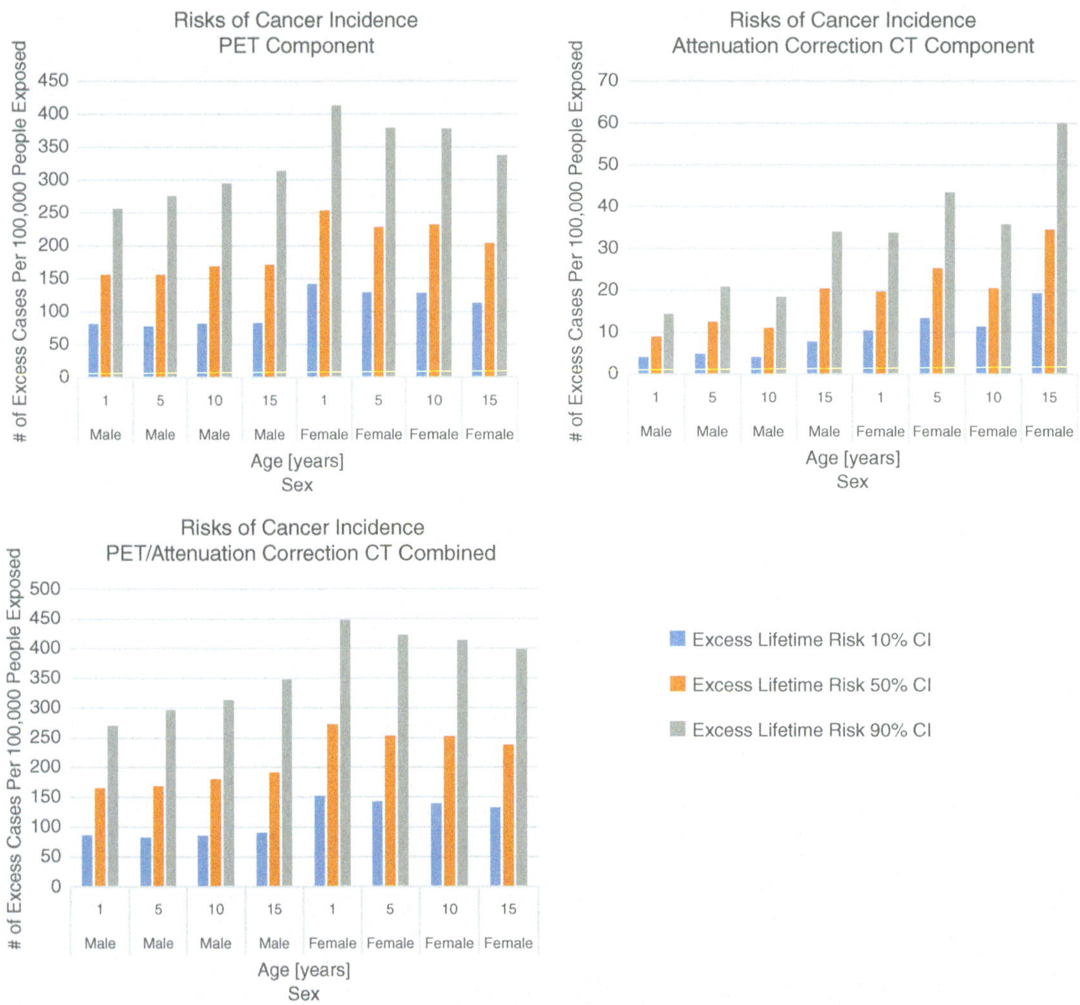

Fig. 5.3 PET, AC CT, and combined excess lifetime risk of cancer *incidence* at the 10%, 50%, and 90% confidence levels for reference patients at ages 1, 5, 10, and 15 years for both males and females

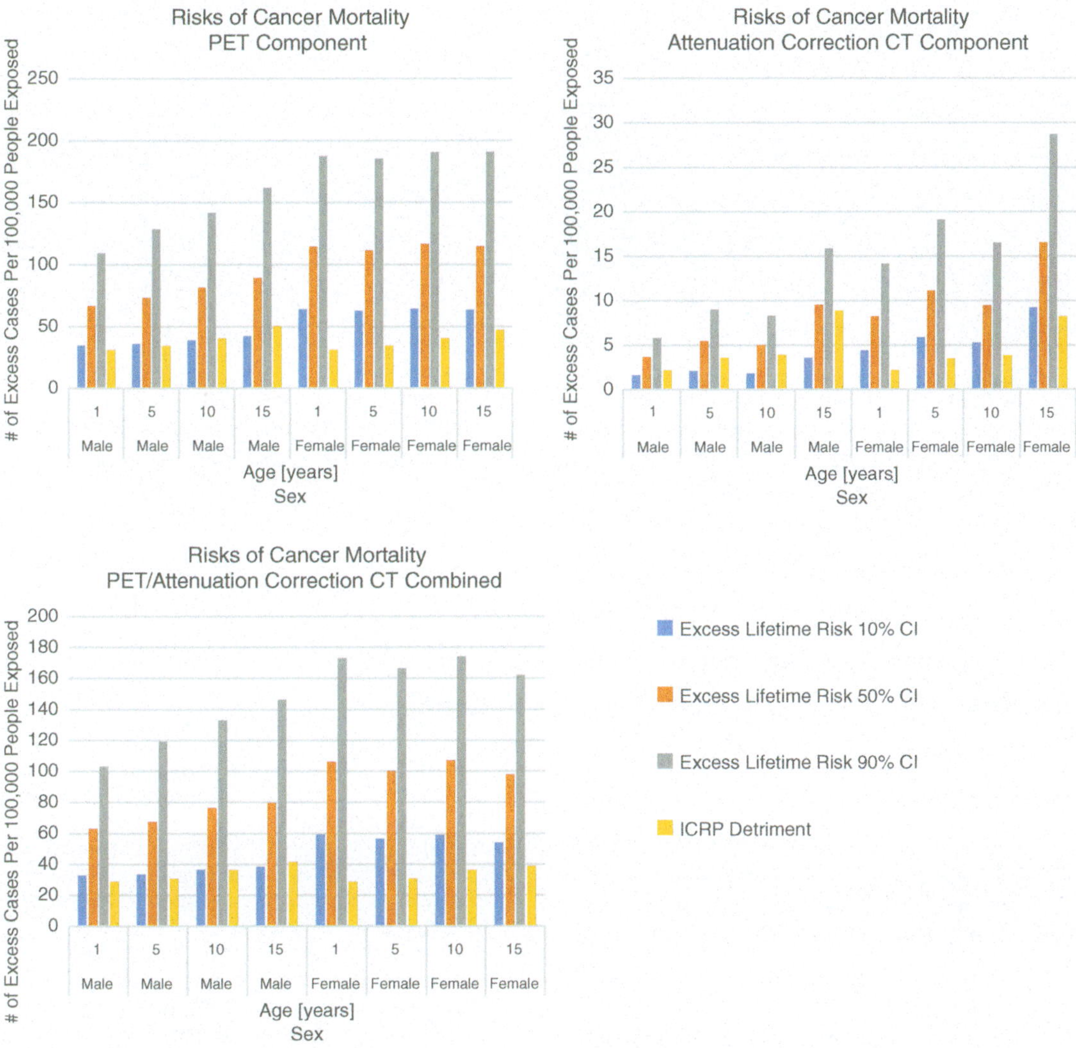

Fig. 5.4 PET, AC CT, and combined excess lifetime risk of cancer *mortality* at the 10%, 50%, and 90% confidence levels, as well as radiation detriment, for reference patients at ages 1, 5, 10, and 15 years for both males and females

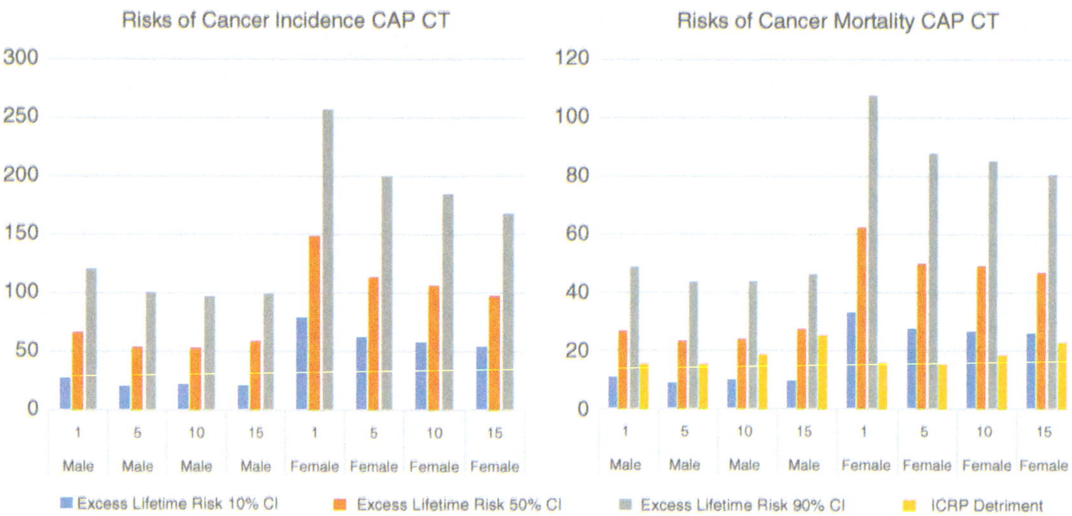

Fig. 5.5 Diagnostic chest-abdomen-pelvis CT scan excess lifetime risk of cancer incidence and mortality at the 10%, 50%, and 90% confidence levels, along with ICRP radiation detriment, for reference patients of ages 1, 5, 10, and 15 years for both males and females

Conclusions

In almost all cases, the radiation harm incurred following CT imaging is vastly outweighed by the medical benefit of timely and accurate image-based diagnostics. Nevertheless, imaging protocols should be medically justified and optimized. The latter entails exploration of trade-offs of image quality – tailored to the diagnostic information sought – and the radiation risk to the patient. These risks can never be assessed on an individual patient basis, but nominal values of radiation cancer risk following CT imaging may be inferred for patient subpopulations (e.g., females between birth and 2 years or male adults over 55 years) using radiation risk models for cancer incidence or mortality derived from radiation epidemiological studies. These measures of nominal patient subpopulation risk can be considered as improvements over estimates of radiation detriment as defined by the ICRP in its protection quality effective dose. In both cases, however, estimates of individual organ dose are required and are most accurately assessed using patient morphometry-matched computational human phantoms and Monte Carlo-based radiation transport modeling of the CT imaging system and patient imaging exam.

References

1. ICRP. ICRP Publication 102: managing patient dose in multi-dector computed tomography (MDCT). Ann ICRP. 2007;37(1):1–79.
2. AAPM. AAPM Report No. 204 – Size-specific dose estimates (SSDE) in pediatric and adult body CT examinations. American Association of Physicists in Medicine: college Park; 2011.
3. AAPM. AAPM Report No. 220 – Use of water equivalent diameter for calculating patient size and size-specific dose estimates (SSDE) in CT. American Association of Physicists in Medicine: college Park; 2014.
4. BEIR. Health risks from exposure to low levels of ionizing radiation: BEIR VII – phase 2. Washington, DC: National Research Council; 2005.
5. UNSCEAR. In: U.N.S.C.o.t.E.o.A. Radiation, editor. Effects of Ionizing Radiation - Annex A: Epidemiological Studies of Radiation and Cancer. New York: United Nations; 2006.
6. Pawel D, Puskin J. U.S. Environmental Protection Agency radiogenic risk models and projections for the U.S. population. Health Phys. 2012;102(6):646–56.
7. Hintenlang DE, Moloney W, Winslow J. Physical phantoms for experimental radiation dosimetry. In: Xu XG, Eckerman KF, editors. Handbook of anatomical models for radiation dosimetry. London: Taylor & Francis Group; 2009.
8. Cristy M. Mathematical phantoms representing children of various ages for use in estimates of internal dose. Oak Ridge: Oak Ridge National Laboratory; 1980.
9. Han EY, Bolch WE, Eckerman KF. Revisions to the ORNL series of adult and pediatric computational

phantoms for use with the MIRD schema. Health Phys. 2006;90(4):337–56.
10. ICRP. ICRP Publication 110: adult reference computational phantoms. Ann ICRP. 2009;39(2):1–165.
11. Kim C, et al. The reference phantoms: voxel vs. polygon. Ann ICRP. 2016;45:188–201.
12. Furuta T, et al. Implementation of tetrahedral-mesh geometry in Monte Carlo radiation transport code PHITS. Phys Med Biol. 2017;62(12):4798–810.
13. ICRP ICRP publication 23: report on the task group on reference man. In: Annals of the ICRP. Oxford: International Commission on Radiological Protection: Pergamon Press; 1975. p. 1–480.
14. ICRP. ICRP publication 89: basic anatomical and physiological data for use in radiological protection – reference values. Ann ICRP. 2002;32(3–4):1–277.
15. Segars WP, et al. Population of anatomically variable 4D XCAT adult phantoms for imaging research and optimization. Med Phys. 2013;40(4):043701.
16. Geyer AM, et al. The UF/NCI family of hybrid computational phantoms representing the current US population of male and female children, adolescents, and adults – application to CT dosimetry. Phys Med Biol. 2014;59(18):5225–42.
17. Johnson P, et al. Hybrid patient-dependent phantoms covering statistical distributions of body morphometry in the US adult and pediatric population. Proc IEEE. 2009;97(12):2060–75.
18. Sands MM, et al. Comparison of methods for individualized astronaut organ dosimetry: morphometry-based phantom library versus body contour autoscaling of a reference phantom. Life Sci Space Res (Amst). 2017;15:23–31.
19. DeMarco JJ, et al. A Monte Carlo based method to estimate radiation dose from multidetector CT (MDCT): cylindrical and anthropomorphic phantoms. Phys Med Biol. 2005;50(17):3989–4004.
20. Li X, et al. Patient-specific radiation dose and cancer risk estimation in CT: part I. development and validation of a Monte Carlo program. Med Phys. 2011;38(1):397–407.
21. Li X, et al. Patient-specific radiation dose and cancer risk estimation in CT: part II. Application to patients. Med Phys. 2011;38(1):408–19.
22. Khatonabadi M, et al. The feasibility of a regional CTDIvol to estimate organ dose from tube current modulated CT exams. Med Phys. 2013;40(5):051903.
23. Stepusin EJ, et al. Physical validation of a Monte Carlo-based phantom-derived approach to computed tomography organ dosimetry under tube current modulation. Med Phys. 2017;44:5423–32.
24. Stepusin EJ, et al. Assessment of different patient-to-phantom matching criteria applied to a Monte Carlo-based CT organ dose library. Med Phys. 2017;44:5498–508.
25. Turner AC, et al. A method to generate equivalent energy spectra and filtration models based on measurement for multidetector CT Monte Carlo dosimetry simulations. Med Phys. 2009;36(6):2154–64.
26. NCRP. NCRP commentary no. 27: implications of recent epidemiological studies for the linear non-threshold model and radiation protection. Bethesda: National Council on Radiation Protection and Measurement; 2018. p. 1–210.
27. ICRP. ICRP publication 103: recommendations of the international commission on radiological protection. Ann ICRP. 2007;37(2–4):1–332.
28. de Gonzalez AB, et al. RadRAT: a radiation risk assessment tool for lifetime cancer risk projection. J Radiol Prot. 2012;32(3):205–22.
29. Lee C, et al. The UF family of reference hybrid phantoms for computational radiation dosimetry. Phys Med Biol. 2010;55(2):339–63.
30. ICRP. ICRP publication 128: radiation dose to patients from radiopharmaceuticals – a compendium of current information related to frequently used substances. Ann ICRP. 2015;44(2S):1–321.

CT Image Quality Characterization

6

Ke Li and Guang-Hong Chen

Introduction

In CT imaging processes, the x-ray attenuation coefficient (μ) of an image object is evaluated as a function of spatial location, energy, and/or time. If such processes are perfect, this chapter shouldn't be written. It is the imperfect representation of μ in typical CT imaging situation that motivated the scientific discussion and research on the topic of CT image quality. Typical imperfections include stochastic deviation of the recorded μ from the true μ (noise), deterministic deviation of the recorded μ from the true μ (bias or certain artifacts), deterministic deformation of the spatial distribution of the recorded μ (spatial resolution loss), and so forth. These imperfections usually can't be avoided due to the upper limits in radiation dose budget, system cost, and data acquisition time, among many other practical considerations. Actually, they don't have to be completely eliminated as long as the prescribed CT imaging task(s) can be carried out with acceptable performance. The subject of CT image quality assessment concerns the physical characteristics and origin of these imperfections as well as their relationships with CT system parameters, so that CT systems can be developed, operated, and maintained to meet the minimal requirements set for the CT imaging tasks.

To help understand the physical characteristics of image imperfections, a set of objective quality metrics such as noise variance, contrast-to-noise ratio (CNR), noise power spectrum (NPS), and modulation transfer function (MTF) have been formulated and widely used in CT imaging community. Guidelines on how to measure these image quality metrics have been extensively reported in multiple review articles [1, 2], ACR publications [3, 4], AAPM task group reports [5, 6], and even CT scanner manuals. As a result, we will not present the methodology and work flow of CT image quality assessment in this chapter. Instead, we will focus on analyzing the physical origins of commonly observed CT image imperfections and quantitative relationships between objective CT image quality metrics and CT system parameters which were scattered in literature and hard to find a systematics and comprehensive discussion for graduate students, researchers, and clinical medical physicists.

The plan for this chapter is given as follows. In the next section (Section "Idealized Linear CT Systems") of this chapter, linear systems theory and a toy model CT system will be used to derive some of the fundamental relationships in CT image quality metrics in order to help readers pinpoint the underlying assumptions of these seemingly familiar relations. As one will see in the discussion of these chapter and in your practice, these assumptions are often mildly violated in realistic CT systems, even for those employing the

K. Li · G.-H. Chen (✉)
Department of Medical Physics and Department of Radiology, School of Medicine and Public Health, University of Wisconsin-Madison, Madison, WI, USA
e-mail: ke.li@wisc.edu; gchen7@wisc.edu

© Springer Nature Switzerland AG 2020

E. Samei, N. J. Pelc (eds.), *Computed Tomography*, https://doi.org/10.1007/978-3-030-26957-9_6

linear filtered backprojection (FBP) algorithm. To enable one to still use the model developed for an idealized CT system to a realistic CT system, we will present a compensation technique using the concept of virtual image object such that the image quality models established based on ideal linear systems can still be applicable to the FBP-based quasi-linear CT systems.

The true challenge in understanding CT image quality came after the commercialization and clinical use of model-based iterative reconstruction (MBIR-based CT systems) [7–17]. For the majority of the implemented MBIR methods, their nonlinear nature spoils the overall quasi-linearity of CT systems. Losing their theoretical foundation, classical CT image quality models often find themselves no longer valid for MBIR-based systems. What is worse is that CT users might not realize the inapplicability of these classical models and thus keep relying on them to guide the development and operation of MBIR-based CT systems. If that is the case, CT image imperfections may not be adequately controlled within the acceptable range, neither may CT imaging tasks be carried out with desired performance standard. To prevent these undesirable consequences and facilitate wider clinical adoptions of MBIR, a plethora of research efforts have been spent in the last few years to advance knowledge about image quality of MBIR-based systems [18–32]. New image quality estimation methods that are not based on the premise of system linearity and stationarity have been developed, and new image quality properties have been identified. Section "Nonlinear CT Systems with Model-Based Iterative Reconstruction" of this chapter will use examples to showcase these new properties and more importantly to justify the necessity of task-directed image quality estimation and modeling for MBIR-based CT systems.

Idealized Linear CT Systems

This section discusses noise, spatial resolution, and CT number accuracy of "toy model" CT systems (Fig. 6.1). Although these systems are quite idealized and rarely encountered in practice, a

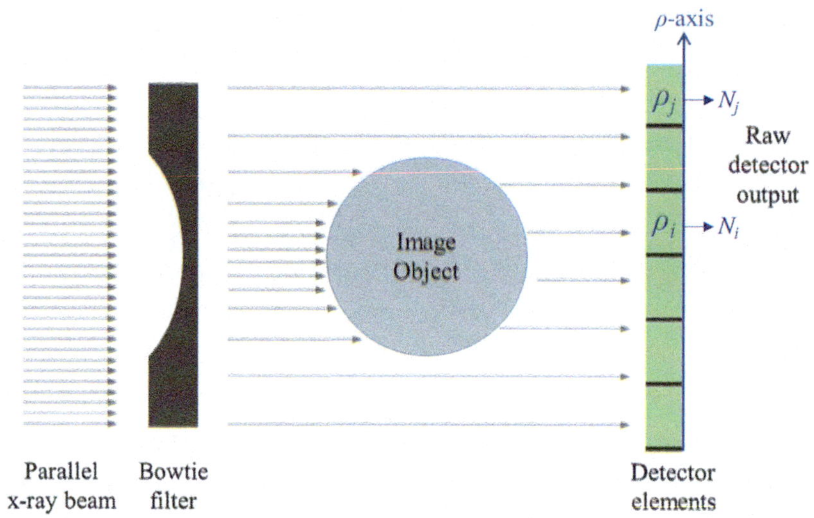

Fig. 6.1 In the illustrated CT system, the x-rays are generated from a parallel array of pencil sources with infinitely small focal spot size and infinitely high-temporal coherence (i.e., monoenergetic). The cylindrical image object has a diameter of D and is placed at the isocenter. The post-object x-ray fluence is uniform due to the use of a beam-flattening bowtie filter. Scattered x-rays that do not travel forwardly are completely rejected. The detector has a uniform response along the ρ axis. Except its finite quantum absorption efficiency, the detector does not introduce any other noise or signal-blurring mechanism. The CT system uses the linear filtered backprojection (FBP) algorithm to perform tomographic reconstruction. Image quality models presented in section "Idealized Linear CT Systems" used these idealized conditions

thorough understanding of image quality properties of ideal systems would inspire subsequent discussions of realistic CT systems that are all certain variants of the idealized systems.

Noise Properties of Raw Detector Outputs

At a given projection angle θ, the raw output of a CT detector element located at ρ can be modeled as

$$N(\rho,\theta)=\langle N(\rho,\theta)\rangle+\Delta N(\rho,\theta), \quad (6.1)$$

where $\langle N\rangle$ denotes the expected value of the output, and ΔN denotes the stochastic deviation of the measured N from $\langle N\rangle$. Based on the Beer-Lambert law, $\langle N\rangle$ is related to the input x-ray flux $\langle n_0\rangle$ (expected number of input x-ray photons per unit area per unit time) by

$$\langle N(\rho,\theta)\rangle=\langle n_0\rangle \Delta t\bar{\varepsilon}\Delta z\Delta\rho e^{-\int_{L(\rho,\theta)} u dl} \quad (6.2)$$

$$=\langle n_0\rangle \Delta t\bar{\varepsilon}\Delta z\Delta\rho e^{-uD}. \quad (6.3)$$

where Δz and $\Delta\rho$ are the detector pixel size along the detector column and row direction, respectively; Δt is the detector integration time per projection view; and $\bar{\varepsilon}$ is the x-ray absorption efficiency of the detector. Under the conditions shown in Fig. 6.1, the right-hand side of Eq. (6.2) is independent of ρ and θ, which enables the simplification of (6.2) to (6.3).

For a given CT system operated at a given tube potential (kV), the x-ray flux $\langle n_0\rangle$ is linearly proportional to the tube current (mA), and the integration time per projection angle (Δt) is linearly proportional to the gantry rotation time per revolution (s). Therefore, Eq. (6.2) can also be written as

$$\langle N(\rho,\theta)\rangle=a(mAs)\ \bar{\varepsilon}\Delta z\Delta\rho e^{-uD}, \quad (6.4)$$

where a is a numerical scaling factor.

For an ideal CT system that uses a photon-counting detector, the probability mass density function (PDF) of N follows the Poisson distribution:

$$p(N|\langle N\rangle)=e^{-\langle N\rangle}\frac{\langle N\rangle^N}{N!}, \quad (6.5)$$

where $p(N|\langle N\rangle)$ denotes the PDF of N given its expected value of $\langle N\rangle$. Based on this PDF, the noise variance of N is related to $\langle N\rangle$ by

$$\begin{aligned}\sigma_N^2&=\langle(\Delta N)^2\rangle=\langle(N-\langle N\rangle)^2\rangle\\&=\langle N^2\rangle-\langle N\rangle^2\\&=\left(\sum_{N=0}^{+\infty}N^2e^{-\langle N\rangle}\frac{\langle N\rangle^N}{N!}\right)-\langle N\rangle^2\\&=\langle N\rangle(\langle N\rangle+1)-\langle N\rangle^2\\&=\langle N\rangle.\end{aligned} \quad (6.6)$$

In addition to noise variance, one may also be interested in the autocovariance of the raw projection data defined as follows:

$$C_N(\rho_i,\theta_m;\rho_j,\theta_n)=\langle\Delta N(\rho_i,\theta_m)\Delta N(\rho_j,\theta_n)\rangle. \quad (6.7)$$

Due to the use of inter-pixel septa and an anti-scatter grid, correlation of noise between discrete detector pixels can be considered negligible for an idealized system. Similarly, assuming the detector used in the idealized CT system has negligible temporal lag, noise correlation between different view angles can also be considered negligible. Under these conditions, C_N is given by

$$\begin{aligned}C_N(\rho_i,\theta_m;\rho_j,\theta_n)&=\sigma_N^2(\rho_i,\theta_m)\delta_{i,j}\delta_{m,n}\\&=a(mAs)\ \bar{\varepsilon}\Delta z\Delta\rho e^{-uD}\delta_{i,j}\delta_{m,n},\end{aligned} \quad (6.8)$$

where $\delta_{i,j}$ and $\delta_{m,n}$ denote Kronecker delta functions and are related to the corresponding Dirac delta functions by

$$\delta_{i,j}=\Delta\rho\delta(\rho_i-\rho_j),\quad \delta_{m,n}=\Delta\theta\delta(\theta_m-\theta_n). \quad (6.9)$$

In summary of the noise properties of the raw projection data generated from idealized linear CT systems, its noise variance is proportional to mAs, detector width ($\Delta\rho$), detector height (Δz), and detector absorption efficiency ($\bar{\varepsilon}$); it is *inversely* proportional to the exponential of the radiological path length of the object exp(μD). For idealized systems, noise of the raw projection data can be considered uncorrelated (i.e., "white") along the ρ and θ directions.

Noise Properties of Post-log Projection Data

To reconstruct a CT image, the following logarithmic transform is usually applied to the raw projection data:

$$R(\rho,\theta)=\ln\left[\frac{\langle N_0(\rho,\theta)\rangle}{N(\rho,\theta)}\right], \quad (6.10)$$

where $\langle N_0\rangle$denotes the expected detector output in the absence of a patient or image object. As shown in Appendix I, the autocovariance of R is related to noise of the raw projection data by

$$\begin{aligned} C_R(\rho_i,\theta_m;\rho_j,\theta_n) &= \langle \Delta R(\rho_i,\theta_m)\Delta R(\rho_j,\theta_m)\rangle \\ &= \frac{\sigma_N^2(\rho_i,\theta_m)}{\langle N(\rho_i,\theta_m)\rangle^2}\delta_{i,j}\delta_{m,n} \\ &= \frac{1}{\langle N(\rho_i,\theta_m)\rangle}\delta_{i,j}\delta_{m,n}. \end{aligned} \quad (6.11)$$

Alternatively, based on the relationship between the Kronecker delta function and Dirac delta function, Eq. (6.11) can also be written as

$$\begin{aligned} & C_R(\rho_i,\theta_m;\rho_j,\theta_n) \\ &= \frac{\Delta\rho\Delta\theta}{\langle N(\rho_i,\theta_m)\rangle}\delta(\rho_i-\rho_j)\delta(\theta_m-\theta_n). \end{aligned} \quad (6.12)$$

The noise variance of R is related to C_R as

$$\begin{aligned} \sigma_R^2(\rho_i,\theta_m) &= C_R(\rho_i,\theta_m;\rho_j=\rho_i,\theta_n=\theta_m) \\ &= \frac{1}{\langle N(\rho_i,\theta_m)\rangle} \\ &= \frac{e^{uD}}{a(mAs)\,\bar{\varepsilon}\Delta z\Delta\rho}. \end{aligned} \quad (6.13)$$

In summary of the noise properties of the post-log projection data (R) for idealized CT systems, noise of R is still white along both ρ and θ directions; the noise variance of R is proportional to the exponential of the radiological path length of the object exp.(μD); it is *inversely* proportional to mAs, detector width ($\Delta\rho$), detector height (Δz), and detector absorption efficiency ($\bar{\varepsilon}$).

Noise Properties of CT Images

Brief Review of Filtered Backprojection Reconstruction Algorithm

As described in detail in [33, 34], the first step in performing a CT reconstruction is to filter the post-log projection data as follows:

$$\tilde{R}'(k,\theta)=\tilde{R}(k,\theta)\,|k|\,G(k), \quad (6.14)$$

where k denotes spatial frequency along the detector row direction, $|k|$ is the ramp kernel, $G(k)$ is a reconstruction window function, and $\tilde{R}$ denotes the one-dimensional (1D) Fourier transform of R along the ρ axis, namely,

$$\tilde{R}(k,\theta)=\int d\rho R(\rho,\theta)e^{-i2\pi k\rho}. \quad (6.15)$$

By backprojecting the filtered post-log projection data as described in the following equation, a tomographic image of the object's linear attenuation coefficient can be estimated:

$$\begin{aligned} \hat{\mu}(x,y) &= \int_0^{\pi} d\theta \int_{-\infty}^{+\infty} \mathrm{d}k\, \tilde{R}'(k,\theta)e^{i2\pi k(x\cos\theta+y\sin\theta)} \\ &= \int_0^{\pi} \mathrm{d}\theta \int_{-\infty}^{+\infty} \mathrm{d}k\, \tilde{R}(k,\theta)G(k)\,|k|\,e^{i2\pi k(x\cos\theta+y\sin\theta)}. \end{aligned} \quad (6.16)$$

Equation (6.16) is applicable to parallel beam FBP reconstructions for half-rotation scans. For full rotation scans, a scaling factor of ½ needs to be applied to account for data redundancy:

$$\begin{aligned} \hat{\mu}(x,y) &= \frac{1}{2}\int_0^{2\pi} d\theta \int_{-\infty}^{+\infty} \mathrm{d}k\, \tilde{R}(k,\theta) \\ & G(k)\,|k|\,e^{i2\pi k(x\cos\theta+y\sin\theta)}. \end{aligned} \quad (6.17)$$

With the estimated linear attenuation coefficient $\hat{\mu}(x,y)$, the final CT image with units of HU is given by

$$f(x,y)=\frac{\hat{\mu}(x,y)-\mu_w}{\mu_w}\times 1000, \quad (6.18)$$

where μ_w denotes the expected linear attenuation coefficient of water.

CT Noise Variance

By definition, the noise variance of a CT image is given by

$$\begin{aligned}\sigma_f^2(x,y)&=\left\langle\left[f(x,y)-f\langle(x,y)\rangle\right]^2\right\rangle\\&=\left(\frac{1000}{\mu_w}\right)^2\left\langle\left[\hat{\mu}(x,y)-\langle\hat{\mu}(x,y)\rangle\right]^2\right\rangle\\&=\left(\frac{1000}{\mu_w}\right)^2\sigma_{\hat{\mu}}^2(x,y),\end{aligned} \quad (6.19)$$

where $\sigma_{\hat{\mu}}^2$ denotes the noise variance of the estimated linear attenuation coefficient. As derived in Appendix II, $\sigma_{\hat{\mu}}^2(x,y)$ is related to the noise variance of R and reconstruction parameters as

$$\begin{aligned}\sigma_{\hat{\mu}}^2(x,y)&=\sigma_R^2\pi\Delta\rho\Delta\theta\int_{-\infty}^{+\infty}\mathrm{d}k\left|G(k)\right|^2|k|^2\\&=\frac{\pi\Delta\theta e^{uD}}{a(mAs)\,\bar{\varepsilon}\Delta z}\int_{-\infty}^{+\infty}\mathrm{d}k\left|G(k)\right|^2|k|^2.\end{aligned} \quad (6.20)$$

Accordingly, CT noise variance $\sigma_f^2(x,y)$ is given by

$$\begin{aligned}\sigma_f^2(x,y)&=\left(\frac{1000}{\mu_w}\right)^2\sigma_{\hat{\mu}}^2(x,y)\\&=\left(\frac{1000}{\mu_w}\right)^2\frac{\pi\Delta\theta e^{uD}}{a(mAs)\,\bar{\varepsilon}\Delta z}\int_{-\infty}^{+\infty}\mathrm{d}k\left|G(k)\right|^2|k|^2.\end{aligned} \quad (6.21)$$

The integration $\int_{-\infty}^{+\infty}\mathrm{d}k\left|G(k)\right|^2|k|^2$ in Eq. (6.21) may be further simplified for specific reconstruction kernels. As an example, for one of the most widely used kernels, the Ram-Lak kernel, its window function is given by

$$G(k)=\mathrm{rect}\left(\frac{k}{2k_N}\right), \quad (6.22)$$

where rect denotes the rectangular function, $k_N = 1/(2\Delta\rho)$ denotes the Nyquist frequency along the direction row direction. With this window function

$$\begin{aligned}\sigma_f^2&=\left(\frac{1000}{\mu_w}\right)^2\frac{\pi\Delta\theta e^{uD}}{a(mAs)\,\bar{\varepsilon}\Delta z}\int_{-k_N}^{+k_N}\mathrm{d}k|k|^2\\&=\left(\frac{1000}{\mu_w}\right)^2\frac{\pi\Delta\theta e^{uD}}{a(mAs)\,\bar{\varepsilon}\Delta z}\frac{2k_N^3}{3}\\&=\frac{1}{12}\left(\frac{1000}{\mu_w}\right)^2\frac{\pi\Delta\theta e^{uD}}{a(mAs)\,\bar{\varepsilon}\Delta z(\Delta\rho)^3}.\end{aligned} \quad (6.23)$$

As another example, if the reconstruction uses the low-pass cosine kernel, the corresponding window function is given by

$$G(k)=\mathrm{rect}\left(\frac{k}{2k_N}\right)\cos\left(\pi\frac{k}{2k_N}\right). \quad (6.24)$$

CT noise variance that corresponds to this window function is given by

$$\begin{aligned}\sigma_{\hat{\mu}}^2&=\left(\frac{1000}{\mu_w}\right)^2\frac{\pi\Delta\theta e^{uD}}{a(mAs)\,\bar{\varepsilon}\,\Delta z}\int_{-k_N}^{+k_N}\mathrm{d}k\cos^2\left(\pi\frac{k}{2k_N}\right)|k|^2\\&=\left(\frac{1000}{\mu_w}\right)^2\frac{\pi\Delta\theta e^{uD}}{a(mAs)\,\bar{\varepsilon}\,\Delta z}\int_{-k_N}^{+k_N}\mathrm{d}k\left[\frac{1}{2}+\frac{1}{2}\cos\left(\pi\frac{k}{k_N}\right)\right]|k|^2\\&=\frac{\pi^2-6}{24\pi^2}\left(\frac{1000}{\mu_w}\right)^2\frac{\pi\Delta\theta e^{uD}}{a(mAs)\,\bar{\varepsilon}\,\Delta z(\Delta\rho)^3},\end{aligned} \quad (6.25)$$

which is approximately 20% of the CT noise variance given by the Ram-Lak kernel in Eq. (6.23). Therefore, compared with the Ram-Lak kernel, the low-pass cosine kernel can effectively reduce CT noise magnitude. Meanwhile, for both reconstruction kernels, the CT noise variance is inversely proportional to the cube of $\Delta\rho$ (in-plane detector pixel size).

In summary of theoretical analysis on CT noise variance, it is related to the following CT system parameters:

- Reconstruction kernel (examples are provided in Fig. 6.2)
- Inversely proportional to mAs (an example is provided in Fig. 6.3)
- Inversely proportional to detector height Δz (an example is provided in Fig. 6.3)
- Inversely proportional to cube of detector width $\Delta\rho$
- Inversely proportional to detector absorption efficiency $\overline{\varepsilon}$
- Proportional to the exponential of patient radiological path length exp.(μD) (examples can be found in reference [35])

CT Noise Power Spectrum

NPS of dimension n is defined as the n-dimensional Fourier transform of the autocovariance function of the same dimension. As shown in Appendix III, the 2D autocovariance between two spatial points (x_i, y_i) and (x_j, y_j) in a CT image is given by

$$C_f\left(x_i, y_i; x_j, y_j\right) = \int_{-\infty}^{+\infty}\int_{-\infty}^{+\infty} \mathrm{d}k_x \mathrm{d}k_y \left(\frac{1000}{\mu_w}\right)^2 \frac{\Delta\rho\Delta\theta |k| \left|G(k)\right|^2}{\langle N \rangle} e^{i2\pi\left[(x_i - x_j)k_x + (y_i - y_j)k_y\right]}. \tag{6.26}$$

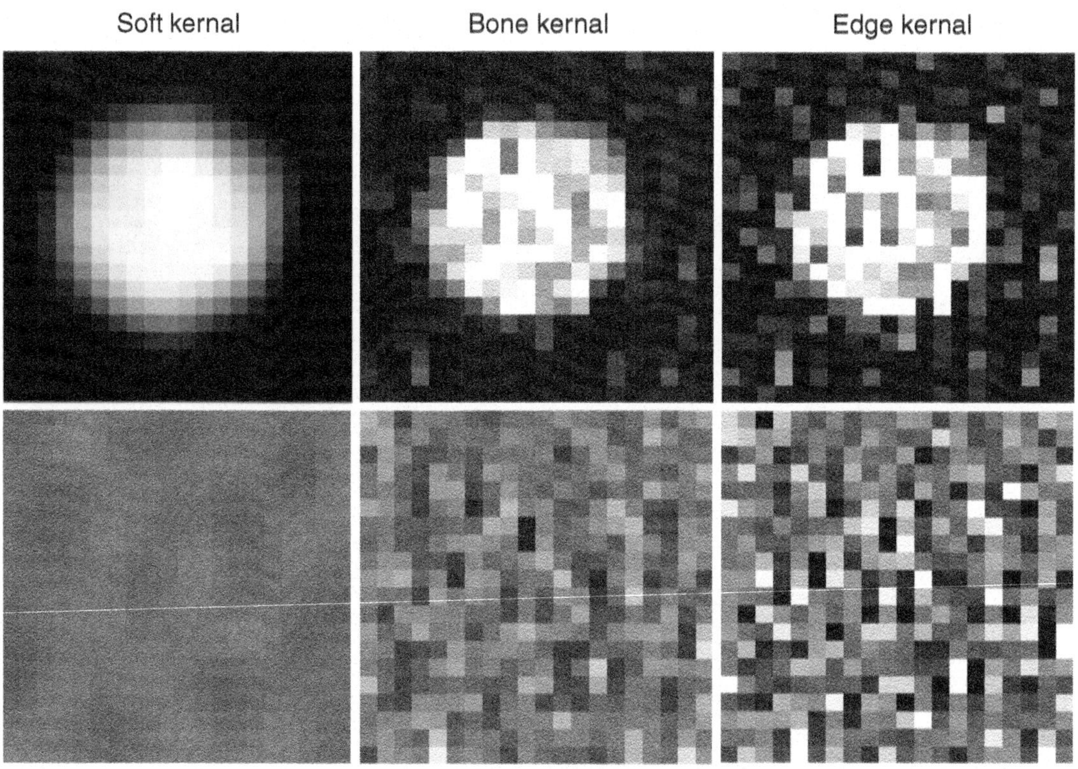

Fig. 6.2 Example images illustrating the dependence of CT noise variance, noise texture, and edge sharpness on reconstruction kernels. Top row: images of a Teflon rod reconstructed from the same set of projection data. Bottom row: noise only images that correspond to images in the top row

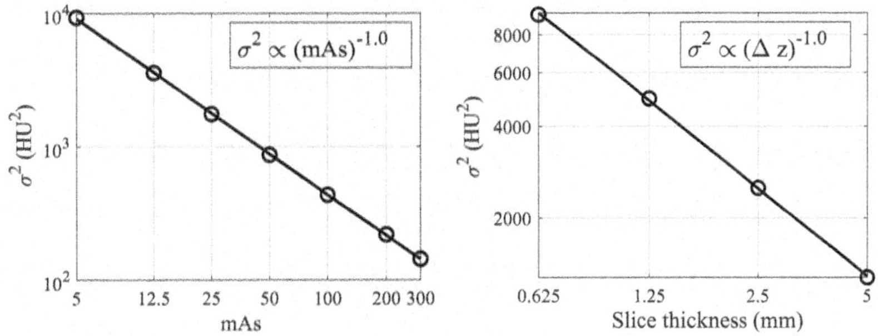

Fig. 6.3 (Left): Plot of CT image noise variance experimentally measured at different mAs levels. (Right): Plot of CT noise variance measured with different Δz values. Circles are experimental data points; solid lines are power-law fits

For an idealized linear CT system, the right-hand side of Eq. (6.26) depends on the relative distance between (x_i, y_i) and (x_j, y_j) instead of their absolute spatial locations. Therefore, by defining $x' = x_i - x_j$, $y' = y_i - y_j$, C_f can be written as a function of x' and y' as follows

$$
\begin{aligned}
C_f(x', y') &= \int_{-\infty}^{+\infty}\int_{-\infty}^{+\infty} \mathrm{d}k_x \mathrm{d}k_y \left(\frac{1000}{\mu_w}\right)^2 \frac{\Delta\rho\Delta\theta |k| |G(k)|^2}{\langle N \rangle} e^{i2\pi(x'k_x + y'k_y)} \\
&= \mathrm{IFT}_{2\mathrm{D}}\left\{\left(\frac{1000}{\mu_w}\right)^2 \frac{\Delta\rho\Delta\theta |k| |G(k)|^2}{\langle N \rangle}\right\},
\end{aligned}
\tag{6.27}
$$

where $\mathrm{IFT}_{2\mathrm{D}}$ stands for 2D inverse Fourier transform. Based on its definition, the 2D NPS of CT images is related to $C_f(x', y')$ by

$$
\begin{aligned}
\mathrm{NPS}_f(k_x, k_y) &= \int_{-\infty}^{+\infty}\int_{-\infty}^{+\infty} \mathrm{d}x' \mathrm{d}y' C_f(x', y') e^{-i2\pi(x'k_x + y'k_y)} \\
&= \mathrm{FT}_{2\mathrm{D}}\left\{\mathrm{IFT}_{2\mathrm{D}}\left\{\left(\frac{1000}{\mu_w}\right)^2 \frac{\Delta\rho\Delta\theta |k| |G(k)|^2}{\langle N \rangle}\right\}\right\},
\end{aligned}
\tag{6.28}
$$

where $\mathrm{FT}_{2\mathrm{D}}$ denotes the 2D Fourier transform. Based on the properties of Fourier and inverse Fourier transform, the 2D NPS of CT is simply

$$
\begin{aligned}
\mathrm{NPS}_f(k_x, k_y) &= \left(\frac{1000}{\mu_w}\right)^2 \frac{\Delta\rho\Delta\theta |k| |G(k)|^2}{\langle N \rangle} \\
&= \left(\frac{1000}{\mu_w}\right)^2 \frac{\Delta\theta e^{uD} |k| |G(k)|^2}{a(mAs)\, \overline{\varepsilon}\, \Delta z}.
\end{aligned}
\tag{6.29}
$$

Note that the integration of NPS of f over the frequency space is equal to the noise variance of f, namely,

$$\begin{aligned}
\int_{-\infty}^{+\infty}\int_{-\infty}^{+\infty} dk_x dk_y \mathrm{NPS}_f(k_x,k_y) &= \int_{-\infty}^{+\infty}\int_{-\infty}^{+\infty} dk_x dk_y \mathrm{NPS}_f(k_x,k_y) e^{-i2\pi(0\cdot k_x+0\cdot k_y)} \\
&= \mathrm{IFT}_{2D}\left\{\mathrm{NPS}_f(k_x,k_y\right\}_{(x'=0,y'=0)} \\
&= C_f(x'=0,y'=0) \\
&= \sigma_f^2 \\
&= \left(\frac{1000}{\mu_w}\right)^2 \frac{\pi\Delta\theta e^{uD}}{a(mAs)\,\bar{\varepsilon}\,\Delta z}\int_{-\infty}^{+\infty} dk\left|G(k)\right|^2\left|k\right|^2.
\end{aligned} \tag{6.30}$$

Therefore, if the NPS is normalized by its area under the curve, it becomes

$$\begin{aligned}
\mathrm{NNPS}_f(k_x,k_y) &= \frac{\mathrm{NPS}_f(k_x,k_y)}{\int_{-\infty}^{+\infty}\int_{-\infty}^{+\infty} dk_x dk_y \mathrm{NPS}_f(k_x,k_y)} \\
&= \frac{\mathrm{NPS}_f(k_x,k_y)}{\sigma_f^2} \\
&= \frac{|k|\,|G(k)|^2}{\pi\int_{-\infty}^{+\infty} dk\left|G(k)\right|^2|k|^2}
\end{aligned} \tag{6.31}$$

In other words, for idealized CT systems, the normalized NPS (NNPS) is solely determined by the reconstruction kernel; it is independent of mAs, slice thickness, detector absorption efficiency, and object attenuation ($e^{\mu D}$). Figure 6.4 shows the corresponding example.

In summary of the above analysis on CT NPS [36, 37]:

- NPS magnitude
  - Inversely proportional to mAs, detector thickness Δz, and detector absorption efficiency $\bar{\varepsilon}$
  - Proportional to exponential of patient radiological path length exp.(μD)
- NPS shape
  - Rotationally symmetric
  - Proportional to $|k|$ at relatively low frequencies
  - Jointly determined by $|k|$ and $|G(k)|^2$at relatively high frequencies

CT Spatial Resolution

Spatial resolution of a CT system can be estimated by imaging a point-like object and analyzing the *expected* CT signal of this object along each spatial dimension. Mathematically, a two-dimensional point-like object can be described as

$$\mu(x,y) = \mu_0\Delta x\Delta y\delta(x-x_0)\delta(y-y_0), \tag{6.32}$$

where μ_0 is the linear attenuation coefficient of the object material, and $\delta(x)$ and $\delta(y)$ are one-dimensional Dirac delta functions. As derived in Appendix II, the expected signal value of this point-like object in the attenuation image is given by

$$\langle\hat{\mu}(x,y)\rangle = \mu_0\Delta x\Delta y\, g(x-x_0,y-y_0), \tag{6.33}$$

where g denotes the reconstruction window function in the spatial domain. Based on the relationship between CT number and the attenuation coefficient in Eq. (6.33), the expected CT signal of this object is given by

$$\begin{aligned}
\langle f(x,y)\rangle &= \frac{\langle\hat{\mu}(x,y)\rangle-\mu_w}{\mu_w}\times 1000 \\
&= \frac{1000}{\mu_w}u_0\Delta x\Delta y\, g(x-x_0,y-y_0)-1000.
\end{aligned} \tag{6.34}$$

The calculation of PSF requires the "background" signal in the image to be removed, namely,

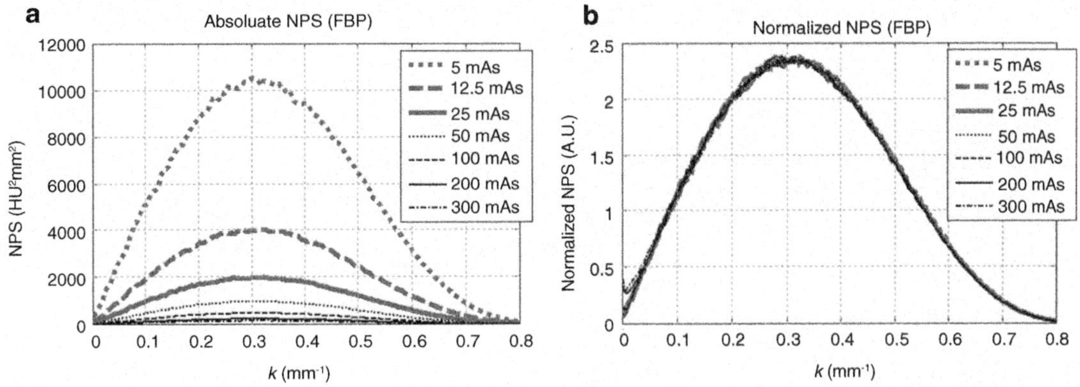

Fig. 6.4 Radial profiles of 2D NPS (**a**) and NNPS (**b**) of a FBP-based CT system measured at different mAs levels. The same reconstruction kernel was used throughout the measurements. The NPS magnitude increased with higher mAs. Once normalized, the NPS shape was independent of mAs. (Modified from [20], with permission)

$$\begin{aligned}\langle f(x,y)\rangle' &= \langle f(x,y)\rangle - \text{background}\\ &= \langle f(x,y)\rangle - \lim_{x\to\infty,y\to\infty}\langle f(x,y)\rangle\\ &= \langle f(x,y)\rangle - (-1000)\\ &= \frac{1000}{\mu_w}u_0\Delta x\Delta y\, g(x-x_0,y-y_0).\end{aligned} \tag{6.35}$$

The 2D point spread function (PSF) is given by normalizing $\langle f(x,y)\rangle'$ as follows:

$$\begin{aligned}\text{PSF}(x,y) &= \frac{\langle \hat{u}(x,y)\rangle}{\iint \langle \hat{u}(x,y)\rangle dxdy}\\ &= \frac{(1000/\mu_w)u_0\Delta x\Delta y g(x-x_0,y-y_0)}{(1000/\mu_w)u_0\Delta x\Delta y\iint g(x-x_0,y-y_0)dxdy}\\ &= \frac{g(x-x_0,y-y_0)}{\iint g(x-x_0,y-y_0)dxdy}.\end{aligned} \tag{6.36}$$

By convention, the window function g is a normalized function. Therefore, the denominator in (6.36) is unity, and this equation can be further simplified as

$$\text{PSF}(x,y) = g(x-x_0,y-y_0). \tag{6.37}$$

The optical transfer function (OTF) is related to PSF by

$$\begin{aligned}\text{OTF}(k_x,k_y) &= \text{FT}_{2\text{D}}\{\text{PSF}(x,y)\}\\ &= \int_{-\infty}^{+\infty}\int_{-\infty}^{+\infty} \text{d}x\text{d}y g(x-x_0,y-y_0)e^{-i2\pi(k_x x+k_y y)}.\end{aligned} \tag{6.38}$$

With a variable change of $x' = x - x_0$, $y' = y - y_0$, OTF in (6.38) becomes

$$\begin{aligned}\text{OTF}(k_x,k_y) &= \int_{-\infty}^{+\infty}\int_{-\infty}^{+\infty} \text{d}x'\text{d}y' g(x',y')e^{-i2\pi[k_x(x'+x_0)+k_y(y'+y_0)]}\\ &= e^{-i2\pi(k_x x_0+k_y y_0)}\int_{-\infty}^{+\infty}\int_{-\infty}^{+\infty} \text{d}x'\text{d}y' g(x',y')e^{-i2\pi(k_x x'+k_y y')}\\ &= e^{-i2\pi(k_x x_0+k_y y_0)}G(k).\end{aligned} \tag{6.39}$$

The modulation transfer function (MTF) is defined as the modulus of OTF, namely,

$$\begin{aligned}\mathrm{MTF}\left(k_x,k_y\right)&=\left|\mathrm{OTF}\left(k_x,k_y\right)\right|\\&=\left|e^{-i2\pi\left(k_x x_0+k_y y_0\right)}G\left(k\right)\right|\\&=\left|G\left(k\right)\right|.\end{aligned}\tag{6.40}$$

In summary, the MTF of an idealized linear CT system is equal to the window function $|G(k)|$ used in the FBP reconstruction. It is *independent* of:

- The ramp kernel $|k|$
- mAs [an example is provided in Fig. 6.5a]
- Attenuation coefficient or image contrast of the point-like object [an example is provided in Fig. 6.5b]
- Image background [because of the background removal step in Eq. (6.35)]

Properties of OTF are similar to those of MTF, except that the spatial location of the point-like object introduces a phase shift factor as shown in Eq. (6.39).

Strictly speaking, the estimation of CT spatial resolution requires a large number of repeated measurements to knock out the influence of noise in individual $f(x,y)$ through ensemble averaging. However, if SNR of $f(x,y)$ is high enough, the requirement for repeated measurement can be relaxed, since in the limit of $\mathrm{SNR}_f\to+\infty$, the PDF of $f(x,y)$ can be approximated by

$$\begin{aligned}\lim_{\mathrm{SNR}_f\to+\infty}p\left(f\,|\langle f\rangle\right)&\approx\lim_{\mathrm{SNR}_f\to+\infty}\frac{1}{\sqrt{2\pi\sigma_f^2}}e^{-\frac{(f-\langle f\rangle)^2}{2\sigma_f^2}}\\&=\lim_{\mathrm{SNR}_f\to+\infty}\frac{1}{\sqrt{2\pi\sigma_f^2}}e^{-\frac{1}{2}\left(\frac{f}{\sigma_f}-\mathrm{SNR}_f\right)^2}\\&=\delta\left(f-\langle f\rangle\right).\end{aligned}\tag{6.41}$$

In other words, in the limit of $\mathrm{SNR}_f\to+\infty$

$$\lim_{\mathrm{SNR}_f\to+\infty}f\left(x,y\right)=\left\langle f\left(x,y\right)\right\rangle.\tag{6.42}$$

Therefore, spatial resolution estimation can get away from repeated measurements if the SNR of the point-like object is high enough. In practice, this condition is usually met by (1) building the point-like object using highly x-ray attenuating material to boost image signal or (2) by scanning the object at a high mAs level to reduce image noise or using both (1) and (2). These measurement strategies are based on the assumption that spatial resolution of idealized CT system is independent of mAs and material attenuation level, which can justify the generalizability of MTF/PSF measured at high attenuation and mAs levels

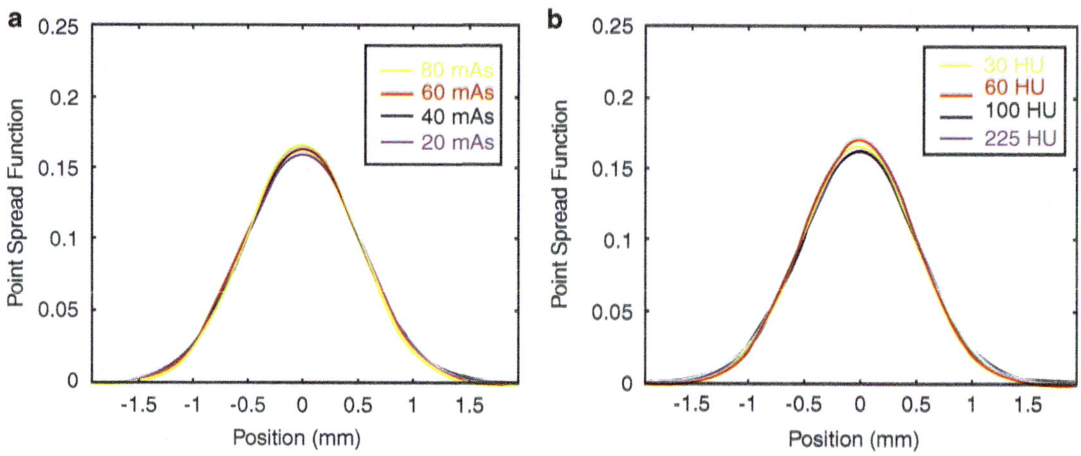

Fig. 6.5 (a) Radial profile of 2D PSFs of a CT system. (**a**) Measurements were performed at four mAs levels. (**b**) Measurements were performed with four materials of different attenuation levels

to other conditions with lower mAs and material attenuation levels. While the assumption is valid for idealized linear CT system, it may be severely violated in nonlinear systems as shown later in section "Nonlinear CT Systems with Model-Based Iterative Reconstruction". Correspondingly, alternative strategy needs to be employed when estimating CT spatial resolution performance.

CT Number Accuracy

CT number accuracy can be quantified by CT number bias, which is essentially the difference between the expected value of the measured CT number and the true CT number of the image object:

$$\text{Bias}(f) = \langle f \rangle - f_{\text{true}}, \tag{6.43}$$

where

$$f = \frac{\hat{\mu} - \mu_w}{\mu_w} \times 1000, \quad f_{\text{true}} = \frac{\mu - \mu_w}{\mu_w} \times 1000. \tag{6.44}$$

Based on (6.44), CT number bias is related to the estimated attenuation coefficient ($\hat{\mu}$) and true attenuation coefficient (μ) by

$$\begin{aligned} \text{Bias}(f) &= \frac{1000}{\mu_w}\left(\langle \hat{\mu} \rangle - \mu\right) \\ &= \frac{1000}{\mu_w}\text{Bias}(\hat{\mu}). \end{aligned} \tag{6.45}$$

As derived in detail in [38, 39], $\text{Bias}(\hat{\mu})$ is given by

$$\text{Bias}(\hat{\mu}) \approx \frac{e^{\mu D}}{\kappa D(mAs)}, \tag{6.46}$$

where $\kappa = 2a\bar{\varepsilon}\Delta\rho\Delta z$ is a numerical scaling factor. If a small "nodule" with a different attenuation coefficient of μ_1 is introduced to the uniform image background, bias of $\hat{\mu}_1$ can be approximated by [38]

$$\text{Bias}(\hat{\mu}_1) \approx \frac{e^{\mu D}}{\kappa D(mAs)}\left(1 + D\Delta\mu\right), \tag{6.47}$$

where $\Delta\mu$ is the difference between the nodule attenuation coefficient (μ_1) and background attenuation coefficient (μ). Based on Eqs. (6.45) and (6.47), CT number bias is provided by [38]

$$\begin{aligned} \text{Bias}(f_1) &= \frac{1000}{\mu_w}\text{Bias}(\hat{\mu}_1) \\ &\approx \frac{1000}{\mu_w}\frac{e^{\mu D}}{\kappa D(mAs)}\left(1 + D\Delta\mu\right) \\ &= \frac{\alpha}{mAs}\left(1 + \beta\Delta HU\right), \end{aligned} \tag{6.48}$$

where α and β are two scaling factors and ΔHU is the CT number contrast between the nodule and the background, namely,

$$\Delta HU = \frac{1000}{\mu_w}\Delta\mu. \tag{6.49}$$

Equation (6.48) states that CT number bias is inversely proportional to mAs; it is also linearly related to the contrast of material of interest: for a given CT system operated at a given mAs level, material with higher contrast tends to generate higher CT number bias. Experimental data that validated this quantitative relationship between CT number bias, mAs, and contrast can be found in Fig. 6.6.

Realistic Quasi-linear CT Systems

The toy model CT system used in section "Idealized Linear CT Systems" enabled key factors and mechanisms governing CT imaging performance to be identified. Building upon the toy model, this section will append other physical factors encountered in realistic CT systems to the image quality models presented in the previous section, leading to more comprehensive understanding of image quality properties of realistic CT systems.

Noise Properties of Realistic Systems

Impacts of Bowtie Filter and Patient Position

Surprisingly (or not), bowtie-shaped beam flattening filters commonly used in modern MDCT

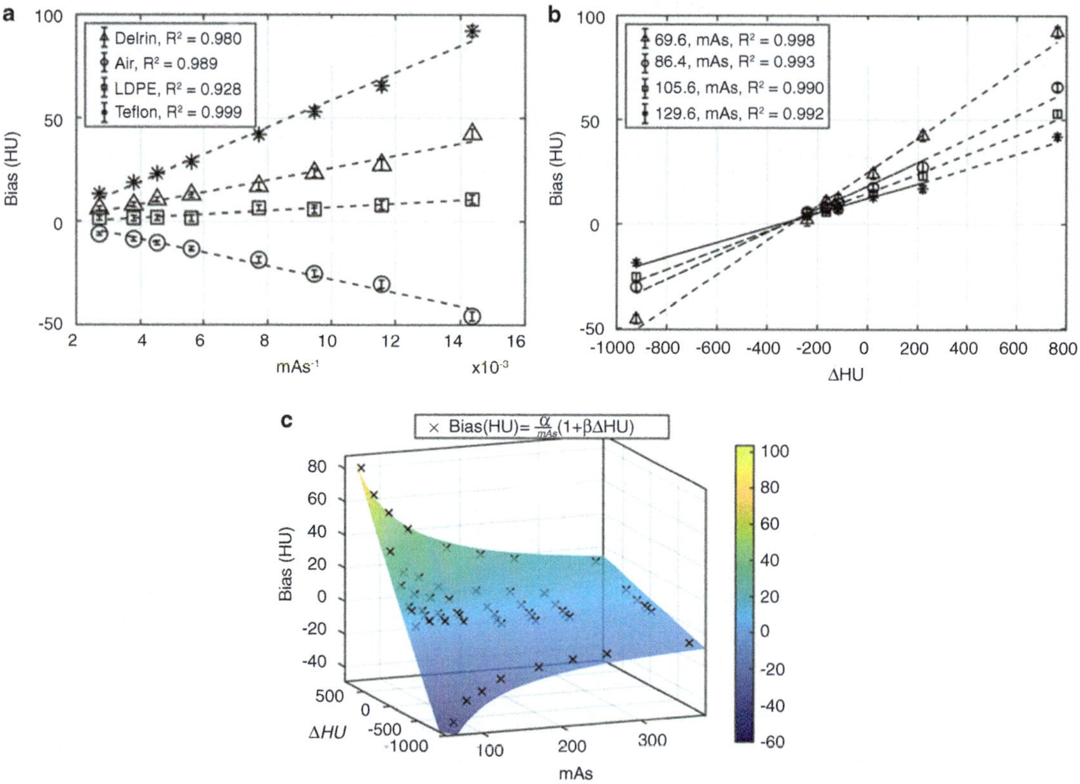

Fig. 6.6 Comparison of experimental and theoretical data of CT number bias. (**a**) Bias as a function of mAs^{-1}. (**b**) Bias as a function of CT number contrast (ΔHU). (**c**) Summary of the joint dependence of CT number bias on mAs and ΔHU. (Modified from [38], with permission)

systems exert considerable influence on CT noise performance [40]. As shown in Fig. 6.7, depending on the bowtie filter size, object position, and location within an image object, the topography of the 2D NPS may deviate from the well-known "*s*" symmetry and demonstrate a "*p*" symmetry or even a "*d*" symmetry that looks like a clover leaf [40].

To help pinpoint the impacts of a bowtie filter on CT noise performance, let's first analyze its impact on the projection data. Let $P_{\text{bf}}(\rho)$ denote the attenuation profile (i.e., radiological path length) of the bowtie filter projected on to a detector pixel located at ρ. Compared with the native x-ray flux $\langle n_0 \rangle$ in the absence of the bowtie filter, the post-bowtie flux is given by

$$\langle n_0 \rangle' = \langle n_0 \rangle \mathrm{e}^{-P_{\text{bf}}(\rho)}. \tag{6.50}$$

When the bowtie filter was designed, the goal was to flatten the post-object flux when imaging a reference cylindrical image object, namely,

$$\langle n_0 \rangle e^{-P_{\text{bf}}(\rho)} \mathrm{e}^{-P_{\text{ref}}(\rho,\theta)} = \text{constant}. \tag{6.51}$$

Note that P_{ref} is independent of projection angle θ since the reference object is assumed to be rotationally invariant and positioned at the isocenter of the CT gantry. The condition in Eq. (6.51) requires

$$P_{\text{bf}}(\rho) + P_{\text{ref}}(\rho) = P_0, \tag{6.52}$$

where P_0 is constant across the detector plane.

When the reference object is replaced by a patient with attenuation profile of $P(\rho,\theta)$, the post-patient flux is given by

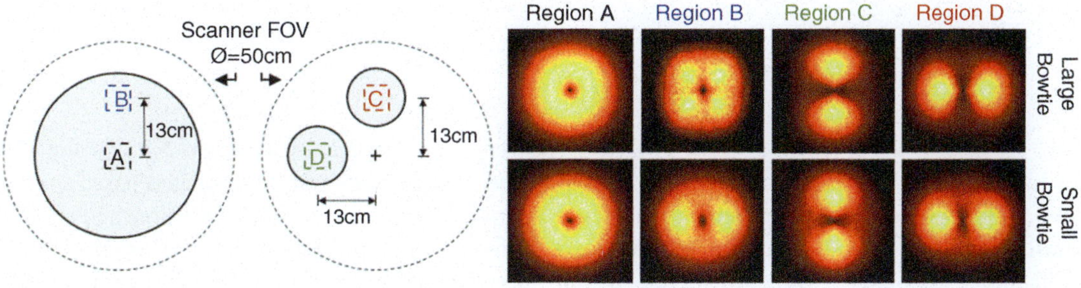

Fig. 6.7 Impacts of bowtie filter and spatial location on 2D CT NPS. NPS of a diagnostic MDCT system was experimentally measured at four locations: Region A is a 5×5 cm^2 area at the center of a 39-cm-diameter cylinder positioned at the isocenter of the scanner. Region B was 13 cm above Region A in the same object. Region C is a centered region in a vertically off-centered object; Region D is a centered region in a laterally off-centered object. For each of the four regions, the 2D NPS was measured with two different bowtie filters: one designed to compensate the attenuation of large adult body and the other one for small adult body. (Modified from [40], with permission)

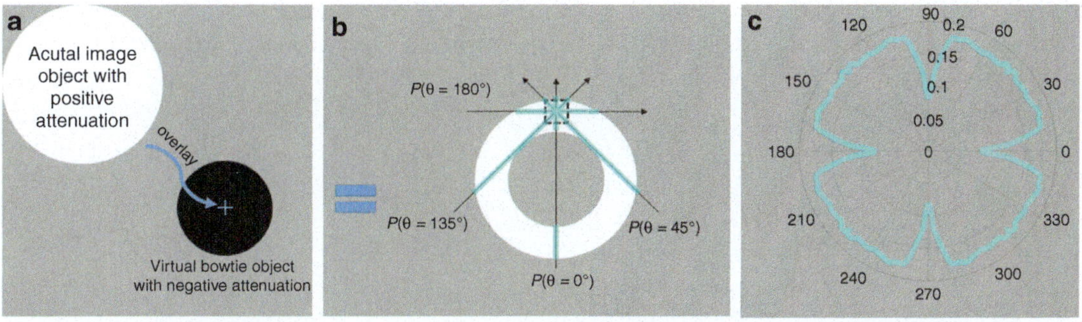

Fig. 6.8 (**a**) For the purpose of noise analysis, when a CT system with a bowtie filter images a patient, it can be considered a bowtie-free system that images a combination of a virtual "negative" object and the patient. Since the virtual object has a negative attenuation coefficient, the central region of the composited object is empty due to the cancellation of positive and negative attenuations. As shown in (**b**), x-rays intercepting a peripheral region in the composite object may have radiological path length that is strongly θ-dependent. In this particular case, the path length reaches its minimum at $\theta = 0$ and 90° and demonstrates a "d" symmetry. (**c**) Plot of the radiological path length of this region as a function of θ

$$\begin{aligned}\left\langle n_0''(\rho,\theta)\right\rangle &= \left\langle n_0'(\rho)\right\rangle \mathrm{e}^{-P(\rho,\theta)} \\ &= \left\langle n_0\right\rangle \mathrm{e}^{-P_{\mathrm{bf}}(\rho)-P(\rho,\theta)} \\ &= \left\langle n_0\right\rangle \mathrm{e}^{-P_0}\,\mathrm{e}^{-\left[P(\rho,\theta)-P_{\mathrm{ref}}(\rho)\right]}.\end{aligned} \tag{6.53}$$

Correspondingly, the expected detector output is given by

$$\begin{aligned}\left\langle N(\rho,\theta)\right\rangle &= \left\langle n_0''\right\rangle \Delta t\varepsilon\Delta z\Delta\rho \\ &= \left(\left\langle n_0\right\rangle \mathrm{e}^{-P_0}\Delta t\varepsilon\Delta z\Delta\rho\right)\mathrm{e}^{-\left[P(\rho,\theta)-P_{\mathrm{ref}}(\rho)\right]}.\end{aligned} \tag{6.54}$$

A comparison between Eq. (6.54) and Equation (6.2) suggests that, for the sake of noise analysis, the bowtie filter can be considered as a virtual image object placed at the isocenter with a negative attenuation profile of $-P_{\mathrm{ref}}(\rho)$ (Fig. 6.8). This virtual object is cylindrical in shape since $-P_{\mathrm{ref}}(\rho)$ is independent of θ. Overall speaking, the image object can be considered as a superposition of the bowtie-induced virtual object and the actual patient, having an attenuation profile of $P(\rho,\theta) - P_{\mathrm{ref}}(\rho)$.

The introduction of the virtual object concept can facilitate the discussion on the impacts of bowtie filter and patient position on CT NPS. For example, if the patient has an identical attenuation profile as the reference object used for designing the bowtie filter and if the patient is centered at the isocenter,

$$\langle N(\rho,\theta)\rangle = \langle n_0\rangle e^{-P_0}\Delta t\varepsilon\Delta z\Delta\rho e^{-[P_{ref}(\rho)-P_{ref}(\rho)]} = \langle n_0\rangle e^{-P_0}\Delta t\varepsilon\Delta z\Delta\rho. \quad (6.55)$$

In this case, the expected detector output $\langle N\rangle$ is independent of ρ and θ, which makes the uniform noise assumption in section "Idealized Linear CT Systems" valid. However, if the patient attenuation profile is different from $P_{ref}(\rho)$ or if the patient is off-centered, $\langle N\rangle$ may become ρ- and θ-dependent. If CT auto-covariance C_f is defined within a local region-of-interest whose projection corresponds to a finite area in the detector plane, the ρ-dependence of $\langle N\rangle$ is generally much weaker than the θ-dependence. Consequentially, term $\langle N\rangle$ in the C_f formula in Eq. (6.27) needs to be replaced by $\langle N(\theta)\rangle$, and the corresponding CT NPS formula is given by

$$\mathrm{NPS}_f^L(k,\theta) = \left(\frac{1000}{\mu_w}\right)^2 \frac{\sigma_N^2(\theta)\Delta\rho\Delta\theta|k||G(k)|^2}{\langle N(\theta)\rangle^2}, \quad (6.56)$$

where NPS_f^L denotes the **local** NPS of the CT image and $\langle N(\theta)\rangle$ can be estimated based on the virtual bowtie object, patient position, and attenuation profile using Eq. (6.54). The concept of the virtual bowtie object could greatly facilitate the understanding of how a bowtie filter influences local CT NPS. An example is provided in Fig. 6.8.

Impacts of Polychromatic Source and Energy-Integrating Detector

Unlike the idealized photon counting and monoenergetic CT system used in section "Idealized Linear CT Systems", the majority of realistic CT systems use energy-integrating detectors and polychromatic x-ray sources. For these systems, the expected number of detector output is given by

$$\langle N(\rho,\theta)\rangle = \langle n_0\rangle \Delta z\Delta\rho\Delta t \int_0^{E_{max}} dE\,\Omega(\rho,E)\varepsilon(E)g(E)e^{-P(\rho,\theta,E)} \quad (6.57)$$

$$= \langle n_0\rangle \Delta z\Delta\rho\Delta t\varepsilon(\xi)g(\xi)e^{-P(\rho,\theta,\bar{E})}, \quad (6.58)$$

where $\Omega(\rho, E)$ denotes the channel-dependent normalized x-ray spectrum that includes the contribution of the bowtie filter, $g(E)$denotes the expected energy weighting factor, and ξ is an energy level within the range of (0, E_{max}). In simplifying Eqs. (6.57 and 6.58), we used the mean value theorem in calculus. With energy integration, the PDF of detector output $N(\rho,\theta)$ no longer follows the Poisson distribution. Instead, a previous study showed that the PDF of $\langle N(\rho,\theta)\rangle$ is a compound Poisson distribution function [41]. Correspondingly, the noise variance of $N(\rho,\theta)$ can be modeled as [42, 43].

$$\sigma_N^2(\rho,\theta) \approx \langle n_0\rangle \Delta z\Delta\rho\Delta t \int_0^{E_{max}} dE\,\Omega(E,\rho)\varepsilon(E)[g(E)]^2 e^{-P(\rho,\theta,E)}, \approx \langle n_0\rangle \Delta z\Delta\rho\Delta t\varepsilon(\xi)[g(\xi)]^2 e^{-P(\rho,\theta,\bar{E})}. \quad (6.59)$$

Based on Eqs. (6.58) and (6.59), σ_N^2 is proportional to$\langle N\rangle$, namely,

$$\sigma_N^2(\rho,\theta) \approx \kappa\langle N(\rho,\theta)\rangle, \quad (6.60)$$

where κ is a scaling factor. In addition to quantum noise, due to electronic noise introduced by the detector readout system, the compound Poisson PDF in [41] needs to be further convolved with the PDF of the electronic noise, resulting in an additional term in the expression of σ_N^2:

$$\sigma_N^2(\rho,\theta) \approx \kappa\langle N(\rho,\theta)\rangle + \sigma_e^2. \quad (6.61)$$

With this detector noise model, the local CT NPS formula in Eq. (6.56) needs to be further revised as

$$\begin{aligned} \mathrm{NPS}_f^L(k,\theta) &= \left(\frac{1000}{\mu_w}\right)^2 \Delta\rho\Delta\theta \frac{\left[\kappa\langle N(\theta)\rangle + \sigma_e^2\right]|k||G(k)|^2}{N(\theta)^2} \\ &= \left(\frac{1000}{\mu_w}\right)^2 \frac{\Delta\rho\Delta\theta}{\langle N(\theta)\rangle}\left[\kappa + \frac{\sigma_e^2}{\langle N(\theta)\rangle}\right]|k||G(k)|^2. \end{aligned} \quad (6.62)$$

Based on Eq. (6.62), when the CT system is operated at lower mAs, the magnitude of $\langle N\rangle$ decreases, which may increase the contribution of electronic noise σ_e^2 to the CT noise. Therefore, an important technical requirement for ultralow-dose CT imaging is to control or suppress electronic noise [44].

Impacts of Discrete Sampling

The discussion of idealized CT systems in section "Idealized Linear CT Systems" does not take the influence of discrete samplings into consideration. In realistic CT systems, sampling operations are present at multiple stages in the imaging chain, including samplings along ρ introduced by the discrete detector elements, along θ introduced by the finite detector readout rate, and along (x,y) introduced by the discrete representation of the reconstructed CT image. Take the sampling in the (x,y) domain as an example: because the acquired projection data is a discrete array of data instead of a continuous function of $R(\rho,\theta)$ and because the to-be-reconstructed CT image is a discrete grid of data points instead of a continuous function $f(x,y)$, the backprojection process usually involves a data interpolation process. If the backprojection is pixel-driven, the interpolation can be described by a 1D convolution of the filtered projection data with a interpolation kernel $g_{\mathrm{int}}(\rho)$; if the backprojection is ray-driven, the interpolation can be described by a 2D convolution of $f(x,y)$ with a 2D kernel $g_{\mathrm{int}}(x,y)$. Correspondingly, the CT NPS formula in Eq. (6.62) needs to be further modified to [37, 45]

$$\mathrm{NPS}_f^L(k,\theta) = \left(\frac{1000}{\mu_w}\right)^2 \Delta\rho\Delta\theta\left[\frac{\kappa}{\langle N(\theta)\rangle} + \frac{\sigma_e^2}{\langle N(\theta)\rangle^2}\right]|k||G(k)|^2|G_{\mathrm{int}}(k)|^2. \quad (6.63)$$

In addition to data interpolation, spatial and angular samplings involved in the data acquisition and reconstruction process may also lead to noise aliasing. As a result, the autocovariance of the projection data (C_R) shown in Eq. (6.11) needs to be revised by multiplying a 2D comb function $\Delta\rho\mathrm{comb}(\rho/\Delta\rho) \cdot \Delta\theta\mathrm{comb}(\theta/\Delta\theta)$. Consequently, noise in the projection data may be aliased along both ρ and θ directions. To reduce noise aliasing along these two directions, x-ray focal spot wobbling/deflection/flying techniques and detectors with a faster sampling rate [46–52] have been applied to increase the actual or effective sampling rate along ρ and θ.

Similarly, 2D sampling in the CT image domain replicates the NPS along k_x and k_y as follows [37, 53]:

$$\mathrm{NPS}_f^{L,S}\left(k_x,k_y\right)=\sum_{m=-\infty}^{\infty}\sum_{n=-\infty}^{\infty}\mathrm{NPS}_f^{L}\left(k_x-\frac{n}{\Delta x},k_y-\frac{n}{\Delta y}\right)$$
$$=\mathrm{NPS}_f^{L}\left(k_x,k_y\right)\otimes\mathrm{comb}\left(\Delta x\,k_x\right)\otimes\mathrm{comb}\left(\Delta y\,k_y\right). \tag{6.64}$$

Letter "S" in $\mathrm{NPS}_f^{L,S}$ denotes "sampling." As shown in Eq. (6.64), replications of the presampled NPS are along two orthogonal directions (k_x and k_y). Therefore, the radial symmetry of the 2D NPS for idealized CT system indicated in Eq. (6.29) may break down due to image domain sampling. In addition, the distance between two replicas in the frequency space is proportional to the reciprocals of Δx and Δy. When Δx and Δy are too large, severe overlap between neighboring replicas of NPS_f^{L} may lead to a strong noise aliasing effect, which destroys the rotational symmetry of the CT NPS. To illustrate this point, an example is provided in Fig. 6.9.

Other Considerations

In realistic CT detector systems, stochastic spatial spreading of secondary quanta [54], finite apertures of the photodiodes [55], detector lag [56–58], residue-scattering signal passing through the anti-scatter grid [59, 60], and low-signal correction algorithms [61, 62] often introduce certain noise correlation along both the ρ and θ directions, resulting in violations of the white noise assumption made behind Eq. (6.8). Correspondingly, the CT NPS formula in Eq. (6.63) needs to be further revised to [45, 63]

$$\mathrm{NPS}_f^{L}\left(k,\theta\right)=\left(\frac{1000}{\mu_w}\right)^2\frac{\tilde{C}_R\left(k,\theta\right)}{\left\langle N\left(\theta\right)\right\rangle^2}\left|k\right|\left|G\left(k\right)\right|^2\left|G_{\mathrm{int}}\left(k\right)\right|^2, \tag{6.65}$$

where $\tilde{C}_R\left(k,\theta\right)$ denotes the 1D Fourier transform of the general form of the projection autocovariance function C_R.

Different from the parallel beam geometry used by the idealized systems, realistic CT systems have fan-beam or cone-beam geometries, and the associated parallel beam and divergent beam reconstruction algorithms may further alter the NPS model derived based on idealized parallel beam systems. As an example, Figure 6.10 shows NPS of CT images of a uniform cylindrical object placed at the isocenter of an experimental CT system. Based on models presented in the previous sections, the NPS of this object should be rotationally invariant. However, when a fan-beam reconstruction algorithm with a Parker weighting [64] was applied, the 2D NPS inherited the θ-dependence of the Parker weighting. This example suggests that NPS models of realistic system may also need to consider differences between parallel and divergent beam reconstruction algorithms. The corresponding analysis and modeling can be found in [65, 66].

Spatial Resolution Properties of Realistic Systems

The spatial resolution model derived for idealized systems in Equations (6.32)–(6.40) assumed an array of pencil beam sources and ideal CT detector systems that do not introduce spatial resolution loss. In realistic systems, the finite focal spot size, finite detector aperture, and stochastic spreading of primary x-ray photons and secondary optical photons in the scintillator modify the projection signal of a point-like object originally presented in Eq. (6.106) of Appendix III as follows:

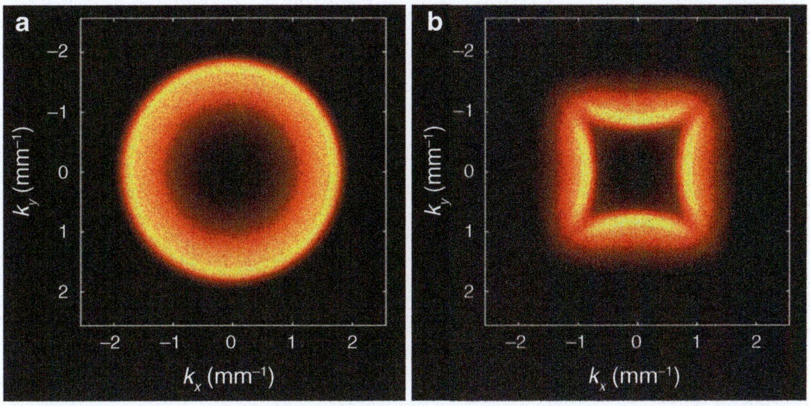

Fig. 6.9 2D CT NPS of a cylindrical and uniform object placed at the isocenter of a diagnostic MDCT system (GE Discovery CT750 HD). A high-definition edge-enhancing reconstruction kernel (HD Edge) provided by the system was selected for image reconstruction. NPS in (**a**) was measured using images with a reconstruction pixel size ($\Delta x \times \Delta y$) of 0.2×0.2 mm. NPS in (**b**) was measured using images with a reconstruction pixel size of 0.4×0.4 mm. (According to Eq. (6.64), larger Δx corresponded to stronger noise aliasing, which led to an NPS in (**b**) that is no longer rotational invariant)

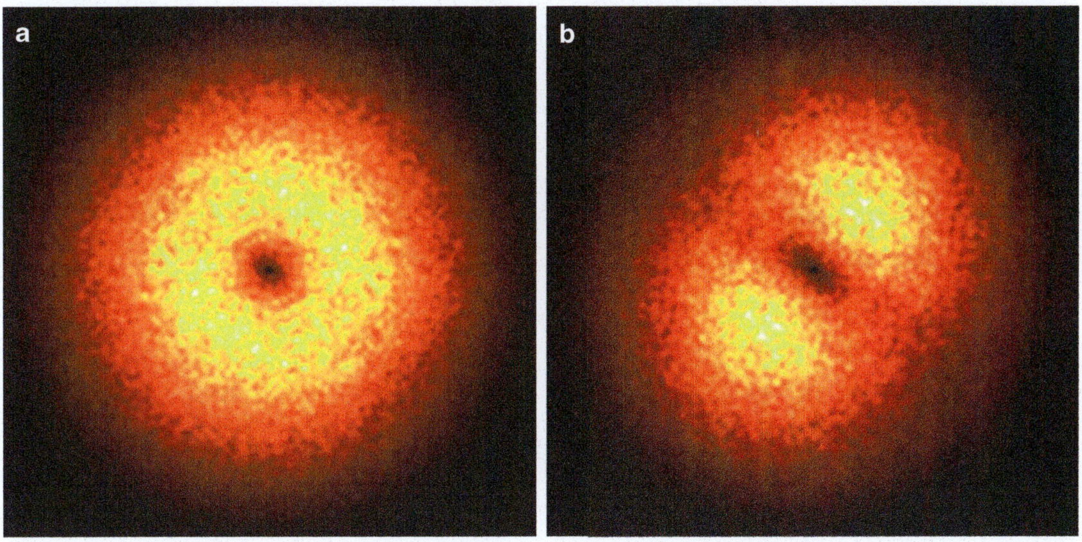

Fig. 6.10 2D CT NPS of a cylindrical and uniform object place at the isocenter of an experimental system. (**a**) NPS of images reconstructed with equal angular weighting. (**b**) NPS of images reconstructed with the Parker weighting. (Figure courtesy of Dr. John Hayes)

$$\begin{aligned}\langle R'(\rho,\theta)\rangle &= \langle R(\rho,\theta)\rangle \otimes g_{\mathrm{FS}}(\rho) \otimes g_{\mathrm{SS}}(\rho) \otimes g_{\mathrm{Aper}}(\rho) \\ &= u_0 \Delta x \Delta y \delta(\rho - x_0 \cos\theta - y_0 \sin\theta) \otimes g_{\mathrm{FS}}(\rho) \otimes g_{\mathrm{SS}}(\rho) \otimes g_{\mathrm{Aper}}(\rho) \\ &= u_0 \Delta x \Delta y \left[g_{\mathrm{FS}}(\rho) \otimes g_{\mathrm{SS}}(\rho) \otimes g_{\mathrm{Aper}}(\rho) \right]_{\rho = x_0 \cos\theta - y_0 \sin\theta},\end{aligned} \tag{6.66}$$

where g_{FS}, g_{ss}, and g_{Aper} denote signal transfer functions introduced by the x-ray focal spot, spatial spreading of secondary quanta, and finite aperture of each detector cell, respectively.

Using similar deviations as those in Appendix III, it can be shown that the expected CT image signal of the point object reconstructed from projection data R' in Eq. (6.66) is given by

$$\begin{aligned}\left\langle \hat{u}'(x,y)\right\rangle &= u_0 \Delta x \Delta y \int_{-\infty}^{+\infty}\int_{-\infty}^{+\infty} \mathrm{d}k_x \mathrm{d}k_y G_{\mathrm{FS}}(k) G_{\mathrm{SS}}(k) G_{\mathrm{Aper}}(k) G(k) \mathrm{e}^{\mathrm{i}2\pi\left[k_x(x-x_0)+k_y(y-y_0)\right]} \\ &= u_0 \Delta x \Delta y \, \mathrm{IFT}_{2\mathrm{D}}\left\{G_{\mathrm{FS}}(k) G_{\mathrm{SS}}(k) G_{\mathrm{Aper}}(k) G(k)\right\},\end{aligned} \tag{6.67}$$

where G_{FS}, G_{ss}, and G_{Aper} denote the Fourier pairs of g_{FS}, g_{ss}, and g_{Aper}, respectively. By definition, the 2D CT MTF that corresponds to the CT signal in Eq. (6.67) is

$$\mathrm{MTF}(k) = G_{\mathrm{FS}}(k) G_{\mathrm{SS}}(k) G_{\mathrm{Aper}}(k) G(k). \tag{6.68}$$

Up until Eq. (6.68), analysis of CT spatial resolution properties assumed a parallel beam geometry. In realistic systems predominantly of divergent beam geometries, *if the point-like object is positioned at the isocenter*, the influence of geometric magnification m can be incorporated as [67]

$$\mathrm{MTF}(k) = G_{\mathrm{FS}}\left((m-1)k/m\right) G_{\mathrm{SS}}(k/m) G_{\mathrm{Aper}}(k/m) G(k). \tag{6.69}$$

Similar to the case of CT NPS, the use of interpolation introduces an additional transfer function G_{int} to the CT MTF as

$$\mathrm{MTF}(k) = G_{\mathrm{FS}}\left((m-1)k/m\right) G_{\mathrm{SS}}(k/m) G_{\mathrm{Aper}}(k/m) G(k) G_{\mathrm{int}}(k). \tag{6.70}$$

At positions away from the isocenter, change in the projected focal spot along the detector plane and influence of the continuous gantry motion need to be considered. The first factor impacts spatial resolution along the radial direction [34, 68], while the second factor contributes to spatial resolution degradation along the tangential direction. As discussed in [34, 69], the continuous focal spot and detector rotation introduces tangential blurring at spatial locations away from the isocenter. Consequentially, spatial resolution accessed at off-centered locations is generally inferior to that of the isocenter (Fig. 6.11). To mitigate spatial resolution degradation loss at off-centered locations, techniques have been developed to reduce the detector integration time per view angle and therefore the motion of the gantry as seen by an object at off-centered locations [51].

Other considerations when modeling spatial resolution of realistic CT systems include patient scattering, beam hardening, image display field of view and matrix size, helical pitch (influencing spatial resolution along the z direction), focal spot blooming, etc. [69]. Contribution of scattered x-ray photons to CT spatial resolution has been empirically modeled as [67]

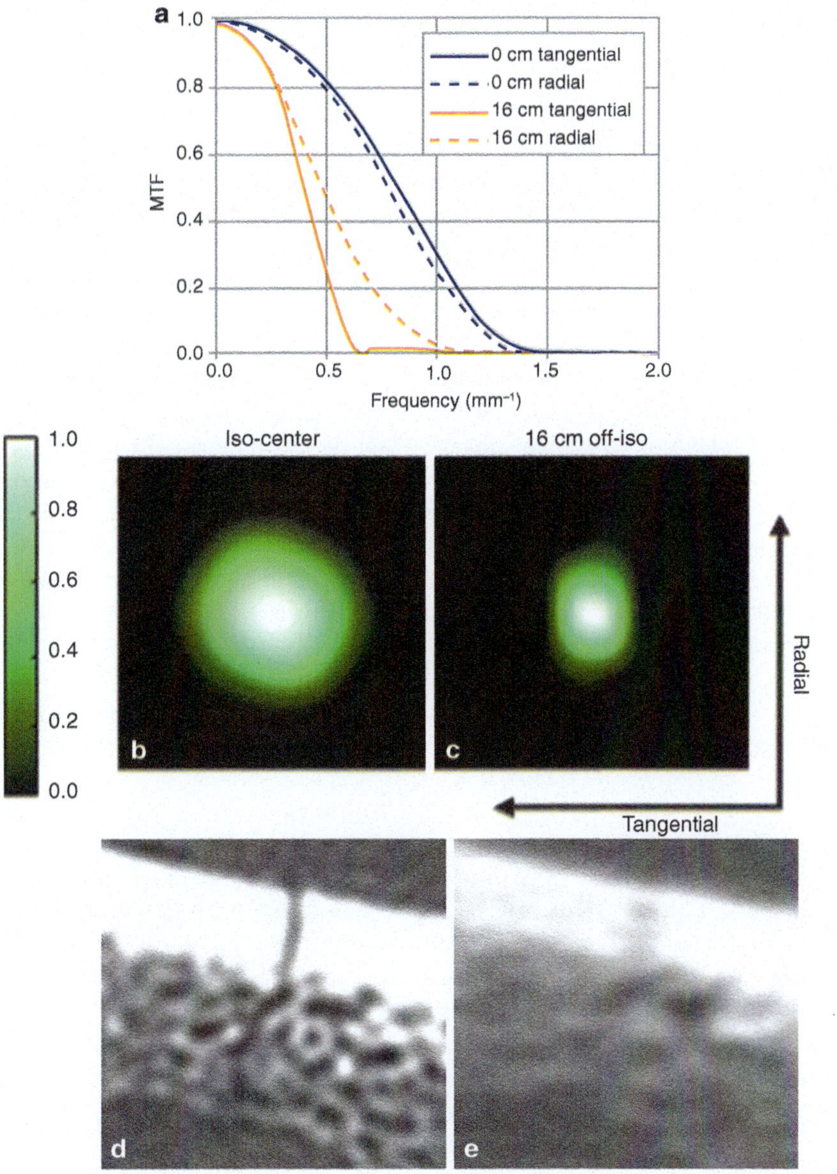

Fig. 6.11 Location and orientation dependence of CT MTF for a realistic diagnostic MDCT system (GE Discovery CT750 HD). (**a**) Line profiles of 2D MTF along radial and tangential directions measured at isocenter (0 cm) and 16 cm off isocenter. (**b**, **c**) Comparison of 2D MTF measured at isocenter and 16 cm off isocenter. The MTF at iso is much more isotropic compared with the off-centered MTF, which suffered much stronger resolution loss along the tangential direction compared than along the radial direction. (**d**, **e**) Example CT images of a bone fracture model acquired at the two locations. (Modified from [51], with permission)

$$\mathrm{MTF}(k)=(1-\mathrm{SF})G_{\mathrm{FS}}((m-1)k/m)+\mathrm{SF}\,G_{\mathrm{Scatter}}(k/m)G_{\mathrm{SS}}(k/m)G_{\mathrm{Aper}}(k/m)G(k)G_{\mathrm{int}}(k),\quad(6.71)$$

where G_{Scatter} denotes an empirical kernel that takes into account spatial resolution loss induced by scattering, and SF denotes the scatter fraction as seen by the detector. Based on the empirical model in Eq. (6.71), CT spatial resolution may have certain dependence on the image object and x-ray energy through terms G_{Scatter} and SF. Similarly, the measured MTF may also slightly depend on the attenuation level of the point-like object because of (1) scattering and (2) beam hardening, both of which may change the shape of the measured PSF [see Fig. 6.5b as an example]. Finally, the actual focal spot size may vary with tube current (mA) and tube potential (kV), making the measured PSF and MTF slightly dependent on these scan parameters (see Fig. 6.5a as an example).

Summary of Realistic Quasi-linear CT Systems

This section highlighted key differences between realistic FBP-based CT systems and idealized CT systems in terms of noise and spatial resolution characteristics. The section also provides examples on how spatial resolution and noise models of idealized systems can be revised so that they embrace realistic systems. As a matter of fact, all of the data and figures shown in section "Idealized Linear CT Systems" on idealized systems were generated from realistic CT systems, indicating that many models such as the inverse scaling law between mAs and CT noise variance are directly applicable under certain conditions. These conditions include no or minor off-centering for the image object and region-of-interest, moderately high-tube current to reduce the influence of electronic noise, relatively small reconstruction field of view to reduce the impact of aliasing, etc. Because these conditions are widely met in routine CT image quality assessments, differences between idealized and realistic systems are often neglected (and even totally forgotten).

Because a major component of the imaging chain—the tomographic reconstruction algorithm—is linear and because of the applicability of linear systems theory in the "routine" conditions, conventional CT systems are often referred to as quasi-linear CT systems. However, as the term "quasi" suggests, a quasi-linear system is not perfectly linear, nor is linear system theory perfectly applicable. Caution needs to be taken when estimating CT image quality under conditions deviating from routine conditions: the NPS and MTF at off-centered positions epitomize the breakdown of idealized system models.

Nonlinear CT Systems with Model-Based Iterative Reconstruction

This section will use one of several commercialized versions of MBIR (Veo, GE Healthcare) installed in a diagnostic MDCT system (Discovery CT750 HD, GE Healthcare) to demonstrate how linear CT systems models can be severely violated. Unlike quasi-linear CT systems for which replenishments of ideal linear system theory would suffice in providing much needed quantitative relationships between image quality metrics and system parameters, the nonlinear nature of the MBIR algorithm fundamentally rejects the applicability of linear systems theory. In addition, nonstationary signal and noise properties of MBIR reported in literature raised concern about whether several Fourier-domain image quality metrics such as NPS can still be well defined. This section will provide scientific argument to address this concern, and it will also present several strategies to estimate signal and noise characteristics of the MBIR system without resorting to linear systems models shown in the previous two sections.

Challenges Introduced by MBIR

Unconventional Noise Characteristics

As shown in Fig. 6.12, a noise-only MBIR image demonstrated a peculiar pattern: the noise magnitude elevated abruptly at locations corresponding to high-contrast gradients (e.g., the jelly bean-air interface). This local noise nonstationarity is fundamentally different from the location dependence of noise performance discussed in section "Realistic Quasi-linear CT Systems" on conventional CT systems, where noise may not be uniform across the entire field of view but is quasi-stationary within a finite local region. The corresponding example can be found in the FBP noise-only image shown in Fig. 6.12. The strong nonstationarity of noise magnitude in MBIR images is unexpected according to linear systems models of conventional CT scanners.

Note that it is important to recognize the difference between the concepts of noise stationarity (defined across pixels) and noise uniformity (defined across different regions). Although MBIR introduces noise nonstationarity, globally speaking, noise performance of different local regions in an object can be quite similar in MBIR images. As shown by an example in Fig. 6.13, the MBIR NPS measured at five different local regions in a water tank were more or less the same in terms of both magnitude and shape. In comparison, the magnitude of the FBP NPS measured at the center (Region C) of the water tank

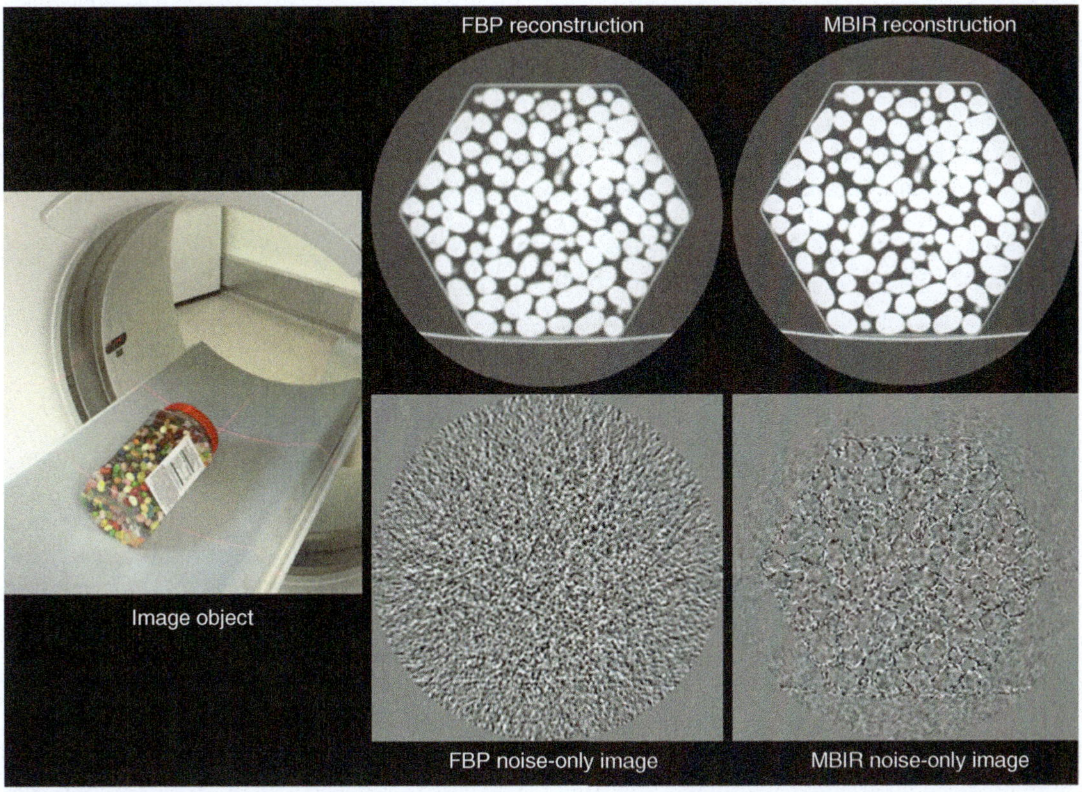

Fig. 6.12 To showcase a difference in noise characteristics between FBP and MBIR, two back-to-back CT scans of a jar of jelly beans were performed, and two reconstruction algorithms (FBP with Standard kernel vs. MBIR) were applied to each set of scan data. By subtracting CT images generated from the back-to-back scans, noise-only images were generated for each algorithm. Compared with the relatively stationary FBP noise pattern, the MBIR noise-only image showed strong noise nonstationarity: the noise magnitude elevated at spatial locations corresponding to large contrast gradients (e.g., edge of each jelly bean)

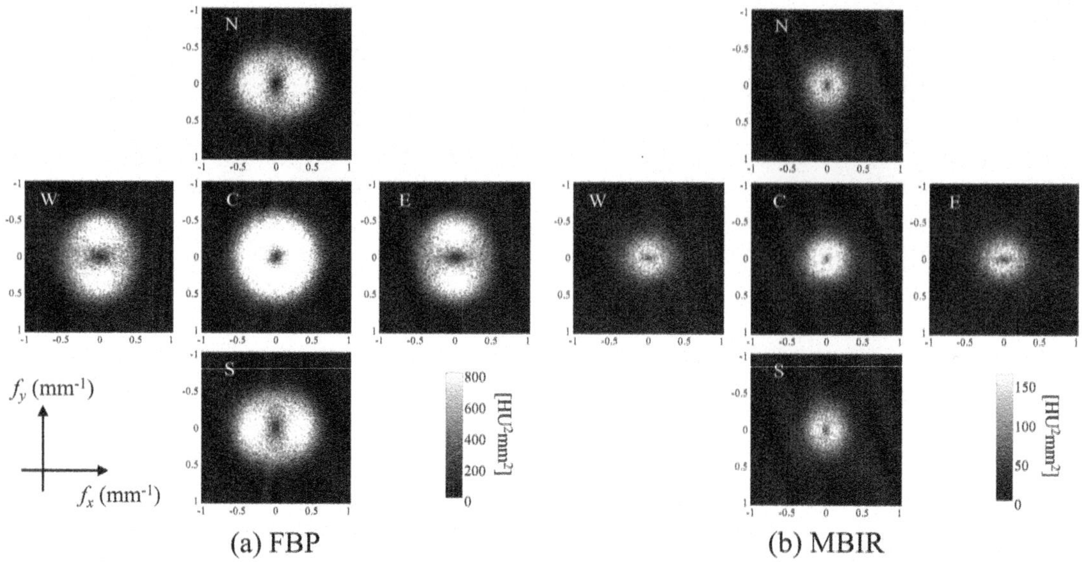

Fig. 6.13 NPS measured locally in five 4×4 cm^2 regions in a uniform water cylinder. Locations of the five regions (denoted by C, N, E, S, W, respectively) are illustrated in Fig. 6.2 of Reference [20]. (Modified from [20], with permission)

was visibly higher than those measured at four peripheral regions. In addition, FBP NPS at these four regions are not radially symmetric due to the reason described in section "Impacts of Bowtie Filter and Patient Position". In contrast, all of the MBIR NPS were quite isotropic, which is another unexpected behavior.

To further demonstrate the violation of linear systems theory in MBIR, three sets of CT images were acquired at 120 kV and the following mAs levels: 100, 200, and 300. Under these conditions, the effect of electronic noise can be considered negligible, and based on Eq. (6.29), NPS of the three image sets should be related by

$$100\cdot \mathrm{NPS}_{100\,\mathrm{mAs}} = 200\cdot \mathrm{NPS}_{200\,\mathrm{mAs}} = 300\cdot \mathrm{NPS}_{300\,\mathrm{mAs}}. \tag{6.72}$$

If we generate a composite image f_{comp} from 100 to 200 mAs images as follows

$$f_{\mathrm{comp}} = \frac{100}{100+200} f_{100\,\mathrm{mAs}} + \frac{200}{100+200} f_{200\,\mathrm{mAs}} = \frac{1}{3} f_{100\,\mathrm{mAs}} + \frac{2}{3} f_{200\,\mathrm{mAs}}, \tag{6.73}$$

Based on Eq. (6.72), NPS of this composite image should be

$$\begin{aligned}\mathrm{NPS}_{\mathrm{comp}} &= \left(\frac{1}{3}\right)^2 \mathrm{NPS}_{100\,\mathrm{mAs}} + \left(\frac{2}{3}\right)^2 \mathrm{NPS}_{200\,\mathrm{mAs}} \\ &= \left(\frac{1}{3}\right)^2 \frac{300}{100}\mathrm{NPS}_{300\,\mathrm{mAs}} + \left(\frac{2}{3}\right)^2 \frac{300}{100}\mathrm{NPS}_{300\,\mathrm{mAs}} \\ &= \mathrm{NPS}_{300\,\mathrm{mAs}}.\end{aligned} \tag{6.74}$$

In other words, if the linear CT systems model is valid, NPS of the composite CT image should equal that of the 300 mAs image. As shown in Fig. 6.14, the NPS equality in Eq. (6.74) was indeed valid for FBP images, but it was no longer the case for MBIR-based results: not only was the NPS magnitude of the composite MBIR image lower than that of the 300 mAs MBIR image but also the NPS peak shifted toward lower-spatial frequency. This observation suggested that noise of MBIR-based CT systems has unconventional dependence on mAs levels.

Noise of MBIR images also demonstrated very weak dependence on slice thickness (Δz), which is unexpected according to the linear systems model in Eq. (6.21). As shown in Fig. 6.15, slice thicknesses of 0.625 mm and 5.0 mm generated quite similar noise-only MBIR images. In contrast, FBP images demonstrated the expected noise-Δz dependence, as the 0.625 mm image was visibly noisier than the 5.0 mm image.

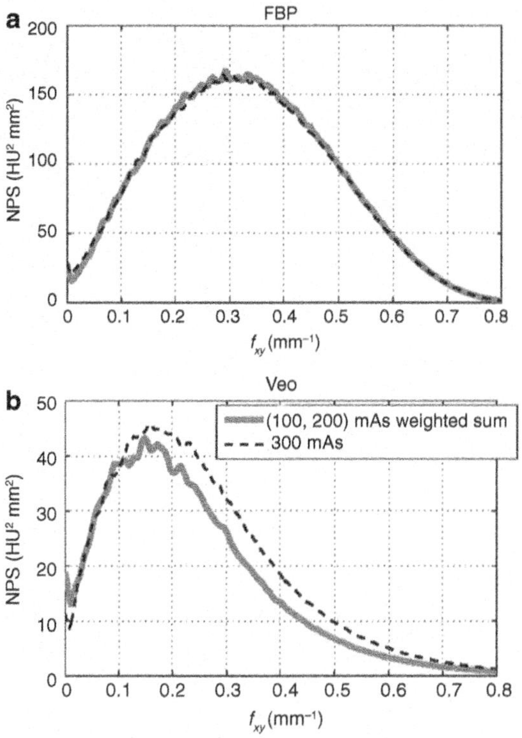

Fig. 6.14 NPS of a composite image described in Eq. (6.73) and a 300 mAs image reconstructed by FBP (**a**) and MBIR (**b**). The legend applies to both (**a**, **b**). (Modified from [20], with permission)

Unconventional Spatial Resolution Characteristics

The spatial resolution performance of MBIR-based systems also demonstrated unconventional spatial resolution characteristics [18, 21, 25, 26]. For example, the PSF of a MBIR system showed strong dependence on object contrast and mAs level (Fig. 6.16). Such strong dependences cannot be explained by the spatial resolution models presented in section "CT Spatial Resolution" (ideal systems) and section "Spatial Resolution Properties of Realistic Systems" (realistic systems), highlighting another breakdown of linear CT system theory.

These unconventional spatial resolution and noise characteristics have introduced significant challenge to the clinical use of MBIR-based CT systems, as the prescription of scan and reconstruction parameters can no longer rely on the well-known relationships between these parameters and CT image quality. Further, the frequent violation of system stationarity in MBIR-based systems brought doubts about whether certain Fourier-domain image quality metrics (e.g., NPS) can still be rigorously defined. How to address these challenges is the focus of the remaining content of this section.

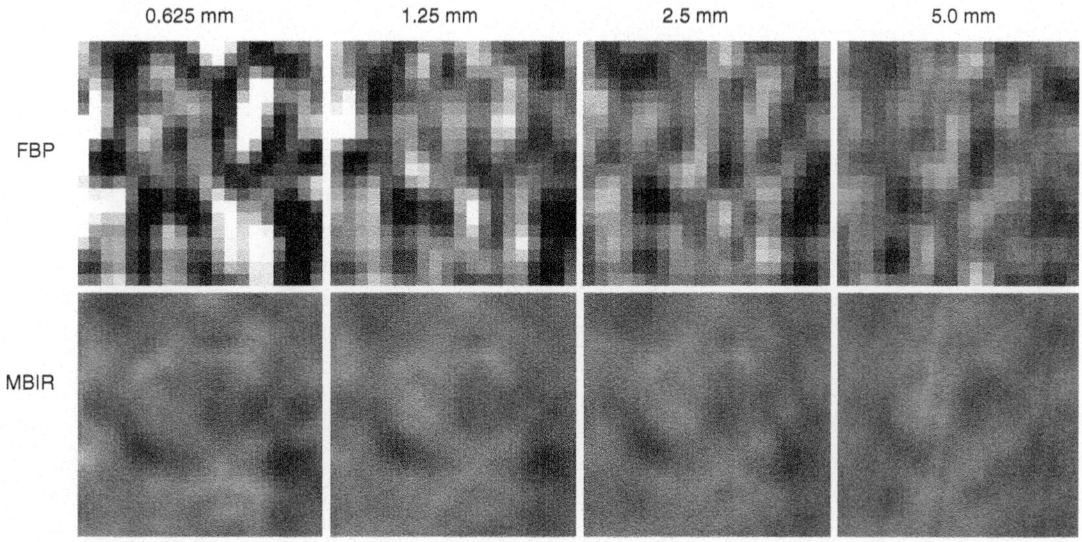

Fig. 6.15 Noise-only FBP (top row) and MBIR images (bottom row) acquired at the same kV and mAs level but with four different reconstruction slice thicknesses

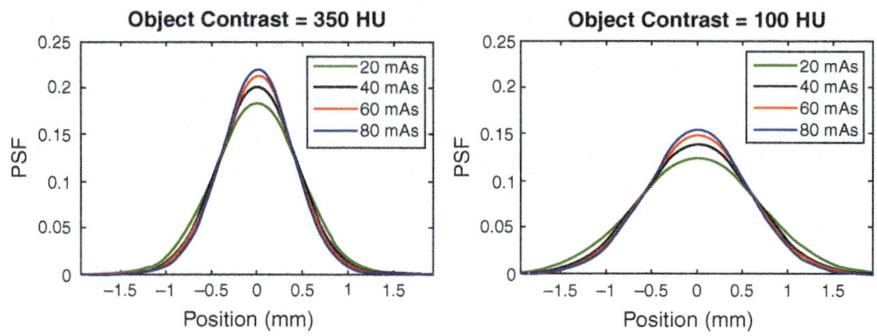

Fig. 6.16 PSF of a MBIR-based CT system measured at two object contrast levels (left figure, 350 HU; right figure, 100 HU) and four mAs levels. (Modified from [21], with permission)

Image Quality Estimation for MBIR-Based CT Systems

Estimation of Noise Performance

To estimate the noise performance of MBIR-based CT systems in a quantitative fashion, one needs to examine whether one of the most widely employed quantitative noise performance metrics—the noise power spectrum—is still well defined for these nonstationary systems. Recall that a 2D NPS is given by 2D Fourier transform of 2D autocovariance function C_f. The general definition of C_f is given by

$$\begin{aligned} C_f\left(x_i,y_i;x_j,y_j\right) &= \left\langle\left[f\left(x_i,y_i\right)-\left\langle f\left(x_i,y_i\right)\right\rangle\right]\left[f\left(x_j,y_j\right)-\left\langle f\left(x_j,y_j\right)\right\rangle\right]\right\rangle \\ &= \left\langle\Delta f\left(x_i,y_i\right)\Delta f\left(x_j,y_j\right)\right\rangle. \end{aligned} \tag{6.75}$$

where (x_i, y_i) and (x_j, y_j) denote two spatial locations in the 2D CT image domain. By substituting x_j with $x_i + x'$ and y_j with $y_i + y'$, where x' and y' quantify the relative spatial distance between (x_i, y_i) and (x_j, y_j), Eq. (6.75) can also be written as

$$C_f\left(x_i,y_i;x_i+x',y_i+y'\right)=\left\langle\Delta f\left(x_i,y_i\right)\Delta f\left(x_i+x',y_i+y'\right)\right\rangle. \tag{6.76}$$

Apparently, the general form of the 2D autocovariance is a function of four variables (x_i, y_i, x', y'). For systems with stationary noise, shift-invariance dictated that C_f does not depend on the absolute spatial location (x_i, y_i), which reduces the number of free variables to two (x', y'). For MBIR systems with nonstationary noise, the loss of shift-invariance due to nonlinearity dictates that C_f may depend on all four parameters. Since a 2D Fourier transform can be taken only with respect to two variables (e.g., x' and y'), the other two variable (e.g., x_i and y_i) will be left in the result of the 2D Fourier transform. As an example,

$$\begin{aligned}\mathrm{NPS}\left(k_x,k_y;x_i,y_i\right)&=\iint C_f\left(x_i,y_i;x_i+x',y_i+y'\right)\mathrm{e}^{-\mathrm{i}2\pi\left(x'k_x+y'k_y\right)}\mathrm{d}x'\mathrm{d}y'\\&=\iint\left\langle\Delta f\left(x_i,y_i\right)\Delta f\left(x_i+x',y_i+y'\right)\right\rangle\mathrm{e}^{-\mathrm{i}2\pi\left(x'k_x+y'k_y\right)}\mathrm{d}x'\mathrm{d}y'.\end{aligned} \tag{6.77}$$

In this example, the Fourier transform of C_f is taken with respect to x' and y'; therefore the left-hand side depends on not only (k_x, k_y) but also (x_i, y_i). A 2D spatial average of $\mathrm{NPS}(k_x, k_y; x_i, y_i)$ will eliminate its dependence on $(x_i, y_i)$and lead to the following formula:

$$\begin{aligned}\overline{\mathrm{NPS}}\left(k_x,k_y\right)&=\frac{\iint\mathrm{NPS}\left(k_x,k_y;x_i,y_i\right)\mathrm{d}x_i\mathrm{d}y_i}{\iint\mathrm{d}x_i\mathrm{d}y_i}\\&=\frac{1}{L_xL_y}\iint\left[\iint\left\langle\Delta f\left(x_i,y_i\right)\Delta f\left(x_i+x',y_i+y'\right)\right\rangle\mathrm{e}^{-\mathrm{i}2\pi\left(x'k_x+y'k_y\right)}\mathrm{d}x'\mathrm{d}y'\right]\mathrm{d}x_i\mathrm{d}y_i,\end{aligned} \tag{6.78}$$

where L_xL_y is the area of the region where the integration is taken. Based on the fact that Δf is real and with variable changes of $x = x_i + x'$, $y = y_i + y'$, Eq. (6.78) can be simplified to

$$\begin{aligned}\overline{\mathrm{NPS}}\left(k_x,k_y\right)&=\frac{1}{L_xL_y}\left\langle\iint\Delta f\left(x,y\right)\mathrm{e}^{-\mathrm{i}2\pi\left(xk_x+yk_y\right)}\mathrm{d}x\mathrm{d}y\iint\Delta f^*\left(x_i,y_i\right)\mathrm{e}^{+\mathrm{i}2\pi\left(x_ik_x+y_ik_y\right)}\mathrm{d}x_i\mathrm{d}y_i\right\rangle\\&=\frac{1}{L_xL_y}\left\langle\left|\mathrm{FT}\left\{\Delta f\left(x,y\right)\right\}\right|^2\right\rangle.\end{aligned} \tag{6.79}$$

The corresponding digital form of Eq. (6.79) is given by

$$\begin{aligned}\overline{\mathrm{NPS}}\left(m\Delta k,n\Delta k\right)&=\frac{1}{L_xL_y}\left\langle\left|\Delta x\Delta y\mathrm{DFT}\left\{\Delta f\left(i\Delta x,j\Delta y\right)\right\}\right|^2\right\rangle\\&=\frac{\left(\Delta x\Delta y\right)^2}{L_xL_y}\left\langle\left|\mathrm{DFT}\left\{\Delta f\left(i\Delta x,j\Delta y\right)\right\}\right|^2\right\rangle\\&=\frac{\Delta x\Delta y}{N_xN_y}\left\langle\left|\mathrm{DFT}\left\{\Delta f\left(i\Delta x,j\Delta y\right)\right\}\right|^2\right\rangle,\end{aligned} \tag{6.80}$$

where $N_x = L_x/\Delta x$, $N_y = L_y/\Delta y$. In terms of mathematical expression, $\overline{\mathrm{NPS}}$ in Eq. (6.79) (analog case) or Eq. (6.80) (digital case) appears to be similar to the classical NPS formulas derived for stationary systems [70], except the following two key differences:

1. *Derivation of* Eqs. (6.79) and (6.80) *never used the condition of noise stationarity*. For nonstationary systems such as those using MBIR, the introduction of the concept of $\overline{\mathrm{NPS}}$ in Eq. (6.78) provides rigorously defined physical meaning to results calculated using

these classical formulas: it is a spatially averaged noise power spectrum.

2. Operator ⟨⟩ in Eqs. (6.79) and (6.80) denotes the statistically defined expected value. It should not be replaced by the operation of spatially shifting the ROI locations in an image, which implicitly requires noise stationarity. Instead, the ⟨⟩ operation must be implemented through *repeated and independent* image acquisitions and ensemble averaging to make $\overline{\text{NPS}}$ meaningful for nonstationary systems.

After justifying the use of $\overline{\text{NPS}}$ as a metric to estimate the noise performance of nonstationary systems, its measurement was performed for a commercial MDCT systems (Discovery CT750 HD, GE Healthcare) with MBIR (Veo, GE Healthcare). To help understand the dependence of MBIR noise performance on mAs level, $\overline{\text{NPS}}$ was measured at seven mAs levels (5, 12.5, 25, 50, 100, 200, 300), which corresponded to CTDI_{vol} values of (1.0, 2.5, 5.0, 10.0, 20.0, 40.0, 60.0) mGy, respectively. At each mAs level, 50 repeated scans were performed, with an inter-scan delay time of at least 10 seconds being enforced to help maintain mutual independence of the data. Radial profiles of the 2D $\overline{\text{NPS}}$ are shown in Fig. 6.17. Compared with the corresponding FBP NPS shown earlier in Fig. 6.4, $\overline{\text{NPS}}$ of MBIR demonstrated significantly lower magnitudes. In addition, the shape of the NPS demonstrated strong dependence on the mAs, as peak of NPS measured at lower mAs level shifted toward lower frequencies. This behavior is a direct violation of the linear systems model, which states that the shape of the CT NPS, once normalized by the noise magnitude, should be independent of the mAs level. Consequently, extensive experimental studies need to be conducted for a given MBIR method in order to obtain relatively comprehensive understanding of its noise characteristics. As an example of this approach, the frequency that corresponds to the NPS peak (referred to as peak frequency or k_{peak}) was measured for all the NPS data in Fig. 6.17 and then plotted as a function of mAs. As shown in Fig. 6.18a, k_{peak} of MBIR monotonically decreased when mAs was reduced. By presenting the results using a log-log plot, k_{peak} seemed to be related to mAs through a power-law relationship, and a power-law fit showed it was indeed the case: k_{peak} was found to be proportional to

$$k_{\text{peak}} \propto (\text{mAs})^{0.16}. \qquad (6.81)$$

Although no theoretical model is available yet to explain the origin of this phenomenon, at least the empirical relationship provides a means to reasonably extend results estimated at one mAs level to other mAs levels for MBIR systems.

The philosophy of empirical modeling also helps toward understanding the dependence of noise magnitude on mAs. As shown in Fig. 6.18b, a log-log plot of MBIR noise variance vs. mAs suggested another power-law relationship, and a power-law fit confirmed it was indeed the case [20]:

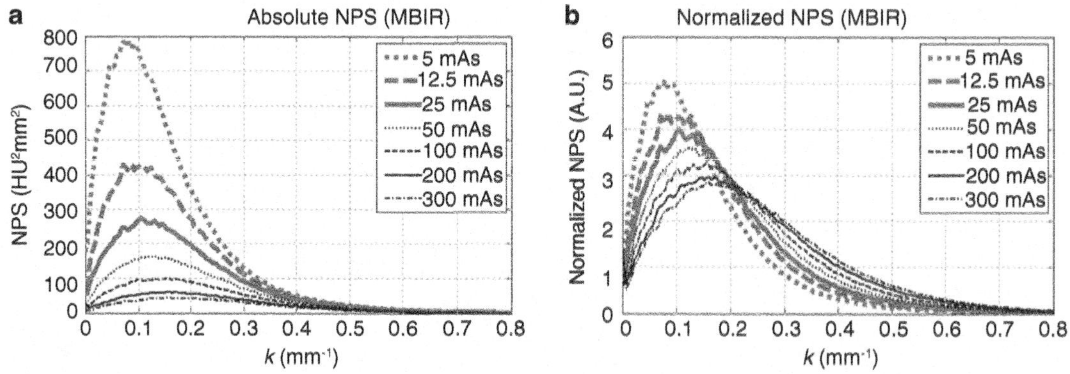

Fig. 6.17 Radially averaged profile of the 2D NPS of MBIR images. (**a**) Absolute NPS. (**b**) NPS normalized by the area under the NPS curve. (Modified from [20], with permission)

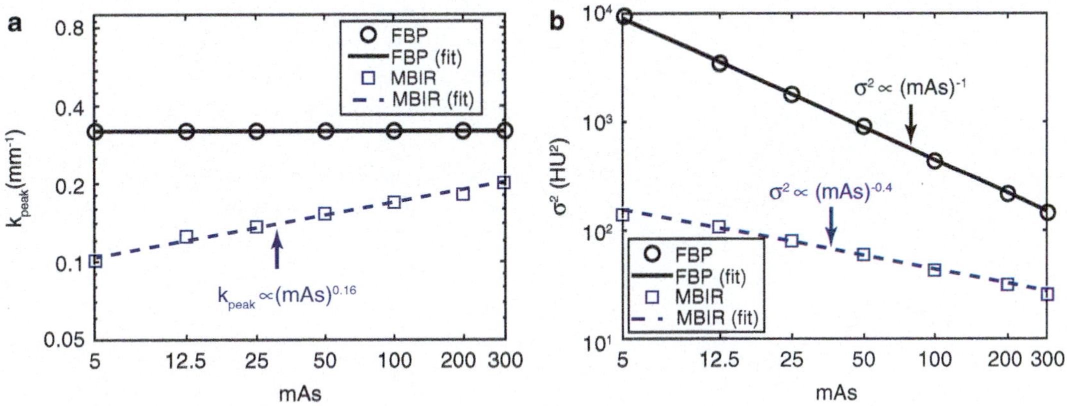

Fig. 6.18 (**a**) Dependence of NPS peak frequency on mAs for both FBP- and MBIR-based CT systems. (**b**) Dependence of CT noise variance σ^2 (i.e., zero-dimensional NPS) on mAs. (Modified from [20], with permission)

$$\sigma^2_{\text{MBIR}} \propto \frac{1}{(\text{mAs})^{0.4}}. \tag{6.82}$$

This is different from the noise model of FBP-based linear systems in Eq. (6.21), which showed

$$\sigma^2_{\text{FBP}} \propto \frac{1}{(\text{mAs})^{1.0}}. \tag{6.83}$$

A comparison between Eqs. (6.82) and (6.83) tells that noise variance of MBIR image has much weaker dependence on mAs level, and therefore a reduction in mAs do not come with much penalty in noise magnitude; there is, however, change in noise texture when mAs is lowered according to Eq. (6.81).

The empirical power-law relationship between MBIR noise variance and mAs in Eq. (6.82) has provided important guidance toward employing MBIR in routine clinical practice. In a prospective trial of reduced dose abdominal CT imaging with MBIR [32], the power-law relationship was used to predict the noise variance of reduced dose (RD) CT scan once the standard dose (SD) scan was finished. Based on Eq. (6.82), noise variances of the two scans should be related by

$$\sigma^2_{\text{MBIR,RD}} = \left(\frac{\text{mAs}_{\text{SD}}}{\text{mAs}_{\text{RD}}}\right)^{0.4} \sigma^2_{\text{MBIR,SD}}. \tag{6.84}$$

Once the RD scan was actually performed, its noise variance $\sigma^2_{\text{MBIR,RD}}$ was experimentally measured in two relatively uniform anatomical regions (the liver and the subcutaneous fat). This process was repeated for each of the 110 human subject enrolled in the trial, and the measured noise variances of RD and SD scans were plotted against the mAs levels of the two scans. The power-law exponent of the plot was estimated for each subject, and the exponents of the study population were compared with the exponent of 0.4 in Eq. (6.82). As shown in Fig. 6.19, the experimental data followed very well with the power-law relationships in Eqs. (6.82) and (6.83), with the population mean ± standard deviation of the power-law exponent to be 0.41 ± 0.12 (liver region) and 0.37 ± 0.12 (fat region) for MBIR, 1.04 ± 0.10 (liver region) and 0.97 ± 0.12 (fat region) for FBP. These results suggested that the power-law relationship observed through phantom-based studies can be decently generalized to in vivo human studies for MBIR, providing a viable approach to estimate noise magnitude when classical theoretical noise model is no longer valid.

Empirical power-law relationship between MBIR noise variance and slice thickness (Δz) was also observed [20]. As shown in Fig. 6.20, noise variance of MBIR images demonstrated a weaker dependence on Δz as

$$\sigma^2_{\text{MBIR}} \propto \frac{1}{(\Delta z)^{0.5}}. \tag{6.85}$$

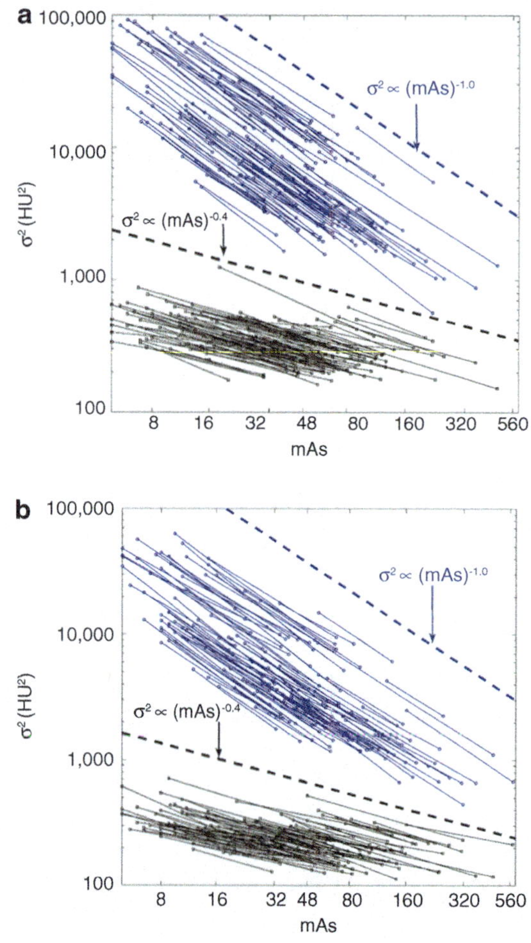

Fig. 6.19 CT noise variances of standard dose and reduced dose series of 110 human subjects. Circles are experimental data points, and each line represents power-law fit for each subject. Blue data were generated from FBP reconstructions, while black data were from MBIR reconstructions. To benchmark the shape of the lines, two reference lines ($\sigma^2 \propto (\text{mAs})^{-0.4}$ and $\sigma^2 \propto (\text{mAs})^{-1.0}$) were added to the figures. (**a**) Measurements were performed in the livers of the subjects. (**b**) Measurements were performed in the subcutaneous fat of the subjects. (Modified from [32], with permission)

This is different from the noise model of FBP-based linear systems in Eq. (6.21), which showed

$$\sigma_{\text{FBP}}^2 \propto \frac{1}{(\Delta z)^{1.0}}. \tag{6.86}$$

Based on Eq. (6.85), reducing slice thickness in MBIR does not come with too much penalty in noise magnitude, which permits thin slice acquisition and reconstruction that enjoy higher through-plane resolution with less blooming artifacts. A corresponding example of this advantage of MBIR is provided in Fig. 6.21.

Task-Based Estimation of Spatial Resolution Performance

As shown earlier in Fig. 6.16, the spatial resolution of an MBIR-based system depends on both radiation dose level and object contrast level. Therefore, spatial resolution assessed under high-contrast and high-dose condition should not be arbitrarily generalized to other conditions. Instead, spatial resolution performance should be estimated separately for each feature of clinical interest at clinically relevant radiation dose levels [18, 21, 25, 26]. *In other words, the estimation should be done in the context of each specific CT imaging task.* For certain imaging tasks such as detection of a low-contrast nodules at a relative low-dose level, the estimation of spatial resolution performance can be quite challenging due to extremely low signal-to-noise ratio (Fig. 6.22): in this case, the estimation result can be contaminated by image noise.

To reliably estimate task-based spatial resolution performance, repeated data acquisitions and ensemble averaging are necessary, especially for low contrast imaging tasks [21, 25]. As shown in Fig. 6.23, ensemble averaging not only helps to knock out the influence of noise in spatial resolution assessment but also provide a background image to help produce noise-only images for estimating $\overline{\text{NPS}}$. Using this work flow, axial PSF was assessed at four contrast levels (ranging from 10 to 1280 HU) and four radiation dose levels (ranging from 4 to 16 mGy), and the width (w) of the PSF was plotted against contrast and dose levels in Fig. 6.24a. For MBIR, w increased monotonically when either contrast or dose was reduced. For example, at 100% dose (16 mGy) and 1280 HU, w was 0.33 mm, which was only 37% of the w value measured at 25% dose and 13 HU. In comparison, w of FBP was independent of radiation dose and contrast level; it stayed around 0.52 mm, with 95% confidence interval

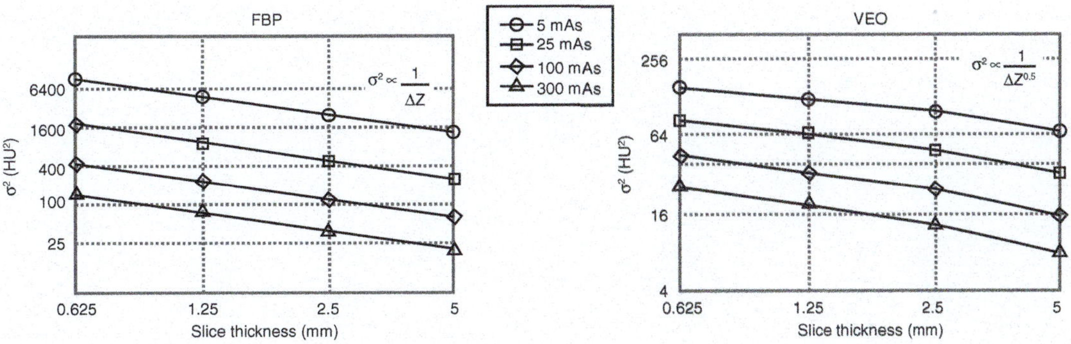

Fig. 6.20 Noise variance-slice thickness (Δz) plots measured at different mAs levels. All plots are displayed using log-log scales. (Modified from [20], with permission)

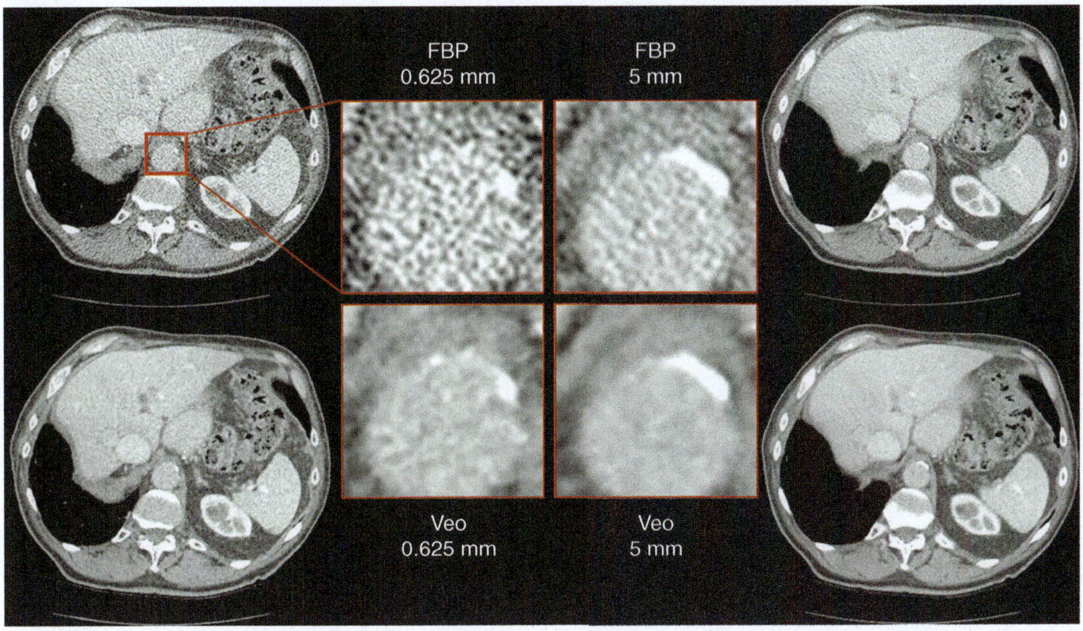

Fig. 6.21 Abdominal CT images of a human subject generated with two reconstruction slice thicknesses (0.625 vs. 5 mm) and two algorithms (FBP vs. Veo). Although all four images showed calcium deposition(s) in the descending aorta, the thin slice (0.625 mm) Veo image provided clearer rendering of size and location of individual calcification, potentially enabling more accurate calcium scoring. Although the thin FBP image also demonstrated less blooming, it suffered much higher noise penalty because of the severe trade-off between slice thickness and noise variance

(CI) of [0.49, 0.55 mm]. In addition, Fig. 6.24b showed the "crossover" contrast level at which spatial resolutions of Veo and FBP became equivalent. The crossover contrast was strongly dose-dependent: it was 300 HU at 25% dose, 174 HU at 50% dose, 127 HU at 75% dose, or 78 HU at 100% dose [21].

Spatial resolution along the z (through-plane) direction demonstrated similar contrast and dose dependences. As shown in Fig. 6.25, the through-plane PSF of MBIR assessed at a contrast level of 270 HU was narrower than that at 120 HU; the width of the through-plane PSF also increased monotonically with decreasing dose level. As a sanity check, through-plane PSF was also measured for FBP images. As expected, the results were independent of contrast and dose level.

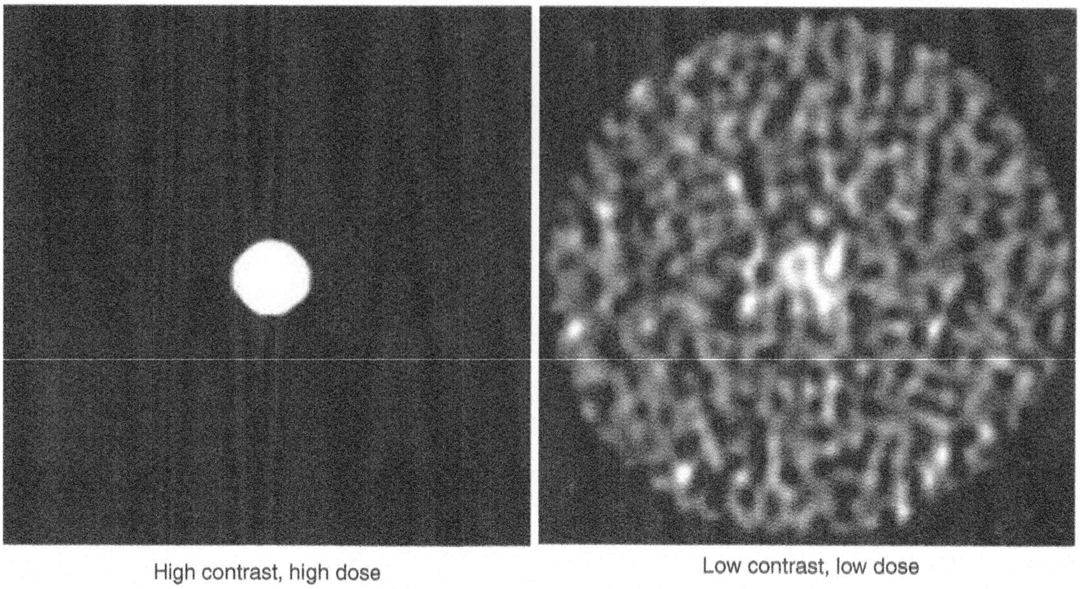

Fig. 6.22 (Left): Image of a high-contrast cylinder acquired at relatively high-radiation dose level. (Right): Image of a low-contrast cylinder acquired at relatively low-dose level

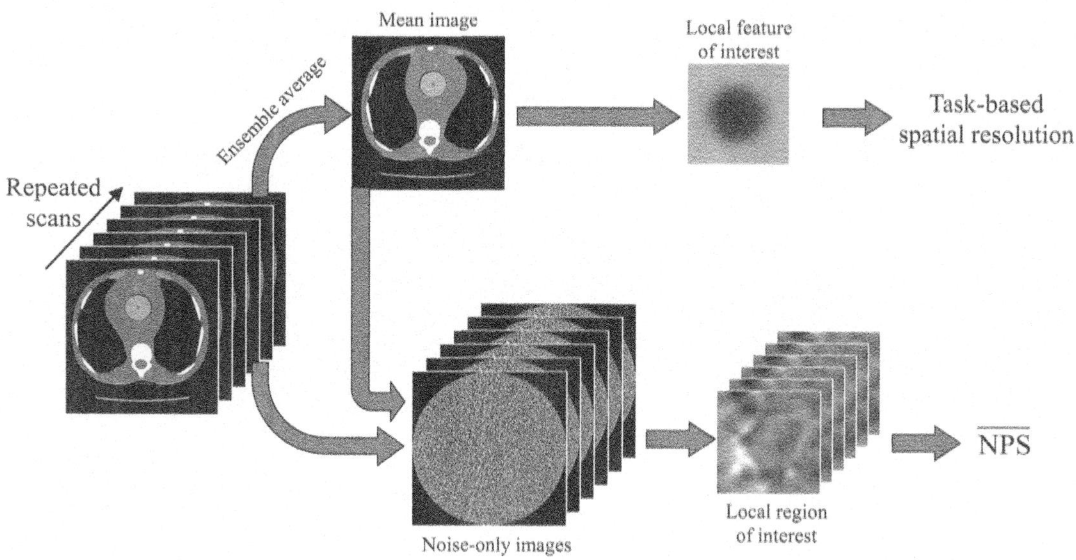

Fig. 6.23 Work flow for estimating task-based spatial resolution and $\overline{\text{NPS}}$ performance from an ensemble of image data. (Modified from [21], with permission)

CT Number Accuracy in MBIR-Based Systems

The task- and ensemble statistics-based approach can also be applied to estimate the CT number accuracy performance of MBIR-based systems [71, 72]. As an example, Fig. 6.26 shows CT biases of a diagnostic MDCT systems (GE Discovery CT750 HD) equipped with both FBP and MBIR. At each mAs level, 50 repeated image acquisitions were performed, and an image-

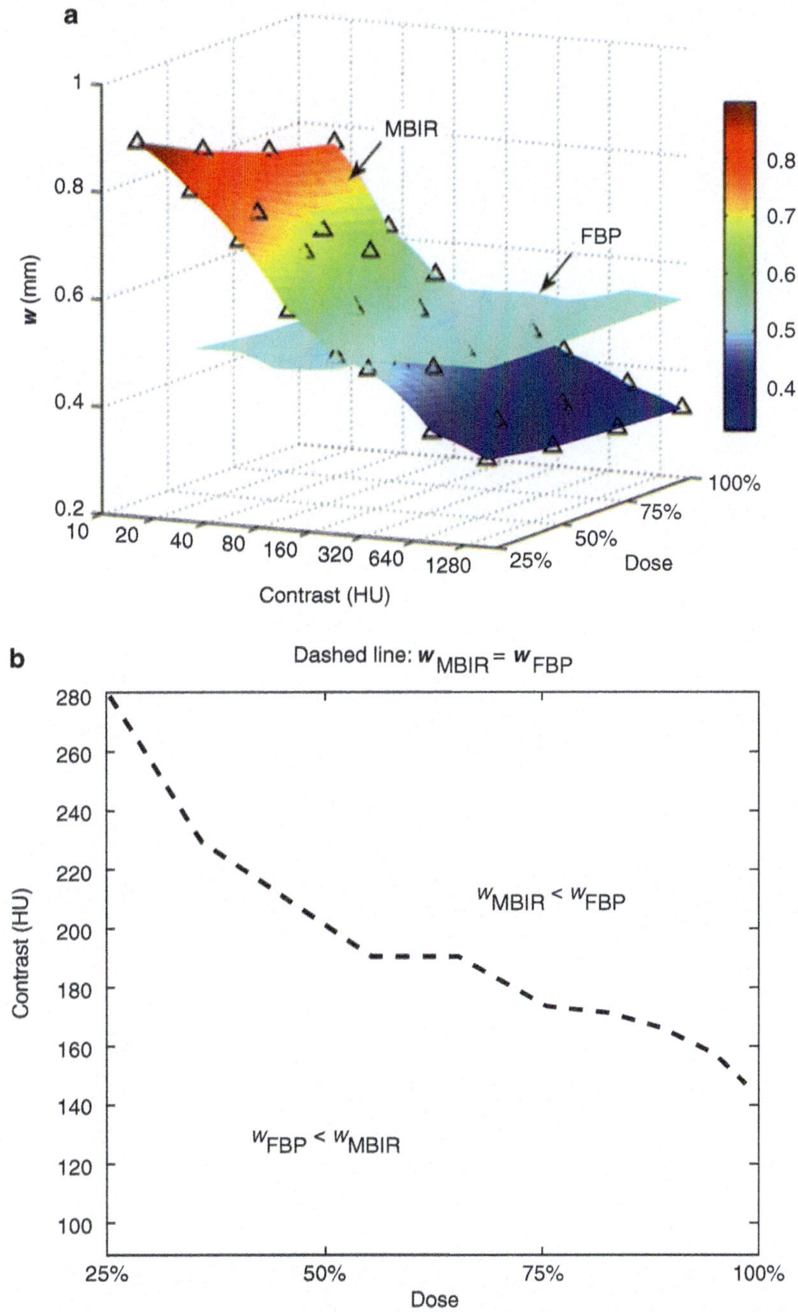

Fig. 6.24 (**a**) Summary of the contrast and dose dependence of in-plane PSF. *w* denotes the width of PSF. The triangles represent the experimental data points, from which other data points were estimated via two-dimensional linear interpolation. (**b**) Crossover contrast-dose pairs at which the PSFs of MBIR and FBP were found to be equivalent. (Modified from [21], with permission)

domain ensemble averaging of the MBIR images provided an estimation of the expected signal $\langle f_{\mathrm{MBIR}} \rangle$. Next, repeated scans were performed at the highest mAs level provided by the CT system, and a projection-domain ensemble averaging was performed to obtain an estimation of the expected projection signal, which was fed into the linear FBP reconstruction engine to produce an estimation of the true CT image signal f_{true}. CT number bias of the MBIR system was estimated by sub-

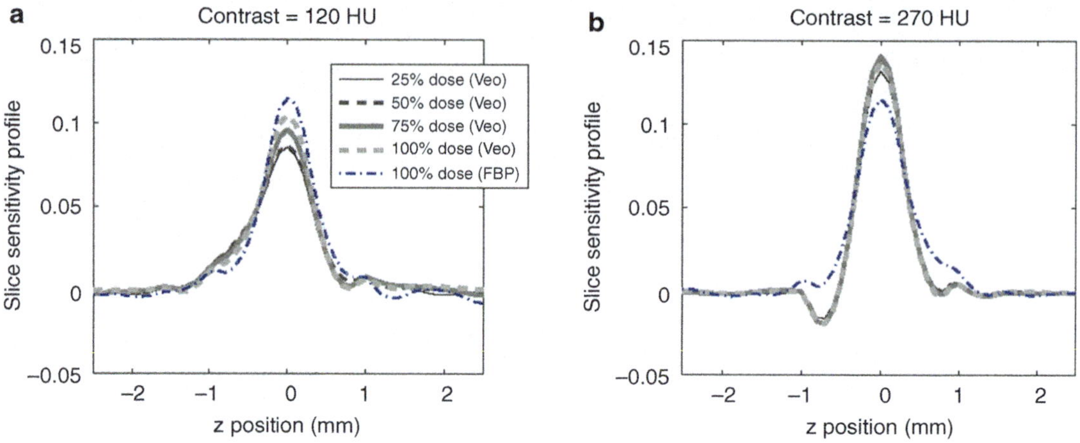

Fig. 6.25 Through-plane PSF (i.e., slice sensitivity profile) assessed at four radiation contrast levels of (**a**) 120 HU and (**b**) 270 HU. (Modified from [21], with permission)

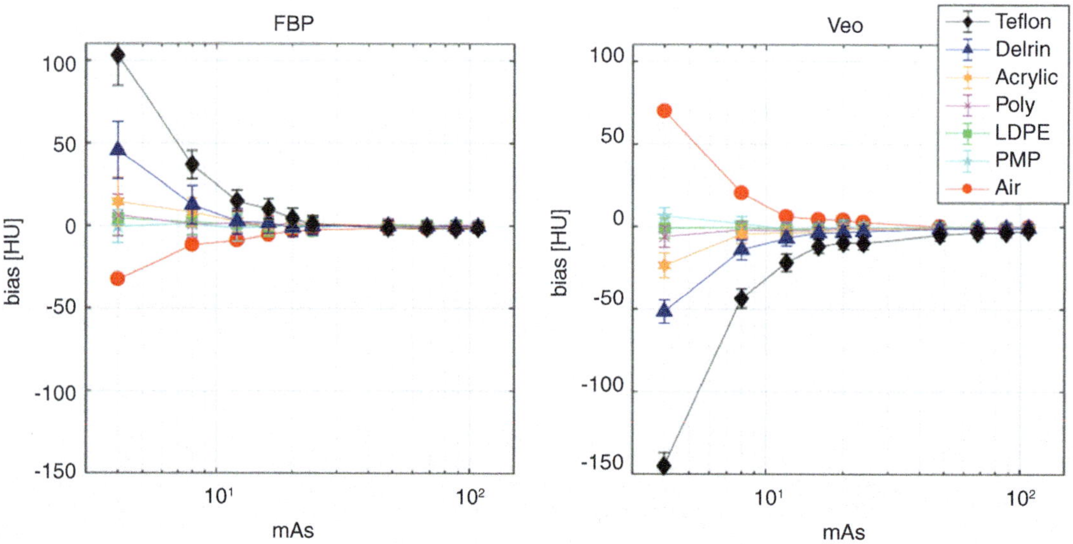

Fig. 6.26 Comparison of CT number biases of FBP- and MBIR (Veo)-based CT systems experimentally measured at different contrast and mAs levels

tracting $\langle f_{\text{MBIR}} \rangle$ and f_{true}. As shown in Fig. 6.26, for a given mAs level and contrast material, bias was flipped from positive in FBP images to negative in MBIR images and vice versa, suggesting that the bias model derived for ideal linear systems [Eq. (6.48)] may not be applicable to nonlinear MBIR systems. One of the ongoing research efforts is to build up better understanding of the signal accuracy properties of nonlinear MBIR-based system so that CT number bias can be controlled or even eliminated in the future.

Summary

For an idealized CT system, its noise is stationary, its axial NPS is rotationally invariant, its NPS magnitude is inversely proportional to mAs, its NPS shape is independent of mAs, its spatial resolution is independent of contrast and mAs, and its CT number bias is linearly related to mAs. These properties can be derived using linear systems theory under the assumptions such as a centered, uniform, and cylindrical image object; a perfectly designed bowtie filter that flattens the post-object flux; negligible beam hardening and scattering effect; ideal photon counting detector; no discrete sampling involved in any stage of the imaging chain; linear tomographic reconstruction algorithm, etc.

For a realistic CT system that uses the linear FBP algorithm, some of the assumptions may be violated. Nevertheless, its image quality performance can be modeled and understood by revising and supplementing theories that were established for ideal systems. The chapter provided examples on how to incorporate realistic tube and detector characteristics, object position, and discrete sampling into image quality models of realistic quasi-linear systems.

For CT systems that use nonlinear MBIR algorithms, the majority of the well-known image quality "laws" are no longer valid. Among evidences for the breakdown of linear systems theory are the contrast- and radiation-dose dependence of spatial resolution, relaxed trade-off between noise magnitude and mAs, strong noise nonstationarity even within local regions, and strong dependence of NPS shape on mAs. The chapter showed that when linear systems theory is no longer valid, task-based image quality estimation methods combined with empirical modeling provide viable means toward understanding the image quality characteristics of nonlinear MBIR-based CT systems.

Appendix I: Autocovariance of Post-log Projection Data

Based on its definition, the autocovariance of R is given by

$$\begin{aligned} C_R(\rho_i,\theta_m;\rho_j,\theta_n) &= \langle \Delta R(\rho_i,\theta_m)\Delta R(\rho_j,\theta_n)\rangle \\ &= \left[\ln N(\rho_i,\theta_m)-\langle \ln N(\rho_i,\theta_m)\rangle\right]\left[\ln N(\rho_j,\theta_n)-\langle \ln N(\rho_j,\theta_n)\rangle\right] \\ &= \langle \ln N(\rho_i,\theta_m)\ln N(\rho_j,\theta_n)\rangle-\langle \ln N(\rho_i,\theta_m)\rangle\langle \ln N(\rho_j,\theta_n)\rangle \\ &= \text{term}_1-\text{term}_2. \end{aligned} \tag{6.87}$$

To facilitate the calculation of term_1 and term_2, we can perform a Taylor expansion of ln N around $\langle N\rangle$:

$$\begin{aligned} \ln N &= \sum_{j=0}^{+\infty}\frac{\left.(\ln N)^{(j)}\right|_{N=\langle N\rangle}}{j!}(N-\langle N\rangle)^j \\ &= \ln\langle N\rangle+\frac{1}{\langle N\rangle}(N-\langle N\rangle)-\frac{1}{2\langle N\rangle^2}(N-\langle N\rangle)^2+\text{L} \end{aligned} \tag{6.88}$$

Based on Eq. (6.88), the expected value of ln N can be expressed as

$$\begin{aligned} \langle \ln N\rangle &= \ln\langle N\rangle+\frac{1}{\langle N\rangle}\langle N-\langle N\rangle\rangle-\frac{1}{2\langle N\rangle^2}\langle (N-\langle N\rangle)^2\rangle+\text{L} \\ &= \ln\langle N\rangle+0-\frac{\sigma_N^2}{2\langle N\rangle^2}+\text{L} \end{aligned} \tag{6.89}$$

With the expanded form of ln$N$ and $\langle \ln N\rangle$, term_1 in Eq. (6.87) can be approximated by

$$\begin{aligned} &\langle \ln N(\rho_i,\theta_m)\ln N(\rho_j,\theta_n)\rangle \\ &= \Bigg\langle \left\{\ln\langle N(\rho_i,\theta_m)\rangle+\frac{1}{\langle N(\rho_i,\theta_m)\rangle}\left[N(\rho_i,\theta_m)-\langle N(\rho_i,\theta_m)\rangle\right]-\frac{1}{2\langle N(\rho_i,\theta_m)\rangle^2}\left[N(\rho_i,\theta_m)-\langle N(\rho_i,\theta_m)\rangle\right]^2+\text{L}\right\} \\ &\quad\times\left\{\ln\langle N(\rho_j,\theta_n)\rangle+\frac{1}{\langle N(\rho_j,\theta_n)\rangle}\left[N(\rho_j,\theta_n)-\langle N(\rho_j,\theta_n)\rangle\right]-\frac{1}{2\langle N(\rho_j,\theta_n)\rangle^2}\left[N(\rho_j,\theta_n)-\langle N(\rho_j,\theta_n)\rangle\right]^2+\text{L}\right\}\Bigg\rangle \\ &\approx \ln\langle N(\rho_i,\theta_m)\rangle\ln\langle N(\rho_j,\theta_n)\rangle-\ln\langle N(\rho_i,\theta_m)\rangle\frac{\sigma_N^2(\rho_j,\theta_n)}{2\langle N(\rho_j,\theta_n)\rangle^2}-\ln\langle N(\rho_j,\theta_n)\rangle\frac{\sigma_N^2(\rho_i,\theta_m)}{2\langle N(\rho_i,\theta_m)\rangle^2}+\frac{C_N(\rho_i,\theta_m;\rho_j,\theta_n)}{\langle N(\rho_i,\theta_m)\rangle\langle N(\rho_j,\theta_n)\rangle}. \end{aligned} \tag{6.90}$$

where we ignored terms higher than the second order since they are much smaller than the zeroth and first order terms. Using similar method, term$_2$ in Eq. (6.87) can be approximated by

$$\begin{aligned}\langle \ln N(\rho_i,\theta_m)\rangle\langle \ln N(\rho_j,\theta_n)\rangle &= \left[\ln\langle N(\rho_i,\theta_m)\rangle - \frac{\sigma_N^2(\rho_i,\theta_m)}{2\langle N(\rho_i,\theta_m)\rangle^2} + \mathrm{L}\right]\left[\ln\langle N(\rho_j,\theta_n)\rangle - \frac{\sigma_N^2(\rho_j,\theta_n)}{2\langle N(\rho_j,\theta_n)\rangle^2} + \mathrm{L}\right] \\ &\approx \ln\langle N(\rho_i,\theta_m)\rangle \ln\langle N(\rho_j,\theta_n)\rangle - \ln\langle N(\rho_i,\theta_m)\rangle\frac{\sigma_N^2(\rho_j,\theta_n)}{2\langle N(\rho_j,\theta_n)\rangle^2} - \ln\langle N(\rho_j,\theta_n)\rangle\frac{\sigma_N^2(\rho_i,\theta_m)}{2\langle N(\rho_i,\theta_m)\rangle^2}.\end{aligned} \tag{6.91}$$

By subtracting term$_2$ in Eq. (6.91) from term$_1$ in Eq. (6.90), majority of the common terms can be cancelled, leading to a much simplified expression for C_R:

$$C_R(\rho_i,\theta_m;\rho_j,\theta_n) \approx \frac{C_N(\rho_i,\theta_m;\rho_j,\theta_n)}{\langle N(\rho_i,\theta_m)\rangle\langle N(\rho_j,\theta_n)\rangle}. \tag{6.92}$$

Using the formula for C_N in Eq. (6.8), formula above can be written as

$$\begin{aligned}C_R(\rho_i,\theta_m;\rho_j,\theta_n) &\approx \frac{\sigma_N^2(\rho_i,\theta_m)\delta_{i,j}\delta_{m,n}}{\langle N(\rho_i,\theta_m)\rangle\langle N(\rho_j,\theta_n)\rangle} \\ &= \frac{\sigma_N^2(\rho_i,\theta_m)\delta_{i,j}\delta_{m,n}}{\langle N(\rho_i,\theta_m)\rangle^2} \\ &= \frac{\delta_{i,j}\delta_{m,n}}{\mathrm{SNR}^2_{N(\rho_i,\theta_m)}}.\end{aligned} \tag{6.93}$$

Appendix II: CT Autocovariance

The autocovariance of $\hat{\mu}$ is defined as

$$C_{\hat{\mu}}(x_i,y_i;x_j,y_j) = \langle \Delta\hat{\mu}(x_i,y_i)\Delta\hat{\mu}(x_j,y_j)\rangle. \tag{6.94}$$

Since $\Delta\hat{\mu}$ is a real number, Eq. (6.94) can also be written as

$$C_{\hat{\mu}}(x_i,y_i;x_j,y_j) = \langle \Delta\hat{\mu}(x_i,y_i)\Delta\hat{\mu}^*(x_j,y_j)\rangle. \tag{6.95}$$

According to the FBP reconstruction formula in Eq. (6.16), $\Delta\hat{\mu}$ is related to the projection data by

$$\begin{aligned}\Delta\hat{\mu}(x,y) &= \hat{\mu}(x,y) - \langle\hat{\mu}(x,y)\rangle \\ &= \int_0^{\pi}\mathrm{d}\theta\int_{-\infty}^{+\infty}\mathrm{d}k\,\tilde{R}(k,\theta)G(k)|k|\,\mathrm{e}^{\mathrm{i}2\pi k(x\cos\theta+y\sin\theta)} \\ &\quad -\left\langle\int_0^{\pi}\mathrm{d}\theta\int_{-\infty}^{+\infty}\mathrm{d}k\,\tilde{R}(k,\theta)G(k)|k|\,\mathrm{e}^{\mathrm{i}2\pi k(x\cos\theta+y\sin\theta)}\right\rangle \\ &= \int_0^{\pi}\mathrm{d}\theta\int_{-\infty}^{+\infty}\mathrm{d}k\left[\tilde{R}(k,\theta)-\left\langle\tilde{R}(k,\theta)\right\rangle\right]G(k)|k|\,\mathrm{e}^{\mathrm{i}2\pi k(x\cos\theta+y\sin\theta)} \\ &= \int_0^{\pi}\mathrm{d}\theta\int_{-\infty}^{+\infty}dk\Delta\tilde{R}(k,\theta)G(k)|k|\,\mathrm{e}^{\mathrm{i}2\pi k(x\cos\theta+y\sin\theta)}.\end{aligned} \tag{6.96}$$

Based on Eq. (6.96), the autocovariance of $\Delta\hat{\mu}$ in Eq. (6.95) can be expanded as

$$\begin{aligned} C_{\hat{\mu}}\left(x_i,y_i;x_j,y_j\right) &= \left\langle \int_0^{\pi} d\theta_1 \int_{-\infty}^{+\infty} dk_1 \Delta\tilde{R}\left(k_1,\theta_1\right) G\left(k_1\right) |k_1| e^{i2\pi k_1\left(x_i\cos\theta_1+y_i\sin\theta_1\right)} \right. \\ &\quad \left. \times \int_0^{\pi} d\theta_2 \int_{-\infty}^{+\infty} dk_2 \Delta\tilde{R}^*\left(k_2,\theta_2\right) G^*\left(k_2\right) |k_2| e^{-i2\pi k_2\left(x_j\cos\theta_2+y_j\sin\theta_2\right)} \right\rangle \\ &= \int_0^{\pi} d\theta_1 \int_{-\infty}^{+\infty} dk_1 G\left(k_1\right) |k_1| \int_0^{\pi} d\theta_2 \int_{-\infty}^{+\infty} dk_2 G^*\left(k_2\right) |k_2| \Delta\tilde{R}\left(k_1,\theta_1\right) \Delta\tilde{R}^*\left(k_2,\theta_2\right) \\ &\quad \times e^{i2\pi\left[x_i k_1\cos\theta_1 - x_j k_2\cos\theta_2 + y_i k_1\sin\theta_1 - y_j k_2\sin\theta_2\right]}, \end{aligned} \tag{6.97}$$

The term $\Delta\tilde{R}\left(k_1,\theta_1\right)\Delta\tilde{R}^*\left(k_2,\theta_2\right)$ in Eq. (6.97) is given by

$$\begin{aligned} \left\langle \Delta\tilde{R}\left(k_1,\theta_1\right)\Delta\tilde{R}^*\left(k_2,\theta_2\right)\right\rangle &= \left\langle \int d\rho_1 \Delta R\left(\rho_1,\theta_1\right) e^{-i2\pi k_1\rho_1} \int d\rho_2 \Delta R^*\left(\rho_2,\theta_2\right) e^{i2\pi k_2\rho_2} \right\rangle \\ &= \int d\rho_1 \int d\rho_2 \left\langle \Delta R\left(\rho_1,\theta_1\right)\Delta R^*\left(\rho_2,\theta_2\right)\right\rangle e^{-i2\pi\left(k_1\rho_1-k_2\rho_2\right)} \\ &= \int d\rho_1 \int d\rho_2 C_R\left(\rho_1,\theta_1;\rho_2,\theta_2\right) e^{-i2\pi\left(k_1\rho_1-k_2\rho_2\right)} \\ &= \int d\rho_1 \int d\rho_2 \frac{\Delta\rho\Delta\theta\delta\left(\rho_1-\rho_2\right)\delta\left(\theta_1-\theta_2\right)}{\langle N\rangle} e^{-i2\pi\left(k_1\rho_1-k_2\rho_2\right)} \\ &= \frac{\Delta\rho\Delta\theta\delta\left(\theta_1-\theta_2\right)}{\langle N\rangle} \int d\rho_1 e^{-i2\pi\rho_1\left(k_1-k_2\right)} \\ &= \frac{\Delta\rho\Delta\theta}{\langle N\rangle}\delta\left(\theta_1-\theta_2\right)\delta\left(k_1-k_2\right). \end{aligned} \tag{6.98}$$

Based on Eq. (6.98), $C_{\hat{\mu}}\left(x_i,;y_i,;x_j,;y_j\right)$ in Eq. (6.97) can be simplified as follows:

$$\begin{aligned} C_{\hat{\mu}}\left(x_i,y_i;x_j,y_j\right) &= \frac{\Delta\rho\Delta\theta}{\langle N\rangle} \int_0^{\pi} d\theta_1 \int_{-\infty}^{+\infty} dk_1 G\left(k_1\right) |k_1| \int_0^{\pi} d\theta_2 \int_{-\infty}^{+\infty} dk_2 G^*\left(k_2\right) |k_2| \delta\left(\theta_1-\theta_2\right)\delta\left(k_1-k_2\right) \\ &\quad \times e^{i2\pi\left[x_i k_1\cos\theta_1 - x_j k_2\cos\theta_2 + y_i k_1\sin\theta_1 - y_j k_2\sin\theta_2\right]} \\ &= \frac{\Delta\rho\Delta\theta}{\langle N\rangle} \int_0^{\pi} d\theta_1 \int_{-\infty}^{+\infty} dk_1 \left|G\left(k_1\right)\right|^2 \left|k_1\right|^2 \int_0^{\pi} d\theta_2 \delta\left(\theta_1-\theta_2\right) e^{i2\pi k_1\left[\left(x_i\cos\theta_1 - x_j\cos\theta_2\right)+\left(y_i\sin\theta_1 - y_j\sin\theta_2\right)\right]} \\ &= \frac{\Delta\rho\Delta\theta}{\langle N\rangle} \int_0^{\pi} d\theta_1 \int_{-\infty}^{+\infty} dk_1 \left|G\left(k_1\right)\right|^2 \left|k_1\right|^2 e^{i2\pi k_1\left[\left(x_i-x_j\right)\cos\theta_1+\left(y_i-y_j\right)\sin\theta_1\right]} \\ &= \frac{\Delta\rho\Delta\theta}{\langle N\rangle} \int_0^{\pi} d\theta \int_{-\infty}^{+\infty} dk \left|G(k)\right|^2 |k|^2 e^{i2\pi k\left[\left(x_i-x_j\right)\cos\theta+\left(y_i-y_j\right)\sin\theta\right]}. \end{aligned} \tag{6.99}$$

By switching from polar coordinate system to Cartesian coordinate system, Eq. (6.99) can be written in the following form:

$$\begin{aligned} C_{\hat{\mu}}(x_i,y_i;x_j,y_j) &= \frac{\Delta\rho\Delta\theta}{\langle N\rangle}\int_{-\infty}^{+\infty}\int_{-\infty}^{+\infty} dk_x dk_y J|G(k)|^2|k|^2 e^{i2\pi[(x_i-x_j)k_x+(y_i-y_j)k_y]} \\ &= \frac{\Delta\rho\Delta\theta}{\langle N\rangle}\int_{-\infty}^{+\infty}\int_{-\infty}^{+\infty} dk_x dk_y \frac{1}{|k|}|G(k)|^2|k|^2 e^{i2\pi[(x_i-x_j)k_x+(y_i-y_j)k_y]} \\ &= \frac{\Delta\rho\Delta\theta}{\langle N\rangle}\int_{-\infty}^{+\infty}\int_{-\infty}^{+\infty} dk_x dk_y |G(k)|^2 |k| e^{i2\pi[(x_i-x_j)k_x+(y_i-y_j)k_y]}, \end{aligned} \tag{6.100}$$

where $k_x = k\cos\theta$, $k_y = k\sin\theta$, and $J = 1/|k|$ are the Jacobian factor introduced by the polar-to-Cartesian coordinate system change.

The noise variance of $\hat{\mu}$ is related to $C_{\hat{\mu}}$ by

$$\begin{aligned} \sigma_{\hat{\mu}}^2 &= C_{\hat{\mu}}(x_i,y_i;x_j=x_i,y_j=y_i) \\ &= \frac{\Delta\rho\Delta\theta}{\langle N\rangle}\int_{-\infty}^{+\infty}\int_{-\infty}^{+\infty} dk_x dk_y |G(k)|^2 |k|. \end{aligned} \tag{6.101}$$

Alternatively, the integration in Eq. (6.101) can be written in the polar coordinate system as

$$\begin{aligned} \sigma_{\hat{\mu}}^2 &= \frac{\Delta\rho\Delta\theta}{\langle N\rangle}\int_0^{\pi} d\theta \int_{-\infty}^{+\infty} dk\, J^{-1}|G(k)|^2 |k| \\ &= \frac{\Delta\rho\Delta\theta}{\langle N\rangle}\int_0^{\pi} d\theta \int_{-\infty}^{+\infty} dk |k|\,|G(k)|^2 |k| \\ &= \frac{\pi\Delta\rho\Delta\theta}{\langle N\rangle}\int_{-\infty}^{+\infty} dk |G(k)|^2 |k|^2. \end{aligned} \tag{6.102}$$

Appendix III: CT Image of a Point-Like Object Generated from an Idealized Linear System

According to [33, 34], the radiological path length of an image object $\mu(x,y)$ along the (ρ,θ) ray is given by

$$\int_{L(\rho,\theta)} u(x,y)dl = \iint u(x,y)\delta(\rho - x\cos\theta - y\sin\theta)dxdy \tag{6.103}$$

For the point object in Eq. (6.32), the radiological path length is

$$\begin{aligned} &\iint u(x,y)\delta(\rho - x\cos\theta - y\sin\theta)dxdy \\ &= \iint u_0\Delta x\Delta y\delta(x-x_0)\delta(y-y_0)\delta(\rho - x\cos\theta - y\sin\theta)dxdy \\ &= u_0\Delta x\Delta y\int dx\delta(x-x_0)\int dy\delta(y-y_0)\delta(\rho - x\cos\theta - y\sin\theta) \\ &= u_0\Delta x\Delta y\int dx\delta(x-x_0)\delta(\rho - x\cos\theta - y_0\sin\theta) \\ &= u_0\Delta x\Delta y\delta(\rho - x_0\cos\theta - y_0\sin\theta). \end{aligned} \tag{6.104}$$

Based on (6.104) and the Beer-Lambert law, the expected number of photons is

$$\langle N(\rho,\theta)\rangle = \langle n_0\rangle \Delta t \Delta z \Delta \rho e^{-u_0 A\delta(\rho - x_0\cos\theta - y_0\sin\theta)}. \quad (6.105)$$

Expected value of the post-log projection data is given by

$$\begin{aligned}\langle R(\rho,\theta)\rangle &= \left\langle \ln\frac{N_0(\rho,\theta)}{N(\rho,\theta)}\right\rangle \\ &= \langle \ln N_0(\rho,\theta)\rangle - \langle \ln N(\rho,\theta)\rangle \\ &\approx \ln\langle N_0(\rho,\theta)\rangle - \ln\langle N(\rho,\theta)\rangle \\ &= u_0\Delta x\Delta y\delta(\rho - x_0\cos\theta - y_0\sin\theta).\end{aligned} \quad (6.106)$$

With $\langle R(\rho,\theta)\rangle$, the following FBP reconstruction can be performed to get $\hat{u}(x,y)$:

$$\langle \hat{u}(x,y)\rangle = \int d\theta \int dk|k|G(k)\left\langle \tilde{R}(k,\theta)\right\rangle e^{i2\pi k(x\cos\theta + y\sin\theta)}, \quad (6.107)$$

where $\tilde{R}(k,\theta)$ is given by

$$\begin{aligned}\tilde{R}(k,\theta) &= \int d\rho \langle R(\rho,\theta)\rangle e^{-i2\pi k\rho} \\ &= u_0\Delta x\Delta y \int d\rho\delta(\rho - x_0\cos\theta - y_0\sin\theta)e^{-i2\pi k\rho} \\ &= u_0\Delta x\Delta y e^{-i2\pi k(x_0\cos\theta + y_0\sin\theta)}.\end{aligned} \quad (6.108)$$

By putting (6.108) into (6.107), we have

$$\begin{aligned}\langle \hat{u}(x,y)\rangle &= u_0\Delta x\Delta y \int d\theta \int dk|k|G(k)e^{-i2\pi k(x_0\cos\theta + y_0\sin\theta)}e^{i2\pi k(x\cos\theta + y\sin\theta)} \\ &= u_0\Delta x\Delta y \int d\theta \int dk|k|G(k)e^{i2\pi[(x-x_0)k\cos\theta + (y-y_0)k\sin\theta]}.\end{aligned} \quad (6.109)$$

By switching from polar-to-Cartesian coordinate system, Eq. (6.109) becomes

$$\begin{aligned}\langle \hat{u}(x,y)\rangle &= u_0\Delta x\Delta y \int_{-\infty}^{+\infty}\int_{-\infty}^{+\infty} dk_x dk_y G(k) e^{i2\pi[k_x(x-x_0) + k_y(y-y_0)]} \\ &= u_0\Delta x\Delta y\, \mathrm{IFT}_{2D}\{G(k)\} \\ &= u_0\Delta x\Delta y\, g(x - x_0, y - y_0),\end{aligned} \quad (6.110)$$

where $g(x - x_0, y - y_0)$ denotes the 2D Fourier transform of the window function $G(k)$.

References

1. Verdun FR, Racine D, Ott JG, Tapiovaara MJ, Toroi P, Bochud FO, et al. Image quality in CT: from physical measurements to model observers. Phys Med. 2015;31(8):823–43.
2. Goldman LW. Principles of CT: radiation dose and image quality. J Nucl Med Technol. 2007;35(4):213–25; quiz 26–8. Epub 2007/11/17.
3. Radiology ACo. CT Accreditation Program Requirements. 2018.
4. Radiology ACo. CT Accreditation Program Testing Instructions. 2018.
5. #2 DX-RICTG. AAPM Report No. 39 Specification and acceptance testing of computed tomography scanners. AAPM, 1993.
6. #12 DX-rICTG. AAPM Report No. 74 Quality control in diagnostic radiology. 2002.
7. Sauer K, Bouman C. A local update strategy for iterative reconstruction from projections. Ieee T Signal Process. 1993;41(2):534–48.
8. Fessler JA, Hero AO. Penalized maximum-likelihood image-reconstruction using space-alternating generalized Em algorithms. Ieee T Image Process. 1995;4(10):1417–29.
9. Lange K, Fessler JA. Globally convergent algorithms for maximum a-posteriori transmission tomography. Ieee T Image Process. 1995;4(10):1430–8.
10. Bouman CA, Sauer K. A unified approach to statistical tomography using coordinate descent optimization. Ieee T Image Process. 1996;5(3):480–92.
11. Thibault JB, Sauer KD, Bouman CA, Hsieh J. A three-dimensional statistical approach to improved image quality for multislice helical CT. Med Phys. 2007;34(11):4526–44.
12. Chen GH, Tang J, Leng SH. Prior image constrained compressed sensing (PICCS): a method to accurately reconstruct dynamic CT images from highly undersampled projection data sets. Med Phys. 2008;35(2):660–3.
13. Lauzier PT, Chen GH. Characterization of statistical prior image constrained compressed sensing. I. Applications to time-resolved contrast-enhanced CT. Med Phys. 2012;39(10):5930–48.
14. Yu Z, Thibault JB, Bouman CA, Sauer KD, Hsieh JA. Fast model-based X-ray CT reconstruction using spatially nonhomogeneous ICD optimization. Ieee T Image Process. 2011;20(1):161–75.
15. Pickhardt PJ, Lubner MG, Kim DH, Tang J, Ruma JA, del Rio AM, et al. Abdominal CT with model-based iterative reconstruction (MBIR): initial results of a prospective trial comparing ultralow-dose with standard-dose imaging. Am J Roentgenol. 2012;199(6):1266–74.
16. Yasaka K, Katsura M, Akahane M, Sato J, Matsuda I, Ohtomo K. Model-based iterative reconstruction for reduction of radiation dose in abdominopelvic CT: comparison to adaptive statistical iterative reconstruction. Springerplus. 2013;2:209.
17. Smith EA, Dillman JR, Goodsitt MM, Christodoulou EG, Keshavarzi N, Strouse PJ. Model-based iterative reconstruction: effect on patient radiation dose and image quality in pediatric body CT. Radiology. 2014;270(2):526–34.
18. Richard S, Husarik DB, Yadava G, Murphy SN, Samei E. Towards task-based assessment of CT performance: system and object MTF across different reconstruction algorithms. Med Phys. 2012;39(7):4115–22.
19. Pal D, Kulkarni S, Yadava G, Thibault JB, Sauer K, Hsieh J. Analysis of noise power spectrum for linear and non-linear reconstruction algorithms for CT. 2011 Ieee Nuclear Science Symposium and Medical Imaging Conference (Nss/Mic). 2011:4382–5.
20. Li K, Tang J, Chen GH. Statistical model based iterative reconstruction (MBIR) in clinical CT systems: experimental assessment of noise performance. Med Phys. 2014;41(4):041906.. Epub 2014/04/04
21. Li K, Garrett J, Ge Y, Chen GH. Statistical model based iterative reconstruction (MBIR) in clinical CT systems. Part II. Experimental assessment of spatial resolution performance. Med Phys. 2014;41(7):071911.. Epub 2014/07/06
22. Li K, Gomez-Cardona D, Hsieh J, Lubner MG, Pickhardt PJ, Chen GH. Statistical model based iterative reconstruction in clinical CT systems. Part III. Task-based kV/mAs optimization for radiation dose reduction. Med Phys. 2015;42(9):5209–21.
23. Solomon J, Samei E. Are uniform phantoms sufficient to characterize the performance of iterative reconstruction in CT? Medical Imaging 2013: Physics of Medical Imaging. 2013;8668.
24. Solomon J, Mileto A, Ramirez-Giraldo JC, Samei E. Diagnostic performance of an advanced modeled iterative reconstruction algorithm for low-contrast detectability with a third-generation dual-source multidetector CT scanner: potential for radiation dose reduction in a multireader study. Radiology. 2015;275(3):735–45.
25. Yu LF, Vrieze TJ, Leng S, Fletcher JG, McCollough CH. Technical note: measuring contrast- and noise-dependent spatial resolution of an iterative reconstruction method in CT using ensemble averaging. Med Phys. 2015;42(5):2261–7.
26. Chen BY, Christianson O, Wilson JM, Samei E. Assessment of volumetric noise and resolution performance for linear and nonlinear CT reconstruction methods. Med Phys. 2014;41(7):071909.
27. Chen BY, Giraldo JCR, Solomon J, Samei E. Evaluating iterative reconstruction performance in computed tomography. Med Phys. 2014;41(12):121913.
28. Solomon J, Samei E. Quantum noise properties of CT images with anatomical textured backgrounds across reconstruction algorithms: FBP and SAFIRE. Med Phys. 2014;41(9):091908.
29. Vaishnav JY, Jung WC, Popescu LM, Zeng R, Myers KJ. Objective assessment of image quality and dose reduction in CT iterative reconstruction. Med Phys. 2014;41(7):071904.

30. Gang GJ, Stayman JW, Zbijewski W, Siewerdsen JH. Task-based detectability in CT image reconstruction by filtered backprojection and penalized likelihood estimation. Med Phys. 2014;41(8):260–78.
31. Hsieh SS, Pelc NJ. Improvements in low contrast detectability with iterative reconstruction and the effect of slice thickness. Medical Imaging 2017: Physics of Medical Imaging. 2017;10132.
32. Gomez-Cardona D, Li K, Hsieh J, Lubner MG, Pickhardt PJ, Chen GH. Can conclusions drawn from phantom-based image noise assessments be generalized to in vivo studies for the nonlinear model-based iterative reconstruction method? Med Phys. 2016;43(2):687–95.
33. Kak AC, Slaney M. Principles of computerized tomographic imaging. New York: IEEE Press; 1988.
34. Hsieh J. Computed tomography principles, design, artifacts, and recent advances. 2nd ed. Hoboken: Wiley; 2009.
35. Szczykutowicz TP, Bour RK, Rubert N, Wendt G, Pozniak M, Ranallo FN. CT protocol management: simplifying the process by using a master protocol concept. J Appl Clin Med Phys. 2015;16(4):228–43.
36. Riederer SJ, Pelc NJ, Chesler DA. The noise power spectrum in computed X-ray tomography. Phys Med Biol. 1978;23(3):446–54.. Epub 1978/05/01
37. Kijewski MF, Judy PF. The noise power spectrum of Ct images. Phys Med Biol. 1987;32(5):565–75.
38. Zhang R, Cruz-Bastida JP, Gomez-Cardona D, Hayes JW, Li K, Chen GH. Quantitative accuracy of CT numbers: theoretical analyses and experimental studies. Med Phys. 2018;45(10):4519–28.. Epub 2018/08/14
39. Fessler JA. Hybrid Poisson/polynomial objective functions for tomographic image reconstruction from transmission scans. IEEE Trans Image Process: Publ IEEE Signal Process Soc. 1995;4(10):1439–50.. Epub 1995/01/01
40. Gomez-Cardona D, Cruz-Bastida JP, Li K, Budde A, Hsieh J, Chen GH. Impact of bowtie filter and object position on the two-dimensional noise power spectrum of a clinical MDCT system. Med Phys. 2016;43(8):4495.. Epub 2016/08/05
41. Whiting BR, editor. Signal statistics in x-ray computed tomography. Medical Imaging 2002. SPIE; 2002.
42. Mandel L. Image fluctuations in Cascade intensifiers. Brit J Appl Phys. 1959;10(5):233–4.
43. Tapiovaara MJ, Wagner RF. SNR and DQE analysis of broad-Spectrum X-ray-imaging. Phys Med Biol. 1985;30(6):519–29.
44. Duan X, Wang J, Leng S, Schmidt B, Allmendinger T, Grant K, et al. Electronic noise in CT detectors: impact on image noise and artifacts. AJR Am J Roentgenol. 2013;201(4):W626–32.. Epub 2013/09/26
45. Tward DJ, Siewerdsen JH. Cascaded systems analysis of the 3D noise transfer characteristics of flat-panel cone-beam CT. Med Phys. 2008;35(12):5510–29.. Epub 2009/01/30
46. Sohval AR, Freundlich D, inventors. Plural source computed tomography device with improved resolution 1986.
47. Lonn AH, inventor. Computed tomography system with translatable focal spot 1990.
48. Hsieh J, Gard M, Gravelle S. A reconstruction technique for focal spot wobbling. Proc Soc Photo-Opt Ins. 1992;1652:175–82.
49. Hsieh J, Saragnese EL, Stahre JE, Dorri B, Kaufman J, Senzig RF, inventors. Methods and apparatus for x-ray imaging with focal spot deflection 2008.
50. Kachelriess M, Knaup M, Penssel C, Kalender WA. Flying focal spot (FFS) in cone-beam CT. Ieee T Nucl Sci. 2006;53(3):1238–47.
51. Cruz-Bastida JP, Gomez-Cardona D, Li K, Sun HY, Hsieh J, Szczykutowicz TP, et al. Hi-Res scan mode in clinical MDCT systems: experimental assessment of spatial resolution performance. Med Phys. 2016;43(5).
52. Cruz-Bastida JP, Gomez-Cardona D, Garrett J, Szczykutowicz T, Chen GH, Li K. Modified ideal observer model (MIOM) for high-contrast and high-spatial resolution CT imaging tasks. Med Phys. 2017;44(9):4496–505.
53. Tward DJ, Siewerdsen JH. Noise aliasing and the 3D NEQ of flat-panel cone-beam CT: effect of 2D/3D apertures and sampling. Med Phys. 2009;36(8):3830–43.
54. Rabbani M, Shaw R, Vanmetter R. Detective quantum efficiency of imaging-systems with amplifying and scattering mechanisms. J Opt Soc Am A. 1987;4(5):895–901.
55. Giger ML, Doi K, Metz CE. Investigation of basic imaging properties in digital radiography .2. Noise wiener Spectrum. Med Phys. 1984;11(6):797–805.
56. Siewerdsen JH, Antonuk LE, ElMohri Y, Yorkston J, Huang W, Boudry JM, et al. Empirical and theoretical investigation of the noise performance of indirect detection, active matrix flat-panel imagers (AMFPIs) for diagnostic radiology. Med Phys. 1997;24(1):71–89.
57. Baek J, Pelc NJ. Effect of detector lag on CT noise power spectra. Med Phys. 2011;38(6):2995–3005.
58. Pineda AR, Tward DJ, Gonzalez A, Siewerdsen JH. Beyond noise power in 3D computed tomography: the local NPS and off-diagonal elements of the Fourier domain covariance matrix. Med Phys. 2012;39(6):3240–52.
59. Yang K, Kwan A, Huang S, Boone J. Noise power properties of a cone-beam CT system for breast Cancer detection. Med Phys. 2008;35(6):2977.. –+
60. Melnyk R, Boudry J, Liu X, Adamak M. Anti-scatter grid evaluation for wide-cone CT. Medical imaging. Phys Med Imaging. 2014;2014:9033.
61. Hayes JW, Gomez-Cardona D, Zhang R, Li K, Cruz-Bastida JP, Chen GH. Low-dose cone-beam CT via raw counts domain low-signal correction schemes: performance assessment and task-based parameter optimization (part I: assessment of spatial resolution

and noise performance). Med Phys. 2018;45(5):1942–56.. Epub 2018/03/14
62. Gomez-Cardona D, Hayes JW, Zhang R, Li K, Cruz-Bastida JP, Chen GH. Low-dose cone-beam CT via raw counts domain low-signal correction schemes: performance assessment and task-based parameter optimization (part II. Task-based parameter optimization). Med Phys. 2018;45(5):1957–69.. Epub 2018/03/14
63. Barrett HH, Gordon SK, Hershel RS. Statistical limitations in transaxial tomography. Comput Biol Med. 1976;6(4):307–23.. Epub 1976/10/01
64. Parker DL. Optimal short scan convolution reconstruction for Fan beam Ct. Med Phys. 1982;9(2):254–7.
65. Baek J, Pelc NJ. The noise power spectrum in CT with direct fan beam reconstruction. Med Phys. 2010;37(5):2074–81.
66. Baek J, Pelc NJ. Local and global 3D noise power spectrum in cone-beam CT system with FDK reconstruction. Med Phys. 2011;38(4):2122–31.
67. Kyprianou LS, Rudin S, Bednarek DR, Hoffmann KR. Generalizing the MTF and DQE to include x-ray scatter and focal spot unsharpness: application to a new microangiographic system. Med Phys. 2005;32(2):613–26.
68. Budde A, Hsieh J, Chen GH. Impact of the distortion of focal spot shape on spatial resolution in MDCT. Med Phys. 2018;45(6):E153.
69. Kalender WA. Computed tomography: fundamentals, system technology, image quality, applications. 3rd ed. Paris: Publicis; 2011.
70. Cunningham IA. Chapter 2. Applied linear-systems theory. In: Beutel J, Kundel HL, Van Metter RL, editors. Handbook of medical imaging volume ! Physics and psychophysics. Bellingham: SPIE Press; 2000. p. 79–160.
71. Gomez-Cardona D, Budde A, Hayes J, Li K, Chen GH. CT number bias in low dose MDCT with Model Based Iterative Reconstruction (MBIR). Radiological Society of North America 2017 Scientific Assembly and Annual Meeting. Chicago, 2017.
72. Hayes J, Zhang R, Gomez-Cardona D, Cruz Bastida JP, Chen GH. Modified model based iterative reconstruction method to improve CT number accuracy in low-dose CT. Radiological Society of North America 2018 Scientific Assembly and Annual Meeting, Chicago, 2018.

Clinical CT Performance Evaluation

7

Nicole Lafata and Christopher J. MacLellan

Performance Evaluation Preparation

There are several steps a physicist should take before entering the CT facility to facilitate an appropriate and efficient CT performance evaluation. The physicist should work with technical and administrative staff to obtain basic information about the unit and facility as well as to schedule time to test the unit. This includes technical details such as the vendor, model, and capabilities (e.g., dual energy, cardiac mode, gantry tilt, etc.) as well as an understanding of the manner in which the scanner is used clinically (e.g., dedicated interventional scanner, therapy simulator, etc.). The technical staff should help to identify the routine protocols for each relevant application and patient population to ensure appropriate protocols are used during the evaluation. The physicist should also be aware of the regulatory and accreditation standards that are applicable to the scanner. While regulatory requirements are typically defined by geography, accreditation requirements can vary significantly between scanners and sites. With this information, the physicist should adjust the performance evaluation accordingly. For example, the evaluation of an American College of Radiology (ACR) accredited general purpose dual energy scanner in a radiology department will differ significantly from a non-accredited hybrid CT in a nuclear medicine department. If the performance evaluation is an acceptance test, the physicist may seek additional technical specifications from the vendor and adjust the test accordingly. The physicist should also ensure that they obtain any login information or service keys that are required to conduct testing.

N. Lafata (✉) · C. J. MacLellan
Clinical Imaging Physics Group, Duke University Health System, Durham, NC, USA
e-mail: nicole.lafata@duke.edu; christopher.maclellan@duke.edu

Safety and Operational Inspection

A safety and operational inspection includes several key safety components, such as (1) a pretest inspection checking for radiation safety measures, proper mechanical operation, and appropriate dosimetric capabilities, (2) ensuring a well-run quality control (QC) program, and (3) inspecting acquisition display monitors.

Pretest Inspection

The safe use of CT imaging systems is defined and enforced at different levels. While the Code of Federal Regulations (CFR) defines specific administrative law regarding CT radiation safety, there are often additional regulations defined by state governments, institutions, and third-party accreditation agencies. Accordingly, it is imperative to verify which safety rules and regulations

© Springer Nature Switzerland AG 2020

E. Samei, N. J. Pelc (eds.), *Computed Tomography*, https://doi.org/10.1007/978-3-030-26957-9_7

are applicable when testing a CT system. Below is a list of checks that – regardless of whether or not they are mandated – are important for a proper performance evaluation. Many of these recommendations have been adopted from the Code of Federal Regulations and AAPM Task Group 233 [1, 2]. These recommended assessments fall into three categories: radiation safety, CT system operation, and dosimetric capabilities.

The pretest inspection includes a list of technical assessments and testing procedures that are performed to ensure radiation safety to both patients and staff. First, proper signage should be present outside of the CT room, ensuring that personnel know they are entering an area where there may be radiation. At a minimum, this may include warning signs posted at all access points stating, "Caution Radiation Area." However, individual states and/or accrediting bodies may have more specific posting regulations. Of particular interest are X-ray beam-on indication lights. If an X-ray indication light is installed at the CT room entry, one should verify the sign illuminates when a scan is performed. Next, it is recommended to consult local regulations and guidelines to determine if CT room doors are required to be shut during exposures. If required and/or intended in the room design, one needs to check for compliance. Another important task is verification that emergency stops are operable and available to operators. In accordance with CRF 21CFR1020.30 (j), control panels shall contain the following warning statement: "Warning: This x-ray unit may be dangerous to patient and operator unless safe exposure factors, operating instructions and maintenance schedules are observed" [2]. A signal shall be produced – either audible or visual – when X-rays are generated. If a system is undergoing acceptance testing, it is important to make sure the shielding in the room has been inspected and surveyed. NCRP 147 provides sufficient recommendations on how to properly evaluate shielding adequacy [3].

For exam rooms that are used for interventional procedures, lead aprons should be available for staff. It may also be informative for the physicist to measure the exposure from X-ray scatter at different locations in the CT room that may be occupied by interventional staff during procedures. This can be performed using a large attenuator (i.e., the CTDI 32 cm phantom) and a survey meter setup to measure the cumulative dose at a defined points of interest in the room. For a known tube current and rotation time, the scatter exposure at each location can be calculated in μR/mA. A diagram of dose rates can be created to display in the room for a commonly used protocol(s).

To ensure patient safety, several different CT system operation checks should be evaluated as follows. The physicist should verify that [1] technologists working at the acquisition workstation have a direct line of sight to the patient and oral communication with the patient is easily achievable; [2] the table movement is smooth and operates properly; and [3] the gantry and acquisition console controls, lights, and indicators function as intended.

Finally, to ensure patients are receiving appropriate doses, it is imperative to check basic capabilities of the CT system. For example, the scanner should have a visual reference plane (e.g., lasers) that corresponds to the principal imaging planes. Prior to an acquisition, the system should be capable of displaying all of the technique factors. While an acquisition utilizing tube current modulation may not show the exact mA, the scanner should be capable of displaying the minimum and maximum mA. Finally, the CTDI, dose length product (DLP), and estimated maximum CTDI at a single slice location should be visible to the user prior to image acquisition. The National Electrical Manufacturers Association (NEMA) has developed a standard requiring scanners to incorporate different "Smart Dose" features to be considered compliant with the XR-29 Standard [4]. This initiative is also known as MITA Smart Dose, and required features include that the scanner is capable of automatic exposure control, DICOM-compliant radiation dose structured reporting, and dose check features and contains reference pediatric and adult protocols. Physicists should ensure (by contacting the vendor) that a CT system has the proper software upgrades to be compliant with XR-29. Finally, the system should be capable of sending the dosimetry information, preferably to a software environment that is capable of monitoring, tracking, and analyzing doses.

Quality Control Program

It is the responsibility of medical physicists to implement, teach, and monitor a quality control (QC) program. At a minimum, a site should be compliant with the QC practices recommended by their accrediting bodies and CT system manufacturer. Prior to scanner use, daily QC programs typically start with a tube warm-up, followed by an air calibration. Next, a water phantom is scanned in either axial or helical mode. Thin image slices should be acquired to check for artifacts, while thicker image slices may be reconstructed to measure the mean and standard deviation of the water CT number.

Ideally, the QC program will be monitored routinely. This ensures any potential problems with QC can be addressed more frequently than once a year. Methods for how to monitor this data are broad in both scope and practice. At some facilities the QC data may simply be recorded on sheets of paper; at others, a technologist is able to enter the QC data into a structured web application database for a physicist to review. Preferably, a QC program will also include a periodic review of the QC images by the physicist. The physicist should review the images for proper setup, acquisition parameters, and artifacts. A more sophisticated approach, however, would include QC images sent to a server where they would be automatically analyzed for CT number, uniformity, noise properties, and artifacts.

While still important, it may be more appropriate to perform other tests on a less frequent or monthly basis. These include items that the ACR recommends on their monthly checklist including checking the proper functioning of the gantry, ensuring the control console is working as it is supposed to, and running an artifact check on a large phantom [5].

It is essential that technologists completing QC procedures and using CT systems appreciate that they are the first line of defense in ensuring both patient safety and exam quality. If they consider images to be unsatisfactory, technologists should feel enabled and comfortable to repeat QC scans, run calibration tests, and contact physics or engineering support.

Display Monitor

CT technologists rely on the display at the scanner console throughout an exam to assess images as they are reconstructed. These displays are an important part of the clinical workflow and should be evaluated on a regular basis. Some key aspects of display integrity include the maximum brightness, grayscale calibration, and the absence of artifacts. Many of these features can be tested qualitatively by evaluating specially designed test patterns on the display. Quantitative evaluations require luminance and illuminance meters that measure the light emitted from or incident on the display, respectively. Displays that are located within interventional suites should also be evaluated since they are used to guide patient procedures. Special care should be taken to make these evaluations in the typical ambient lighting conditions as this can have a significant impact on the ability to resolve the lowest gray levels. Resources for display technical specifications, testing procedures, and test patterns can be found in the reports of AAPM Task Groups 18 [6] and 270 [7].

System Geometry

System geometry evaluation requires testing many of the constituent subsystems of the scanner: laser accuracy, table movement, gantry tilt, and collimation. If any of these subsystems are in misalignment, they could degrade the image quality or affect patient dose.

Laser Alignment Accuracy

Accurate laser alignment ensures optimal patient positioning. Axial lasers ensure proper coverage in localizer views, while sagittal and coronal lasers ensure the patient is properly centered in the field of view. Collectively, this helps ensure appropriate patient dose and image quality. Several methods exist to verify laser alignment. These generally rely on placing small radiopaque markers at each of the visible laser locations. The scanner is landmarked and a series of thin axial slices are prescribed at the landmark position. The table position where the marker is most prominent represents the axial laser position. The accuracy of the sagittal and coronal lasers can be found by measuring the orthogonal distance from the markers in the image to the appropriate axis in the image. This measurement is easily performed with the aid of a grid overlay or by recording the coordinates of each fiducial in the image at the scanner console. Common approaches are to use a phantom with multiple markers known to be embedded in the same plane (e.g., ACR phantom) or place a thin wire-like object (e.g., staples) along each laser on an existing phantom prior to scanning (Fig. 7.1).

Scout Prescription Accuracy

In routine clinical imaging, the scan extent is defined using the localizer image. Thus, it is important to ensure that the location prescribed from the localizer is faithfully acquired during a given acquisition. To verify the prescription accuracy, a radiopaque marker should be placed at a known table location, and a localizer should be acquired. A series of axial images centered on the marker should be prescribed using the localizer. The marker should be most visible at the slice corresponding to the known table location.

Table Movement

Accurate table movement is critical to the performance of any CT scanner and can be evaluated by recording the table position indicated on the scanner and comparing it with an independent measure of position. A simple approach is to place a tape measure in the center of the scanner table and move the table into and out of the gantry at predefined increments. The distance traveled on the tape measure and on the scanner should match at every position including when the table is returned to the original location. Alternatively,

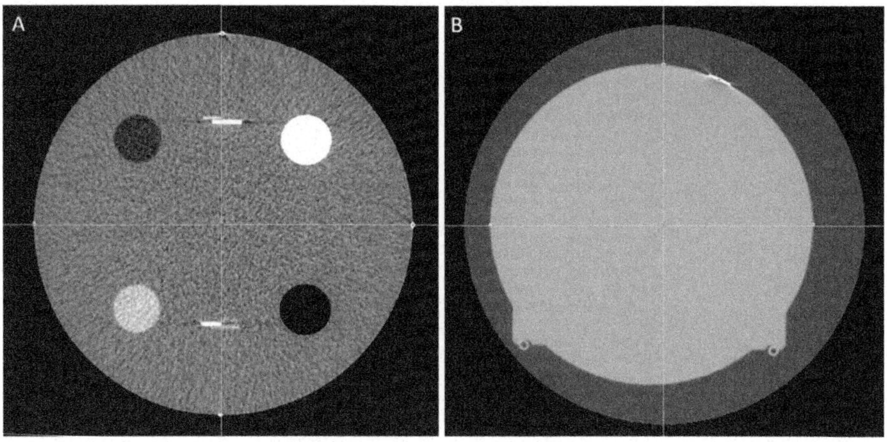

Fig. 7.1 Axial laser alignment. Two examples of laser accuracy measurement with crosshairs placed at the isocenter for reference. The ACR phantom has fiducial markers embedded in the phantom that are aligned with the lasers (**a**). Fiducial markers can also be attached to a phantom to align with the lasers (**b**). The sagittal and coronal laser accuracy is measured by finding the coordinates of the fiducials in the image. Axial laser alignment is measured by verifying the markers are most prominent at the table position corresponding to the axial laser

the same information can be measured using a phantom with two sets of fiducials that are a known distance apart. Regardless of the method, it is important to evaluate table motion over the maximum range of table motion.

Gantry Tilt

Scanners with tilting gantries should be evaluated to ensure angular accuracy. This can be measured using a computed radiography (CR) plate or a piece of film placed perpendicular to the table in the sagittal plane. The table should be positioned such that the isocenter is located within the plate or film. Rigid objects with low-to-moderate attenuation properties (e.g., foam blocks) and/or tape can be used to ensure the plate or film stays in position. Using the thinnest collimation, axial acquisitions should be acquired throughout the available range of gantry tilt angles with a technique that is appropriate for the measuring device. The angles should be measured either virtually on the digital images (CR) or using a protractor (film). An alternative approach is to perform the axial acquisitions described above on a cylindrical water phantom of known diameter (Fig. 7.2). The apparent diameter of the phantom in the anterior/posterior direction can be used to calculate the actual gantry tilt using the following trigonometric relationship.

$$\theta_{\text{measured}} = \cos^{-1}\left(\frac{d_{\text{true}}}{d_{\text{apparent}}}\right) \tag{7.1}$$

Axial Slice Thickness

The true reconstructed slice thicknesses should be in agreement with the thickness selected at the scanner console. This is typically measured using a phantom with a specialized insert containing objects of known size and geometry designed specifically for this purpose. Common methods include counting a series of specially placed high-attenuating targets or measuring the full width half maximum of highly attenuating cross ramps of a known angle (Fig. 7.3). The actual calculation of the slice thickness will depend on the size and arrangement of ramps/targets within the specific phantom.

Helical Slice Thickness

All modern CT scanners are capable of acquiring images in helical mode where the tube is rotated while the table is moving, which allows the

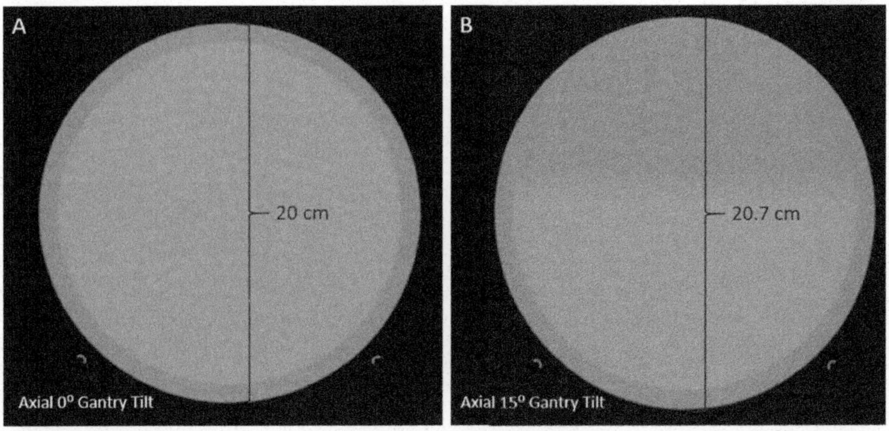

Fig. 7.2 Gantry tilt accuracy. An approach to measure gantry tilt when a CR plate or film is not available. A phantom of known diameter is measured with and without tilting the gantry, and the apparent length in the anterior/posterior direction is compared using trigonometry to verify the gantry angle

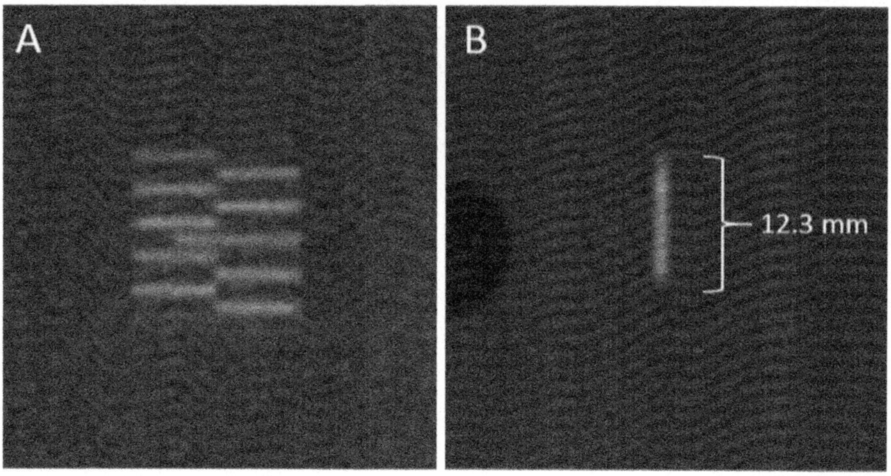

Fig. 7.3 Axial slice thickness. Two ways to measure axial slice thickness. In the ACR phantom, highly attenuating objects are placed in the superior inferior direction such that they can be easily counted to calculate the slice thickness (**a**). In this case each bar represents 0.5 mm. The Catphan phantom contains highly attenuating cross ramps (**b**). The length can be used to calculate the slice thickness. In this case the angle is 23^0 from the superior/inferior axis

reconstruction of arbitrary slice thicknesses. The effective slice thickness of a helical acquisition is best evaluated by measuring full width at half maximum of the impulse response of the system [6, 7]. This requires a phantom with a small (0.05–0.1 mm) highly attenuating disk or bead or a small air hole embedded in an attenuating medium. Helical reconstruction should be performed with small intervals (<10% of the nominal slice thickness) between slices for each acquisition of interest. Practically, the extent of the scan should be limited due to the number of images produced by this type of acquisition. The impulse response can be found by plotting the maximum (or minimum for an air hole) CT number in each image as a function of table position. The full width at half maximum of this impulse response is representative of the effective slice thickness for a given acquisition [8–10].

Radiation Beam Width

Like other imaging modalities that utilize ionizing radiation, it is imperative to ensure the size of the radiation field emitted from a CT scanner is consistent with the nominal size. Modern CT scanners have several beam collimations that can be used during acquisition. These can be verified using either film or a CR plate placed at the isocenter of the scanner. When using film, the full width half max of the exposed region may be evaluated visually or electronically if an image of the film is obtained. While there is substantial uncertainty using film, it is generally sufficient to meet vendor's tolerances. Theoretically, using a CR plate can provide a more accurate and precise measurement provided the pixel values are properly converted to exposure [11–13].

Radiation Output Performance

Accurate and reliable radiation output is an important aspect of CT performance. However, making meaningful measurements of radiation output is nontrivial due to the unique rotational geometry found in CT. For this reason, a standardized measurement called the computed tomography dose index (CTDI) is customarily used to assess the radiation output of CT scanners. To measure the CTDI, a physicist will need an ionization chamber and two CTDI phantoms. These phantoms are made of polymethyl methacrylate (PMMA) and are either 16 cm or 32 cm in diameter for use in head and abdomen protocols, respectively. Each phantom contains five holes for insertion of the ionization chamber. One hole is located at the center of the phantom and four at different locations around the periphery. The CTDI is most commonly measured using a 100-mm-long cylindrical ionization chamber, and this special case is referred to as $CTDI_{100}$:

$$\mathrm{CTDI}_{100} = \frac{E * f * 100}{N * T} \tag{7.2}$$

where E is the exposure measured in a 100 mm ion chamber, f is a conversion factor from exposure to dose in air, N is the number of data channels used in the acquisition, and T is the thickness of each channel. Due to the nonuniform energy deposition, CTDI measurements are performed at both a central and a peripheral location in the phantom. Each value can be based on a single measurement, but best practice is to take an average of multiple measurements. Based on Eq. 7.2, CTDI_w is defined as a linear combination of the central and the peripheral measurements:

$$\mathrm{CTDI}_w = \frac{1}{3}\mathrm{CTDI}_{100,\text{center}} + \frac{2}{3}\mathrm{CTDI}_{100,\text{periphery}} \tag{7.3}$$

where $\mathrm{CTDI}_{100,\text{ center}}$ and $\mathrm{CTDI}_{100,\text{ periphery}}$ are the CTDI_{100} measurements taken from the center and periphery, respectively. To adapt this model to helical scans, $\mathrm{CTDI}_{\mathrm{vol}}$ is used. This model allows the measurement of the CTDI in a single axial rotation; however, it accounts for the pitch in a prescribed protocol:

$$\mathrm{CTDI}_{\mathrm{vol}} = \mathrm{CTDI}_w \frac{N * T}{I} \tag{7.4}$$

where I is the travel distance of the table per rotation of a helical scan. Although modern CT systems display CTDI values, it is important to verify the reliability of such readings. Beyond checking the accuracy of the reported CTDI, the output reproducibility and linearity should also be characterized. It is also important to note that the CTDI measurements are simply a characterization of the output of a CT system under standardized conditions and do not represent the dose delivered to a patient.

Exposure and Timer Characterization

Using the CTDI measurement setup defined in the previous section, it is possible to characterize the exposure and timer of a CT system. This includes testing for accuracy, reproducibility, and linearity. Given a set of acquisition parameters, it is essential to verify a scanner will produce a consistent exposure output that is linearly proportional to the tube current. Exposure should also respond linearly to an increase in rotation time. Furthermore, testing for timer accuracy helps ensure the tube is rotating at the expected speed.

A variety of methods can be used to measure the linearity, accuracy, and reproducibility of the CT system, the simplest of which is as follows: (1) acquire multiple datasets to test for reproducibility; (2) acquire data for at least two additional mA settings to test for linearity; and (3) acquire data at different tube rotation times with a constant mA to test for rotation timer accuracy. Each acquisition should be performed with the ion chamber in the same location. The exposure and exposure time should be recorded for each acquisition to evaluate (a) exposure linearity and reproducibility and (b) timing accuracy and linearity.

Following the characterization of system linearity and reproducibility, it is helpful to characterize the system at different tube voltages. This can be accomplished by repeating the same scanning protocol at different tube voltages. Prior to the acquisitions, one should record the manufacturer displayed $\mathrm{CTDI}_{\mathrm{vol}}$ so that it can be compared to the measurement $\mathrm{CTDI}_{\mathrm{vol}}$. In addition, it is worthwhile to compare the results to historical data to check for deviations from the prior evaluation.

Bow-Tie Filter Characterization

Another aspect of CT system dose characterization is the accuracy of CTDI measurements with different bow-tie filters. In general, accurate CTDI measurements with all available bow-tie filters, along with the above radiation output tests, signify a robust system output to within user-acceptable tolerance. However, bow-tie filter response characterization may not be a necessary test to perform apart from acceptance testing and/or after relevant system repairs.

Displayed $CTDI_{vol}$ Accuracy for Clinical Protocols

As it is not possible to measure image quality and verify dosimetry at each machine setting that could be used clinically, it is important to verify the accuracy of the displayed $CTDI_{vol}$ for a few select clinical protocols. Different accrediting bodies and states require the CTDI to be measured for a variety of protocols. Most commonly, the following protocols are evaluated: (1) adult head, (2) adult abdomen, (3) pediatric head, and (4) pediatric abdomen. However, additional protocol evaluation may be required. In North Carolina, for example, the radiation output and dose indices must also be evaluated for brain perfusion studies [14].

In order to measure the $CTDI_{vol}$ for a helical protocol, it must first be converted into that of a single axial slice. In most cases, three measurements are taken at the center position, and three measurements are taken in a periphery position. Subsequently, these measurements can be used in Eqs. 7.2, 7.3, and 7.4 to calculate the $CTDI_{vol}$.

Half-Value Layer and kVp

Half-value layer (HVL) and kVp measurements are not needed for the routine testing of a CT system unless required by regulation or done as part of a comprehensive physics evaluation or troubleshooting [9]. The HVL can be derived by measuring the change in exposure for added aluminum filters of different thicknesses and then calculating the thickness which reduces the exposure by a factor of one-half. This can be done with aluminum rings around an ionization chamber or with aluminum plates and the tube in a stationary position (e.g., localizer mode) [15]. Tube potential accuracy can also be tested noninvasively with a kV meter calibrated for CT or invasively with a high voltage divider [1].

Localizer Dose

While a CT localizer has lower dose than the diagnostic scans that follow, a physicist may nonetheless be interested in exposure measurements resulting from these low-dose scans. The simplest way to quantify the exposure from a CT localizer is to measure it in a similar fashion to a projection radiograph [16]. Although this test may be beneficial to perform during a CT system acceptance, it may not be necessary to perform on an annual basis.

Tube Current Modulation

A growing percentage of clinical CT acquisitions utilize tube current modulation (TCM). Although TCM has a large impact on dose and image quality, most traditional annual testing procedures do not address this aspect of a CT system. The goal of TCM is to provide consistent image quality by changing the tube current based on the attenuation of the patient. It is therefore important to characterize (a) how the tube output responds to different amounts of beam attenuation and (b) how TCM may affect changes in image quality.

It is essential to be able to characterize both the output of the tube and the resultant image quality when tube current modulation is activated. While there are many ways to simulate different patient thicknesses, the simplest way is to use a phantom that gradually changes in thickness. Another option is to place phantoms of differing sizes next to each other (e.g., the 32 cm and 16 cm CTDI phantoms). Ideally the phantom would also encapsulate image quality inserts so metrics beyond the noise can be measured.

Currently, there is no global standard for TCM. A simple TCM evaluation is to plot the CTDIvol (or effective mAs) and the water-equivalent diameter of the phantom as a function of slice location (Fig. 7.4). These values can be compared to historical data, as well as to other CT systems, to search for consistent trends and detect a potential anomaly. A simple image quality test is to take a noise measurement from an ROI in the center of each slice to evaluate the noise level as a function of the water-equivalent diameter of the phantom. Alternatively, a more advanced approach would be to incorporate image quality metrics beyond a noise measurement if a phantom with appropriate inserts is available [1, 17, 18].

Image Quality

Image quality assessment is an essential step of a CT system evaluation. A physicist needs to ensure that the images coming from a CT system are of appropriate quality for their designated task. Below, traditional measures of image quality are discussed as well as more advanced methods that are tailored specifically to clinical tasks.

CT Number Accuracy

A critical part of any CT performance evaluation is to ensure the accuracy of CT number values under typical imaging conditions. This is measured by imaging phantoms containing inserts with known CT numbers and measuring the mean and standard deviation of their CT number values (Fig. 7.5). The quantity of inserts and tolerances varies by phantom but should always include a water-equivalent insert. This should be repeated at different tube potentials to verify the CT numbers of water and air remain within the relevant tolerances.

CT Number Uniformity

CT numbers should also be uniform across the image. This can be tested by measuring the mean CT number in several ROIs distributed throughout a uniform section of a phantom. Given the radial nature of the CT acquisition and reconstruction, it is best practice to ensure that the measurement is performed at least two different radii (Fig. 7.6). Alternatively, the uniformity can be assessed by measuring the variation in CT number in profiles taken throughout the uniform section of the phantom.

Spatial Resolution

The spatial resolution of a CT scanner can be assessed using several different methods. A simple and common approach is to use a phantom with a series of high-contrast line pairs with progressively increasing spatial frequency. A human observer can assess the last resolvable insert and can obtain an estimate of the spatial resolution of that acquisition (Fig. 7.7). While this approach is simple, its interpretation is subjective, and its precision is fundamentally limited by the

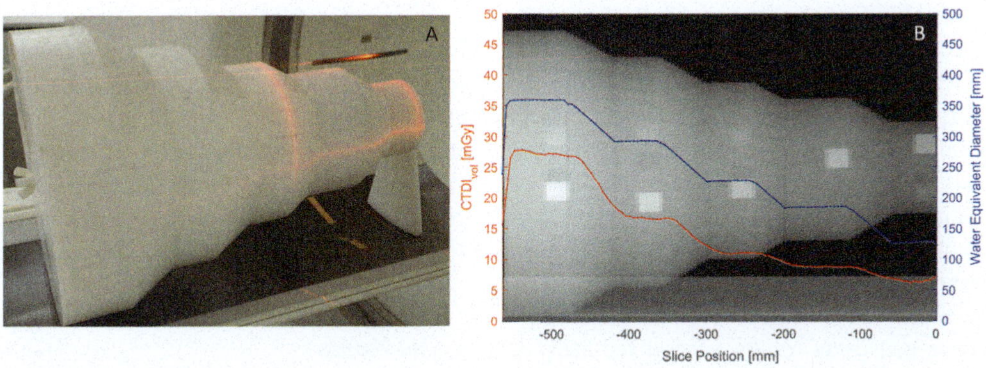

Fig. 7.4 Assessment of tube current modulation. The Mercury Phantom is used to evaluate the tube current modulation that contains sections of varying diameters made from polyethylene and image quality inserts (**a**). An example of the CTDI$_{vol}$ and water-equivalent diameter graphed as a function of slice position overlaid on the CT lateral localizer produced by ImQuest [19], a publicly available computer program (**b**)

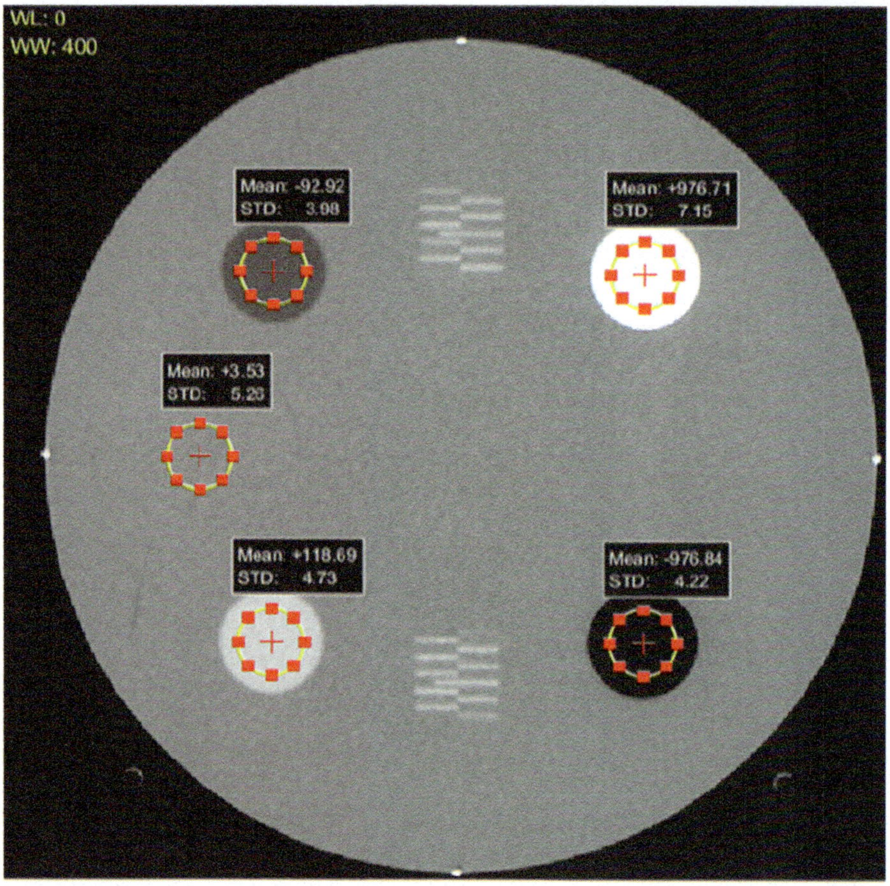

Fig. 7.5 CT number accuracy. CT number accuracy measurement. CT numbers are measured in phantom inserts made of various materials with known CT numbers. This phantom contains polyethylene, Teflon (bone equivalent), acrylic, and water-equivalent inserts as well as a cutout for air

finite number of inserts. A more comprehensive method is to measure the modulation transfer function (MTF) of the image. This is typically achieved by measuring the point spread function (PSF) [20], edge spread function (ESF) [21–23], or line spread function (LSF) [24, 25] of an object with known properties and applying Fourier analysis. A specialized phantom can be used, or an existing phantom can be repurposed provided it has a suitable geometry. While simple in principle, performing an MTF measurement requires special attention to phantom alignment and image noise. For consistent results, specialized analysis software is advised [22] (Fig. 7.8). When the MTF is used to characterize an imaging system, there is an implicit assumption that the system is linear and space invariant. This assumption is violated when iterative reconstruction techniques are used. In such cases, additional information such as the contrast, noise, and radial position of the measurement should be reported to complement the MTF. This method of characterizing the spatial resolution, also known as the task-transfer function or target transfer function [26, 27], provides a more comprehensive measure of CT performance when linearity assumptions are violated.

Image Noise

Similar to spatial resolution, there are several ways to measure noise during a performance evaluation. The simplest approach is to take

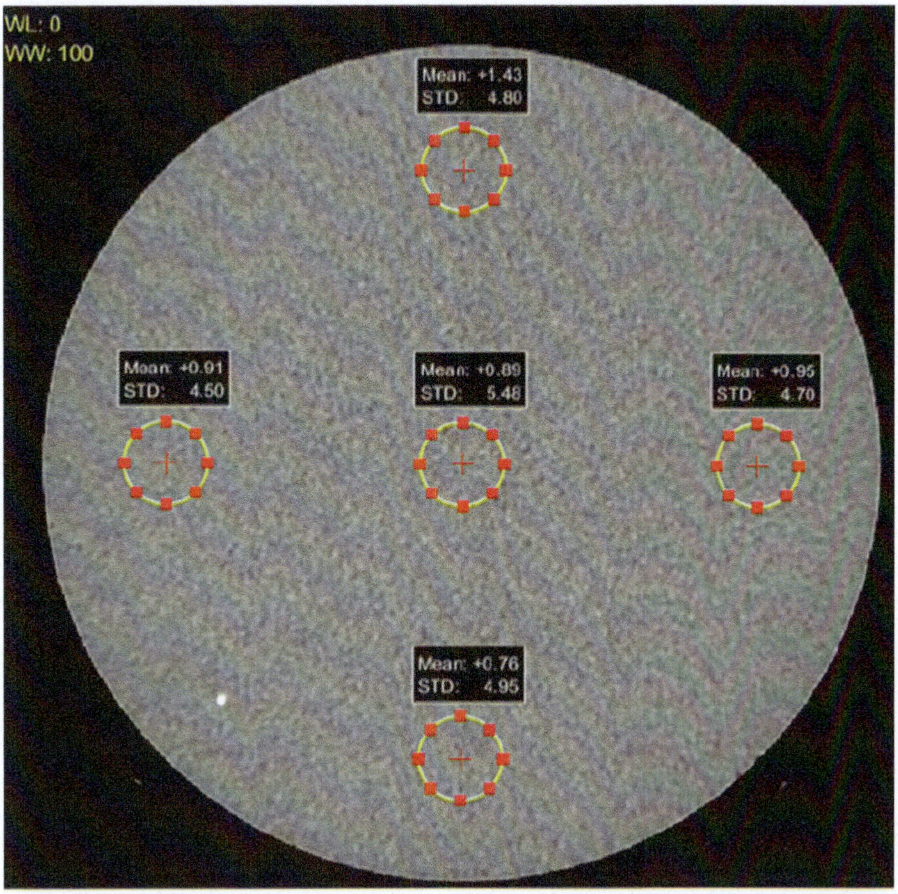

Fig. 7.6 CT number uniformity. CT number uniformity measurement. Five ROIs are placed throughout a uniform section of the phantom, and the ROI means are used to assess uniformity

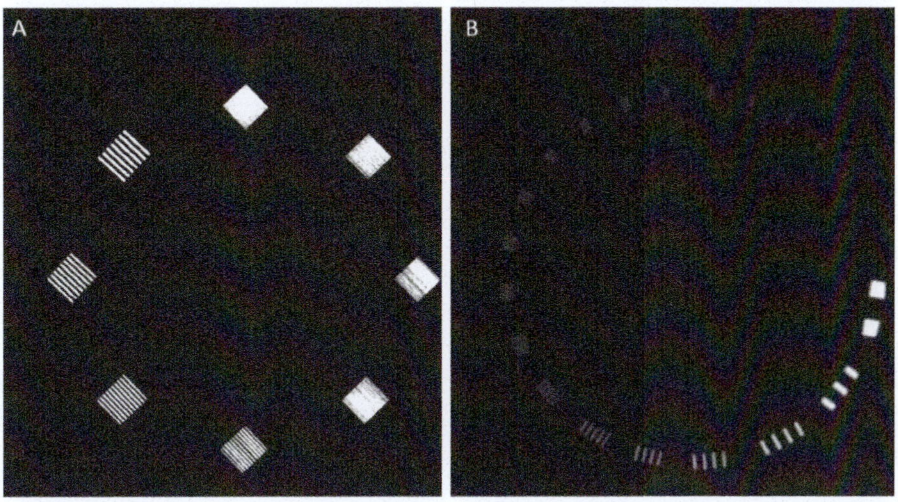

Fig. 7.7 Assessment of spatial resolution using line pair inserts. Two examples of high-contrast resolution measurement using line pair objects. A human observer assesses the last resolvable set of pairs which corresponds to the limiting spatial resolution

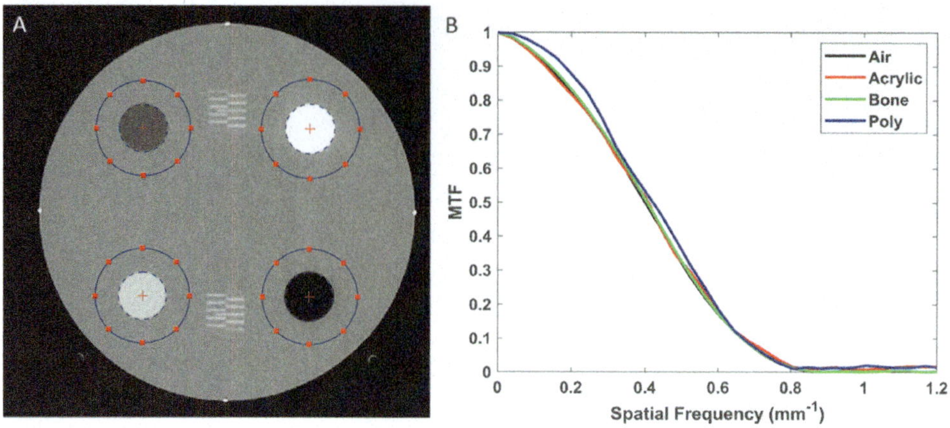

Fig. 7.8 Calculation of modulation transfer function. Measurement of the modulation transfer function (MTF). ROIs are placed around inserts at different contrast levels, and a computer program (ImQuest) [19] measures the edge spread function by exploiting the rotational symmetry of the inserts. (**a**) Fourier analysis is used to calculate the MTF for each insert (**b**)

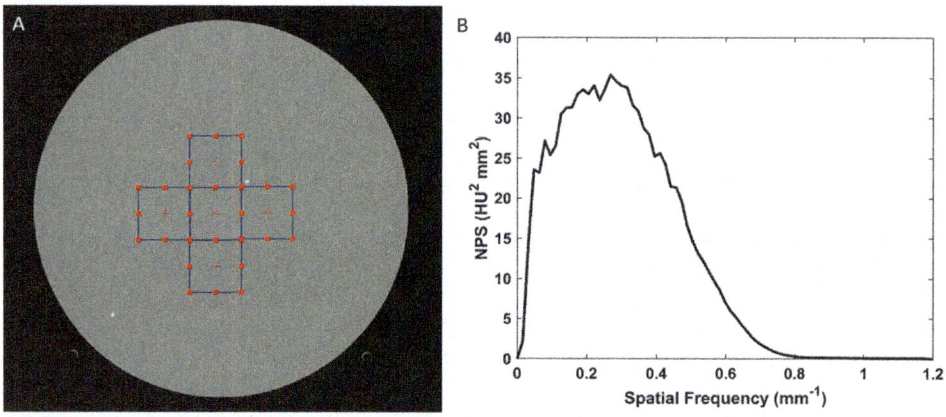

Fig. 7.9 Noise power spectrum. Measurement of the noise power spectrum (NPS). Five ROIs are placed in a uniform section of the phantom (the high-contrast fiducial is intentionally avoided) to average any rotational dependence (**a**). The Fourier transform is used to calculate the average NPS (**b**)

a large ROI in a uniform section of a phantom and calculate the standard deviation. While this is a simple and straightforward measurement, it only measures the magnitude of the noise without providing any information about the noise texture. With the increasing adoption of iterative reconstruction, the noise texture has taken on increased importance in clinical CT. Noise texture can be evaluated by calculating a noise power spectrum. This can be achieved by isolating the stochastic noise in a uniform section of phantom and taking the Fourier transform in as many dimensions as desired. This provides an assessment of noise texture (in areas with uniform signal) which better demonstrates the noise characteristics of iterative reconstructions (Fig. 7.9).

Low-Contrast Resolution

Another fundamental aspect of image quality is the ability to discern low-contrast objects. A basic assessment can be made by measuring the contrast to noise ratio in phantom inserts of known CT numbers. A more robust assessment can be made by performing the same measurement and qualitatively assessing visibility in a contrast-detail phantom containing a series of objects with different sizes and or contrast levels. For a given protocol and phantom, the low-contrast resolution should remain stable over time and meet the limits defined by the manufacturer, regulation, or accreditation program.

Artifact Evaluation

Artifact evaluation is naturally performed throughout the CT performance evaluation as the physicist reviews the images generated by the system. However, this assessment is best performed in a uniform section of phantom where there are no objects that may obfuscate the artifacts. The physicist should seek as large a phantom as is practical in order to assess the entire SFOV for artifacts (particularly in the case of ring artifacts). If a large phantom is not available, the physicist may consider scanning the smaller one off isocenter or acquiring an air scan. Dedicated acquisitions for artifact detection should be performed at the minimum slice thickness to increase the conspicuity of artifacts arising from faulty detector elements.

Task-Based Performance

One drawback of traditional measures of image quality is that they are independent of the clinical task for which an imaging study is designed. Without the context of specific clinical task, the concept of optimizing image quality is poorly defined. For example, it is clear that low-contrast detectability should be prioritized when trying to detect low-contrast liver lesions. However, it's unclear how important acquisition parameters – such as the dose, type of reconstruction, and reconstruction kernel – affect the ability of the human reader to perform this specific imaging task in a quantitative way. To allow for quantitative assessment of the effects that image quality has on the ability to perform clinical tasks, it is important for the physicist to consider evaluating task-based measures of scanner performance.

One approach to task-based performance is to calculate a metric which correlates well with increased performance of a task. For the task of low-contrast detectability, a common metric is called the detectability index, d'. The detectability index is a quantitative measure of an observer's ability to detect a particular signal, such as a low-contrast lesion, in a given image. The significance of d' can be understood by imagining a study where observers are presented many images where half contain the signal of interest and half do not. If the observers are asked to provide a score for each image that represents their confidence that the signal is present, two distributions can be constructed, one for images containing the signal and one for images not containing the signal. One can calculate d' from this data by taking the differences between the means divided by the square of their average variance:

$$d' = \frac{\mu_{\text{signal}} - \mu_{\text{no signal}}}{\sqrt{\frac{1}{2}\left(\sigma_{\text{signal}}^2 + \sigma_{\text{no signal}}^2\right)}} \tag{7.5}$$

Another way to conceptualize d' is to think of it as signal-to-noise ratio for the observer's ability to detect the signal. Similar to SNR, d' is a unitless quantity where high values indicate better detection task performance (Fig. 7.10).

Closer analysis of the hypothetical observer study reveals the three key components that are required for measuring d': a signal or detection task, an observer, and a model of the imaging chain. The observer study is logistically challenging because it requires construction of a physical phantom that represents the imaging task, substantial time commitment from human observers, and repeated imaging to build what is essentially a stochastic model of the imaging chain. This can be simplified by defining a mathematical model of the signal or task which is often referred to as the task function, W_{Task}, and utilizing a theoretical model of the imaging chain to synthesize images. A simple example of W_{Task} for the detection of a low-contrast mass may be the equation for a disk scaled for the appropriate size and contrast level. If one assumes a linear

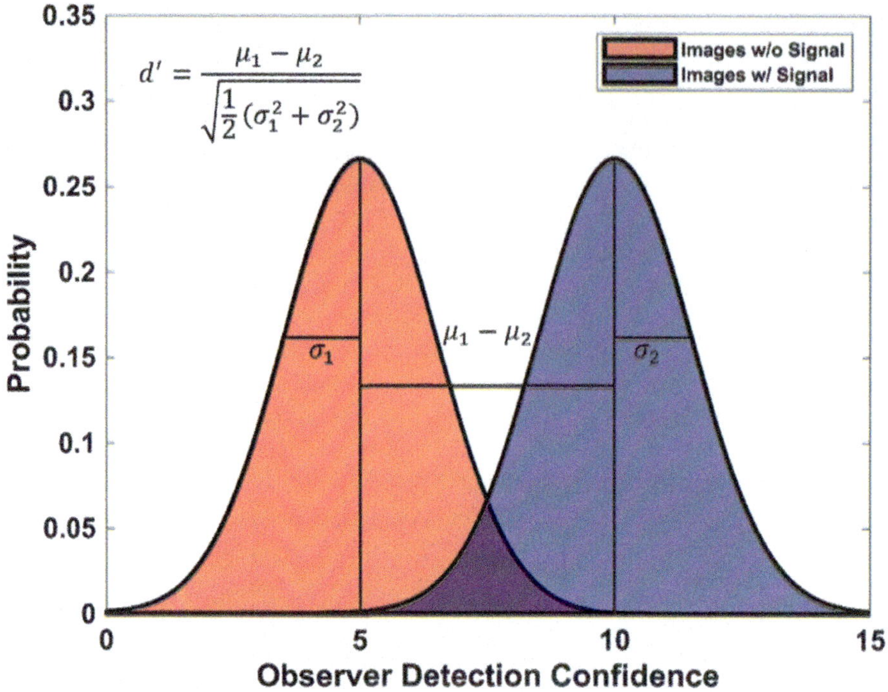

Fig. 7.10 Illustration of d'. In a hypothetical observer study where images are presented with and without a signal that is to be detected. The distance between the distributions of the observer's confidence in detecting the signal scaled by their variance is used to calculate d'. This value is used to quantify the detectability of the signal under specific imaging conditions

and space-invariant imaging system, the effects of the imaging chain can be modeled using only the modulation transfer function and noise power spectrum. The process of measuring d' can be further simplified by replacing the human observer with a machine observer. One straightforward machine observer model is the non-prewhitening matched filter which essentially performs a cross correlation or inner product between the image and the task function to provide a quantitative measure of the observer's ability to detect a signal. Using this approach, the equation for d' can be written in closed form as [28]:

$$d'^{2}_{\mathrm{NPW}} = \frac{\left[\iint \left|\hat{W}(u,v)\right|^{2} \cdot \mathrm{MTF}^{2}(u,v)\,\mathrm{dudv}\right]^{2}}{\iint \left|\hat{W}(u,v)\right|^{2} \cdot \mathrm{MTF}^{2}(u,v) \cdot \mathrm{NPS}(u,v)\,\mathrm{dudv}}. \quad (7.6)$$

where $\hat{W}(u,v), \mathrm{MTF}(u,v), \mathit{and}\ \mathrm{NPS}(u,v)$ are the Fourier transform of the task function, modulation transfer function, and noise power spectrum, respectively.

This approach is formulated entirely in the frequency domain using known transfer properties of the imaging system and eliminates the need to acquire images provided that the NPS and MTF are known. This makes measuring d' in this way a practical option for a physicist performing a CT evaluation if they elect to make MTF and NPS measurements and utilize freely available software for making the relevant calculations [19]. However, one should make sure to make the MTF and NPS measurements under conditions that closely match the task of interest as possible to minimize the effects of any nonlinearities that are not accounted for in the modeling of the imaging chain [28, 29].

One drawback of using this frequency-domain approach to calculating d' is that it is not well suited to spatially based tasks. For example, consider the case where an observer must detect a signal that could be located anywhere in an image. This is more representative of a real-life imaging task but precludes the use of single, simple task function and requires images to be acquired or synthesized. Specialized phantoms exist for these types of studies that typically contain a series of low-contrast objects to be identified and/or localized by a human or machine observer such as a template matching algorithm. Numerous study designs and analysis methods exist for these tasks depending on the complexity of the task. These range from something as simple as the localization success rate to a full analysis of free response operating characteristic curve [30, 31]. While inherently more complicated, assessing task-based performance in the spatial domain is more flexible and allows more realistic tasks. Like d', freely available software exists to assist with these analyses [19].

While assessing task-based performance is more complicated than many first-order measures of image quality, it provides valuable information for optimizing and comparing the performance of scanners, particularly when supporting a fleet of scanners from multiple vendors that contain variable technology.

Dual Energy

Dual energy CT is an advanced application that warrants special consideration by a physicist during a performance evaluation. In a dual energy exam, two distinct X-ray spectra are used to extract information about the energy dependence of the attenuation of materials. Several types of images can be calculated using post-processing techniques that are distinct from routine single energy images. For example, dual energy data can be used to quantify the density of pairs of materials provided that their energy-dependent X-ray absorption is sufficiently different (e.g., water vs. iodine). This material density data can be exploited for classification tasks, such as discrimination of urinary stone compositions [32–34], or quantification tasks, such as measuring iodine concentrations to aid in differential diagnosis [35–37]. Spectral information has also been used to synthesize virtual monoenergetic images at arbitrary keVs [38–41] that seek to remove polyenergetic spectral effects from images. Many vendors have also implemented virtual non-contrast images [42, 43] by reducing or removing the effects of iodine from contrast-enhanced acquisitions.

In general, there is considerable heterogeneity in the methods and hardware configurations used by different vendors to acquire dual energy data. A physicist should be familiar with the specific hardware and acquisition configuration on the scanner being evaluated and how this impacts protocol design. The frequency and clinical use of the dual energy protocols used at a particular site should also be well known. This information helps to inform additional evaluations that will need to be made for radiation output and image quality. Traditional image quality testing can be applied to both polyenergetic images and monoenergetic images. However, special attention should be given to the monoenergetic images since the additional image processing may significantly alter traditional image quality measures [44, 45].

A specialized phantom is required to properly evaluate the image quality of each of material density image. This phantom should contain inserts that mimic relevant materials (e.g., water, fat, iodine, etc.) at physiological concentrations. Many of the previously described image quality metrics can be evaluated using the same methods described in the previous section, albeit with different limits. Several types of phantoms meeting these criteria are commercially available.

The extent of the material density evaluation should be protocol specific. For protocols that require classification tasks, such as bone and iodine separation for angiography, one should verify that the relevant inserts are properly differentiated. For protocols that require accurate material quantification, the concentration of relevant elements should be accurate over the range of physiological concentrations. Given that dual energy CT is an emerging technology, there are currently no consensus standards for limits on associated tests. Ultimately, the physicists need to use their judgment in conjunction with vendor specifications and available scientific literature [45–47].

Theoretically, dosimetry data can be acquired in the typical manner for many of the dual energy implementations due to the energy independence of ionization chambers. However, physicists should familiarize themselves with the user interface to ensure that they are able to utilize dual energy functionality in axial mode. Additionally, if the scanner has a two-tube configuration, one may consider working with vendor-specific service engineers to test the tubes independently to verify all of the radiation output data is consistent with expectations.

Posttest Responsibilities

After completing a CT system evaluation, it is essential that the results are appropriately reported. If any problems are identified on the CT system rendering it unsafe, the appropriate staff members should be notified prior to the physicist leaving the site. Key personnel involved will vary depending on institutional regulations and guidelines.

While preparing the report, it is important to be mindful of the audience. While the bulk of the report should contain the data collected during the testing, it is important to provide a concise summary so hospital administrators and/or other laypersons can quickly understand the state of the CT system. If artifacts or image quality issues arise, it is appropriate to include relevant images in the report. If there are problems with the system, the report should include enough details so the engineering team can fully comprehend and reproduce the issue. A time frame indicating how soon the issue needs to be fixed should also be included for completeness. In addition to appropriate reporting, the report itself should be archived so it may be referenced for future regulatory or accreditation efforts. The physicist should also keep a copy to reference when performing future evaluations.

Clinical physics duties are not complete after the annual system evaluation. In particular, the physicist should also be actively involved in patient dose monitoring and protocol review. This can involve monitoring outliers or any dose alerts as well as analyzing general trends. This role should also involve regularly reviewing and updating clinical protocols to ensure proper dose levels and appropriate image quality to the population they serve.

References

1. Samei E, Bakalyar D, Boedeker K, Brady S, Fan J, Leng S, et al. Performance Evaluation of Computed Tomography Systems. American Association of Physicists in Medicine; Under Review. Report No.: 233.
2. Performance Standard for Ionizing Radiation Emitting Products. 21CFR. Sect. 1020.
3. Archer BR, Gray JE, Dixon R, Elde Jr. W, Hubbard L, Kearsely E, et al. Structural shielding design for diagnostic imaging facilities. NCRP; Report No.: 147.
4. Standard attributes on CT equipment related to dose optimization and management. NEMA. 2013. Report No.: XR-29.
5. Dillon C, Breeden III W, Clements J, Cody D, Gress D, Kanal K, et al. ACR CT quality control manual 2017. American College of Radiology; 2017.
6. Polacin A, Kalender WA, Brink J, Vannier MA. Measurement of slice sensitivity profiles in spiral CT. Med Phys. 1994;21(1):133–40.
7. Wang G, Vannier MW. Stair-step artifacts in three-dimensional helical CT: an experimental study. Radiology. 1994;191(1):79–83.
8. Greene TC, Rong XJ. Evaluation of techniques for slice sensitivity profile measurement and analysis. J Appl Clin Med Phys. 2014;15(2):4042.
9. Quality Assurance Programme for Computed Tomography: Diagnostic and Therapy Applications. International Atomic Energy Agency. 2016. (IAEA Human Health Series). Report No.: 19.
10. Evaluation and routine testing in medical imaging departments – part 3–5: acceptance tests – imaging performance of computed tomography X-ray equipment. International Electrotechnical Comission; 2004. (IEC Standards). Report No.: 61223–3.
11. Liu H-L, Liu RR, Reeve DM, Shepard SJ, Willis CE. Measurement of CT radiation profile width using CR imaging plates. Med Phys. 2005;32(9):2881–7.

12. Jackson SR, Ahmad S, Hu Y, Ruan C. Evaluation of different techniques for CT radiation profile width measurement. J Appl Clin Med Phys. 2013;14(4):4122.
13. Bjarnason TA, Yang CJ. CT radiation profile width measurement using CR imaging plate raw data. J Appl Clin Med Phys. 2015;16(6):501–7.
14. Computed tomography (CT) x-ray systems. NCAC. Sect. 15.0611.
15. Kruger RL, McCollough CH, Zink FE. Measurement of half-value layer in x-ray CT: a comparison of two noninvasive techniques. Med Phys. 2000;27(8):1915–9.
16. O'Daniel JC, Stevens DM, Cody DD. Reducing radiation exposure from survey CT scans. Am J Roentgenol. 2005;185(2):509–15.
17. International Commission on Radiation Units and Measurements. ICRU report no. 87: radiation dose and image-quality assessment in computed tomography. J ICRU. 2012;12(1):1–149.
18. Wilson JM, Christianson OI, Richard S, Samei E. A methodology for image quality evaluation of advanced CT systems. Med Phys. 2013;40(3):031908.
19. TG233 Resources [Internet]. [cited 2019 May 8]. Available from: http://deckard.mc.duke.edu/~samei/tg233.html.
20. Cruz-Bastida JP, Gomez-Cardona D, Li K, Sun H, Hsieh J, Szczykutowicz TP, et al. Hi-res scan mode in clinical MDCT systems: experimental assessment of spatial resolution performance. Med Phys. 2016;43(5):2399–409.
21. Chen B, Christianson O, Wilson JM, Samei E. Assessment of volumetric noise and resolution performance for linear and nonlinear CT reconstruction methods. Med Phys. 2014;41(7):071909.
22. Friedman SN, Fung GSK, Siewerdsen JH, Tsui BMW. A simple approach to measure computed tomography (CT) modulation transfer function (MTF) and noise-power spectrum (NPS) using the American College of Radiology (ACR) accreditation phantom. Med Phys. 2013;40(5):051907.
23. Cunningham IA, Fenster A. A method for modulation transfer function determination from edge profiles with correction for finite-element differentiation. Med Phys. 1987;14(4):533–7.
24. Boone JM. Determination of the presampled MTF in computed tomography. Med Phys. 2001;28(3):356–60.
25. Judy PF. The line spread function and modulation transfer function of a computed tomographic scanner. Med Phys. 1976;3(4):233–6.
26. Richard S, Husarik DB, Yadava G, Murphy SN, Samei E. Towards task-based assessment of CT performance: system and object MTF across different reconstruction algorithms. Med Phys. 2012;39(7):4115–22.
27. Robins M, Solomon J, Richards T, Samei E. 3D task-transfer function representation of the signal transfer properties of low-contrast lesions in FBP- and iterative-reconstructed CT. Med Phys. 2018;45(11):4977–85.
28. Monnin P, Marshall NW, Bosmans H, Bochud FO, Verdun FR. Image quality assessment in digital mammography: part II. NPWE as a validated alternative for contrast detail analysis. Phys Med Biol. 2011;56(14):4221–38.
29. Ott JG, Becce F, Monnin P, Schmidt S, Bochud FO, Verdun FR. Update on the non-prewhitening model observer in computed tomography for the assessment of the adaptive statistical and model-based iterative reconstruction algorithms. Phys Med Biol. 2014;59(15):4047–64.
30. Verdun FR, Racine D, Ott JG, Tapiovaara MJ, Toroi P, Bochud FO, et al. Image quality in CT: from physical measurements to model observers. Phys Med. 2015;31(8):823–43.
31. Nonparametric signal detectability evaluation using an exponential transformation of the FROC curve – Popescu – 2011 – Medical Physics – Wiley Online Library [Internet]. [cited 2019 May 5]. Available from: https://aapm.onlinelibrary.wiley.com/doi/full/10.1118/1.3633938.
32. Primak AN, Fletcher JG, Vrtiska TJ, Dzyubak OP, Lieske JC, Jackson ME, et al. Noninvasive differentiation of uric acid versus non–uric acid kidney stones using dual-energy CT. Acad Radiol. 2007;14(12):1441–7.
33. Eiber M, Holzapfel K, Frimberger M, Straub M, Schneider H, Rummeny EJ, et al. Targeted dual-energy single-source CT for characterisation of urinary calculi: experimental and clinical experience. Eur Radiol. 2012;22(1):251–8.
34. Boll DT, Patil NA, Paulson EK, Merkle EM, Simmons WN, Pierre SA, et al. Renal stone assessment with dual-energy multidetector CT and advanced postprocessing techniques: improved characterization of renal stone composition—pilot study. Radiology. 2009;250(3):813–20.
35. Mileto A, Marin D, Alfaro-Cordoba M, Ramirez-Giraldo JC, Eusemann CD, Scribano E, et al. Iodine quantification to distinguish clear cell from papillary renal cell carcinoma at dual-energy multidetector CT: a multireader diagnostic performance study. Radiology. 2014;273(3):813–20.
36. Zarzour JG, Milner D, Valentin R, Jackson BE, Gordetsky J, West J, et al. Quantitative iodine content threshold for discrimination of renal cell carcinomas using rapid kV-switching dual-energy CT. Abdom Radiol. 2017;42(3):727–34.
37. Kaza RK, Caoili EM, Cohan RH, Platt JF. Distinguishing enhancing from nonenhancing renal lesions with fast kilovoltage-switching dual-energy CT. Am J Roentgenol. 2011;197(6):1375–81.
38. Pomerantz SR, Kamalian S, Zhang D, Gupta R, Rapalino O, Sahani DV, et al. Virtual monochromatic reconstruction of dual-energy unenhanced head CT at 65–75 keV maximizes image quality compared with conventional polychromatic CT. Radiology. 2013;266(1):318–25.
39. Wichmann JL, Nöske E-M, Kraft J, Burck I, Wagenblast J, Eckardt A, et al. Virtual monoenergetic dual-energy computed tomography: optimization of kiloelectron volt settings in head and neck cancer. Investig Radiol. 2014;49(11):735–41.

40. Schneider D, Apfaltrer P, Sudarski S, Nance JW, Haubenreisser H, Fink C, et al. Optimization of kiloelectron volt settings in cerebral and cervical dual-energy CT angiography determined with virtual monoenergetic imaging. Acad Radiol. 2014;21(4):431–6.
41. Yu L, Leng S, McCollough CH. Dual-energy CT–based monochromatic imaging. Am J Roentgenol. 2012;199(5_supplement):S9–15.
42. Graser A, Johnson TRC, Hecht EM, Becker CR, Leidecker C, Staehler M, et al. Dual-energy CT in patients suspected of having renal masses: can virtual nonenhanced images replace true nonenhanced images? Radiology. 2009;252(2):433–40.
43. Ferda J, Novák M, Mírka H, Baxa J, Ferdová E, Bednářová A, et al. The assessment of intracranial bleeding with virtual unenhanced imaging by means of dual-energy CT angiography. Eur Radiol. 2009;19(10):2518–22.
44. Yu L, Christner JA, Leng S, Wang J, Fletcher JG, McCollough CH. Virtual monochromatic imaging in dual-source dual-energy CT: radiation dose and image quality. Med Phys. 2011;38(12):6371–9.
45. Jacobsen MC, Schellingerhout D, Wood CA, Tamm EP, Godoy MC, Sun J, et al. Intermanufacturer comparison of dual-energy CT iodine quantification and monochromatic attenuation: a phantom study. Radiology. 2017;287(1):224–34.
46. Nute JL, Jacobsen MC, Stefan W, Wei W, Cody DD. Development of a dual-energy computed tomography quality control program: characterization of scanner response and definition of relevant parameters for a fast-kVp switching dual-energy computed tomography system. Med Phys. 2018;45(4):1444–58.
47. Jacobsen MC, Cresssman EN, Tamm EP, Baluya D, Duan X, Cody DD, et al. Dual-energy CT: lower limits of iodine detection and quantification. Radiology. 2019;292:414–9.

CT Performance Optimization

8

Justin Solomon and Ehsan Samei

Introduction

From a mathematical perspective, optimization is the process of finding the minimum or maximum value of a function of several variables subject to a set of constraints. This definition should be familiar to anyone working in artificial intelligence (i.e., machine learning). The training process of a machine learning model is an optimization problem in which the parameters of the model are iteratively updated until the "utility function" (e.g., percent correctly classified) is maximized. For radiology, a useful definition of "optimize" is to maximize the utility of the imaging examination across a population of patients. The utility of an imaging examination is maximized if the patients receive the greatest possible net benefit of the examination considering the probabilities of all positive and negative outcomes. Their long-term benefit depends on a number of factors including:

- Appropriateness – How well are patients indicated to receive the imaging examination in question?
- Image quality – How much information is encoded in the images about the disease state of the patients?
- Risk – What negative consequences could the patient experience as a result of undergoing the imaging examination?
- Interpretation – How well do the radiologists (and/or automated image analysis systems) extract the information provided by the images?
- Management – How well are the findings from the imaging examination communicated to and utilized by the broader healthcare team to care for the patient?

Based on the above definition of optimization, we can think of the utility function of an imaging examination as being some appropriately weighted combination of all these listed factors (Fig. 8.1). For example, as the image quality increases, you would expect the utility of the examination to also increase, and conversely as the risk increases, you would expect the utility to decrease. Therefore, to truly optimize an imaging examination, we need to know precisely how the entire process of ordering, acquiring, and interpreting the images affects each of these factors and how the factors should be combined to compute a final measure of utility.

In practice, because of the high-dimensional, complex, and uncertain nature of the problem, this holistic optimization process is never formally performed. Most of the radiology scientific literature on this topic focuses on just the balance between

J. Solomon
Department of Radiology, Duke University Health System, Durham, NC, USA
e-mail: justin.solomon@duke.edu

E. Samei (✉)
Department of Radiology, Duke University, Durham, NC, USA
e-mail: ehsan.samei@duke.edu

© Springer Nature Switzerland AG 2020

E. Samei, N. J. Pelc (eds.), *Computed Tomography*, https://doi.org/10.1007/978-3-030-26957-9_8

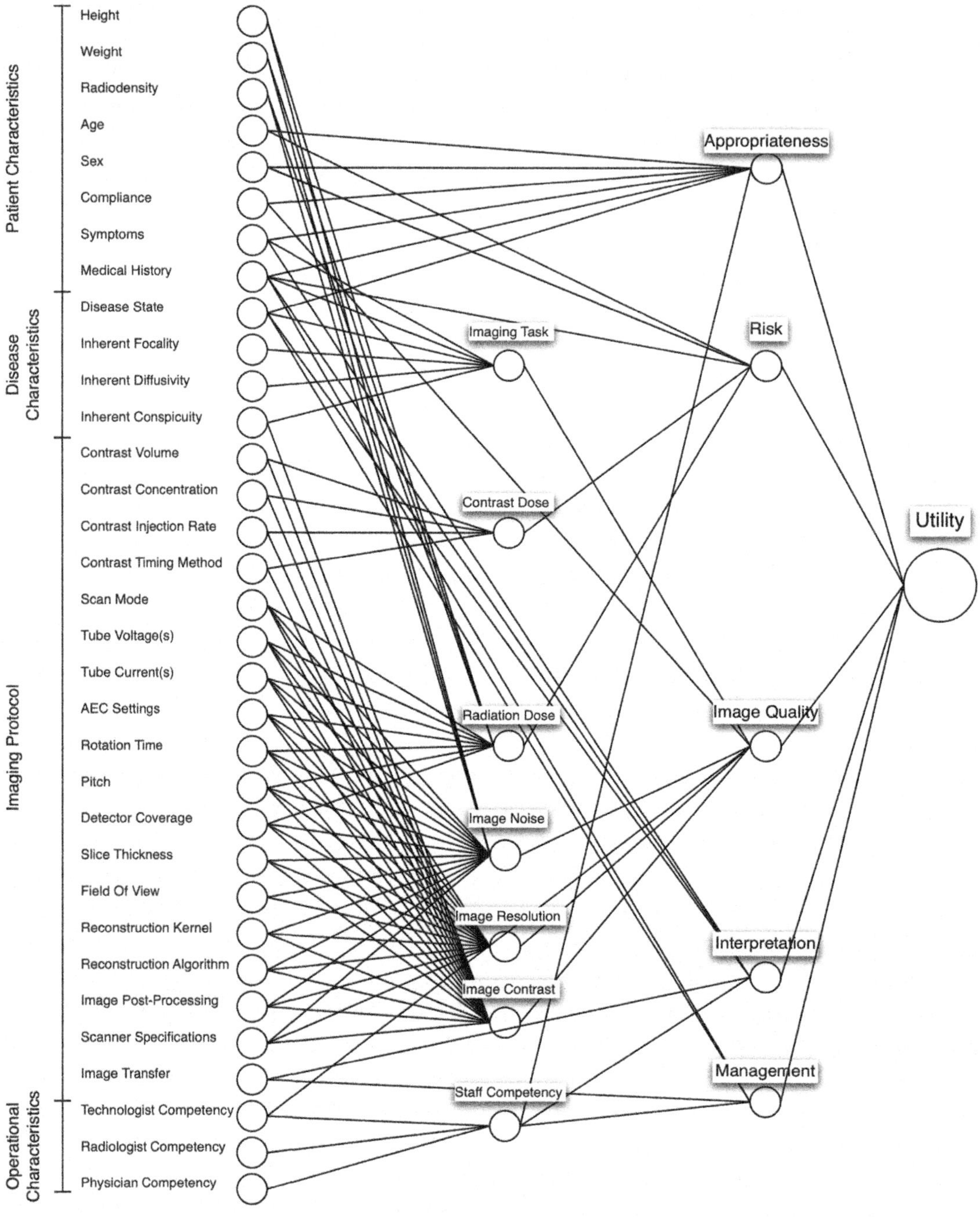

Fig. 8.1 A hypothetical neural network demonstrating how the final utility of an imaging examination is highly dependent on many factors. Note that this diagram is not meant to be comprehensive but rather an example

image quality and the risk from radiation exposure, and it is generally understood that increasing the radiation dose improves image quality but also increases risk. Thus, a balance must be found. The term "optimize" is found in many CT-related journal articles and conference abstracts but is most often used in a more colloquial sense to mean that some balance of imaging settings was found that

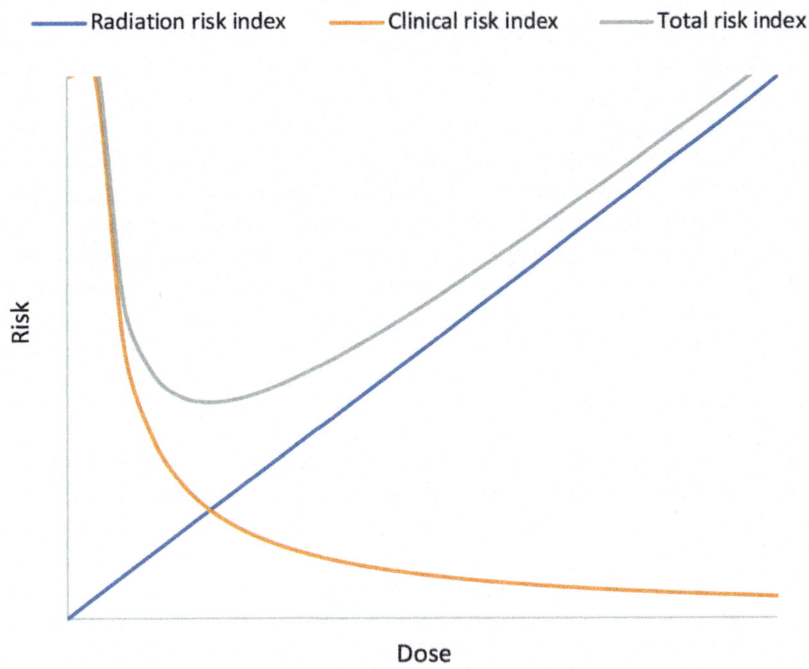

Fig. 8.2 Hypothetical plot of risk vs radiation dose. The minimum of the total risk index would be the optimal operating point

produced acceptable image quality at radiation dose levels that were also considered acceptable [1–4]. In other words, what is deemed as acceptable is often described as optimal. In some papers, a utility function is implied and/or discussed as a benefit-to-risk ratio (or conversely as a risk-to-benefit cost function), but a true benefit-to-risk analysis is never really performed in practice. This chapter follows this tradition and focuses primarily on the trade-offs between image quality and dose. However, it should be acknowledged that this focus is fundamentally incomplete and there is a need for a more holistic mathematical framework which allows for true optimization of the entire imaging examination process. In a recent paper, Barrett et al. laid out the mathematical framework needed to truly optimize imaging settings with respect to image quality and radiation dose [5]. This chapter builds on that framework with a more applied/practical focus.

Framework for CT Optimization

CT optimization is best to be understood not simply in terms of dose reduction or even the balance between dose and quality, rather as a balance between radiation safety and safety in not acquiring an image that provides compromised diagnostic performance. In approaching optimization, one useful concept is to think of a plot of total risk as a function of radiation dose (Fig. 8.2) [6]. In this case the total risk is composed of a "clinical risk index" and a "radiation risk index." The clinical risk index encodes image quality and describes unwanted patient outcomes that could occur if the examination is either not performed or the images aren't of sufficient quality to make a diagnosis. It could also include other non-radiation risks from the examination such as an adverse reaction to iodine contrast. The radiation risk index includes potential adverse effects from the radiation exposure. The total risk index is the combination of the radiation and clinical risk indices. Figure 8.2 shows an example of what such a plot might look like and the optimal operating point would be at the minimum of the total risk index.

To begin to construct such a plot, we need task-based measurements of image quality that are related to how well the images can be used for their diagnostic purpose, and we also need measures of radiation dose and derived indices that are related to the potential risk of adverse effects. Both of these topics are discussed in more detail in other chapters of this book and thus will only be discussed superficially in this chapter. In practice, both measures of image quality and radiation dose can be estimated prospectively from phantom data and/or retrospectively from monitoring systems. Both prospective and retrospective analysis are needed to perform any robust optimization.

Ascertaining the dependencies of image quality and dose provide the knowledge of how the associated risks relate to one another, and thus how the two may need to be balanced in the context of an individual patient care. That knowledge enables one to make informed decisions and adjustments to the acquisition parameters or CT techniques to achieve certain desired goals or operating points. This enables the practitioner to minimize the dose for any given examination while simultaneously safeguarding its clinical utility.

Radiation Risk Quantification

The simplest metrics of dose in CT are CTDI and DLP. Their dependency on scan parameters is reasonably established as that is currently part of the expected setup for literally all fan-beam CT systems; changes in mA, for example, involves a linear effect on CTDI and DLP, the slope of which is dependent on kV and pitch. However, as convenient as that might be, these widely used scanner output dose indices reflect only dose in specific-sized cylindrical phantoms and are naïve to patient specifics (e.g., size, age, anatomy, gender), scatter dose properties, and protocol [7].

The newer metric of size-specific dose estimate (SSDE) addresses the size limitation of CTDI [8]. With the established relationship between the scanner factors and CTDI, SSDE can be readily derived by applying a nonlinear size correction factor. A more complete metrology, taking into consideration of the actual patient volume being exposed, is imparted energy [9], which, while being more patient representative and modality-generic than CTDI or SSDE, does not account for varying tissue sensitivities. Taking tissue sensitivities into consideration, effective dose (E) can be used in optimization approaches [10]. A significant advantage of E is its applicability to the radiation burden to the entire body and its cross-modality applicability. However, it is only applicable to a reference patient, estimated using DLP to E conversion factors (the k factors) derived for specific-sized body habitus. In this way, the inherent limitations of CTDI, propagated to the SSDE, DLP, and E, would still persist, while E still offers improvements over CTDI and DLP for optimization purposes.

While the above metrics conveniently offer a single value reflection of dose, they are far removed from the actual radiation burden to the patient. An ideal metric should be reflective of the complexity of dose distribution, be more directly related to the dose burden, and offer an indication of image safety in communicating relevance of dose in numbers that are intuitive and meaningful to the majority of stakeholders: patients, clinicians, regulators, and manufacturers. Organ dose provides a patient-centric indicator of the radiation burden to the patient. The dependency of scan factor to organ dose can be established by relating CTDI to organ dose conversion factor (so-called h-indices) [11]. Those factors are highly protocol and size dependent, which should be taken into consideration. One key limitation of organ dose, however, is that for the purpose of optimization, a singular metric need to be identified, either through risk estimation methods or through identifying dose to a single organ as the limiting metric for optimization purposes (e.g., breast dose in female patients undergoing chest CT).

A given CT examination naturally involves the irradiation of multiple organs (which vary in size and position in patients). The multiplicity of organs and organ doses suggest a need for a supra-organ indicator that incorporates all the organ doses into a single metric of radiation burden for the entire body. E, calculated from organ doses, can serve that function, with the acknowledged limitation that E is technically defined for a reference human model and does

	CTDI or DLP	SSDE	Organ Dose	Effective Dose	Imparted Energy	Effective Risk
Physical quantity	●	⊙	⊙		●	
Derived quantity				●		●
Accounting for:						
Scanner model	●	●	●	●	●	●
Protocol parameters	●	●	●	●	●	●
Patient Size		●	⊙	⊙	⊙	⊙
Organ-level dose			●	⊙	⊙	⊙
Patient age			⊙			●
Patient gender			⊙			●
Patient total burden				●	●	●

Fig. 8.3 Summary of the attributes and incorporating factors of currently available metrics for CT radiation exposure (KEY: ● = Yes – accounted for; ⊙ = Possibly – depending on the implementation)

not take into consideration patient gender and age [10]. An extension of E has been envisioned, so-called risk index [12], with added dependencies of age and gender. RI can be derived by protocol and size-dependent DLP to RI conversion factors.

All surrogates and their dependencies noted above have their inherent limitations (Fig. 8.3). However, regardless of what metric is used, a surrogate of radiation burden is essential if one is to practically approach the aim of CT dose optimization.

Clinical Risk Quantification

As dose is related to radiation risk, it should also be related to clinical risk through image quality metrics. These metrics fall into multiple categories, performance-based, preference-based, phantom-based, and study-based. In performance-based metrology, CT image quality is characterized in terms of the ability of a group of observers to visualize specific abnormalities of interest in groups of images [13, 14]. While objective, this metric of image quality is inefficient for use for optimization purposes as every scan setting requires multiplicity of images with ground truth, something that is more appropriate for research purposes than clinical settings. Preference-based aesthetic metrics offer a rapid characterization of image quality, which can further be quantified and analyzed with statistical methods. However, this method is fundamentally subjective and prone to bias as it is primarily influenced by the bias of the observer. However, it can readily be ascertained using simple observer feedback to scan factor changes [15, 16].

More quantitative and efficient, the phantom-derived, first-order statistics of contrast and noise magnitude form the CNR. Based on a popular model of lesion detection [17] [8], CNR provides a reflection of image quality [17]. The CNR is directly influenced by mA, but also to a lesser extent by kV and pitch. The reconstruction kernel also has a strong influence on the CNR. These dependencies can readily be evaluated efficiently using phantom measurements. However, CNR does not include texture and sharpness attributes of image quality, which also influence detection. Those attributes, particularly when iterative reconstructions are used, can be captured by second-order metrics of quality [18]. These metrics include noise texture in terms of the NPS [13] and resolution in terms of the TTF [13, 19, 20]. Together along with a definition of a task, NPS and TTF can be used to derive a detectability index. This metrology can accommodate a multiplicity of tasks, ranging from the detection of lesions of different size and morphology to newer ones defined for estimation and classification purposes [21, 22] (Fig. 8.5). Depending on the theories of how human visual system perceives image features against varying backgrounds, a host of such indices has been devised, many of which have been of effective utility for CT dose optimization [21, 23, 24].

	Observer-based Performance	Observer-based Preference	Phantom-based CNR	Phantom-based Detectability	Study-based Detectability
Objective	●		●	●	●
Patient specific	●	●		⊙	●
Indication specific	●	●		●	●
Efficient		●	●	●	⊙

Fig. 8.4 Summary of the attributes and incorporating factors of currently available metrics for CT image quality (KEY: ● = Yes – accounted for; ⊙ = Possibly – depending on the implementation)

Considering the inherent limitation of phantom-based methods [25] and complexity of clinical image-based assessment techniques, there have been recent innovations in measuring image quality based on features of individual patient images [26–29]. This strategy, deriving toward a study-based index of detectability, is highly relevant as it provides a depiction of quality for individual cases, getting closer to a metric that is more reflective of the ideal image quality: clinical-based and relevant to individual images. Such metrics alleviate some of the limitations of other metrics in being cohort-based, subjective, or simplistic. However, it needs a computational resource.

These surrogates of image quality and their attributes are listed in Fig. 8.4. Just as in case of radiation burden, regardless of what metric is used, however, a surrogate of image quality for the benefit region of the optimization framework is essential if one is to practically approach the aim of CT dose optimization.

Optimization Dependency and Operating Points

Ascertaining the risk and benefit dependences, the optimization dependencies can then be established. Figure 8.5 offers a depiction of how image quality and dose surrogates can be related to one another in the context of pediatric patients of varying age and size. The relationships were ascertained for a given size patient based on the 50th percentile size for that age [30]. In this example, a reference task was defined in terms of the detection of a 3–5 mm solitary lesion in the thoracic cavity. The lesion detection was measured thru a performance-based ROC metrology at multiple dose levels and the data fit to analytical equations.

A comprehensive optimization undertaking may include all scan factors that influence the balance of image quality and radiation dose. But for this demonstrative example, it was assumed that all scan parameters other than mA and its governing associated settings (e.g., noise index in GE scanners and reference effective mAs in Siemens) were chosen reasonably optimum based on non-dose constraints: kV set based on the desired contrast, pitch and scan time based on needed acquisition speed, and reconstruction based on the preferred image appearance. The dose variation was achieved through changes in the mA setting of the imaging system (through a validated noise addition software which alleviated the need for repeated exposure of patients). The dose settings were then related to four different surrogates of radiation dose – CTDI, SSDE, effective dose, and risk index.

Certain trends are readily generalizable. Regardless of the metric of dose applied, for each patient group, there is an asymptotic relationship between image quality and dose. As dose increases, the image quality increases as well. However, the rate of increase diminishes with the continued increase in dose, approaching a plateau at higher dose levels. The curves corresponding to larger older patients tend to be lower with the plateau approached at higher dose settings. The curves also tend to be closer to one another when the patient age is taken into consideration in the context of risk index.

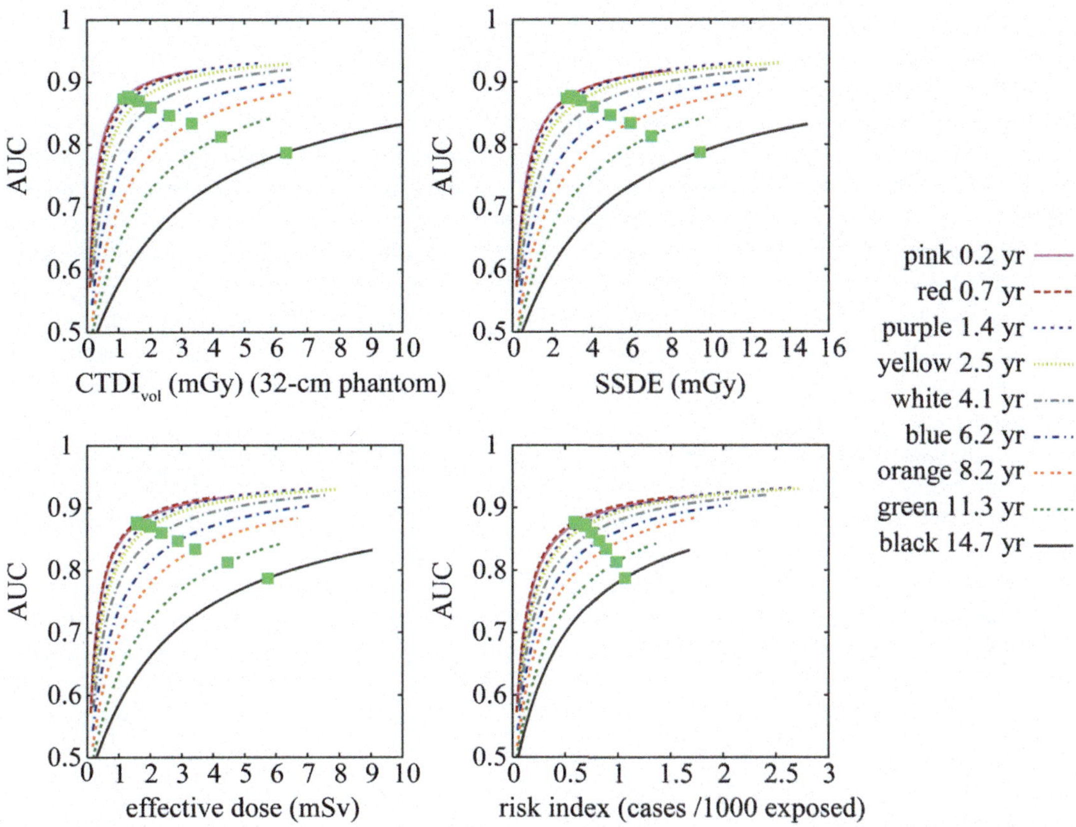

Fig. 8.5 The relationship between image quality and radiation dose indicators across patient sizes. Such dependencies can be the basis of dose/quality optimization by enabling the operator to select an operating point (points shown) defining an optimum ratio of quality per safety surrogate

As the data in Fig. 8.4 show, for a given imaging technique, with any dose reduction, there is a reduction in the inherent quality of the image. The example of Fig. 8.4 provides the necessary knowledge regarding the exact attributes of this dependency. However, once such dependencies are ascertained, establishing the operating points is a necessary follow-up task. The operating point(s) refer to the exact values of the scan factors (i.e., collectively, the protocol) for a given patient that should be used to achieve specific operating targets on the quality-dose continuum.

Discerning the operating targets should be based on the basic principle of dose optimization: reducing dose yet preventing a degradation of image quality that would negatively influence a clinical decision. So certain degrees of degradation are defensible provided there is no negative *clinical* impact. However, that requires the establishment of a minimum level or range of image qualities as a function of indication (e.g., a certain lesion size and contrast to be detectable with a certain degree of statistical significance). This is a clinical task that has not yet been methodically undertaken based on medical evidence.

In lieu of full clinical evidence, the operating points might be selected based on various criteria. One approach is to select protocols based on adherence to targeted diagnostic reference levels, for example a sub-mSv target. This approach is somewhat misguided as it falls short of properly considering the very purpose of imaging-dosing in the first place: achieving image quality for a clinical purpose. Alternatively, one may target adherence to specific diagnostic quality for particular abnormalities. This is perhaps a better strategy. However, as examples of Fig. 8.10 show, this strategy can lead to high doses for larger patients. Furthermore, clinical practice often demonstrates different visibility criteria for different sized patients.

An alternative strategy to the above two extremes is to target operating points in the relatively stable zones of the image quality-dose continuums, where image quality remains relatively stable as dose is varied. This approach is an implementation of the ALARA principles. It can be argued that if the operating point is in the high-slope zone of the continuum, small changes in dose or patient specifics can have marked effect on image quality. Thus such operating points will not lead to robust clinical operation. Conversely, if the points are selected to be in the plateau portions of the continuum, the increase in dose to such a level of quality has marginally limited impact on image quality. Thus such points would also be put an unnecessary burden to the patient for questionable diagnostic gain.

Avoiding the above two extremes, an iso-gradient condition can provide a justifiable balance between image quality and dose, such that image quality is reasonably stable, and dose is not excessively high for marginal improvement in image quality. The operating points in Fig. 8.10 provide a depiction of such iso-gradient optimizations. Exactly what gradient (or slope) one may choose can be operator selected. However, once such "bang-for-the-buck" criterion is established, one may apply justifiably consistent operating points across multiple patient cohorts, protocols, and tasks to achieve optimum performance [23].

The CT Protocol Review Process

What Is a CT Imaging Protocol?

For the purposes of this chapter, a protocol refers to a list of instructions containing *all* the information needed for the technologists to perform the CT examination [31]. This includes:

- Demographics – Clinical indication, age, and body habitus
- Patient setup – Patient positioning (e.g., head-first supine), breathing instructions, anatomical coverage
- IV contrast administration – Volume, concentration, rate, IV gauge, scan delay timing method (e.g., fixed, bolus tracking, or test bolus)
- EKG gating setup – Prospective or retrospective where applicable
- Scan acquisition settings – Scan type, kV, mA/mAs/effective mAs, collimation, pitch, rotation time, automatic exposure control method + settings
- Image reconstruction settings – Slice thickness, field of view, reconstruction algorithm/kernel, special reconstruction processing (e.g., metal artifact reduction)
- Image post processing – Sagittal or coronal reformatted images, maximum intensity projections, 3D volume rendering, quantitative processing (e.g., perfusion maps)
- Image transfer – Network destination (e.g., PACS)
- Expected radiation dose range – Typical and upper limits on the expected radiation dose indices from the examination

The list above may not be fully comprehensive, but most CT protocols should contain at least this information.

Review Process

The American Association of Physicist in Medicine (AAPM), the American College of Radiology (ACR) CT accreditation program, and The Joint Commission (TJC) have all stated that CT protocols should be reviewed by a team of medical physicists, radiologists, and CT technologists. This team is responsible for ensuring that protocols are at least safe, and hopefully optimal. The majority of the work in this review process is done by the medical physicist, and the AAPM has published a practice guideline as a starting point [31]. The ACR and TJC accreditation requirements seem to be largely based on these AAPM guidelines. It is not the intent of this chapter to rehash that content but rather to outline some practical steps that can be taken to work toward more optimal protocols. The author's institution has adopted a process with three major steps:

1. Standard checklist – Review the protocol for overall safety using a checklist of common sense guidelines based on accepted national standards.
2. Achieving consistency – Adjust protocols to achieve consistent performance across the health system's operation.
3. Toward optimality – Adjust the protocols to achieve more optimal performance with respect to radiation dose and image quality.

Note that each step is dependent on the previous step and should be taken in order. For example, it doesn't make sense to do detailed adjustments of a protocol that is a grossly ill-conceived based on accepted national standards for the exam type. It also doesn't make sense to try and optimize a protocol across a fleet of potentially different CT scanner models until you can first ensure that you are getting consistency across the fleet. Each of these steps is discussed in detail below.

Standard Checklists

The checklist below is based on the standards from the ACR CT accreditation program [32] and the TJC accreditation standards [33]. It also calls for a comparison with standard protocols available from the AAPM [34]. These items should be reviewed one by one by the medical physicist, and any suggested changes should be discussed and confirmed with radiologists and technologists.

- TJC
  - Protocol addresses key criteria, including:
    - Clinical indication
    - Contrast administration
    - Age
    - Patient size and body habitus
    - Expected radiation dose index range
  - Input on this protocol has been received from:
    - Interpreting radiologist
    - Medical physicist
    - Lead technologist
- ACR
  - A typical protocol should include the following elements:
    - Indication
    - Phase of respiration
    - Anatomical coverage
    - IV contrast (if applicable):
      - Injection rate
      - Scan delay
    - EKG gating policy
    - Scanner acquisition settings:
      - kV
      - mA/mAs/effective mAs
      - Collimation (NxT)
      - Pitch
      - Rotation time
      - Usage of dose reduction methods (e.g., automatic exposure control)
      - Settings for dose reduction methods (e.g., noise index, quality reference mAs)
    - Reconstruction settings:
      - Slice thickness
      - Slice interval
      - Reconstruction kernel/filter
      - Reconstructed FOV
  - Protocol has been reviewed by:
    - Lead radiologist
    - Lead CT technologist
    - Qualified medical physicist (QMP):
      - This team ensures that image quality and radiation dose are appropriate.
      - No unintended changes have been applied that may degrade image quality or unreasonably increase radiation dose.
      - Attention has been paid to acquisition and reconstruction parameters that should be influenced by the specific requirements of the diagnostic imaging task, including:
        - kV
        - mA
        - Rotation time
        - Pitch

  - Detector configuration (beam collimation)
  - Reconstructed image thickness, interval, and additional reformats (e.g., sagittal plane)
  - Reconstruction algorithm and/or kernels
  - Specific aspects of the acquisition that are demanded by the protocol (e.g., breath hold time)
- ○ Review of the appropriate use of dose reduction methods:
  - Review of appropriate settings for patients of various sizes:
    - Noise index, quality reference mAs, or other TCM settings.
    - Special attention should be paid to how adjustments are made for pediatric patients.
  - Ensure that appropriate CTDI values result from these settings before patients are scanned.
- ○ Clinical scans should be reviewed for:
  - Acceptable image quality for the diagnostic task required.
  - CTDI and/or DLP values should be checked and verified against expected values on patient images.
  - Appropriate centering, especially for AEC and pediatric patients.
- ○ Protocol meets ACR practice standards (where applicable):
  - Reconstructed image thickness for standard adult head and standard abdomen should be ≤5 mm.
  - Appropriate rotation time for pediatric abdomen should be chosen to minimize motion and breath-hold.
  - Meets guidelines in ACR testing instructions (see p. 8) for key protocols (head, chest, abdomen, cardiac, peds, etc.).
- ○ ACR's rules of thumb have been considered:
  - The largest value of the detector configuration or beam collimation (N x T) available for the scan should be used whenever practical, as this improves dose efficiency. For example, 4×5 mm collimation is up to 30% more dose efficient than 2×5 mm in axial mode with no image quality penalty.
  - The facility may wish to be able to reconstruct both conventional thickness (e.g., 3 or 5 mm) and thinner images (e.g., 1 or 1.5 mm) under some circumstances (e.g., to obtain multi-planar reformats, etc.). In this case, the largest value of N x T that allows both to be accomplished should be used for a standard scan.
  - Lower kV settings should be considered for pediatric scans as well as those scans that use intravenous or oral contrast.
  - High-resolution chest (HRC) protocol should incorporate a sharp reconstruction kernel or filter. "Standard" reconstruction kernel or filter (or equivalent) is generally not appropriate.
  - HRC images should be axial, thin images separated by 10–20 mm. If HRC images are extracted from a helical chest scan, it must be verified that the chest scan is used appropriately for diagnosis.
  - Doses should be as low as necessary to accomplish the diagnostic task. For standard head and abdomen protocols, the $CTDI_{vol}$ must not exceed the ACR pass/fail levels and should not exceed ACR reference levels for the stated standard patient sizes (1-year-old head, 23 kg pediatric abdomen, adult head, 70 kg adult abdomen).
  - Develop radiation dose thresholds during any new CT protocol design.
- Compared to AAPM protocols when available [34]

Achieving Consistency

The checklist above represents most of the "low hanging fruit" that can be adjusted when reviewing a protocol. However, it does not address a common issue that healthcare providers face in delivering consistent care. Most providers have multiple CT scanners and often have a diverse fleet of scanners makes/models. Some sites purchase their equipment from a single vendor, but even then, because of upgrade cycles, systems are usually not identical across the entire organization; it is common to have different models from the same manufacturer. Different scanner models have different features, capabilities, strengths, and weaknesses. However, it is expected that most routine CT examinations could be performed similarly on any scanner. Therefore, there is a need to set up the imaging protocols to try and achieve consistent quality across different scanner models (as much as possible). This is a necessary first step toward optimization of the entire organization's delivery of a particular type of CT examination. To achieve consistency, you first need to know to what degree you are currently being inconsistent. This can be determined based on retrospective analysis for radiation dose and image quality data as outlined below.

Retrospective Radiation Dose Data

It is now commonplace (and required for most healthcare providers) to maintain a dose monitoring system to track the radiation dose delivered from CT examinations. There are numerous commercial products available, and also some academic centers have developed their own in-house systems. The dose information for the protocol of interest should be extracted from this database for each scanner that performs the protocol. Typically, the dose monitoring system will keep track of the volumetric CT dose index ($CTDI_{vol}$) and the dose-length product (DLP) and, depending on its sophistication, may also provide other derived metrics such as size-specific dose estimate (SSDE)[8] or effective dose (ED). Because of the strong relationship between patient size and radiation dose, when automatic exposure control (AEC) methods are used, it is also recommended that some measure of patient size (e.g., BMI, water equivalent diameter [35], and/or effective diameter) be recorded. All of these metrics may be useful during the broader optimization process. However, this chapter will focus on CTDI and DLP. Figure 8.6 shows what such data may look like for a single protocol.

It should be mentioned that real-world clinical radiation dose data is often complex and full of idiosyncrasies. In our experience there are two main sources of the complexity. First, inconsistent naming of protocols across the clinical operation leads to data that is often difficult to bin correctly when trying to understand the radiation dose delivered from a particular protocol. In the dose monitoring systems, the protocol name is populated into the dose database based on information in the DICOM headers of the dose reports and/or images coming from the scanner. The protocol name in those DICOM files is based on how the protocol was manually named when it was saved on the scanner console. Very rarely are these names consistent (e.g., "CAP w/Contrast" vs "C_A_P W CON"). As an example, in our dose monitoring system, we have around 3000 unique protocol names in the database (Fig. 8.7), but in reality we only have around 300 unique CT protocols. There are a few non-mutually exclusive solutions to these problems, including manually mapping each "messy" protocol name to a "clean" protocol name, updating the protocol names saved on all the scanners to be more consistent, and developing a machine learning method to automatically map the names based on natural language processing methods. All three of these methods could be utilized to clean up the data and make it easier to meaningfully query the database.

The second source of the data complexity is that the dose data can be formatted in different ways on different scanners. In some cases, the dose monitoring database has to use optical character recognition to parse the dose screen capture images. These images have unique fonts and organizational structures according to each manufacturer. Thus, the parsing code needs to be able to handle many different formats. Preferably the scanners are able to output a structured radiation dose structured report (RDSR) which eliminates the need to parse a dose screen capture image. RDSRs also provide much more information about the radiation events and allow one to more fully reconstruct all the radiation exposures that happened during a CT examination. However, even having RDSRs does not solve all these

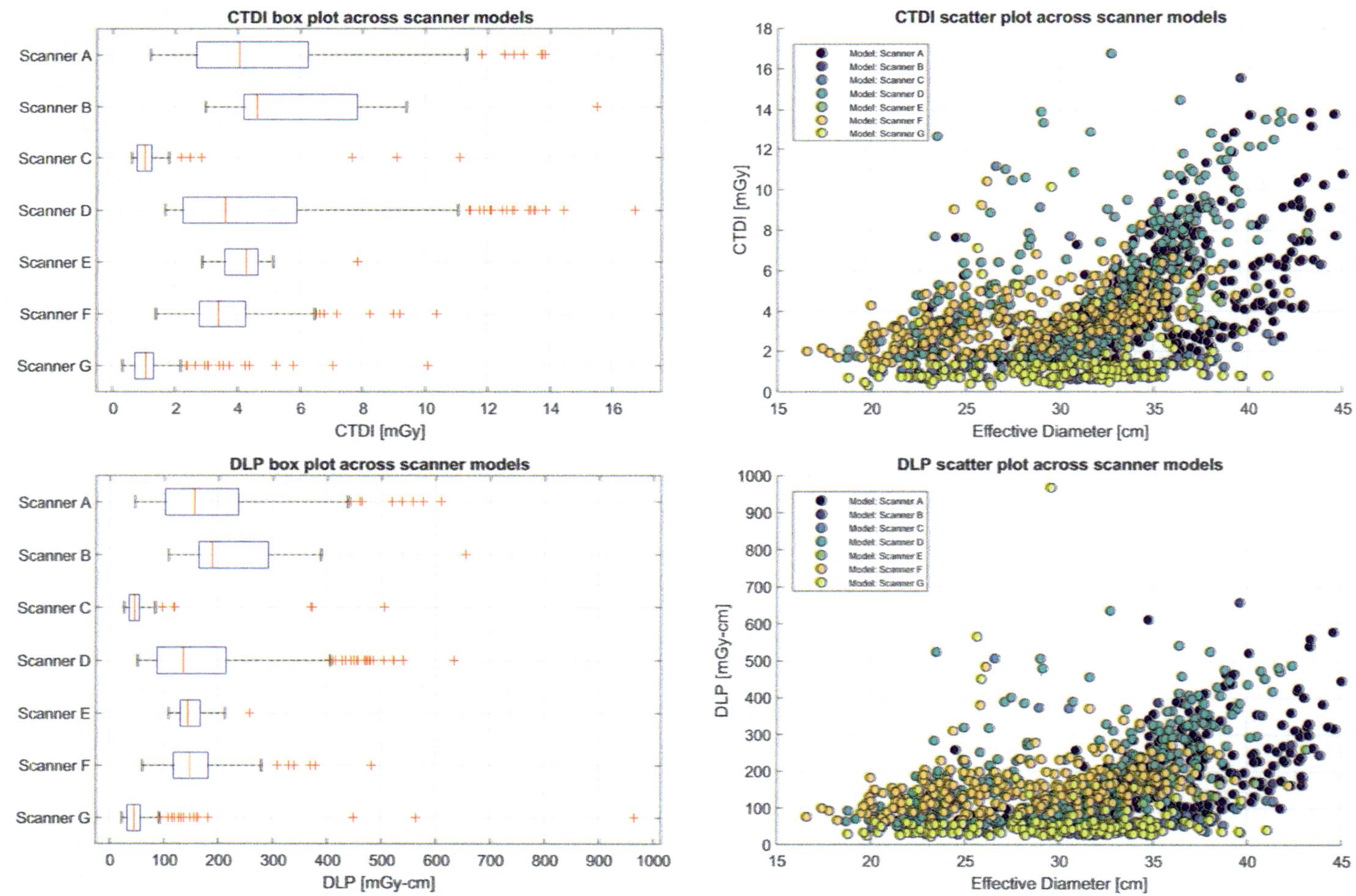

Fig. 8.6 Box plots (left) and scatter plots (right) showing radiation dose across different scanner models for a single CT protocol in terms of CTDI (top) and DLP (bottom)

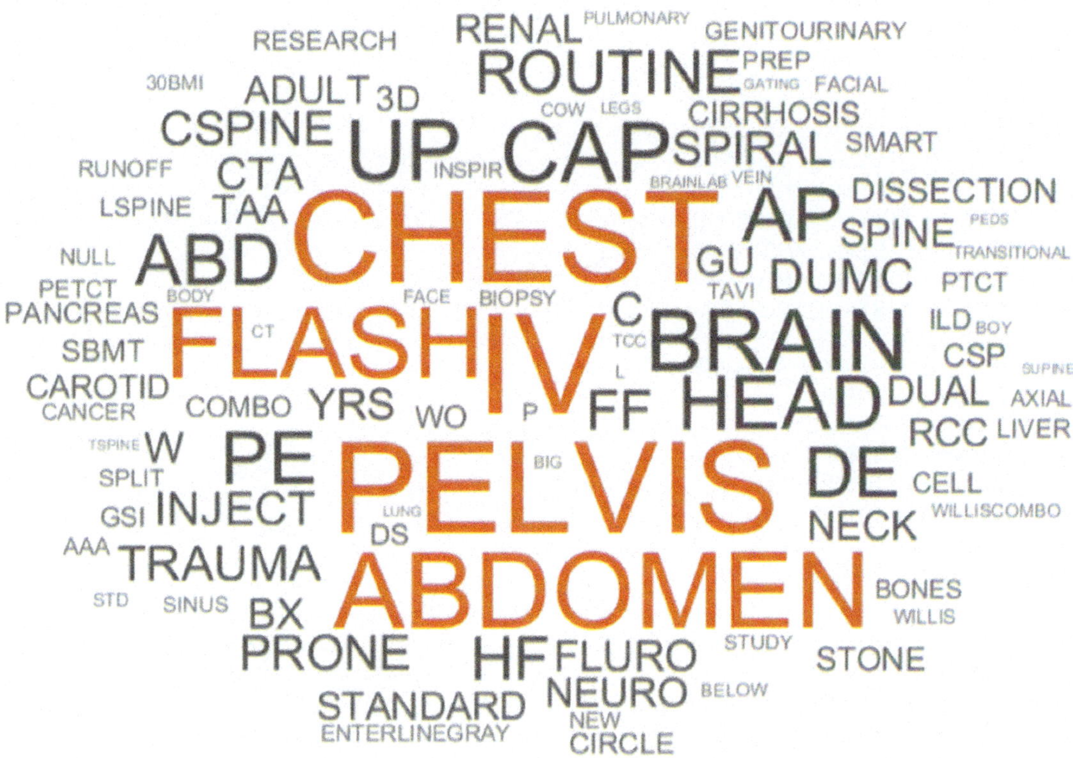

Fig. 8.7 Word cloud showing the words that were present our dose monitoring system under the "ProtocolName" field

problems. For example, it is not uncommon to perform multiple types of CT examinations during a single CT scanning session. When this happens, the technologist will often retrospectively do an "exam split" so that the images from each exam show up as individual studies on PACS. However, when this happens, the RDSR does not get split up along with it. Usually all the dose events will get labeled as having come from the protocol that was run first. This leads to confounding information in the dose database that can be difficult to triage in an automated way. All this being said, these are all solvable problems that will be addressed as dose monitoring systems become smarter and begin to incorporate more artificial intelligence.

Retrospective Image Quality

Large-scale information about image quality is critical to have in order to achieve consistency. After all, the goal is to achieve consistency in quality, not radiation dose. This data could be acquired in multiple ways, two of which are described here. One way is to randomly pick as many examinations as feasible for the protocol of interest and have them reviewed/scored by radiologists for quality. This can be done relatively easily on a small scale but may or may not be feasible on a large scale unless a system can be put in place in which CT studies are periodically evaluated for quality within the normal workflow of a radiologist. The second method is to implement one of several techniques for extracting image quality information directly from the CT images. The technique that was developed and is currently used at the author's institution involves estimating a "global noise index" from each CT series [27]. This method has been further refined by others as well [36]. Another technique takes this a step further and attempts to estimate an "in vivo" detectability index [28]. This in vivo detectability index is still in development, and this chapter will assume that the global noise index technique has been implemented.

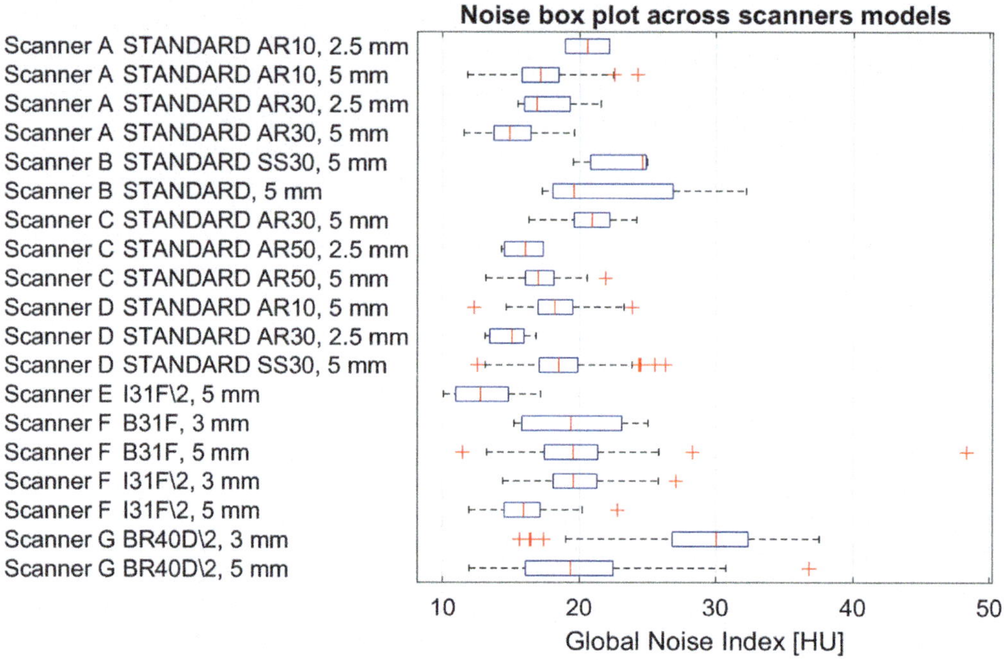

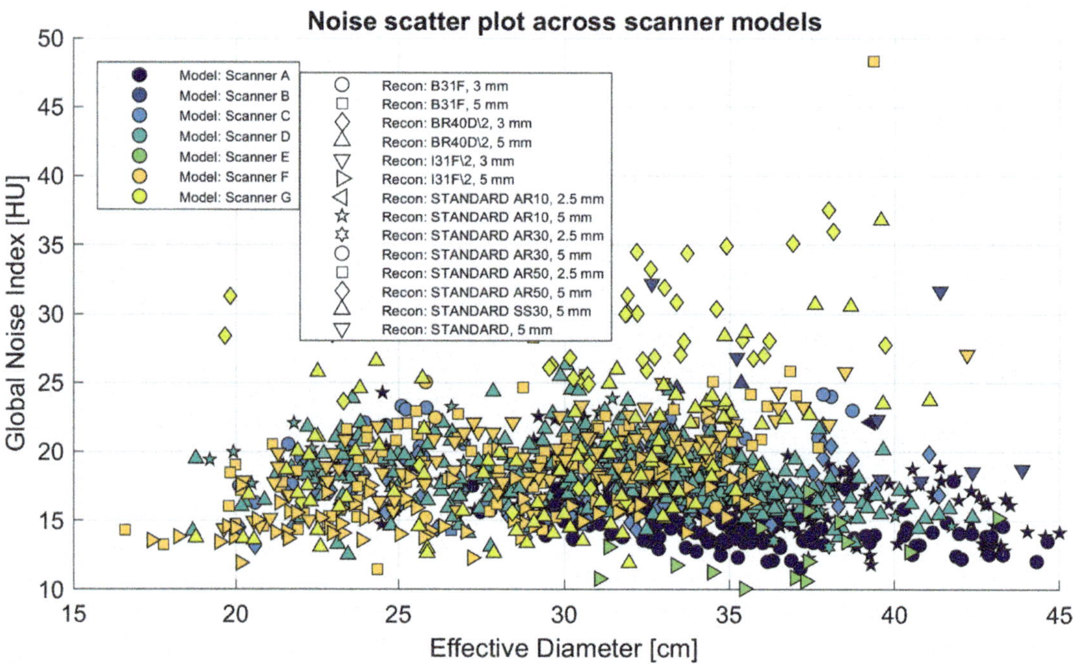

Fig. 8.8 Box plot (top) and scatter plot (bottom) showing the estimated "global noise index" across different scanner models for a single CT protocol

Assuming the dose monitoring database also contains noise information, one can query the database to compare noise across different scanner models for the same protocol (Fig. 8.8). When doing this, it is important to keep in mind that it is common to create multiple reconstructed image series from the same scan data, so it is useful to identify which series contains the primary diagnostic images. Specifically, post-processed images such as maximum intensity projections

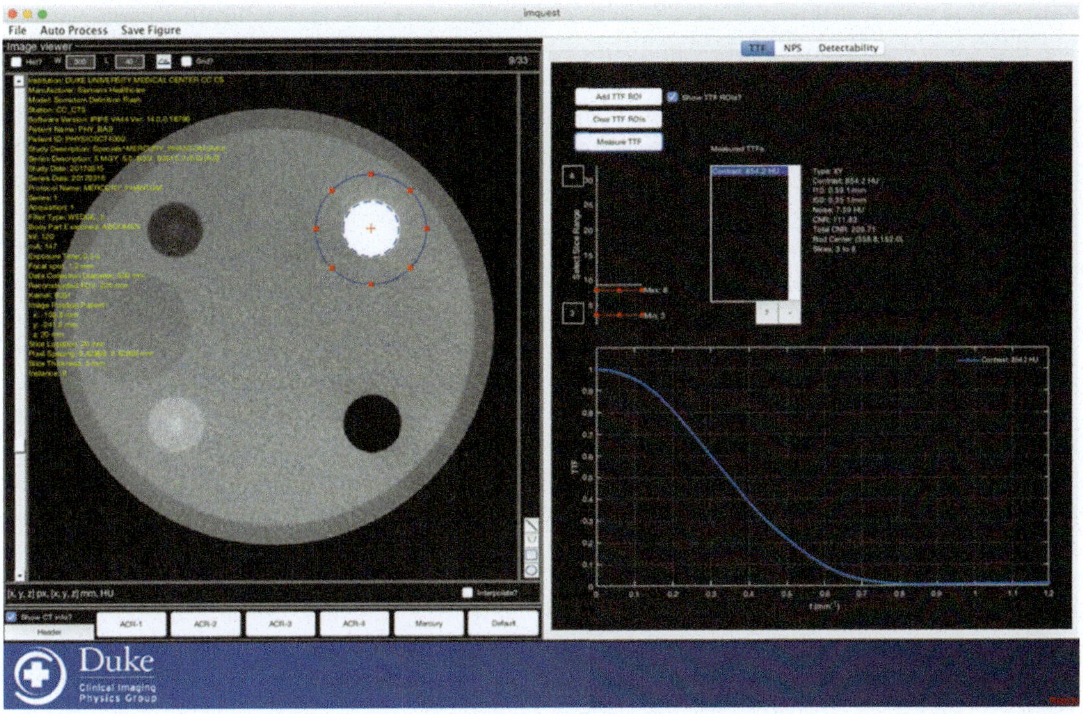

Fig. 8.9 Screen capture image of the imQuest software tool available for free from the AAPM. This tool allows the user to measure noise, resolution, and detectability properties from phantom CT images

(MIPs) and multi-planar reconstructions (MPRs) do not need to be included in these data.

Prospective Image Quality Data from Phantoms

The retrospective data described above is necessary to know the degree of inconsistency currently across different scanner models in terms of image noise. However, image noise is only one aspect of image quality, and thus this retrospective data is not sufficient for the purposes of achieving consistency. One also needs to know how resolution and noise texture vary across scanner models, and what would be the expected effect on noise, noise texture, and resolution if changes to the protocol are made. Phantom images are suitable to gather this information. It is recommended that a standard phantom such as the ACR image quality phantom or the multi-sized Mercury Phantom [37–39] be used. The phantom should be imaged on each scanner of interest using the current protocol and also some potential variations to the protocol. If possible, the phantom should be imaged at a few different radiation dose levels and reconstructed with all available reconstruction kernels/algorithms to create an image quality "lookup" table that will be used in the next step. The image quality metrics of interest for these images are the noise power spectrum (NPS) [40–49] and the task-transfer function (TTF) [49]. A free software tool has been made available from the AAPM as part of the TG-233 report to assist in making such measurements (Figure 8.9) [37]. Once the NPS and TTF of each image series are measured, it is useful to summarize and tabulate those measurements as scalar values such as the average NPS spatial frequency (f_{av}) and the TTF 50% or 10% frequency ($f_{50\%}$ or $f_{10\%}$, respectively). It is also helpful to tabulate the noise magnitude which can be determined from the noise power spectrum.

Adjust Protocols for Consistency

Having gathered all the necessary data, it is now possible to adjust the protocol to achieve consistent image quality in terms of noise magnitude, noise texture, and spatial resolution. The following steps can be followed to accomplish this. First the reconstruction settings should be adjusted to target consistent noise texture and resolution. A method to match noise texture across different reconstruction conditions has been developed based on comparing the NPS curves across scanners and reconstruction kernels [50]. This method was further refined to simultaneously target similar spatial resolution [51]. The method works by considering a 2D metric space of noise texture (f_{av}) and spatial resolution ($f_{50\%}$). A point in this 2D space represents a single reconstruction condition from a single scanner model. Points that are clustered near each other represent reconstruction conditions with similar noise texture and spatial resolution. Thus, if you have a reference reconstruction condition that is acceptable for one reference scanner, you can find the closest matching reconstruction settings from other scanners using a Euclidean distance in this space (Fig. 8.10). Note that when computing this distance, it is possible to weigh differences in f_{av} and $f_{50\%}$ differently depending on how important it is that noise texture or resolution be most similar, respectively. Other types of distances could be used as well.

This matching method can produce images that have overall similar "impression" as the reference scanner images to a human observer. If the overall radiation dose is also properly adjusted, then it is possible to achieve images with overall similar detectability. To determine how much the radiation dose should be adjusted, it is necessary to use the retrospective image quality data and the prospective phantom data. Note that because different scanner models use different AEC methods, it may not be possible to achieve consistent noise magnitude across all patient sizes. Because of this, it is recommended to target consistent noise for a narrow "reference" patient size range. The specific reference size that should be used is dependent on the protocol, but it makes sense to choose a reference size corresponding to the median-sized patient for that protocol, ± 5–10%. Once the reference size range is chosen, the retrospective image quality data should be filtered to only include data for patients within that range. From these filtered retrospective data, calculate the median global noise index for each scanner model. Next, based on prospective phantom data, determine how much relative change in noise magnitude would be expected for each scanner model based on the new reconstruction settings from the previous matching step. This relative change in noise magnitude can be computed for each scanner by taking the ratio of noise magnitude from the original reconstruction settings and the new reference-matched reconstruction settings. Multiplying this relative change by the median noise for each scanner model results in the expected noise magnitude from the new reconstruction settings for each scanner model (before adjusting the dose). Finally, knowing how the noise magnitude changes as a function of radiation dose ($CTDI_{vol}$) for the new reference-matched reconstruction settings allows one to adjust the dose-related scan protocol settings (e.g., noise index, quality reference mAs, etc.) to target a noise magnitude equal to the reference scanner.

The noise-dose relationship can be generally modeled as $\sigma \propto (DT)^{\beta}$ where σ is the image noise (pixel STD), D is the radiation dose index (e.g., $CTDI_{vol}$), T is the slice thickness, and β is a fitting parameter specific to the scanner model and image reconstruction settings. Most commonly β is assumed to be −0.5 resulting in the theoretical relationship that noise is inversely proportional to the square root of dose. However, empirical measurements generally show that β is not exactly −0.5 in practice for real-world CT systems. This is especially true for iterative reconstruction algorithms with strong nonlinear regularization steps. The true β value can be estimated from the phantom scan data if the phantom is scanned at several dose levels (at least three dose levels needed for the fit). If an empirical measurement of β is not available, an assumption of −0.5 is acceptable. The equation above can be inverted to solve for the dose needed to achieve a specific noise level for the scanner and reconstruction condition of interest. If this procedure is followed, one can expect images with similar

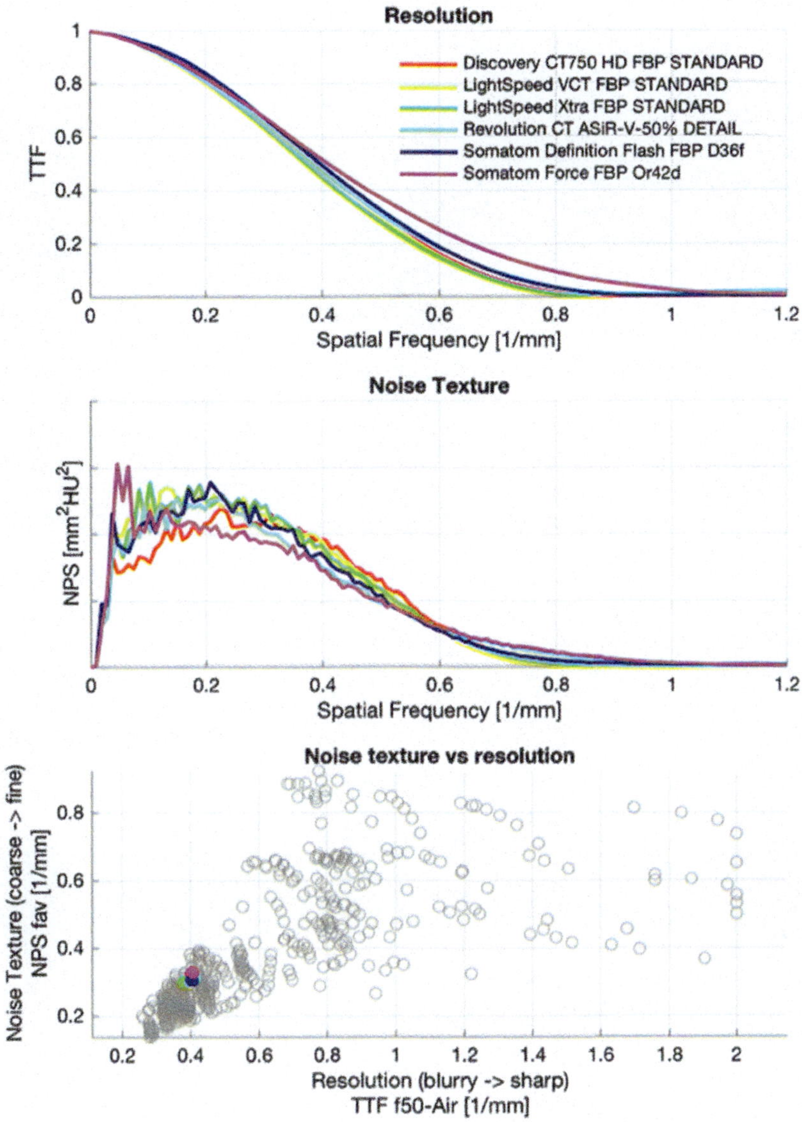

Fig. 8.10 Task transfer function (top), noise power spectrum (middle) and noise texture vs resolution scatter plot (bottom) for six different scanner models. In this example the GE Discovery 750 HD was considered as a reference. In the scatter plot, the gray circles each correspond to a single combination of reconstruction settings (e.g., kernel + iterative strength or FBP). The colored dots correspond to the reconstruction conditions from each scanner that were most similar to the reference scanner. The TTF and NPS plots confirm similar spatial resolution, and noise texture would be expected for those scanners if the recommended reconstruction settings are used

noise magnitude, noise texture, spatial resolution, and therefore detectability for all scanner models (Fig. 8.11). Note that this procedure may result in different dose levels being used on different scanner models, which is acceptable if the dose levels are all within a reasonable range.

Expected Dose and Image Quality Ranges for Revised Protocol

Based on the proposed changes, it will be possible to estimate the expected changes in image quality and dose. It is useful to calculate these ranges

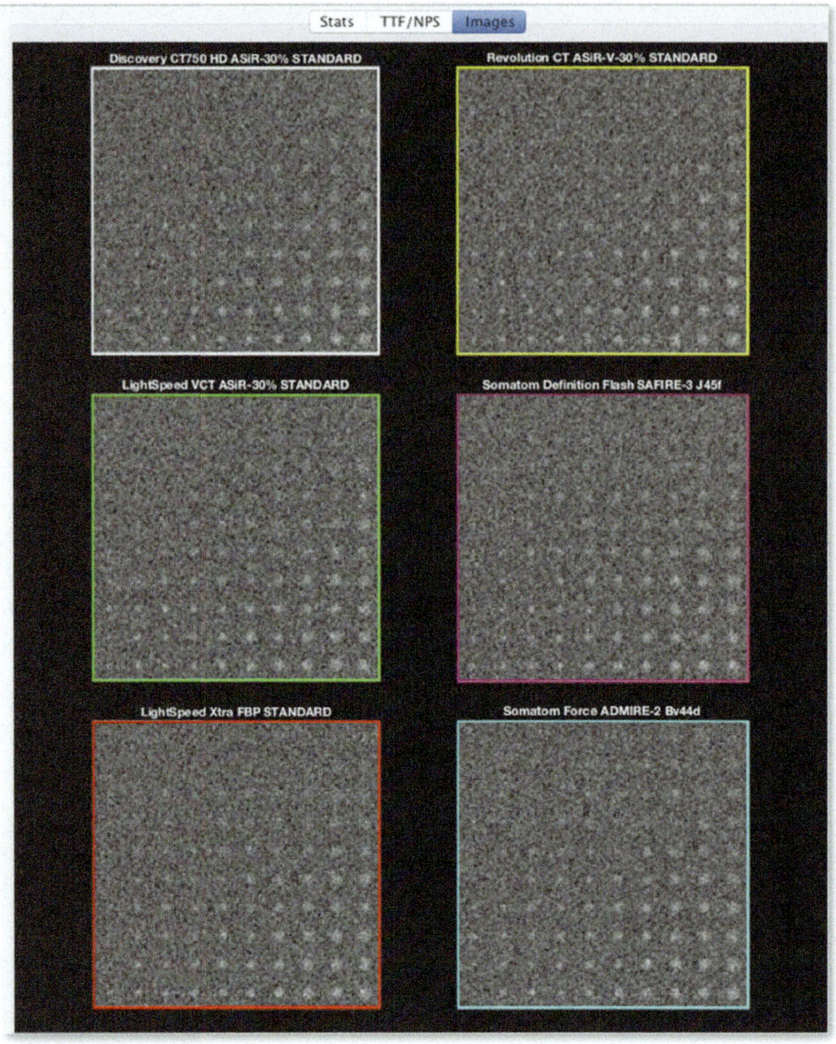

Fig. 8.11 Synthesized contrast detail diagrams demonstrating what CT images would be expected to look like across CT scanner models using the matching method

before implementing the changes and confirm that the new dose levels are within acceptable limits based on national standards. An estimate of the expected changes in image quality is also helpful for the next step when discussing the revised protocol with clinical colleagues. A summary table similar to the example below (Table 8.1) is recommended. If many protocol adjustments are made, it may be difficult to exactly know how radiation dose would be expected to change across the entire patient population. In that scenario, scanning a multi-size image quality phantom [39] is helpful to make the predictions more accurate.

Feedback from Technologists and Radiologists

Before implementing changes to the protocol, it is critical to gather feedback about the proposed changes from technologists and radiologists. They may have insight about a particular setting that was not considered previously. For example, the technologist may know that the user interface for a particular feature is not well designed and implementing that feature may be disruptive without providing detailed training and instructions. Similarly, the radiologist may have com-

Table 8.1 Example of how the expected changes to radiation dose and image quality could be summarized

Scanner model	Radiation dose	Noise STD	Noise texture	In-plane resolution	Z-direction resolution	Contrast
Scanner A	+30%	+24%	No change	No change	Improved	No change
Scanner B	−17%	+24%	Marginally coarser	No change	Improved	No change
Scanner C	−36%	+56%	Marginally coarser	No change	Improved	Potential improvement
Scanner D	+43%	+41%	Finer	No change	Improved	Potential improvement
Scanner E	−15%	+29%	Finer	Improved	Improved	Potential improvement
Scanner F	No change	+36%	Finer	No change	Improved	No change

ments about how the proposed changes could affect aspects of the images besides noise, resolution, and contrast. For example, it may be the case that proposed changes may affect the frequency of motion artifacts. This feedback should be carefully discussed and considered before implementing changes.

Monitor and Adjust if Needed

After the protocol changes have been implemented, it is important to carefully monitor the performance of the protocol shortly thereafter. Gathering another round of feedback from radiologists and technologists is helpful at this stage to confirm that the protocol can be run as designed and that the image quality is judged to be acceptable and consistent across scanner models. After a period of a few months, it is also helpful to redo a condensed version of the analysis above to confirm that the targeted level of radiation dose and noise is being achieved. Slight adjustments may be needed to further refine the protocol and achieve greater consistency.

Relating Consistency to Optimization

The previous section discussed a strategy to achieve consistent images from different scanner models in terms of noise, noise texture, and spatial resolution. However, it is possible to be consistently sub-optimal, and consistency should be considered only the first step toward optimality. As mentioned in the introduction to this chapter, there are many scientific papers that claim to achieve imaging optimality, but that term has traditionally been used to mean "acceptable image quality at a radiation dose that is tolerable."

To truly optimize an imaging protocol requires maximizing its utility, as denoted in the earlier section of this chapter. Ideally we need to think of the goal of the imaging examination as attempting to classify a patient into one of N classes (e.g., healthy, diseased, metastatic, stage X, etc.). For a given patient, there are N possible corresponding decisions based on the image data. You then define (a priori) an NxN utility matrix which assigns an expected utility of the ith decision when the patient belongs to the jth class. For example, the utility of classifying a patient having cancer when they do have cancer would be high, and the utility of a misclassification would be negative. The final utility of the imaging examination is found by summing over this utility matrix weighted by the conditional probabilities of the ith decision being made for patients of the jth class given the image data and the baseline probabilities of the patients in the population belonging to each class. The image quality provided by a given imaging protocol on a given scanner can be encoded into the aforementioned conditional probabilities (e.g., the probability of making the ith decision when the patient belongs to the ith class would be high if the image quality is good). The possible risks from the imaging examination could be further encoded into this formalism by adding an additional protocol/

scanner-specific risk term (e.g., negative utility) to the summation. To do this one needs to make several assumptions about the relationship between radiation dose and risk. It is beyond the scope of this chapter to discuss that topic but suffice to say that reasonable assumptions could be made for the purposes of protocol optimization. The protocol is optimized if the utility is maximized, and this would be expected to happen when the image quality is sufficient for the most important imaging tasks and the risk from radiation is low enough as to not cause undue burden on the population.

The formalism described above depends on (a) assigning sensible utilities to each decision/class pair, (b) understanding how imaging settings affect image quality and clinical decisions, and (c) understanding how imaging settings affect radiation dose and long-term risk. There is a large amount of scholarship available in each of these areas, but it should be noted that there is also still considerable uncertainty, highlighting an opportunity for further research. Unfortunately, the type of research needed to make this optimization possible in practice can be very expensive, time-consuming, and potentially unethical. As such, there is a need going forward to develop realistic imaging simulation tools. Such simulations could be the basis of so-called "virtual clinical trials" (VCT). A VCT is the only way to ethically study the effects of changing imaging settings on dose and image quality in a comprehensive and systematic manner. Tools are currently being developed that will eventually allow for realistic VCTs for the purposes of optimizing CT imaging protocols [52–54].

All that being said, there are some practical methods that can be applied relatively easily and quickly to help move toward more optimal protocols. After the image quality has been made consistent across scanner models (see previous section), then the question is how much should one adjust the dose (up or down) across all scanner models to achieve just good enough image quality. A hybrid approach can be used in which real CT images are modified to simulate reduced dose levels and/or infused with virtual pathology. The hybrid images can then be utilized in a reading study with radiologists to measure clinical performance (which can be different compared to clinical preference). This approach has been used successfully to determine the radiation dose reduction potential of an iterative reconstruction algorithm relative to FBP for liver CT imaging [55, 56]. The tools to do such studies are becoming more and more available over time.

Summary

CT protocol optimization is a complex topic and an area of active research. In most cases, there is currently not enough information available to achieve true optimization when considering the holistic effect of imaging on a population's health. However, it is possible to make sensible assumptions and adjust protocols to be more consistent across scanner models and perhaps more optimal for the primary imaging tasks that are performed by radiologists. This chapter describes the general optimization problem and some practical steps that can be taken to move toward more optimal imaging.

References

1. Demb J, Chu P, Nelson T, Hall D, Seibert A, Lamba R, Boone J, Krishnam M, Cagnon C, Bostani M, Gould R, Miglioretti D, Smith-Bindman R. Optimizing radiation doses for computed tomography across institutions: dose auditing and best practices optimizing radiation doses for computed tomography across institutions optimizing radiation doses for computed tomography across institutions. JAMA Intern Med. 2017;177(6):810–7.
2. Kordolaimi SD, Saradeas I, Ploussi A, Pantos I, Argentos S, Efstathopoulos EP. Introduction of an effective method for the optimization of CT protocols using iterative reconstruction algorithms: comparison with patient data. AJR Am J Roentgenol. 2014;203(4):W434–9.
3. Trattner S, Pearson GDN, Chin C, Cody DD, Gupta R, Hess CP, Kalra MK, Kofler JM Jr, Krishnam MS, Einstein AJ. Standardization and optimization of CT protocols to achieve low dose. J Am Coll Radiol: JACR. 2014;11(3):271–8.
4. Zarb F, McEntee MF, Rainford L. CT radiation dose and image quality optimization using a porcine model. Radiol Technol. 2013;85(2):127–36.

5. Barrett HH, Myers KJ, Hoeschen C, Kupinski MA, Little MP. Task-based measures of image quality and their relation to radiation dose and patient risk. Phys Med Biol. 2015;60(2):R1–R75. PMCID:PMC 4318357.
6. Samei E, Jarvinen H, Kortesniemi M, Simantirakis G, Goh C, Wallace A, Vano E, Bejan A, Rehani M, Vassileva J. Medical imaging dose optimisation from ground up: expert opinion of an international summit. J Radiol Prot. 2018;38(3):967–89.
7. Li X, Samei E, Williams CH, Segars WP, Tward DJ, Miller MI, Ratnanather JT, Paulson EK, Frush DP. Effects of protocol and obesity on dose conversion factors in adult body CT. Med Phys. 2012;39(11):6550–71. PMCID:PMC 3482255.
8. American Association of Physicists in Medicine. AAPM report no. 204: size-specific dose estimates (SSDE) in pediatric and adult body CT examinations. 2011.
9. Sanders J, Tian X, Segars WP, Boone J, Samei E. Automated, patient-specific estimation of regional imparted energy and dose from tube current modulated computed tomography exams across 13 protocols. J Med Imaging (Bellingham). 2017;4(1):013503. PMCID:PMC PMC5260633.
10. International Commission on Radiological Protection. The 2007 Recommendations of the International Commission on Radiological Protection. 2007.
11. Sahbaee P, Segars WP, Samei E. Patient-based estimation of organ dose for a population of 58 adult patients across 13 protocol categories. Med Phys. 2014;41(7):072104. PMCID:PMC PMC4105960.
12. Li X, Samei E, Segars WP, Sturgeon GM, Colsher JG, Frush DP. Patient-specific radiation dose and cancer risk for pediatric chest CT. Radiology. 2011;259(3):862–74. PMCID:PMC 3099041.
13. Samei E, Krupinski EA. The handbook of medical image perception and techniques. Cambridge, UK: Cambridge Press; 2010.
14. International Commission on Radiation Units and Measurements. ICRU report 54: medical imaging- the assessment of image quality. 1995.
15. Solomon J, Mileto A, Ramirez-Giraldo JC, Samei E. Diagnostic performance of an advanced modeled iterative reconstruction algorithm for low-contrast detectability with a third-generation dual-source multidetector CT scanner: potential for radiation dose reduction in a multireader study. Radiology. 2015;275(3):735–45.
16. Månsson LG. Methods for the evaluation of image quality: a review. Radiat Prot Dosim. 2000;90(1–2):89–99.
17. Rose A. The sensitivity performance of the human eye on an absolute scale. J Opt Soc Am. 1948;38(2):196–208.
18. Samei E, Richard S. Assessment of the dose reduction potential of a model-based iterative reconstruction algorithm using a task-based performance metrology. Med Phys. 2015;42(1):314–23.
19. Chen B, Christianson O, Wilson JM, Samei E. Assessment of volumetric noise and resolution performance for linear and nonlinear CT reconstruction methods. Med Phys. 2014;41(7):071909.
20. Li K, Garrett J, Ge Y, Chen GH. Statistical model based iterative reconstruction (MBIR) in clinical CT systems. Part II. Experimental assessment of spatial resolution performance. Med Phys. 2014;41(7):071911. PMCID:PMC 4106476.
21. Solomon JB, Samei E. Correlation between human detection accuracy and observer model-based image quality metrics in computed tomography. J Med Imaging. 2016;3:12.
22. Richard S, Samei E. Quantitative breast tomosynthesis: from detectability to estimability. Med Phys. 2010;37(12):6157–65. PMID: 21302772.
23. Zhang Y, Smitherman C, Samei E. Size-specific optimization of CT protocols based on minimum detectability. Med Phys. 2017;44(4):1301–11.
24. Gang GJ, Siewerdsen JH, Stayman JW. Task-driven optimization of CT tube current modulation and regularization in model-based iterative reconstruction. Phys Med Biol. 2017;62(12):4777–97. PMCID:PMC PMC5738673.
25. Solomon J, Samei E. Quantum noise properties of CT images with anatomical textured backgrounds across reconstruction algorithms: FBP and SAFIRE. Med Phys. 2014;41(9):091908.
26. Samei E, Lin Y, Choudhury KR, McAdams HP. Automated characterization of perceptual quality of clinical chest radiographs: validation and calibration to observer preference. Med Phys. 2014;41(11):111918.
27. Christianson O, Winslow J, Frush DP, Samei E. Automated technique to measure noise in clinical CT examinations. AJR Am J Roentgenol. 2015;205(1):W93–9.
28. Smith TB, Solomon J, Samei E. Estimating detectability index in vivo: development and validation of an automated methodology. J Med Imaging (Bellingham). 2018;5(3):031403. PMCID:PMC PMC5724743.
29. Sanders J, Hurwitz L, Samei E. Patient-specific quantification of image quality: an automated method for measuring spatial resolution in clinical CT images. Med Phys. 2016;43(10):5330.
30. Samei E, Tian X, Paul Segars W, Frush DP. Radiation risk index for pediatric CT: a patient-derived metric. Pediatr Radiol. 2017;47(13):1737–44.
31. Cody DD, Fisher TS, Gress DA, Layman RR Jr, McNitt-Gray MF, Pizzutiello RJ Jr, Fairobent LA. AAPM medical physics practice guideline 1.a: CT protocol management and review practice guideline. J Appl Clin Med Phys. 2013;14(5):3–12.
32. ACR. CT accreditation program requirements. 2019. Available from: https://www.acraccreditation.org/-/media/ACRAccreditation/Documents/CT/Requirements.pdf?la=en.
33. TJC. The Joint Commission Diagnostic Imaging Standards. 2015. Available from: https://www.jointcommission.org/diagnostic_imaging_standards/.
34. AAPM. The Alliance for Quality Computed Tomography: Protocols. 2017. Available from: https://www.aapm.org/pubs/CTprotocols/default.asp.

35. American Association of Physicists in Medicine. AAPM report no. 220: use of water equivalent diameter for calculating patient size and size-specific dose estimates (SSDE) in CT. 2014.
36. Malkus A, Szczykutowicz TP. A method to extract image noise level from patient images in CT. Med Phys. 2017;44(6):2173–84.
37. American Association of Physicists in Medicine. AAPM report no. 233: performance evaluation of computed tomography systems. 2019.
38. Solomon J, Wilson J, Samei E. Characteristic image quality of a third generation dual-source MDCT scanner: noise, resolution, and detectability. Med Phys. 2015;42(8):4941–53.
39. Wilson JM, Christianson OI, Richard S, Samei E. A methodology for image quality evaluation of advanced CT systems. Med Phys. 2013;40(3):031908.
40. Faulkner K, Moores BM. Analysis of x-ray computed tomography images using the noise power spectrum and autocorrelation function. Phys Med Biol. 1984;29(11):1343–52.
41. Boedeker KL, Cooper VN, McNitt-Gray MF. Application of the noise power spectrum in modern diagnostic MDCT: part I. measurement of noise power spectra and noise equivalent quanta. Phys Med Biol. 2007;52(14):4027–46.
42. Boedeker KL, McNitt-Gray MF. Application of the noise power spectrum in modern diagnostic MDCT: part II. Noise power spectra and signal to noise. Phys Med Biol. 2007;52(14):4047–61.
43. Siewerdsen JH, Cunningham IA, Jaffray DA. A framework for noise-power spectrum analysis of multidimensional images. Med Phys. 2002;29(11):2655–71.
44. Yang K, Kwan AL, Huang SY, Packard NJ, Boone JM. Noise power properties of a cone-beam CT system for breast cancer detection. Med Phys. 2008;35(12):5317–27. PMCID:PMC 2736717.
45. Riederer SJ, Pelc NJ, Chesler DA. The noise power spectrum in computed X-ray tomography. Phys Med Biol. 1978;23(3):446–54.
46. Baek J, Pelc NJ. The noise power spectrum in CT with direct fan beam reconstruction. Med Phys. 2010;37(5):2074–81. PMCID:PMC 2871306.
47. Kijewski MF, Judy PF. The noise power spectrum of CT images. Phys Med Biol. 1987;32(5):565–75.
48. Benitez RB, Ning R, Conover D, Liu S. NPS characterization and evaluation of a cone beam CT breast imaging system. J Xray Sci Technol. 2009;17(1):17–40.
49. Chen B, Richard S, Barnhart H, Colsher JG, Maxwell A, Samei E. Volumetric quantification of lung nodule in CT: effects of reconstruction algorithm (FBP, ASiR, and MBiR), dose and slice thickness, RSNA Annual Meeting. Chicago: Radiological Society of North America; 2010.
50. Solomon JB, Christianson O, Samei E. Quantitative comparison of noise texture across CT scanners from different manufacturers. Med Phys. 2012;39(10):6048–55.
51. Winslow J, Zhang Y, Samei E. A method for characterizing and matching CT image quality across CT scanners from different manufacturers. Med Phys. 2017;44(11):5705–17.
52. Segars WP, Veress AI, Sturgeon GM, Samei E. Incorporation of the living heart model into the 4-D XCAT phantom for cardiac imaging research. IEEE Trans Radiat Plasma Med Sci. 2019;3(1):54–60.
53. Abadi E, Segars WP, Sturgeon GM, Harrawood B, Kapadia A, Samei E. Modeling "textured" bones in virtual human phantoms. IEEE Trans Radiat Plasma Med Sci. 2019;3(1):47–53.
54. Segars WP, Mahesh M, Beck TJ, Frey EC, Tsui BM. Realistic CT simulation using the 4D XCAT phantom. Med Phys. 2008;35(8):3800–8. PMCID:PMC PMC2809711.
55. Solomon J, Marin D, Roy Choudhury K, Patel B, Samei E. Effect of radiation dose reduction and reconstruction algorithm on image noise, contrast, resolution, and detectability of subtle hypoattenuating liver lesions at multidetector CT: filtered Back projection versus a commercial model-based iterative reconstruction algorithm. Radiology. 2017;2017:161736.
56. Solomon J, Samei E. A generic framework to simulate realistic lung, liver and renal pathologies in CT imaging. Phys Med Biol. 2014;59(21):6637–57.

Part III

CT Practice

9 CT Practice Management

Timothy P. Szczykutowicz

Introduction: Motivation for Protocol Uniformity

Patients deserve imaging exams specifically tailored to their own unique body characteristics (e.g., coronary output, weight, etc.) and clinical indication. In some cases, if exams are not tailored to patient-specific characteristics or indications, the exam will have no or limited diagnostic utility. For example, a prospectively gated exam performed on a patient with a high and irregular heart rate is likely to be highly contaminated with cardiac motion artifact. One method for achieving patient- and indication-specific imaging would be for a clinical care team to design an exam specifically for each patient. The team would consist of a physician who will ultimately interpret the images, a technologist who will run the scanner, and a technical person (i.e., vendor applications specialist or medical physicist) who can advise their clinical partners on the image quality and dosimetry trade-offs of any parameter decision. This model is not ideal, however, as many patients will present with the same indication and with similar body characteristics. Therefore the work of the team would be repeated again and again as patients presented with the same indication and body characteristics. Additionally, all modern CT scanners have the ability to modulate image quality and contrast enhancement to adapt for changes in patient's body characteristics. In practice, instead of needing to create unique exam instructions for individual patients, we can create sets of exam instructions for specific groups of patients exhibiting similar body characteristics and indications. We refer to a set of exam instructions as a protocol in the world of diagnostic radiology. Creation and management of these protocols will be the focus of this chapter.

Figure 9.1 depicts the ideal situation for an imaging center: harmonized workflows across body section and location. An example of a workflow's facet that can be harmonized across body sections is protocol documentation. A harmonized workflow would use the same template/format to record protocol information across all body sections. CT technologists sitting at one scanner would look in the same place for the same information no matter the body section. For example, the CT technologist would know to look at the end of the protocol for instructions on how to bill the exam, no matter if the exam was a cardiovascular section-owned non-gated chest exam or a pediatric section-owned dynamic 3D airway exam. An example of a workflow facet that can be harmonized across scanner would be recon number/type. For example, if the same indication of gated CTA chest non-coronaries is performed on a cardiology owned scanner and a radiology owned scanner,

T. P. Szczykutowicz (✉)
University of Wisconsin Madison, School of Medicine and Pubic Health Department of Radiology, Madison, WI, USA
e-mail: tszczykutowicz@uwhealth.org

© Springer Nature Switzerland AG 2020

E. Samei, N. J. Pelc (eds.), *Computed Tomography*, https://doi.org/10.1007/978-3-030-26957-9_9

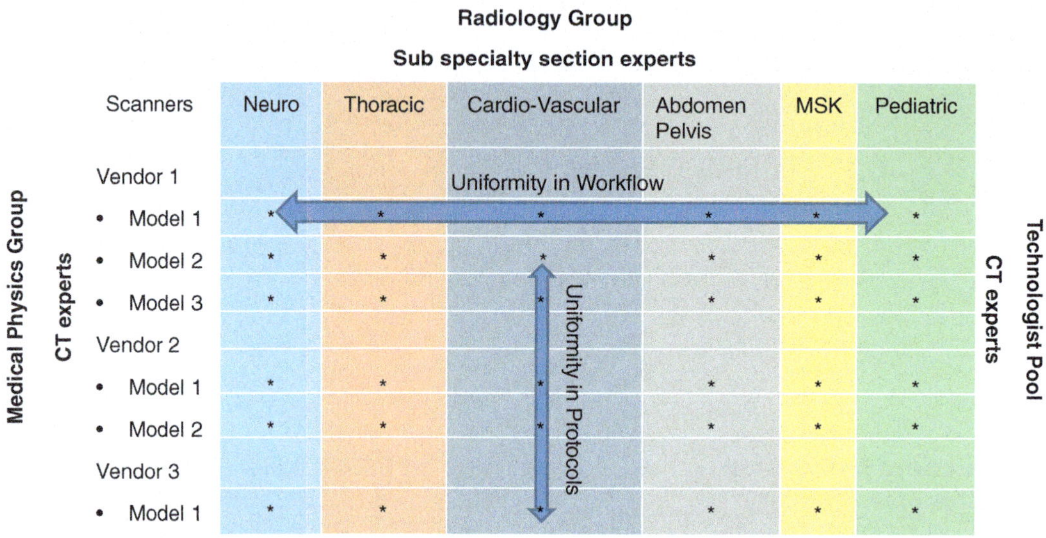

Fig. 9.1 Uniformity of image quality, contrast enhancement, and image presentation (i.e., reconstruction and reformatting options) is important. Uniformity needs to be thought of in two ways: (1) between exams performed on the same scanner but for different clinical indications and (2) between exams performed on different scanners for the same clinical indication. Many practice setting and device-specific differences make these goals of uniformity challenging to realize. This figure was adapted from a slide presented by Professor Mika Kortesniemi at the Prague 2018 CT workshop hosted by EFOMP

one would hope the reconstructions coming from that study to be the same. It may be that a non-harmonized workflow has the cardiology scanner not producing high-resolution wider field of view reconstructions of the lung fields, as the cardiologists are not interested in performing a screening exam for the lung fields. Since prior image comparison is an essential facet of medical image interpretation, harmonization of images is an important goal for an imaging center.

Definition of a Protocol

Executing a medical imaging protocol is not a trivial task [1]. Ordering physicians must weigh the appropriateness of ordering a CT against other imaging modalities and diagnostic tests [2]. The ordering physician must then put in an order for the exam. Radiology will schedule the exam. The ordering and scheduling takes alone can quickly become complicated. For example, if a physician orders an orthopedic implant planning exam, often these exams must be performed only on scanners "commissioned" by the orthopedic implant vendor. This immediately complicates ordering and scheduling as not all CT imaging centers and not all CT scanners within a center will be commissioned for the exam. Other issues with ordering and scheduling can involve the need for cardiac gating (i.e., not all scanners have this option), respiratory gating (not all scanners have this option), bariatric patient (individual scanners have unique limits for patient weight and scanner output), implants (if the implant is known to cause metal artifacts, the patient may have to be scanned only on scanners with metal artifact reduction), etc. All of these limitations should be documented somewhere in one's protocols. Relying on individual schedulers and technologists to remember what indications can be scanned on what scanner may work in a small setting with two scanners, but is not realistic for a large imaging practice. In practice, at our institution, we rely on notes in the protocols and notes in the scheduling teams templates for individual scanners to align patient-specific needs with the option sets on our CT fleet.

Once the patient actually gets to the imaging center, there are hundreds of steps involved in actually performing the exam [1, 3, 4]. Some of these steps will start before the patient even sees the scanner. For example, many sites will place IVs before the patient gets into the scan room, and oral contrast is usually given tens of minutes to hours before the imaging procedure. For cardiac gated exams, sites usually have heart rate and heart rate variability guidelines tied to the administration of beta blockers; workflows that are completed before the patient receives their scan. All of these details are important if the exam is to have maximum diagnostic utility. For example, the amount of gastrointestinal tract opacified by oral contrast is related to the amount of time between when the patient starts drinking and the scan. Different indications will require different parts of the tract to be contrast filled. Relying on individual technologists to remember details like these may work in a small setting that only perform a handful of indications, but is not realistic for a large imaging practice.

Once actually on the scanner, there are literally hundreds of options per irradiation event [5]. From the "breathing lights" to the reconstructed slice thickness, a technologist cannot be expected to program all of the options on a per patient basis. Most sites will have set protocols that require little to no modification at scan time. Post exam, the technologist will have to send the automatically reconstructed images off for interpretation, send some images off for further processing (e.g., TAVR planning), and may be required to perform some custom image creation on the scanner (e.g., aligning head axial images slices to the patients' true anatomical axial plane). A common radiologist complaint is missing image reformats. Missing images means the radiologist either has to interpret the exam with missing views, try to make them on the PACS, or call the scanner to have the technologist send them. Even for sites using the "auto reformat" and/or "auto send" features of their scanners, documenting what protocols and what series/phases within those protocols have these automatic features turned on is needed when setting up new imaging equipment to copy existing equipment. All of these actions, and the parameters that define them, cannot be expected to be remembered for sites realizing hundreds of different indications.

The previous paragraphs have discussed how medical imaging protocols are complex. Protocols in medical imaging involve instructions aimed at technologist, nursing staff, physicians, and imaging devices. Too often protocols are focused on the instructions for the imaging device and are light on the instructions for the personnel interacting with the device. This is evident by looking over many published protocols which are largely made up of tables or lists of technical acquisition and reconstruction parameters that are pre-programmed into an imaging device. Historically, this is due to most CT vendors providing protocols that are just lists of acquisition parameters. Providing just acquisition parameter details limits their liability with respect to practicing medicine. The rest of this section is devoted to providing a robust list of parameters to be captured when documenting a CT protocol.

We cannot ignore the influence of regulation on the need for protocol documentation. Currently, in the USA, requirements from accreditation agencies such as the American College of Radiology (ACR) and The Joint Commission (TJC) require protocols to be documented and changes to be recorded. The Joint Commission has provided an itemized list of requirements they consider necessary to be documented (PC 01.03.01 A 25) [6]: clinical indication, contrast administration, age (i.e., adult or pediatric), patient size, patient body habitus, and the expect radiation dose index. The Joint Commission also requires sites verify (PC.01.02.15 A 10), before scanning a patient, that the patient is properly positioned, that the correct protocol is selected, and that the correct scanner parameters are being used. The verification requirements imply a site is also required to document patient positioning, indication, and technical (i.e., programmable) scanner parameters. We cover all of these accreditation-based requirements in the following tables.

Tables 9.1, 9.2, 9.3, and 9.4 represent all the fields we consider important to document for a clinical CT protocol in the diagnostic setting.

Table 9.1 Compliance components of a CT protocol

Section	Comment
Contributors	Provide the name of the people putting together this protocol. This author list should reflect those individuals responsible for creating the protocol content. If the content of the protocol is novel, refer to the creators of the protocol in the "Design Philosophy" section of this template. You may also list the name of an organization, for example, "University of XXX CT Protocol Optimization Team"
Protocol name	A protocol name should appear in this box. This name should be descriptive of the protocol. The convention usually adopted in CT is to have the name refer to three things: the body part being imaged, the use of contrast, and sometimes the name of the indication commonly or usually associated with the protocol. If your center appends protocol names with the last date they were edited or checked, you may include that information on the share. Dating your protocols in the name field will enable easier sharing of your protocol across a large hospital network and facilitate data analysis from dose monitoring programs
RadLex Playbook name and ID	A valid RPID number and name should appear in this box. The RSNA has published a naming system for CT protocol names. Almost all CT protocols can be mapped to this standard. This mapping is commonly needed for centers with more than one CT scanner who wish to combine dose monitoring data and/or for quality improvement, billing, workflow analysis, or other reasons. Information about the RadLex Playbook can be found here https://www.rsna.org/RadLex Playbook.aspx. RadLex has provided a playbook browser which can be used to quickly find a matching playbook number; this can be accessed here http://playbook.radlex.org/playbook/SearchRadlexAction
Clinical indications	A concise statement of a few sentences should describe for what clinical indications this protocols is to be used for
Design philosophy details	A concise statement (a few sentences to a few paragraphs in length) describing the clinical/workflow/technical thinking guiding the development of the protocol
Academic references	A list of references corresponding to the text given in the design philosophy
Other resources	Links to YouTube or other instruction videos, white papers not indexed online, etc. should be provided here. If a link is provided, please provide a title for the link which clearly describes what the link contains followed by the full (including the http:// or www.) web address
Billing code	Provide a list of CT billing codes (CTP) codes here
Billing notes	Provide any notes pertaining to the billing codes here. Appropriate information to include would be any post-processing steps needed to satisfy billing requirements. For example, "to bill as a CTA, the volume rendered images must be made from the angio phase of the exam"
RSNA reporting template	The title of the template (identical to the one on the www.radreport.org website). Note, the template page provides suggested RPID to be used with this template; please cross-check the RPID you used in the protocol name subsection "RadLex Playbook name and number" with the RPID listed here. If there is a difference, you may want to consider editing the RPIDs you provided, but this is not always appropriate

Table 9.1 (continued)

<table>
<tr><th>Section</th><th colspan="6">Comment</th></tr>
<tr><td rowspan="8">Dose table</td><td colspan="6">Most modern CT protocols will employ automatic exposure control (e.g., tube current modulation) which varies as a function of patient size. Additionally, multiple options for patient dose surrogates are in use today. Because of this, there are many options for reporting dose data</td></tr>
<tr><td colspan="6">The dose metric value for each metric and phantom/patient combination should be placed in a table. Note, for multiphasic exams, the dose from each phase/series/group must be included. Not all of the dose metric and phantom/patient combinations need to be filled out</td></tr>
<tr><td>Series name</td><td></td><td>Dose check value (NV)</td><td></td><td></td><td></td></tr>
<tr><td></td><td>Vendor-supplied water phantom</td><td>Vendor-supplied water phantom diameter</td><td>16 cm CTDI phantom</td><td>32 cm CTDI phantom</td><td>Patient population data</td></tr>
<tr><td>CTDIvol</td><td></td><td></td><td></td><td></td><td></td></tr>
<tr><td>DLP</td><td></td><td></td><td></td><td></td><td></td></tr>
<tr><td>SSDE</td><td></td><td></td><td></td><td></td><td></td></tr>
<tr><td>Effective dose</td><td></td><td></td><td></td><td></td><td></td></tr>
<tr><td>ACR</td><td colspan="6">Compliance with any programs should be documented here by listing the program name, for example, ACR Lung Cancer Screening</td></tr>
<tr><td>OPTN/UNOS</td><td colspan="6">This box should be filled in with the name of the organ covered by the OPTN/UNOS guidelines. OPTN (Organ Procurement and Transportation network) and UNOS (United Network for Organ Sharing) periodically publish guidelines for CT scanning done in conjunction with organ transplants. For example, see http://pubs.rsna.org/doi/full/10.1148/radiol.12121698 for an example of guidelines for HCC liver imaging</td></tr>
<tr><td>Device manufacturer</td><td colspan="6">Compliance with a device manufacturers protocols should be documented here by stating the name of the manufacturer and the specific device or procedure name. For example, if your protocol meets the slice thickness and reconstruction kernel requirements of a robotic orthopedic surgery device company for a knee replacement, you would document the manufacturer name and the specific procedure or device name in the protocol</td></tr>
<tr><td>Software (CAD/surface rendering, etc.)</td><td colspan="6">Compliance with a software manufacturer's recommended protocols should be documented here by stating the name of the manufacturer and the specific software package. For example, if your protocol meets the beam energy and slice thickness requirements mandated by a computer-aided diagnosis company, provide the company's name and specific CAD software package</td></tr>
<tr><td>Trial/study/ publication details</td><td colspan="6">If this protocol is being used or was used for a specific research paper or study, the paper reference should be included</td></tr>
</table>

One may need additional fields for radiation therapy and interventional scanning. One can perform radiation therapy simulation and CT interventional procedures with the same scanners as used in diagnostic radiology. We intend Tables 9.1, 9.2, 9.3, and 9.4 to aid a CT protocol optimization team in defining all of the pieces of information associated with their imaging protocols. It is very likely not all of these fields will or should end up in your sites final protocol documentation. We intend these tables to capture all of the possible clinically relevant information one needs to realize a diagnostic CT exam. Your site may choose to publish a subset of these parameters in your final clinical documentation, an example of which is shown in Fig. 9.2. Interested readers should also review DICOM supplement 121 [9] which details the technical acquisition parameters in a vendor neutral manner needed to fully capture the essential elements defining a CT protocol. The DICOM supplement overlaps greatly with the protocol components presented in Tables 9.1, 9.2, 9.3, and 9.4 but at a higher less clinically approach-

Table 9.2 Clinical components of a CT protocol

Section	Comment
Patient preparation	Patient preparation instructions should be provided. Examples of patient instructions include asking female patients undergoing a chest CT scan to remove their brassier to avoid underwire artifacts. Another example is to have patients undergoing a pelvis CT scan remove their pants if they contain any metal rivets/zippers/buttons. The medication and heart rate monitoring instructions needed for some cardiac gated exams would also be documented here. While the IVC parameters are provided below, the IVC needle placement and gauge details should be provided here
Oral contrast instructions	Provide the total volume, dose per drink, and temporal spacing between drinks. Additionally, provide the contrast agent type (manufacturer), concentration, and dosage and any special mixing instructions
IVC contrast instructions	Provide the total volume, flow rate, contrast agent type (manufacturer), and concentration for both the contrast and saline chaser (if used). If using a power injector protocol, provide the make and model of the injector and the specific protocol
Patient coaching instructions	Provide details on patient coaching. For example, provide details on patient breathing instructions or instructions on how to induce a Valsalva maneuver when needed. While patient coaching details are included in the "Workflow Details" section of the template, this section should contain a more robust version of coaching instructions. The coaching instructions provided in the workflow table are meant to be a reminder to the technologists during the exam; the instructions provided here should fully convey all needed details of the instructions
Physician or nurse monitoring instructions	Patient monitoring details should be provided here. If the monitoring party is expected to make a mid-exam decision based on the results of the exam (e.g., the decision to proceed to the perfusion phase of a stroke protocol may depend on the presence of a bleed detected on the non-contrast series), details on this decision should be provided in this box
Patient positioning	Provide details on patient positioning. For example, for musculoskeletal exams which demand high resolution, a note should be made to ensure the anatomy of interest is positioned as close to the scanner's isocenter as possible to maximize the spatial resolution capabilities of the scanner

Table 9.3 Clinical workflow components of a CT protocol

Exam logistics by series	One should provide technologists with a high-level overview of what the exam includes. Provide them with concise details needed to navigate a CT exam from CT localizer radiographs to exam end
	Series Names: Provide each series name (i.e., series description or reconstruction name). The series name should be as descriptive as possible and usually describes the contrast phase imaged. For example, a routine three-phase abdomen protocol could have series names of "non-con," "wIVC," and "delayed"
	Coaching: Provide a short and concise reminder to the technologist. Provide the full description of the coaching details in the "Clinical Components" section of your template
	Bolus Tracking: Provide the size and placement of the bolus tracking region of interest. Document details on timing delays associated with bolus tracking and enhancement thresholds in the "Technical Acquisition Details" section of this template; do not repeat them here
	Scan Ranges: Provide a pictorial or textual description of the scan range including where to start and stop the scan. For example, a scan of the head may be scanned from the top of the head to the mandible. This could be documented as "start above the head, some air should be included in the image volume, continue down to the level of the mandible"
Reformats	Name: Provide the name of the reformat. Usually, the name consists of the reformat plane and the type of reformat being displayed (recon algorithm/kernel, MIP/minIP, etc.)
	Plane: Provide the anatomical plane name
	Type: Provide the reformat type. For example, maximum intensity project (MIP), average, etc.
	ww/wl: Provide the window width and level of the reformat
	Thickness: Provide the reformat thickness in mm
	Interval: Provide the reformat interval (distance between adjacent reformat slices)
	Source: Provide the source image volume used to create the reformatted view

Table 9.3 (continued)

Networking destinations	Provide a reference to technologists after the exam to facilitate getting the images the right places as quickly as efficiently as possible
	Series Name: Provide the series name. Note, not all series have to be sent to radiologists for review. For example, it may be appropriate to reconstruct thin axial slices for the sole purpose of reformatting into thicker non-axial planes; in such a case, the thin axial slices may not always be sent to radiologists for review. Also note, the destination for networking does not always have to be a PACS; it may also be a computer-aided diagnosis server or a three-dimensional post-processing laboratory
Destination	Destination: Provide the networking destination. Usually, a generic name is all that is needed, like "PACS," "LUNG CAD," or "3D LAB." The actual networking details usually only go into one place on a scanner and to not need to be entered for each exam. Details like AE title/port number and IP address

Table 9.4 Technical acquisition components of a CT protocol

Section	Comment
Scanner platform	Scanner options vary greatly between vendors and even within the same make and model via the different available options within a model line. Providing the make and model will ensure the vendor-specific verbiage is correct. Providing the tube power, detector number, and optional packages will enable you to understand how similar your scanners are to each other and people to whom you share your protocols
Make	Provide the vendor name (i.e., Cannon, GE, etc.)
Model	Provide the model name of the scanner
Tube power	Provide the maximum tube power rating. Usually, vendors report this value on your bid/quote
Detector number	Some scanners report a number double the actual number of detector elements (e.g., 128 instead of 64). If your scanner reports double the actual number of elements, report this "double number" as this is the number that is commonly cited when referring to the scanner in the community
Gating/perfusion, etc. packages	Provide the vendor-specific name of the cardiac or respiratory gating options your scanner has enabled. Provide the vendor-specific name of any special perfusion or cine options your scanner has enabled (e.g., not all scanners ship with a shuttle mode for perfusion imaging). State any other special options needed to perform the protocol. An example of another option would be any special dual-energy processing modes. In general, options included here are options the user has to pay "extra" for when buying a CT scanner
Acquisition details	Due to the complexity of modern automatic exposure control systems and other vendor-specific nuances, many acquisition parameters behave differently based on how other seemingly non-related parameters are set. Therefore, this part of the template aims to capture all possible acquisition and reconstruction options
	Scan type: Provide the scan type. Scan types should be one of the following: CT localizer radiograph, axial, helical/spiral, cine, perfusion, cardiac gated, and respiratory gated. All of these scan types may also need to have a modifier for dual energy
	kV: Provide the beam energy. If the kV is selected by the scanner based on the patient size, the setting for the kV selection should be provided here. For example, list the min and max allowable kV settings and the iodine contrast strength selector
	Pitch: The pitch used for helical/spiral scanning should appear in this box. For scanners that pick the pitch for you at scan time (i.e., some cardiac gated exams), you can list this parameter as "variable"
	Rotation time: Provide the rotation time
	mA/effective mAs: Provide the mA or effective mAs. Some vendors only provide one or the other
	Collimation: Provide the collimation or beam width. Give the value as a distance in mm and, if possible, a detector configuration. For example, 40 mm (0.625 × 64)
	AEC/TCM setting: Provide the AEC or TCM setting(s). Examples include noise index, effective mAs, or standard deviation value
	Acquisition slice thickness: Provide the slice thickness used for the first or primary reconstruction
	Acquisition interval (axial scanning only): Provide the interval used. Note, this interval refers to the distance the scanner will move between axial couch positions
	Acquisition reconstruction filter/kernel: Provide the filter/kernel for the first or primary reconstruction
	Scan FOV: Provide the scan field of view. Note, the scan field of view can differ from the reconstruction field of view. The scan field of view is not an option on all scanners

(continued)

Table 9.4 (continued)

Section	Comment
Recon options	You will need to document recon options for every reconstruction made from the source data described in the acquisition details section above. It is not uncommon for a single acquisition event to have more than two reconstructions. Some protocols may need to have more than ten reconstructions to provide interpreting radiologist the mage they require
	Due to the ever-growing size of new reconstruction options, do not expect this template will accommodate all future reconstruction options. Currently many vendor-specific options are difficult to classify and group together. Therefore, this portion of the template has a few generic spaces left open for the placement of vendor-specific reconstruction options
	Recon name: Provide the reconstruction name. This is the name PACS will label the images with in the series description DICOM field
	Reconstruction filter/kernel: Provide the filter/kernel
	Display FOV: Provide the display or reconstruction field of view
	Slice thickness: Provide the slice thickness
	Slice interval: Provide the interval. Note, do not confuse this value with the spacing between adjacent axial/cine/perfusion/cardiac scans. In general, this value will be equal to or smaller than the slice thickness
	Iterative denoising level: Provide the type and strength/level/percentage of denoising
	Recon options: Provide any reconstruction option not accounted for by another section on this part of the template. For example, you should describe any special beam hardening correction algorithm, motion compensation, registration, dual-energy-specific options, etc. here. More than one box is provided to document multiple options separately (e.g., you would place, on a GE Healthcare scanner, the "IQ enhance" option here)
	WW/WL: Provide the window width and window level used for the reconstruction

able level (i.e., DICOM supplement 121 is a technical document that may not be easy for people unfamiliar with the DICOM standard to understand).

CT Protocol Optimization Team

No practice can cost efficiently have one individual scanning patients, interpreting images, and mastering the technical facets of CT scanner operation. Practices employ CT technologists to run the scanners and guide the patients through the required pre-/during/post-scanning activities. Interpreting radiologists are the recipients of the images created by the CT scanner and post-processed images created by the CT technologists. Auxiliary support people include the CT vendor's application specialists who are usually experts on the latest scanner features and have dose and image quality skills for protocols optimization. Other auxiliary support people include PACS or networking professionals who manage the connectivity of the CT scanner within the informatics environments (i.e., connections to the DICOM modality worklist, PACS, dose repositories, 3D workstations, etc.). Most sites will also either have an in-house service professional or use the services of their CT vendor to provide CT preventative maintenance and troubleshoot scanner errors and malfunctions. Lastly, regulatory bodies are usually required to have a physicist perform annual testing to ensure the scanner is safe with respect to the delivery of ionizing radiation and capable of providing adequate image quality. The physicist should also be a part of protocol optimization as they should be experts in the relationships between image quality and scanner parameters. The actions of each of the individuals described here make up the work of what we refer to as a "CT protocol optimization team" [7, 10–16].

The membership and responsibilities of members can vary widely between centers. Do not take this section's descriptions as the only accepted realization of a CT protocol optimization team. We based these descriptions on the work of the author. They reflect real job roles

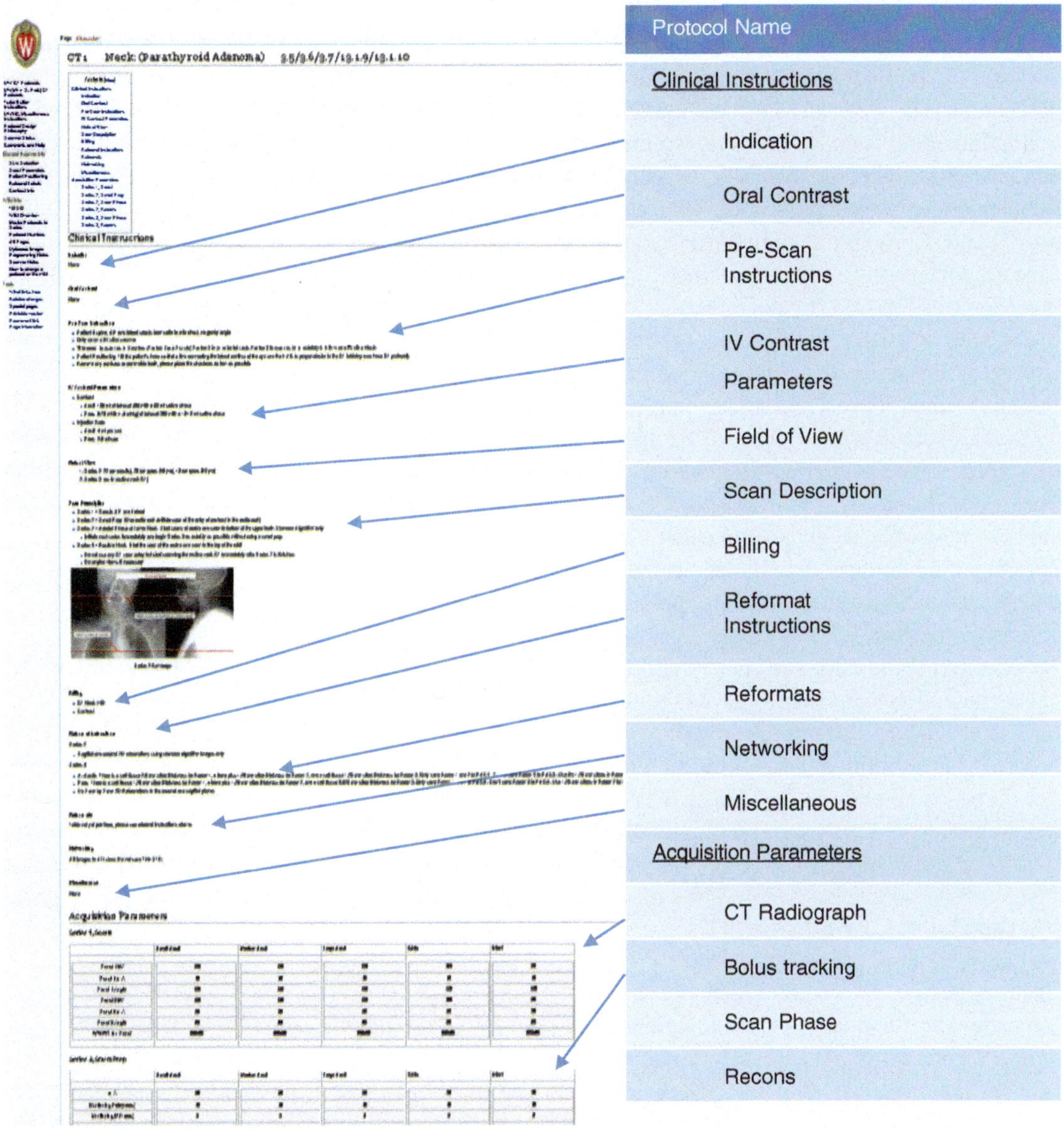

Fig. 9.2 Example protocol layout used by the University of Wisconsin Madison [7]. This layout includes many of the items listed in Tables 9.1, 9.2, 9.3, and 9.4 of this chapter, albeit not all of those protocol components need to be available for technologist or physician references for every protocol. We mean Tables 9.1, 9.2, 9.3, and 9.4 to provide your CT protocol optimization team with all protocol facets to consider documenting. For many sites, you only need a subset of these options recorded for individual protocols as we have done here. Image from TP Szczykutowicz et al. 2015 [8]

and duties as detailed in Szczykutowicz et al. (2015) [16]. A societal guideline has been provided by the AAPM for this task (see [12]). Sites without dedicated lead CT technologist time, without dedicated radiologist time for protocol development, and without onsite medical physicists will likely outsource protocol optimization work to vendor-supplied application specialists or simply copy protocols from other sites. The rest of this section will elaborate on individual team member roles.

Lead CT Radiologist

The lead CT radiologist is responsible for coordinating efforts between all aspects of the CT protocol optimization team. In practice, we have seen administrators take on this role, especially for radiology practice groups who serve multiple hospital centers. Without individual radiologists accepting the result of the CT protocol optimization team's efforts (e.g., by not requesting changes to the scan acquisition parameters at scan time), consistent image quality cannot be obtained. As most individuals have a preference on performing an exam a certain way, which is often backed up by studies from the literature, individual institutions must decide on a uniform way to perform studies, or else CT technologists will be asked to change protocols depending on who is the current attending radiologist in the reading room.

Lastly, the lead CT radiologist is responsible for prioritizing the efforts of the entire CT protocol optimization team. At any given moment, we have at around six different protocol revisions in progress. Determining what order these tasks should be completed is the task of the lead CT radiologist.

Section Lead CT Radiologist

Each section lead CT radiologist is responsible for reviewing the quality of the imaging studies within their section. At our institution, we have six sections: neuro, thoracic, cardiovascular, abdominal, musculoskeletal, and pediatrics. We also have a nuclear medicine section that does read CT when performed in conjunction with a PET study. For large cancer centers with many PET/CT studies, it may make sense to have a dedicated radiologist working on cultivating protocols for PET/CT. For sites with radiology groups that read all studies, we have seen good results when leadership assigns individuals to lead specific body regions.

Quality here can refer to multiple facets of imaging, including but not limited to radiation dose, complexity of the protocol for the technologists, image quality, contrast enhancement quality, oral contrast enhancement quality, etc. The interval for these reviews varies at our institution, but for routine protocols, these reviews occur once per year. Our radiology sections also have regular meetings where individuals may bring up issues to the attention of the group. For new protocols, or protocols with new revisions, we have CT technologists compile lists of patients scanned using the new protocol. These lists then facilitate radiologist review.

Section lead radiologists are also responsible for distilling the wishes of their section and communicating these with the CT protocol optimization team. The section lead radiologists also must settle disagreements on alternate scanning techniques to ensure uniformity of protocols within their section.

CT Physicist

The CT physicist is responsible for making changes to CT protocol acquisition and reconstruction parameters. Changes can be due to optimizing a current protocol, adapting protocols to new scanners, or creating new protocols. At our institution protocol changes are motivated by and guided by data we collect in a quality assurance IT solution [17]. The CT physicist is also responsible for educating radiologists and CT technologists on the function of the various scan options of each scanner. This education usually takes the form of relating the differences between the various options in terms of image quality (resolution, noise level, noise texture, etc.) and any logistical characteristics like time and or tube heating limits. Specifically, the lead CT physicists will reconstruct clinical and/or phantom images using different settings to educate the clinical staff. Changes in scan time can easily be computed, and such numbers are also presented to the clinical staff.

The CT physicist also assists in protocol revision on the scanner (i.e., typing in protocol changes to the scanner console) and checks all protocol parameters within our protocol documents against what is actually programmed into the scanner. At our institution, the physicist also manages the digital repository of protocol information, as described in section "Definition of a

Protocol". Our solution uses a server running Wikimedia software to provide Internet-based access to textual- and pictorial-based protocol information for every scanner and protocol in our fleet [10, 16]. An in-house solution like this is not feasible for most sites. We discuss commercial realizations of our approach for protocol management in section "Management Solutions".

Lead CT Technologist

The lead CT technologist is responsible for notifying the other CT technologists of changes to the protocols, entering protocol changes and new protocols onto the scanner, notifying billing and coding personnel when changes need to be made, notifying the IT personnel that maintain our clinical CT protocoling system when changes have to be made, and most importantly providing "logistical" information to the rest of the CT protocol optimization team. By logistical we refer to information pertaining to realistic patient breath hold times for different age patients and realistic patient breath hold times for patients with different clinical indications.

In addition, our lead CT technologist is responsible for controlling revisions within our actual CT protocol documents and keeping track of the numbering of our protocols. We maintain uniform numbering for all protocols across all of our scanners. We recommend institutions also strive to maintain uniformity in naming and numbering [14, 18, 19] of protocols across all of their scanners as this reduces the chance of error as CT technologists move from scanner to scanner.

IT Support

Failure to recognize the importance of informatics personnel can effectively kill the efforts of a CT protocol optimization team. For sites who have IT policies that restrict use of scanner side computers, posting digital copies of protocols scanner side may be impossible. If protocols changes are dependent on changing ordering sets or billing options, and changing those takes months, protocol updates will suffer.

We currently house our protocol documents on a server with an implementation of Wikimedia's wiki software. We also manage our CT protocol optimization team efforts and document protocol changes on an instance of SharePoint (Microsoft Corporation, Redmond WA). Lastly, we rely on IT support personnel from our hospital EMR's system Radiologist Information Service (RIS) and billing divisions to integrate protocol changes with ordering and billing. We also rely on informatics personnel from our PACS and informatics security teams to assist with getting data to and from our CT scanners. Members of these informatics teams are not present at any regular CT Protocol Optimization meeting; they receive requests via our institutional informatics request ticketing system.

Applications Specialist

The knowledge of an application specialist (apps) should be a valued input to a CT protocol optimization team. The knowledge of apps will reflect the latest product options and instructions from your CT vendor. In our experience, which spans multiple vendors, apps receives training directly from factory sources who are intimately involved with the creation of new scanner features. Therefore, the input of apps in the creation of new CT protocols and the updating of existing protocols is essential. The ability of apps to build protocol varies by country due to local laws regulating the ability of apps to adjust scan settings technologists will use on patients. Therefore you may find some sites that solely rely on apps to build their entire protocols, while others do not let their apps personnel touch their protocols. Apps can also assist in disseminating optimized protocols from site to site. Often, apps will have trialed protocol parameters your CT protocol optimization team may be considering at other sites. Therefore, involving apps may mitigate the need for some in-house optimization work when apps shares optimal scanner settings and scanning workflows learned at other sites.

Management Solutions

Protocol Editing/Disseminating/Reviewing

Figure 9.3 demonstrates two workflows for management CT protocols. In the non-ideal approach, a user is required to maintain physical media of protocol parameters or each unique type of scanner model in their fleet. These physical media must be brought to each scanner to perform protocol save (i.e., copy) and restore (i.e., load) operations. The more ideal workflow presented in Fig. 9.3 depicts a centralized management scheme where the editing, saving, and restoring of protocols can be done remotely. Currently, there are commercial solutions realizing the ideal workflow shown in Fig. 9.3. We will discuss some tasks these protocol administration systems enable in the rest of this section.

There are four steps central to the administration of protocols. One must be able to view, edit, save, and restore protocols. These operations are essential regardless of if users do them via a remote system as described in Fig. 9.3, or locally at the scanner console. The Integrating the Healthcare Enterprise (IHE) has a profile defining all the interactions enabled using the DICOM standard which cover the four basic steps mentioned here [20]. We refer the interested reader to the IHE Management of Acquisition Profile, which provides a modality agnostic presentation of the needed informatics transactions needed to implement a protocol administration system.

In addition to the central steps of protocol administration, the IHE MAP profile combined with the DICOM supplement on CT protocols also allows a user to:

- Approve a protocol change. As a DICOM object, protocols can have states, which are intended to limit their use. For example, a protocol can be approved, but not for use on pregnant patients. Other examples include approving a protocol but only for experimental use. A table of states is available in Section 44.4.1.9 of the MAP profile.
- Track protocol changes. Protocol DICOM objects can contain information about the previous version of the protocol or from which protocol one modified the current protocol. For example, if one edits an adult chest protocol to become a pediatric chest protocol, the pediatric protocol would reference the original adult protocol.
- Constrain protocol parameters. DICOM 121 defines what and how information can be stored in a CT protocol object. The standard allows one to set limits for some parameters instead of fixed values. For example, one may desire to allow the kV to vary between 70 and 100 kV instead of fixing it at 80 kV. In this way, a protocol administration system, via the protocol, can set the limits for how much freedom a technologist has at scan time to adjust parameters.
- Store/retrieve protocols off scanner. Currently, the workflow of saving or storing old versions of protocols is not present on all CT scanners. It is a welcome feature, however, when tasked with reverting to old scan parameters. It is also a useful feature to diagnose image quality issues from scans acquired in the past. The MAP profile defines a means for remotely (i.e., off scanner) storing protocol information.

At the time of this writing, several commercial solutions exist in the space of CT protocol management. The vendors currently offering these solutions are equipment manufacturers and dose monitoring companies. Many other companies like contrast injector and PACS companies have relationships with the OEMs and dose monitoring companies to offer these protocols management and dose monitoring solutions as a part of their product offerings. All of these commercial solutions that involve direct connection to modality units are not vendor agnostic at this time. This means one is currently forced to have a vendor-specific solution for protocol management if direct device connectivity is needed [21].

Here is an itemized list of some product features currently commercially available:

1. Ability to view all the CT scanners one has in their fleet (i.e., a dashboard view)
2. Ability to query protocols of certain type from a scanner or collection of scanners (see Fig. 9.4)

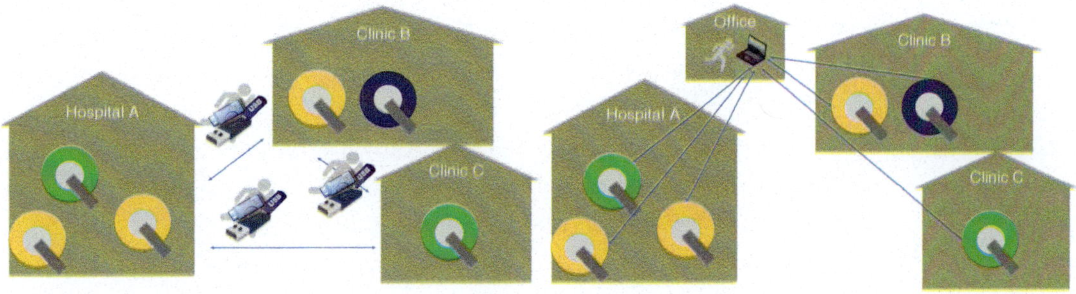

Fig. 9.3 Examples of non-ideal and ideal protocol dissemination practices. On the left, a protocol optimization team member must manually transport protocol between imaging facilities on physical media (i.e., flash drives or CDs). Since most centers have CT scanners of different makes and models, one must transport a unique set of protocols for each scanner make and model. An ideal protocol dissemination practice is shown on the right. In the figure on the right, the CT protocol optimization team can edit protocols, retrieve protocols, and push protocols to other scanners from a single remote location. The workflow shown on the right mitigates the need to physical store or transport any protocol information and commercially available at the time of this writing

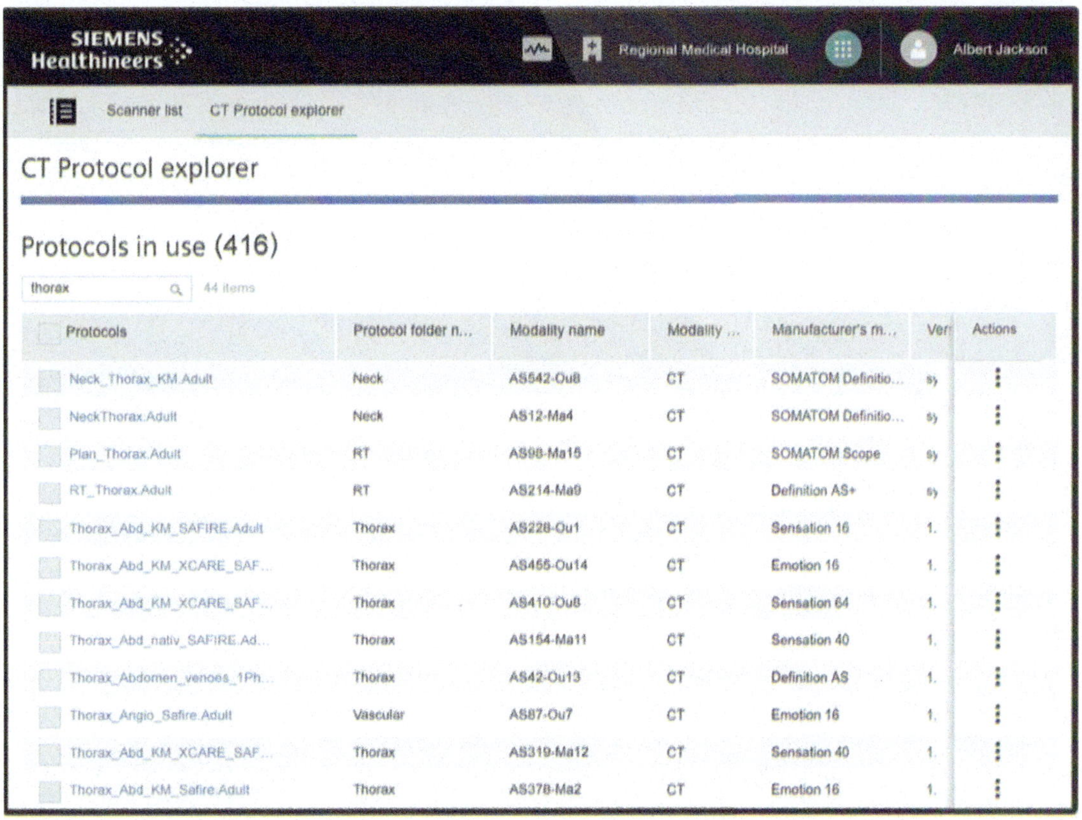

Fig. 9.4 Example of a protocol management solution. In this figure, the user is able to view all of the protocols in use a given facility. The view allows filtering by scanner, location, body region, etc. to facilitate protocol administration tasks. Image provided by Siemens Healthineers. This view demonstrates the aggregation of data across many scanners. Manually obtaining such information would require one to visit each scanner and manually interrogate the on scanner protocol manager

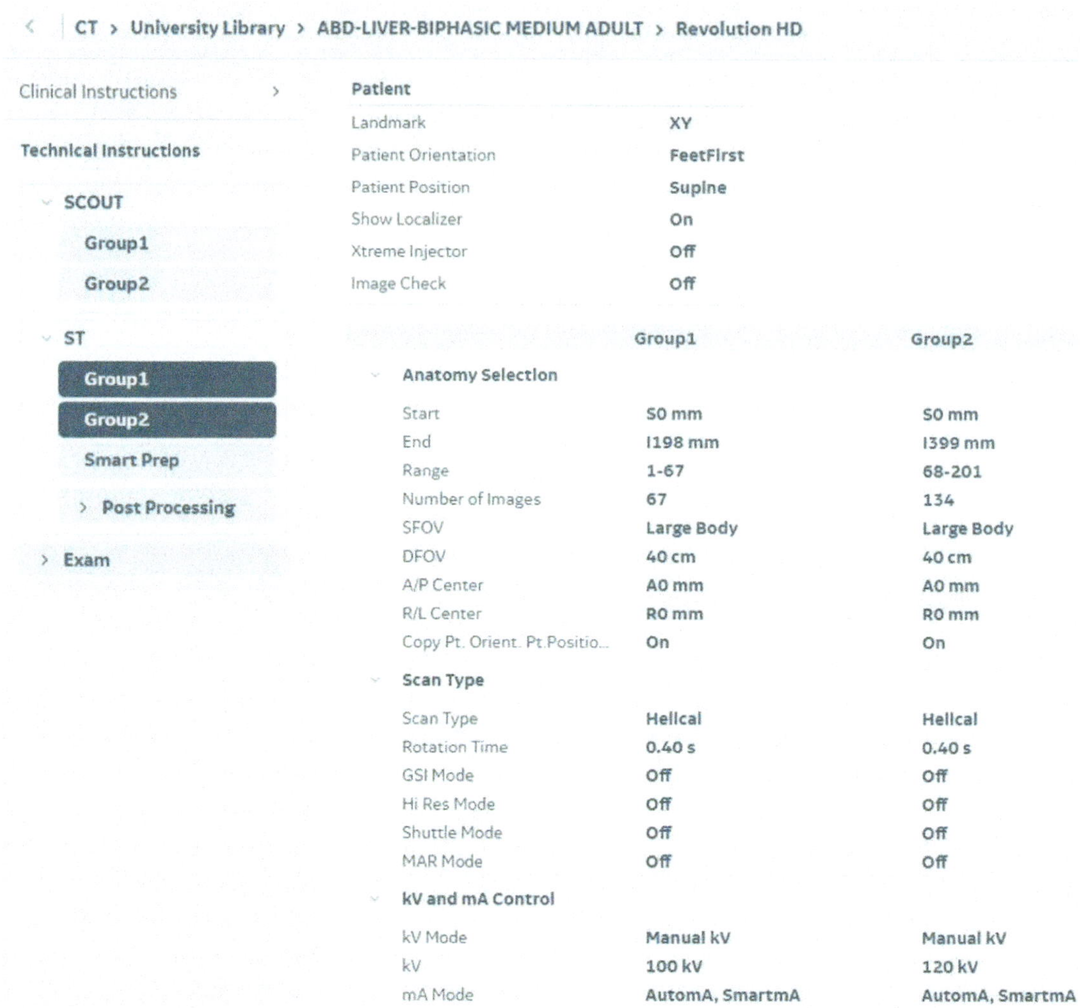
CT > University Library > ABD-LIVER-BIPHASIC MEDIUM ADULT > Revolution HD
Clinical Instructions
Technical Instructions
SCOUT
Group1
Group2
ST
Group1
Group2
Smart Prep
Post Processing
Exam
Patient
Landmark XY
Patient Orientation FeetFirst
Patient Position Supine
Show Localizer On
Xtreme Injector Off
Image Check Off
Group1 Group2
Anatomy Selection
Start S0 mm S0 mm
End I198 mm I399 mm
Range 1-67 68-201
Number of Images 67 134
SFOV Large Body Large Body
DFOV 40 cm 40 cm
A/P Center A0 mm A0 mm
R/L Center R0 mm R0 mm
Copy Pt. Orient. Pt.Positio... On On
Scan Type
Scan Type Helical Helical
Rotation Time 0.40 s 0.40 s
GSI Mode Off Off
Hi Res Mode Off Off
Shuttle Mode Off Off
MAR Mode Off Off
kV and mA Control
kV Mode Manual kV Manual kV
kV 100 kV 120 kV
mA Mode AutomA, SmartmA AutomA, SmartmA

Fig. 9.5 Example of a protocol management solution. In this screenshot, the user is able to view acquisition details for a specific protocol. The protocol manager would display this view by clicking on one of the individual protocols shown in Fig. 9.4, albeit this view is from a different protocol manager realization. Image provided by GE Healthcare

3. Ability to remotely view scan parameters on a scanner (see Fig. 9.5)
4. Ability to push a protocol from one scanner to another
5. Ability to remotely edit a scanner's protocols
6. Ability to define library of protocols that can be pushed to scanners
7. Ability to combine dose data and protocol data in one view
8. Ability to create CT protocol documentation in a digital format
9. Ability to store user created CT protocol documentation
10. Ability to track CT protocol revision history
11. Ability to compare two defined protocols (i.e., from the same or different scanners)
12. Ability to compare defined and performed CT protocols [22, 23]

CT scanners are not the only equipment in the diagnostic (or radiation therapy) environment that require protocols. Modern contrast injectors also allow for programmable combinations of settings to be stored. In other words, contrast injectors also have protocols to manage. The parameters adjustable on an injector may involve parameters like contrast agent strength, target organ group, target contrast imaging phase (i.e., angio versus parenchymal), selection of a weight to contrast volume conversion table, etc. The number of injection protocols is usually much less than the number of imaging protocols. The contrast injection protocols, however, can have a large impact on image quality [24]. Bae 2010 provides an excellent tutorial on CT contrast administration which can serve as a starting point for understanding the vendor-specific offerings provided for contrast administration [24, 25]. Currently, one contrast injector company allows for remote management of contrast protocols. Other companies allow for remote visualization of injection details. A record of the actual injected volume of contrast, chaser, and flow/pressure rates is important for reviewing extravasation events or quantifying your department's use of contrast media.

Access to Protocol Information

The solutions described in Section "Protocol Editing/Disseminating/Reviewing" are explicitly designed to aid in CT protocol management. For years, however, CT vendors and dose monitoring companies have been providing methods for accessing CT protocol information. This section discusses these methods.

Most CT vendors allow for the exporting of CT protocol information. The output of this information was only recently codified by a DICOM standard. Therefore, current CT scanners all output CT protocol information in vendor-specific and in some cases model specific formats. These outputs are usually in a spreadsheet amenable format, for example, a comma-separated value data format. These outputs, in our opinion, are not sufficient for technologist use for performing a CT scan. They are just lists of the technical acquisition parameters described in section "Definition of a Protocol". They do not contain images or clinical details related to the use of the protocol. They are, however, invaluable in that they actually reflect what is defined on the scanner for a given protocol. Access to these protocol "dumps" is usually available via an export or protocol save operation. Some companies have solutions for reading in these data dumps and importing them into their CT protocol documentation software. Technologists are still free to change the parameters seen in these dumps at scan time. Therefore, you should be careful when using this source of protocol information when troubleshooting an image quality or dose complaint as it may not actually reflect how the patient was scanned. In other words, if a CT technologist turns off AEC and lowers the mA to 10 at the time of the scan, image quality may suffer, while the defined protocol on the scanner would not indicate this decrease in technique.

Dose monitoring companies receive a variety of inputs. Depending on the vendor and connection method, these companies may receive one or more of the following inputs: RIS information defining the orderable and patient information (e.g., height, weight, name, etc.), structured dose reports from the CT scanner, dose slides from the CT scanner, CT localizer radiograph images from the CT scanner, and the actual CT image axial slices from the study. Information from these inputs is then extracted by the dose monitoring vendor and stored in a database. Most dose monitoring vendors allow you to export this database. Since the information extracted contains as many parameters relevant for defining image quality and dose as can be obtained, this database contains a majority of the values needed to describe the performed protocol. Therefore, a user can use this database to perform many of the review tasks described in Section "Protocol Editing/Disseminating/Reviewing", albeit a protocol has to actually be performed in order to populate the dose monitoring database.

For troubleshooting specific image quality issues, the information continued in scanner-based data "dumps" is usually limited. The scanner data "dump" reflects what the user defines for the protocol. At scan time, technologists may change the protocol. In DICOM verbiage, the actual protocol used to scan the patient is the performed protocol. The settings for the performed protocol are in the dose monitoring company's database of irradiation event details. They will also be in the DICOM header of the images sent to PACS. Therefore, for patient-specific image quality or dose issues, referring to the performed protocol parameters is essential for troubleshooting issues. For patient agnostic protocol management tasks, the defined protocols will usually suffice.

References

1. Boland GW. Enhancing CT productivity: strategies for increasing capacity. Am J Roentgenol. 2008;191(1):3–10.
2. ACR appropriateness criteria. American College of Radiology Web site. https://www.acr.org/Clinical-Resources/ACR-Appropriateness-Criteria Accessed 23rd Jan 2019.
3. Brunnquell CL, Avey GD, Szczykutowicz TP. Objective evaluation of CT time efficiency in acute stroke response. J Am Coll Radiol. 2018;15(6):876–80.
4. Szczykutowicz TP, Brunnquell CL, Avey GD, Bartels C, Belden DS, Bruce RJ, Field AS, Peppler WW, Wasmund P, Wendt G. A general framework for monitoring image acquisition workflow in the radiology environment: timeliness for acute stroke CT imaging. J Digit Imaging. 2018;31(2):201–9.
5. AAPM CT Lexicon Version 1.3. AAPM Web site. https://www.aapm.org/pubs/CTProtocols/documents/CTTerminologyLexicon.pdf Accessed 23rd Jan 2019.
6. TJC The Joint Commission Diagnostic Imaging Standards. https://www.jointcommission.org/assets/1/18/AHC_DiagImagingRpt_MK_20150806.pdf. Retrieved 18th Jan 2019.
7. Szczykutowicz TP, Pozniak M. A team approach for CT protocol optimization. J Assoc Med Imaging Manag Radiol Manag. 2016. Available at http://www.radiologymanagement-digital.com/radiologymanagement/11122016.
8. Szczykutowicz TP, Rubert N, Belden D, Ciano A, Duplissis A, Hermanns A, Monette S, JanssenSaldivar E. A wiki based CT protocol management system. Radiol Manage. 2015;(6):25–9.
9. DICOM. DICOM Supplement 121: CT Protocol Storage. ftp://medical.nema.org/medical/dicom/final/sup121_ft.pdf Accessed 23rd Jan 2019.
10. Szczykutowicz TP, Rubert N, Belden D, Ciano A, Duplissis A, Hermanns A, Monette S, Saldivar EJ. A wiki-based solution to managing your institution's imaging protocols. J Am Coll Radiol. 2016;13(7):822–4.
11. Sachs PB, Hunt K, Mansoubi F, Borgstede J. CT and MR protocol standardization across a large health system: providing a consistent radiologist, patient, and referring provider experience. J Digit Imaging. 2017;30(1):11–6.
12. Cody DD, Fisher TS, Gress DA, Jr RRL, McNitt-Gray MF, Jr RJP, Fairobent LA. AAPM medical physics practice guideline 1. A: CT protocol management and review practice guideline. J Appl Clin Med Phys. 2013;14(5):3–12.
13. Siegelman JRQW, Gress DA. Radiology stewardship and quality improvement: the process and costs of implementing a CT radiation dose optimization committee in a medium-sized community hospital system. J Am Coll Radiol. 2013;10(6):416–22.
14. Kofler JM, Cody DD, Morin RL. CT protocol review and optimization. J Am Coll Radiol. 2014;11(3):267–70.
15. Trattner S, Pearson GD, Chin C, Cody DD, Gupta R, Hess CP, et al. Standardization and optimization of CT protocols to achieve low dose. J Am Coll Radiol. 2014;11(3):271–8.
16. Szczykutowicz TP, Bour RK, Pozniak M, Ranallo FN. Compliance with AAPM practice Guideline 1. a: CT protocol management and review—from the perspective of a university hospital. J Appl Clin Med Phys. 2015;16(2):443–57.
17. Szczykutowicz TP, Bour RK, Rubert N, Wendt G, Pozniak M, Ranallo FN. CT protocol management: simplifying the process by using a master protocol concept. J Appl Clin Med Phys. 2015c;16(4):228–43.
18. Zhang D, Savage CA, Li X, Liu B. Data-driven CT protocol review and management—experience from a large academic hospital. J Am Coll Radiol. 2015;12(3):267–72.
19. Grimes J, Leng S, Zhang Y, Vrieze T, McCollough C. Implementation and evaluation of a protocol management system for automated review of CT protocols. J Appl Clin Med Phys. 2016;17(5):523–33.
20. IHE Integrating the Healthcare Enterprise: Management of Acquisition Protocols (MAP). https://www.ihe.net/uploadedFiles/Documents/Radiology/IHE_RAD_Suppl_MAP.pdf. Retrieved 18th Jan 2019.
21. Bohl M, Szczykutowicz T. A challenge to radiology and its professional associations: advocate for the implementation of IHE's management of acquisition protocols (MAP) profile. Published in the Radiology Business Management Association (RBMA) Bulletin November–December 2018.
22. Szczykutowicz TP, Siegelman J. On the same page—physicist and radiologist perspectives on protocol management and review. J Am Coll Radiol. 2015;12(8):808–14.
23. Szczykutowicz TP, Malkus A, Ciano A, Pozniak M. Tracking patterns of nonadherence to prescribed CT protocol parameters. J Am Coll Radiol. 2017;14(2):224–30.
24. Bae KT. Intravenous contrast medium administration and scan timing at CT: considerations and approaches. Radiology. 2010;256(1):32–61.
25. Kalra MK, Saini S, Rubin GD, editors. MDCT: from protocols to practice. New York: Springer Science & Business Media; 2009. Chapter 2 by KT Bae.

CT Practice Optimization

10

Mannudeep K. Kalra, Fatemeh Homayounieh, and Ramandeep Singh

Introduction: Defining the Scope

From a clinical perspective, optimization of CT practice enables and empowers interpreting physicians and CT technologists to deliver best services to their patients. From a clinical process improvement standpoint, practice optimization identifies stakeholders in introduction and maintenance of optimum CT services. Ideally, it must detail a framework or method by which appropriateness of clinical indications for CT can be judged using evidence-based likelihood of providing diagnostic information. It must include development of specific CT protocols for appropriate clinical indications with modification of scan parameters to tailor the image quality and radiation dose to as low as reasonably achievable (ALARA principle) to obtain the needed diagnostic information. Practice optimization should also describe surveillance strategies so that image quality issues and those related to outlier radiation doses can be addressed in a timely manner.

In this chapter, we describe the three essential elements of CT practice optimization from a clinical perspective: proper indications, protocol design, and parameter adjustments.

Proper Indication for CT Equals Justification

> The man of science has learned to believe in justification, not by faith, but by verification. Thomas Huxley, 1825–1895.

Justification should get maximum importance when it comes to optimization of CT practice. A low-dose CT for an unjustified or unindicated CT examination is a high-dose exam since the patient could have avoided radiation dose altogether. Indeed, given the sensitivity of CT, beyond the associated radiation dose, an unjustified exam can reveal incidental findings which can add to patient anxiety, trigger additional imaging tests or procedures, and increase healthcare costs.

Fortunately, several guidelines are available through notable organizations such as the American College of Radiology (ACR), Royal College of Radiologists of the United Kingdom, European Commission, and Royal College of Radiologists of Australia and New Zealand [1–6]. These guidelines describe appropriateness and/or diagnostic pathways for clinical indications with imaging examinations including CT. In the United States, ACR Appropriateness Criteria™ are most often cited or used in the online radiology order entry and decision support systems. The ACR Appropriateness Criteria™

M. K. Kalra (✉) · F. Homayounieh · R. Singh
MGH Webster Center for Quality and Safety, Department of Imaging, Massachusetts General Hospital, Boston, MA, USA

Harvard Medical School, Boston, MA, USA
e-mail: mkalra@mgh.harvard.edu; fhomayounieh@mgh.harvard.edu; rsingh17@mgh.harvard.edu

© Springer Nature Switzerland AG 2020

E. Samei, N. J. Pelc (eds.), *Computed Tomography*, https://doi.org/10.1007/978-3-030-26957-9_10

provide diagnostic utility scores for different imaging examinations for a host of clinical indications. The utility scores range from one through nine and represent the probability of obtaining required diagnostic information from an imaging test for a specific clinical indication based on reported evidence. Scores of one to three imply low diagnostic utility of an imaging test for the specific clinical indication or, in other words, the lower probability that the chosen imaging test will provide meaningful information for the clinical indication. Scores seven to nine imply high diagnostic utility, and four to six means intermediate diagnostic utility.

In the early 2000s, the Massachusetts General Hospital introduced an online radiology order entry and decision support system for ordering physicians to request and to schedule imaging tests from their computers [3, 7–9]. After secure login, the system prompts the physician to enter patient's medical record number and, then, select the required imaging test (e.g., chest CT). These steps pre-populate a list of clinical indications (such as a persistent cough, shortness of breath, nodule on chest radiograph, and cancer staging) specific to the selected imaging test (such as for chest CT). If the physician selects persistent cough as an indication for chest CT, the system displays a diagnostic utility score for chest CT (score 9). In addition, the system also displays other pertinent tests for the selected clinical indication and their utility scores (in the current example, chest radiograph also garners a score of 9). The physician can either proceed with the chest CT, change the ordered test (in this case, select chest radiograph), or modify specified clinical indication or indications and redo the diagnostic utility scores. If the ordering physician decides to proceed with CT, the system provides two pieces of information before confirming the order. The first displays a list and date of all previous imaging tests so that repeat, duplicate, or excessive imaging exams can be avoided. Second, a text page with information on appropriate use and associated radiation dose with CT is displayed. Although the procedure seems long, with familiarity, most physicians can place an order in under a minute and directly from within their patients' electronic medical record system.

Several studies have reported a substantial decrease in the use of CT following use of these decision support systems [1, 4, 5, 10–20]. The rules of decision support at our hospital are based on the ACR Appropriateness Criteria™ and recommendations from several internal panels of subspecialty radiologists and physicians. The diagnostic utility scores for different physicians and practices are recorded, audited, and used for reimbursement purposes by the third-party payors.

For institutions without online platforms such as the one described above, radiologists need to serve as gatekeepers for ensuring justification is met before a CT scan is acquired. Though time-consuming and tedious, it is an indispensable part of ensuring the highest level of vigilance in safe and appropriate use of radiation dose. Fortunately, as stated above, justification guidelines through various radiological organizations and bodies are available to aid the process.

CT Protocols: Why, How, Who, and What?

The Why?

Beyond justification, attention to clinical indications helps tailor the exam to answer a specific clinical question(s). Creation of CT protocols enables optimization to answer specific clinical indications from the point of view of the number of scan phases, scan parameters, details of intravenous and oral contrast media, as well as radiation dose (Table 10.1). For example, for follow-up of an incidental lung nodule, no contrast medium injection is needed, and the scan parameters are modified to enable thin sections and lower radiation dose for a single-phase inspiratory acquisition [21–24]. Conversely, if the indication is lung nodule in a patient with primary malignancy in the lungs or elsewhere, a contrast medium injection is often needed for a single inspiratory acquisition. Scan parameters are adjusted to provide sufficient radiation dose to assess regions beyond

Table 10.1 Top reasons for creating formal CT protocols

Adapt CT to answer specific or general clinical questions
Tailor image quality requirement
Establish the number of scan phases required for different indications
Set scan start and end location
Determine need and technique of oral and intravenous contrast administration
Tailor radiation dose in line with as low as reasonably achievable for specific questions
Specify section thickness, reconstruction kernel, and image postprocessing

lungs such as the mediastinum. Tracheal stenosis or tracheomalacia protocol often requires scanning in both inspiratory and expiratory phases although doses for each phase are lower than for patients undergoing CT for cancer staging, surveillance, or treatment response.

In the abdomen, clinical indications should affect the scan range, scan start, and end locations for each phase. For example, the noncontrast kidney stone protocol spans from the top of kidneys to the pubic symphysis; the single, portal venous phase, appendicitis protocol extends from L1 vertebral level to pubic symphysis; and the biphasic liver CT covers just the liver in the arterial phase and the entire abdomen-pelvis for the portal venous phase [25].

Dozens of prior studies have reported CT radiation dose reduction based on specific body regions and clinical indications [21, 22, 25–32]. Implementation of clinical indication-based CT protocols enables users to make full use of these options.

The Who and How?

Having established the need for adapting scanning protocols to clinical indications, the creation of indication-specific scan protocols becomes paramount. Making separate protocols for each clinical indication is neither feasible nor possible given the gamut of things that can go wrong with the same or different patients. Thus, a stratified approach should be adopted.

Scan protocols are divided into different body regions such as the head, neck, chest, abdomen-pelvis, and musculoskeletal regions. Protocols are then created separately for each region; in our institution, a subspecialty radiologist within each division is designated to create, modify, and update the CT protocols with help of a senior CT technology manager or supervisor. Medical physicists may be consulted on specific details of protocols. For each body region, the designated radiologist and CT technologist create different CT protocols using standardized protocol template. Apart from the date and version, each protocol template states the protocol title, clinical indications for its use, scanner name and detector profile, number of phases, scan range (start and end location) for each phase, details of oral and intravenous contrast media, patient instructions (regarding breath hold), and detailed scan, image reconstruction, and postprocessing parameters.

A standardized protocol template helps maintain consistency and avoid errors. Once protocol templates are approved by the rest of the division and/or the division head, they should be created, archived, and locked on the scanner graphic user interface. In our institution, only the approved users (CT technologist manager) with password access can change the saved protocols. In addition, all CT users (technologists and radiologists) should have access to hard and digital copies of all CT protocols for details such as clinical indications, contrast administration, scan range, and image postprocessing.

Beyond clinical indications, users should also create CT protocols specific for bariatric patients with large body habitus which require specific adjustments in scan and contrast injection techniques. Likewise, very small children also require adjustment of scan parameters to obtain motion-free, rapid scanning techniques (faster rotation time, higher pitch, and/or wider beam collimation). For advanced CT scanners, we also create a separate set of scan protocols for adult patients who cannot hold their breath or keep still for the duration of the scan.

To minimize confusion, nomenclature of scan protocols should be consistent across different CT scanners. For example, routine chest CT with contrast should be called the same on different CT scanners. This is especially important in larger institutions with a large number of CT technologists which circulate among multiple CT scanners. These steps also help in monitoring radiation doses and image quality across different CT scanners in institutions with multiple scanners.

The role of CT users does not end with the creation of CT protocols. These protocols should be reviewed at least once every year and, if necessary, updated should there be any change in scanner features (such as new detector assembly, new dose optimization feature, or new iterative reconstruction technique). For new or modified scan protocols, it is advisable to closely monitor image quality and radiation doses in the initial few patients, to avoid too low or too high image quality and radiation doses.

The What?

Before details of scan parameters, every scan protocol should address attributes which affect image quality and the associated radiation dose. These include patient position, centering, oral and intravenous contrast, number of scan phases, their scan ranges, and breathing instructions.

Although most CT procedures are performed in the supine position, certain protocols are performed in the prone position (hematuria protocol CT and prone images for evaluation of diffuse lung diseases).

The position of arms should be dealt with. For chest and abdomen CT, arms should be placed over shoulders to avoid artifacts and excessive radiation dose. When patients cannot place their arms over the shoulders, they should be placed in such as way so that the hands rest on a pad over the abdomen and not by the side of the body. This helps reduce the severity of artifacts. Scanners should be allowed to use higher radiation dose for such patients to decrease the penalty on image quality.

In bariatric patients undergoing chest CT, the head first position of the patient (i.e., head is closer to the CT gantry aperture than the feet) may be more comfortable and safer than feet first, when the abdominal girth exceeds the thoracic girth. For abdominal CT in bariatric patients, if the liver is the organ of interest, patients can be shifted slightly to the left to avoid truncation artifacts in the region of liver.

Patient centering is another factor that should be emphasized in CT protocols. For cardiac CT, the heart should be in the center of gantry aperture, which implies that these patients should be centered slightly lower compared to those having chest CT. Importance of appropriate patient centering should be emphasized for all patients but particularly for smaller adults and children since they are more likely to be off-centered with respect to the gantry isocenter. Mis-centering can result in an inaccurate estimation of patient size and attenuation for automatic exposure control (AEC) technique. It also interferes with the performance of the beam-shaping filters that help reduce surface radiation dose to vulnerable organs such as the breasts.

Tremendous variations exist between the number of scan phases for the same CT protocol and clinical indications. More phases mean greater radiation doses. For routine contrast-enhanced chest or abdominal CT, non-contrast images should not be acquired. Unless clinical indications demand evaluation of arterial and systemic venous anatomy, only one post-contrast scanning phase should be acquired for chest CT.

CT of the abdomen and pelvis often involves scanning patients in multiple phases. While routine non-contrast scanning before post-contrast acquisition should be avoided, in certain protocols multiple phases provide meaningful information. Biphasic or triphasic liver protocol involves post-contrast scanning in arterial, portal venous and/or delayed phases. To reduce radiation dose, in our institution, arterial and delayed phases are limited to the liver only, while portal venous phase spans the entire abdomen. For CT hematuria protocol, low-dose non-contrast images are acquired from the top of the kidneys to the pubic symphysis. Post-contrast images are then acquired with split bolus contrast injection technique, which enables a single scan phase acquisition with combined nephrographic and excretory information. This modified contrast injection technique has been extensively validated in prior publications and results in substantial radiation dose reduction compared to two to three post-contrast scan phases with separate nephrographic and excretory phases. In children, multiphase CT should be avoided, often with the use of ultrasonography or, when feasible, with MR imaging.

Apart from the variations in scan range for different scan phases, anatomic start and end locations should also be stated in all CT protocols based on the clinical indication. This has been discussed in the preceding section of this chapter.

For each scanning phase, CT protocols should mention breathing instructions. Technologists must instruct patient to avoid voluntary motion during scan acquisition. They should inform and demonstrate breath-hold instructions to the patients undergoing chest CT since motion artifacts related to breathing during scan acquisition can destroy the diagnostic usability of acquired CT images and require repeat scanning. Patients should be advised to breathe quietly and hold their breath for CT pulmonary angiography since deep inspiration or Valsalva maneuver can lead to contrast bolus interruption and suboptimal contrast enhancement in the pulmonary arteries. This is not an infrequent issue with CT pulmonary angiography and, therefore, warrants close attention.

CT protocols should also specify details of contrast media for both oral and intravenous routes. For intravenous contrast medium, these details should consider contrast concentration, volume, the rate of injection, injection duration, dilution (if any), and scan triggering technique. Most CT angiography examinations should involve the use of bolus tracking or timing bolus to determine the scan delay from the time of injection of contrast medium. Attention to these details can help avoid suboptimal contrast enhancement, which may require repeat scanning and additional radiation dose.

Both scan type (routine abdomen CT versus CT angiography of the abdomen) and intravenous contrast administration affect the choice of tube potential with or without automatic tube potential selection techniques (Sure KV, Canon; Auto KV, GE; Care KV, Siemens) which in turn determines the radiation dose [REF]. Furthermore, CT protocols with intravenous contrast medium in our institution often employ dual-energy CT techniques when performed on dual-energy capable scanners.

Scan Parameters

The choice of scan parameters depends on patient size, the body region, as well as scan protocol. In this section, we will discuss scan parameters based on body regions and scan protocols. Scan parameters may be arbitrarily classified into acquisition parameters that have some effect on image quality and radiation dose and reconstruction algorithm that do not have a direct effect on the radiation dose associated with scanning (Table 10.2). There is some overlap between parameters such as section thickness and beam pitch which on some scanners (Siemens, Philips) has no effect on radiation dose but may affect radiation dose on other scanners (GE, Canon).

Modern multidetector-row CT scanners are equipped with AEC, which helps adapt radiation dose to differences in patient body habitus. Tweaking of AEC may be necessary for bariatric patients, particularly for abdomen-pelvis CT. Likewise, automatic tube potential selection techniques are available on most modern scanners for selecting tube potential based on patient size and specified exam type (such as non-contrast CT, CT angiography, and routine post-contrast abdomen-pelvis CT).

Iterative reconstruction techniques reduce image noise and artifacts in low radiation dose CT images, and when available, other scan parameters can be adjusted to reduce radiation dose relative to conventional filtered back projection techniques of image reconstruction. Several studies have documented the potential for a substantial decrease in radiation dose with iterative reconstruction techniques [33–52]. Although a few studies have reported a decrease in conspicuity of low-contrast structures with iterative recon-

Table 10.2 Specific acquisition and reconstruction parameters for CT protocols

Acquisition parameters
Scan start location
Scan end location
Number of scan phases or acquisitions
Scan mode (helical or axial)
Scan type (single energy or dual energy)
Tube current (use AEC)
Specify noise index, dose right index, standard deviation, or quality reference mAs
Specify minimum and maximum mA or strength of modulation
Tube potential (use automatic tube potential selection when available)
Beam pitch
Detector configuration
Gantry rotation time
Section thickness (for some scanners, this is a prospective parameter and affects dose)
Reconstruction parameters
Section thickness (for some scanners, this does not affect dose)
Section interval
Reconstruction technique (use iterative reconstruction when available)
Reconstruction algorithms/filters/kernels
Reconstruction field of view
Image postprocessing (plane, thickness, and interval)

struction techniques, the clear majority of evidence supports their use [53, 54]. In our institution, where available, iterative reconstruction techniques are the default technique of image reconstruction. The strength of noise reduction with iterative reconstruction varies between different body regions and protocol types. It is important for institutions not comfortable with the image appearance with iterative reconstruction techniques to start at the lowest strength with minimal dose reduction. Once radiologists get used to the image appearance, the strength of noise reduction can be gradually increased while reducing radiation dose.

Head CT

Users must create at least few different CT protocols for each body region (Table 10.3). While most CT centers use axial mode of scanning for head CT, the helical acquisition mode is becoming popular as it is faster, causes fewer artifacts, and can deliver similar dose to axial scanning mode. Scanners with wide area detector array (GE and Canon) that span 16 cm per rotation can scan the entire head in one rotation. On those scanners, a single body part with scan lengths of less than 16 cm is often scanned in axial scanning mode. Several studies have reported the use of AEC for head and neck CT studies to reduce radiation dose while maintaining diagnostic confidence [46, 55–59]. Thus, we use AEC techniques for all such CT studies in our institution. Compared to the other body regions, due to low inherent tissue contrast of brain parenchyma, a higher tube current or a lower noise index or standard deviation is often needed.

Table 10.3 Common CT protocols in the head and neck

Head trauma CT
Head stroke protocol
CT angiography of head and/or neck
Routine head CT
CT of paranasal sinuses (non-contrast, low-dose)
CT of paranasal sinuses (contrast-enhanced for evaluation of soft tissue evaluation)
CT of cervical spine
CT neck for soft tissue evaluation (with or without contrast enhancement)

CT for assessing brain perfusion should be performed at 80 kV without exception to reduce dose and enhance the conspicuity of intravenous contrast on CT images. Several studies have reported the use of low tube potential (<120 kV) for CT angiography of the head and neck [60–62]. Whether with manually specified tube potential or with the use of automatic tube potential selection technique, lower tube potential (<120 kV) helps increase the contrast enhancement and reduce radiation dose, when compared to a higher tube potential (≥120 kV). When available, automatic tube potential selection technique should be used.

Typically, gantry rotation time of 1–2 s is used for most head CT. For uncooperative or moving patients, faster gantry rotation time (≤0.5 s) can be used to decrease motion artifacts. For CT scanners with less than 16 cm longitudinal length, thinner detector configuration or beam width is employed for head CT. For example, detector configuration of 32×0.625 mm is used for head CT on GE VCT (64-row CT scanner) compared to 64×0.625 mm for body CT examinations. This helps reduce beam hardening artifacts in the posterior fossa. Furthermore, given the shorter scan length, narrow detector configuration is more dose efficient in head CT for such scanners. An exception to this rule would be head and neck CT angiography which requires faster scanning over greater scan length, and thus, a wider detector configuration is desirable (e.g., 64×0.625 mm for GE VCT).

For head CT, patient positioning should involve placement of patient's head in the headrest unless contraindicated or unsafe. Given the smaller dimension of the head relative to the body, CT technologists must pay close attention when centering the head in the gantry isocenter.

Chest CT

Common CT protocols in the chest are summarized in Table 10.4. All chest CT must be performed with AEC and, when available, with automatic tube potential selection technique, to optimize image quality and radiation dose. Most chest CT on modern CT scanners equipped with iterative reconstruction techniques can be and should be performed at ≤100 kV unless the patient is markedly obese.

AEC technique should be modified suitably for different CT protocols. For example, if 100 quality reference mAs (QRM, Care Dose 4D, Siemens) is used for routine chest CT protocol, 30–40 mAs QRM suffices for lung nodule follow-up (Fig. 10.1) or lung cancer screening low-dose CT (Fig. 10.2). Likewise, when iterative reconstruction techniques are available, AEC technique should be modified to reduce dose compared to the conventional filtered back projection [21, 33, 41, 42, 52, 63–69].

Table 10.4 Common CT protocols in the chest

Routine chest CT (with or without contrast)
Chest CT for patients unable to hold their breath (with or without contrast)
CT pulmonary angiography
Diffuse lung disease CT (also called high resolution CT)
CT for airway evaluation (tracheal abnormalities)
Low-dose lung nodule follow-up CT
Low-dose CT for lung cancer screening
CT for chest wall abnormalities

Relative to the abdominal CT of the same patient, AEC should be modified to deliver a lower radiation dose to the chest than to the abdomen. A rule of thumb, which we find useful here, is that radiation dose for routine chest CT must be at least 30–50% lower than for routine abdominal CT in the same patients. There are many reasons for this rule. Firstly, there is higher inherent tissue contrast in the chest than in the abdomen. Secondly, lesions in the chest tend to have higher contrast compared to their background tissues, which means that these lesions can be assessed despite higher noise at much lower doses relative to low-contrast lesions in the liver, pancreas, or kidneys. Thirdly, the air in the lungs causes little attenuation of the X-ray beam, and thus noise content in chest CT at equivalent doses is substantially lower relative to the abdomen. The shoulder region is an exception, and often, AEC will increase the tube current in this region to maintain image quality.

Another unique aspect of chest CT which has been previously stated is the possibility of motion artifacts that can limit evaluation. Thus, a faster scanning speed is preferred for chest CT in addition to good breath-hold instructions to the patients. A wider detector configuration and faster table speed are also used to facilitate faster scanning in the chest.

In our institution, for patients who are unable to hold their breath for chest CT, we employ specific strategies. These patients are preferentially scanned on dual-source CT scanners (such as Siemens Definition Flash and Force) or wide area detector single-source CT (GE Revolution). On the dual-source CT, we use a high, nonoverlapping pitch (up to 3.4:1) and 0.25–0.27 s gantry rotation time. These patients are either instructed to take shallow breaths or given no instruction for breath hold. Chest CT images can

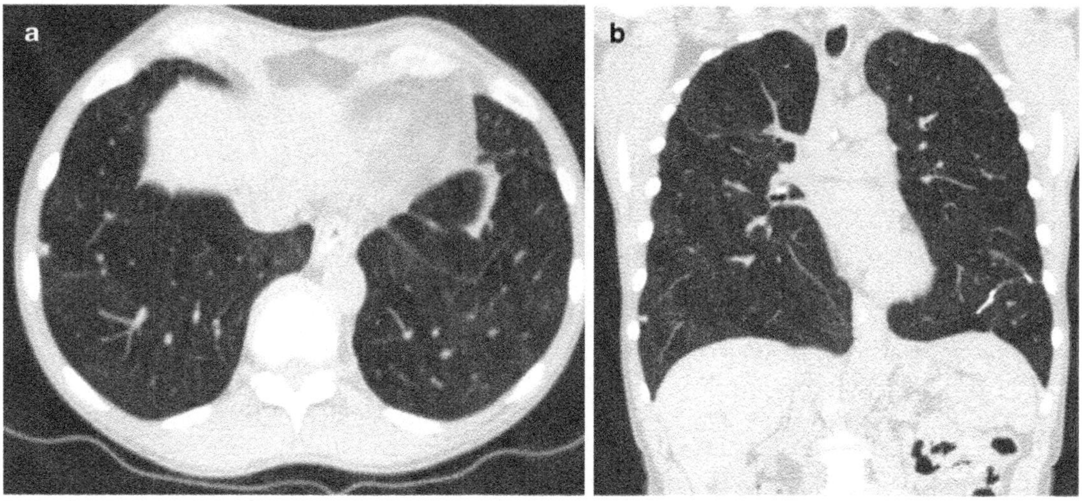

Fig. 10.1 Transverse (**a**) and coronal (**b**) images of a 64-year-old man (49 kg) who underwent low-dose, non-contrast-enhanced chest CT (CTDIvol 1 mGy, DLP 44 mGy.cm) for lung nodule follow-up. There is a 5 mm subpleural nodule in the right lower lobe

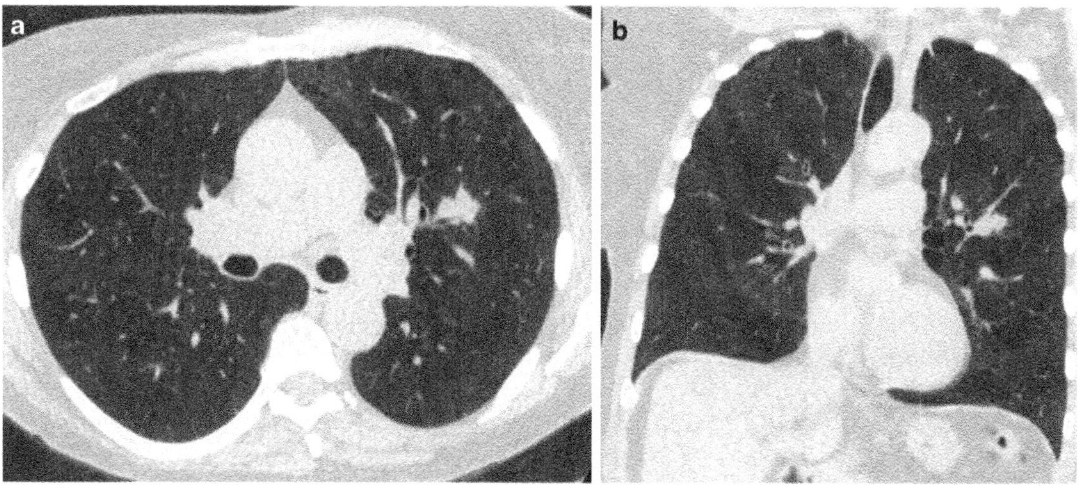

Fig. 10.2 Transverse (**a**) and coronal (**b**) images of a 64-year-old woman (65 kg) who underwent low-dose CT for lung cancer screening (CTDIvol 0.85 mGy, DLP 32 mGy.cm). There is a lobulated 1.5 cm nodule in the left upper lobe with changes of paraseptal emphysema in bilateral lungs

be acquired in about 1 s with this approach. On non-dual-source CT scanners, selection of highest pitch (typically up to 1.6:1), fastest gantry rotation time, and widest available detector configuration can help reduce scan duration. On wide area detector arrays (with 16 cm detector width), a single rotation can cover up to 16 cm scan length in an axial scanning mode which is sufficient in small children. Beyond 16 cm scan length (for older children and all adults), the interscan delay increases the scan duration for axial mode, and helical scanning mode with 8 cm detector configuration is faster and preferable with fast rotation times.

Dual-energy CT is being increasingly used for clinical indications such as CT pulmonary angiography, where it can provide greater contrast enhancement and aid in the evaluation of pulmonary parenchymal perfusion [21, 70–73]. Multiple studies have explored the value of dual-energy CT in the lung and mediastinal lesions for tissue characterization and assessment of treatment response [74, 75]. In our institution, dual energy is used for all contrast-enhanced routine chest CT and CT pulmonary angiography when patients are scanned on dual-energy-capable CT scanners (Fig. 10.3). Dose parity with single-energy CT is important, and studies have demonstrated that it is possible to achieve this parity [73, 76–79]. Recent studies have shown that multiphase dual-energy CT of the chest can help characterize pulmonary and mediastinal lesions [80–82]. However, there is no conclusive evidence at the time of writing this manuscript to recommend multiphase CT protocols for chest in routine clinical practice.

Abdomen-Pelvis CT

CT of the abdomen and pelvis must be performed with AEC and, when available, with automatic tube potential selection technique. When the latter is unavailable, most abdominal CT examinations are performed at 120 kV. For multiphase CT, such as for liver lesions and renal masses, lower tube potential (≤100 kV) can be used for arterial phase images in nonobese patients. This approached coupled with reduced scan length for certain phases help reduce radiation dose for multiphase abdomen-pelvis CT examinations. Lower tube potential (≤100 kV) also helps reduce radiation dose in patients undergoing CT for evaluation of renal colic or urinary calculi.

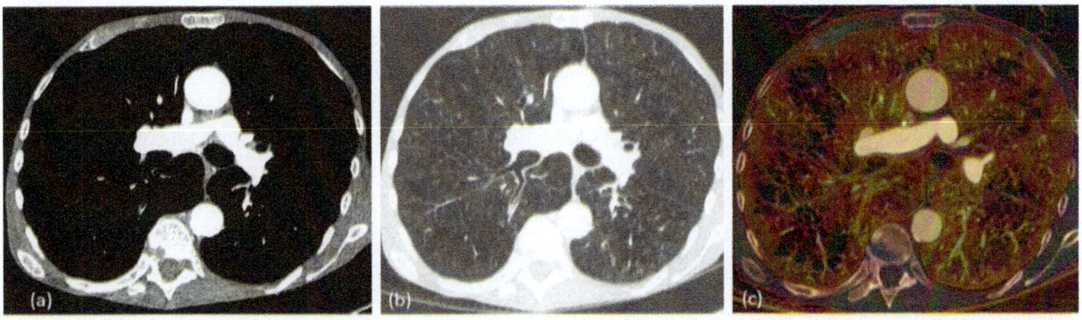

Fig. 10.3 Transverse CT images of a 65-year-old man (33 kg) who underwent dual-source, dual-energy CT pulmonary angiogram (CTDIvol 2.9 mGy, DLP 132 mGy.cm) for shortness of breath. There is optimal contrast enhancement of thoracic vessels on 40 kev virtual monoenergetic image (**a**). The lung window (**b**) demonstrates changes of emphysema, which result in matched perfusion defects on material decomposition image (**c**)

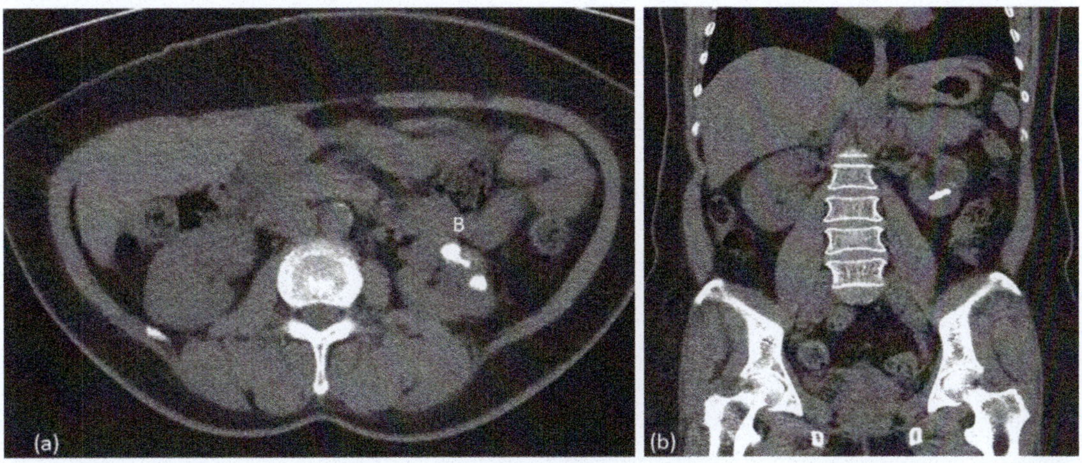

Fig. 10.4 Transverse (**a**) and coronal (**b**) images of a 60-year-old (62 kg) who underwent single-energy, noncontrast-enhanced abdominal CT with kidney stone protocol. There are nonobstructive left renal calculi. The low radiation dose protocol resulted in CTDIvol of 2.5 mGy and DLP of 136 mGy.cm

Table 10.5 Common CT protocols in the abdomen and pelvis

Routine abdomen-pelvis CT (with *or* without contrast enhancement)
Biphasic or triphasic liver
Kidney stone CT (low dose, non-contrast)
CT for hematuria (low dose, non-contrast, followed with single post-contrast phase)
CT for pancreatic mass
CT for adrenal lesion
CT renal mass
CT angiography of abdominal arteries
CT for appendicitis
CT colonography

Like for chest CT, AEC should be modified for different abdomen-pelvis CT protocols. Thus, CT for kidney stone evaluation (Fig. 10.4) and colonography should be performed at lower radiation dose with changes to the AEC as compared to routine abdomen-pelvis CT. Further modifications to AEC and/or automatic tube potential selection technique are required to reduce radiation dose when using iterative reconstruction technique.

Routine abdomen-pelvis CT examinations (Table 10.5) are performed with a gantry rotation time of 0.5–0.8 s, a pitch greater than 1:1, and a wider detector configuration to maintain reasonable scan duration and avoid motion artifacts [25, 29, 83]. Certain modifications may be necessary in bariatric patients such as increasing the applied tube current (by adjusting the image quality metric for AEC), prolonging the gantry rotation time (e.g., from 0.5 to 0.8 to 1 s), and/or decreasing the pitch (to less than 1:1). These steps enable the scanner to use greater tube current and obtain desirable diagnostic quality images of the abdomen and pelvis. Increase in tube potential to 140 or 150 kV also helps decrease the image noise and artifacts in very large patients, although it is associated with a decrease in contrast enhancement. The strength of iterative reconstruction techniques can be increased to decrease image noise. Use of thicker sections (≥5 mm) and/or smoother reconstruction algorithm also reduce image noise.

Dual-energy CT techniques in abdomen-pelvis are being increasingly used for a variety of indications including liver lesion evaluation, kidney stone characterization, and CT angiography [84–91]. As is true for other body regions, unless there is overriding clinical evidence, dose parity between dual-energy and single-energy CT scanners should be maintained for abdomen-pelvis CT as well.

Pediatric CT

Pediatric CT poses special challenges to optimization since children vary substantially in size (1–100 kg) and are also more susceptible to potential risks from radiation dose. The common CT protocols in children are summarized in Table 10.6. As stated in preceding sections, AEC and automatic tube potential selection techniques help select tube current and tube potential for children of various sizes. When these techniques are not available, users should employ a weight- or size-based approach to adapt tube current and tube potential in children of different sizes. These strategies have been described in several publications [6, 37, 92–95].

Small children undergoing contrast-enhanced CT may only receive 2–10 ml of intravenous contrast. Thus, care should be taken to set optimal scan trigger time following contrast injection, ideally with input and presence of an experienced radiologist. This can avoid repeat imaging due to suboptimal contrast enhancement. A test saline injection should help ensure that the intravenous access is patent and there is no risk for extravasation. Extra-long connecting tubes between the site of the intravenous catheter and the injector (whether manual or automatic) should be avoided due to small contrast volume. Likewise, any kinks or obstructions in the connecting tube should be assessed prior to scanning.

Table 10.6 Common CT protocols in children

Routine head CT
Routine chest CT
Routine abdomen-pelvis CT
CT for appendicitis (after inconclusive ultrasonography and MR imaging)
Chest CT for airway evaluation
Chest CT for chest wall deformity

Children who are likely to move during CT scanning may require tight bundling (only works in newborns and small infants), sedation, or anesthesia. To decrease the need for sedation or anesthesia, as well as motion artifacts, CT parameters should be adjusted in line with what has been described in the chest CT section with regard to uncooperative adult patients. Studies have reported that nonoverlapping pitch (up to 3.4:1) on dual-source CT and wide area detector arrays (up to 16 cm detector width) can avoid motion artifacts and, thus, reduce the need for sedation or anesthesia in children [96–99].

Quality Concerns

Creation and implementation of CT protocols are clinical processes that require constant surveillance to ensure that protocols deliver studies that help practicing radiologists answer the clinical questions. Quality issues may arise due to patient factors (such as motion artifacts, arms by the side, suboptimal contrast, and large body habitus) and/or imaging staff (such as wrong scan protocol, wrong or incorrect contrast injection, and too short or too long scan lengths). CT protocols must be updated where possible to address and rectify such errors. In our institution, radiologists can electronically notify the CT protocol team about any issues related to any imaging modality including CT. When corrective strategies can be adopted, an electronic communication is sent to the notifying radiologist within 24 h. These steps help maintain staff confidence and ensure constant vigilance to any serious concerns.

Dose Monitoring

Dose monitoring is an important part of CT practice. It allows for benchmarking of radiation doses for different CT protocols versus local, regional, national, and international dose levels. Although reference dose levels for common CT protocols are available for both adults and children, the less frequently used CT protocols often do not have such levels available [100–106].

In the United States, the American College of Radiology Dose Index Registry (ACR DIR) receives millions of CT dose reports from several hundred CT centers [107, 108]. Each contributing center receives periodic dose summaries which compare the doses from their center with the regional and national median doses. All three metrics, CT dose index volume (CTDIvol), dose length product (DLP), and size-specific dose estimates (SSDE), are reported. The dose data are de-identified prior to their transfer to the ACR DIR.

Several commercial dose monitoring services and software are also available for dose monitoring on the institutional level [104, 109, 110]. These software help monitor radiation doses and find protocols and specific CT examinations that exceed prespecified dose levels. Dose monitoring identifies CT protocols with excessive doses that need attention and modifications.

Conclusions

CT practice optimization for radiation dose optimization begins with ensuring that CT examinations have an appropriate clinical indication. Once appropriateness is established, clinical indication-based CT protocols must be established with a team-based approach. Active surveillance strategies are critical for ensuring the diagnostic quality of performed CT examinations at as low as reasonably achievable radiation doses.

References

1. O'Connor SD, Sodickson AD, Ip IK, Raja AS, Healey MJ, Schneider LI, et al. Journal club: requiring clinical justification to override repeat imaging decision support: impact on CT use. AJR Am J Roentgenol. 2014;203(5):W482–90.
2. Street M, Brady Z, Van Every B, Thomson KR. Radiation exposure and the justification of computed tomography scanning in an Australian hospital emergency department. Intern Med J. 2009;39(11):713–9.
3. Vartanians VM, Sistrom CL, Weilburg JB, Rosenthal DI, Thrall JH. Increasing the appropriateness of out-

patient imaging: effects of a barrier to ordering low-yield examinations. Radiology. 2010;255(3):842–9.
4. Sistrom CL, Weilburg JB, Dreyer KJ, Ferris TG. Provider feedback about imaging appropriateness by using scores from order entry decision support: raw rates misclassify outliers. Radiology. 2015;275(2):469–79.
5. Moriarity AK, Klochko C, O'Brien M, Halabi S. The effect of clinical decision support for advanced inpatient imaging. J Am Coll Radiol: JACR. 2015;12(4):358–63.
6. Frush DP. Deciding why and when to use CT in children: a radiologist's perspective. Pediatr Radiol. 2014;44(Suppl 3):404–8.
7. Sistrom CL, Dang PA, Weilburg JB, Dreyer KJ, Rosenthal DI, Thrall JH. Effect of computerized order entry with integrated decision support on the growth of outpatient procedure volumes: seven-year time series analysis. Radiology. 2009;251(1):147–55.
8. Rosenthal DI, Weilburg JB, Schultz T, Miller JC, Nixon V, Dreyer KJ, et al. Radiology order entry with decision support: initial clinical experience. J Am Coll Radiol: JACR. 2006;3(10):799–806.
9. Morin RL, Rosenthal DI, Stout MB. Radiology order entry: features and performance requirements. J Am Coll Radiol: JACR. 2006;3(7):554–7.
10. Huber T, Gaskin CM, Krishnaraj A. Early experience with implementation of a commercial decision-support product for imaging order entry. Curr Probl Diagn Radiol. 2016;45(2):133–6.
11. Gupta A, Ip IK, Raja AS, Andruchow JE, Sodickson A, Khorasani R. Effect of clinical decision support on documented guideline adherence for head CT in emergency department patients with mild traumatic brain injury. J Am Med Inform Assoc: JAMIA. 2014;21(e2):e347–51.
12. Gupta A, Raja AS, Khorasani R. Examining clinical decision support integrity: is clinician self-reported data entry accurate? J Am Med Inform Assoc: JAMIA. 2014;21(1):23–6.
13. Brink JA. Clinical decision-making tools for exam selection, reporting and dose tracking. Pediatr Radiol. 2014;44(Suppl 3):418–21.
14. Gimbel RW, Fontelo P, Stephens MB, Olsen CH, Bunt C, Ledford CJ, et al. Radiation exposure and cost influence physician medical image decision making: a randomized controlled trial. Med Care. 2013;51(7):628–32.
15. Duszak R Jr, Berlin JW. Utilization management in radiology, part 2: perspectives and future directions. J Am Coll Radiol: JACR. 2012;9(10):700–3.
16. Duszak R Jr, Berlin JW. Utilization management in radiology, part 1: rationale, history, and current status. J Am Coll Radiol: JACR. 2012;9(10):694–9.
17. Rehani MM, Berris T. International atomic energy agency study with referring physicians on patient radiation exposure and its tracking: a prospective survey using a web-based questionnaire. BMJ Open. 2012;2(5).
18. Zafar HM, Mills AM, Khorasani R, Langlotz CP. Clinical decision support for imaging in the era of the patient protection and affordable care act. J Am Coll Radiol: JACR. 2012;9(12):907–18.e5.
19. Yousem DM. Combating overutilization: radiology benefits managers versus order entry decision support. Neuroimaging Clin N Am. 2012;22(3):497–509.
20. Ip IK, Schneider LI, Hanson R, Marchello D, Hultman P, Viera M, et al. Adoption and meaningful use of computerized physician order entry with an integrated clinical decision support system for radiology: ten-year analysis in an urban teaching hospital. J Am Coll Radiol: JACR. 2012;9(2):129–36.
21. Tabari A, Lo Gullo R, Murugan V, Otrakji A, Digumarthy S, Kalra M. Recent advances in computed tomographic technology: cardiopulmonary imaging applications. J Thorac Imaging. 2017;32(2):89–100.
22. Singh S, Kalra MK, Ali Khawaja RD, Padole A, Pourjabbar S, Lira D, et al. Radiation dose optimization and thoracic computed tomography. Radiol Clin N Am. 2014;52(1):1–15.
23. Singh S, Kalra MK, Thrall JH, Mahesh M. Pointers for optimizing radiation dose in chest CT protocols. J Am Coll Radiol: JACR. 2011;8(9):663–5.
24. Tack D. Radiation dose optimization in thoracic imaging. JBR-BTR: Organe Soc R Belge Radiol (SRBR) = Orgaan van de Koninklijke Belgische Vereniging voor Radiologie (KBVR). 2010;93(1):15–9.
25. Kalra MK, Maher MM, Toth TL, Hamberg LM, Blake MA, Shepard JA, et al. Strategies for CT radiation dose optimization. Radiology. 2004;230(3):619–28.
26. Sung MK, Singh S, Kalra MK. Current status of low dose multi-detector CT in the urinary tract. World J Radiol. 2011;3(11):256–65.
27. Kalra MK, Maher MM, Rizzo S, Kanarek D, Shepard JA. Radiation exposure from chest CT: issues and strategies. J Korean Med Sci. 2004;19(2):159–66.
28. Maher MM, Kalra MK, Toth TL, Wittram C, Saini S, Shepard J. Application of rational practice and technical advances for optimizing radiation dose for chest CT. J Thorac Imaging. 2004;19(1):16–23.
29. Kalra MK, Sodickson AD, Mayo-Smith WW. CT radiation: key concepts for gentle and wise use. Radiographics: Rev Publ Radiol Soc N America, Inc. 2015;35(6):1706–21.
30. Padole A, Ali Khawaja RD, Kalra MK, Singh S. CT radiation dose and iterative reconstruction techniques. AJR Am J Roentgenol. 2015;204(4):W384–92.
31. Trattner S, Pearson GD, Chin C, Cody DD, Gupta R, Hess CP, et al. Standardization and optimization of CT protocols to achieve low dose. J Am Coll Radiol: JACR. 2014;11(3):271–8.
32. Tack D, Kalra MK, Gevenois PA. Radiation dose from multidetector CT. 2nd ed. Heidelberg: Springer; 2012.. xviii, 649 p. p
33. Padole A, Digumarthy S, Flores E, Madan R, Mishra S, Sharma A, et al. Assessment of chest CT at CTDIvol

less than 1 mGy with iterative reconstruction techniques. Br J Radiol. 2017;90(1071):20160625.
34. Padole A, Sainani N, Lira D, Khawaja RD, Pourjabbar S, Lo Gullo R, et al. Assessment of sub-milli-sievert abdominal computed tomography with iterative reconstruction techniques of different vendors. World J Radiol. 2016;8(6):618–27.
35. Khawaja RD, Singh S, Blake M, Harisinghani M, Choy G, Karaosmanoglu A, et al. Ultra-low dose abdominal MDCT: using a knowledge-based iterative model reconstruction technique for substantial dose reduction in a prospective clinical study. Eur J Radiol. 2015;84(1):2–10.
36. Khawaja RD, Singh S, Blake M, Harisinghani M, Choy G, Karaosmanoglu A, et al. Ultralow-dose abdominal computed tomography: comparison of 2 iterative reconstruction techniques in a prospective clinical study. J Comput Assist Tomogr. 2015;39(4):489–98.
37. Khawaja RD, Singh S, Otrakji A, Padole A, Lim R, Nimkin K, et al. Dose reduction in pediatric abdominal CT: use of iterative reconstruction techniques across different CT platforms. Pediatr Radiol. 2015;45(7):1046–55.
38. Singh S, Khawaja RD, Pourjabbar S, Padole A, Lira D, Kalra MK. Iterative image reconstruction and its role in cardiothoracic computed tomography. J Thorac Imaging. 2013;28(6):355–67.
39. Kalra MK, Woisetschlager M, Dahlstrom N, Singh S, Lindblom M, Choy G, et al. Radiation dose reduction with Sinogram affirmed iterative reconstruction technique for abdominal computed tomography. J Comput Assist Tomogr. 2012;36(3):339–46.
40. Singh S, Kalra MK, Shenoy-Bhangle AS, Saini A, Gervais DA, Westra SJ, et al. Radiation dose reduction with hybrid iterative reconstruction for pediatric CT. Radiology. 2012;263(2):537–46.
41. Singh S, Kalra MK, Gilman MD, Hsieh J, Pien HH, Digumarthy SR, et al. Adaptive statistical iterative reconstruction technique for radiation dose reduction in chest CT: a pilot study. Radiology. 2011;259(2):565–73.
42. Prakash P, Kalra MK, Ackman JB, Digumarthy SR, Hsieh J, Do S, et al. Diffuse lung disease: CT of the chest with adaptive statistical iterative reconstruction technique. Radiology. 2010;256(1):261–9.
43. Prakash P, Kalra MK, Digumarthy SR, Hsieh J, Pien H, Singh S, et al. Radiation dose reduction with chest computed tomography using adaptive statistical iterative reconstruction technique: initial experience. J Comput Assist Tomogr. 2010;34(1):40–5.
44. Prakash P, Kalra MK, Kambadakone AK, Pien H, Hsieh J, Blake MA, et al. Reducing abdominal CT radiation dose with adaptive statistical iterative reconstruction technique. Investig Radiol. 2010;45(4):202–10.
45. Schmid AI, Uder M, Lell MM. Reaching for better image quality and lower radiation dose in head and neck CT: advanced modeled and sinogram-affirmed iterative reconstruction in combination with tube voltage adaptation. Dentomaxillofac Radiol. 2017;46(1):20160131.
46. Scholtz JE, Wichmann JL, Bennett DW, Leithner D, Bauer RW, Vogl TJ, et al. Detecting intracranial hemorrhage using automatic tube current modulation with advanced modeled iterative reconstruction in unenhanced head single- and dual-energy dual-source CT. AJR Am J Roentgenol. 2017;208(5):1089–96.
47. Soenen O, Balliauw C, Oyen R, Zanca F. Dose and image quality in low-dose CT for urinary stone disease: added value of automatic tube current modulation and iterative reconstruction techniques. Radiat Prot Dosim. 2017;174(2):242–9.
48. Chen CM, Lin YY, Hsu MY, Hung CF, Liao YL, Tsai HY. Performance of adaptive iterative dose reduction 3D integrated with automatic tube current modulation in radiation dose and image noise reduction compared with filtered-back projection for 80-kVp abdominal CT: anthropomorphic phantom and patient study. Eur J Radiol. 2016;85(9):1666–72.
49. Hata A, Yanagawa M, Honda O, Gyobu T, Ueda K, Tomiyama N. Submillisievert CT using model-based iterative reconstruction with lung-specific setting: an initial phantom study. Eur Radiol. 2016;26:4457.
50. Lee S, Kwon H, Cho J. The detection of focal liver lesions using abdominal CT: a comparison of image quality between adaptive statistical iterative reconstruction V and adaptive statistical iterative reconstruction. Acad Radiol. 2016;23(12):1532–8.
51. McLaughlin PD, Murphy KP, Twomey M, O'Neill SB, Moloney F, O'Connor OJ, et al. Pure iterative reconstruction improves image quality in computed tomography of the abdomen and pelvis acquired at substantially reduced radiation doses in patients with active Crohn disease. J Comput Assist Tomogr. 2016;40(2):225–33.
52. Schafer ML, Ludemann L, Boning G, Kahn J, Fuchs S, Hamm B, et al. Radiation dose reduction in CT with adaptive statistical iterative reconstruction (ASIR) for patients with bronchial carcinoma and intrapulmonary metastases. Clin Radiol. 2016;71(5):442–9.
53. Volgyes D, Pedersen M, Stray-Pedersen A, Waaler D, Martinsen AC. How different iterative and filtered Back projection kernels affect computed tomography numbers and low contrast detectability. J Comput Assist Tomogr. 2017;41(1):75–81.
54. Viry A, Aberle C, Racine D, Knebel JF, Schindera ST, Schmidt S, et al. Effects of various generations of iterative CT reconstruction algorithms on low-contrast detectability as a function of the effective abdominal diameter: a quantitative task-based phantom study. Phys Med: PM: Int J Devoted Appl Phys Med Biol: Off J Ital Assoc Biomed Phys (AIFB). 2018;48:111–8.
55. Furuya K, Nambu A, Nakamura K, Watanabe R, Nogata Y, Komiyama T, et al. Modified method for automatic exposure control in pediatric brain CT-application of the standard deviation

value method by use of patient's age and head size. Nihon Hoshasen Gijutsu Gakkai zasshi. 2010;66(4):334–42.

56. Gnannt R, Winklehner A, Goetti R, Schmidt B, Kollias S, Alkadhi H. Low kilovoltage CT of the neck with 70 kVp: comparison with a standard protocol. AJNR Am J Neuroradiol. 2012;33(6):1014–9.
57. Tan JS, Tan KL, Lee JC, Wan CM, Leong JL, Chan LL. Comparison of eye lens dose on neuroimaging protocols between 16- and 64-section multidetector CT: achieving the lowest possible dose. AJNR Am J Neuroradiol. 2009;30(2):373–7.
58. Wallace AN, Vyhmeister R, Bagade S, Chatterjee A, Hicks B, Ramirez-Giraldo JC, et al. Evaluation of the use of automatic exposure control and automatic tube potential selection in low-dose cerebrospinal fluid shunt head CT. Neuroradiology. 2015;57(6):639–44.
59. Tsapaki V, Aldrich JE, Sharma R, Staniszewska MA, Krisanachinda A, Rehani M, et al. Dose reduction in CT while maintaining diagnostic confidence: diagnostic reference levels at routine head, chest, and abdominal CT--IAEA-coordinated research project. Radiology. 2006;240(3):828–34.
60. You J, Dai Y, Huang N, Li JJ, Cheng L, Zhang XL, et al. Low-dose computed tomography with adaptive statistical iterative reconstruction and low tube voltage in craniocervical computed tomographic angiography: impact of body mass index. J Comput Assist Tomogr. 2015;39(5):774–80.
61. Zhang WL, Li M, Zhang B, Geng HY, Liang YQ, Xu K, et al. CT angiography of the head-and-neck vessels acquired with low tube voltage, low iodine, and iterative image reconstruction: clinical evaluation of radiation dose and image quality. PLoS One. 2013;8(12):e81486.
62. Singh S, Kalra MK, Thrall JH, Mahesh M. Pointers for optimizing radiation dose in head CT protocols. J Am Coll Radiol: JACR. 2011;8(8):591–3.
63. Pourjabbar S, Singh S, Kulkarni N, Muse V, Digumarthy SR, Khawaja RD, et al. Dose reduction for chest CT: comparison of two iterative reconstruction techniques. Acta Radiol (Stockholm, Sweden: 1987). 2015;56(6):688–95.
64. Khawaja RD, Singh S, Gilman M, Sharma A, Do S, Pourjabbar S, et al. Computed tomography (CT) of the chest at less than 1 mSv: an ongoing prospective clinical trial of chest CT at submillisievert radiation doses with iterative model image reconstruction and iDose4 technique. J Comput Assist Tomogr. 2014;38(4):613–9.
65. Kalra MK, Woisetschlager M, Dahlstrom N, Singh S, Digumarthy S, Do S, et al. Sinogram-affirmed iterative reconstruction of low-dose chest CT: effect on image quality and radiation dose. AJR Am J Roentgenol. 2013;201(2):W235–44.
66. Pontana F, Billard AS, Duhamel A, Schmidt B, Faivre JB, Hachulla E, et al. Effect of iterative reconstruction on the detection of systemic sclerosis-related interstitial lung disease: clinical experience in 55 patients. Radiology. 2016;279(1):297–305.
67. Barras H, Dunet V, Hachulla AL, Grimm J, Beigelman-Aubry C. Influence of model based iterative reconstruction algorithm on image quality of multiplanar reformations in reduced dose chest CT. Acta Radiol Open. 2016;5(8):2058460116662299.
68. Macri F, Greffier J, Pereira FR, Mandoul C, Khasanova E, Gualdi G, et al. Ultra-low-dose chest CT with iterative reconstruction does not alter anatomical image quality. Diagn Interv Imaging. 2016;97(11):1131–40.
69. Nakajo C, Heinzer S, Montandon S, Dunet V, Bize P, Feldman A, et al. Chest CT at a dose below 0.3 mSv: impact of iterative reconstruction on image quality and lung analysis. Acta Radiol (Stockholm, Sweden: 1987). 2016;57(3):311–7.
70. Otrakji A, Digumarthy SR, Lo Gullo R, Flores EJ, Shepard JA, Kalra MK. Dual-energy CT: Spectrum of thoracic abnormalities. Radiographics: Rev Publi Radiol Soc N Am, Inc. 2016;36(1):38–52.
71. Schenzle JC, Sommer WH, Neumaier K, Michalski G, Lechel U, Nikolaou K, et al. Dual energy CT of the chest: how about the dose? Investig Radiol. 2010;45(6):347–53.
72. Giordano J, Khung S, Duhamel A, Hossein-Foucher C, Bellevre D, Lamblin N, et al. Lung perfusion characteristics in pulmonary arterial hypertension (PAH) and peripheral forms of chronic thromboembolic pulmonary hypertension (pCTEPH): dual-energy CT experience in 31 patients. Eur Radiol. 2017;27(4):1631–9.
73. Godoy MC, Heller SL, Naidich DP, Assadourian B, Leidecker C, Schmidt B, et al. Dual-energy MDCT: comparison of pulmonary artery enhancement on dedicated CT pulmonary angiography, routine and low contrast volume studies. Eur J Radiol. 2011;79(2):e11–7.
74. Sudarski S, Hagelstein C, Weis M, Schoenberg SO, Apfaltrer P. Dual-energy snap-shot perfusion CT in suspect pulmonary nodules and masses and for lung cancer staging. Eur J Radiol. 2015;84(12): 2393–400.
75. Yoo SY, Kim Y, Cho HH, Choi MJ, Shim SS, Lee JK, Baek SY. Dual-energy CT in the assessment of mediastinal lymph nodes: comparative study of virtual non-contrast and true non-contrast images. Korean J Radiol. 2013;14(3):532–9. https://doi.org/10.3348/kjr.2013.14.3.532. Epub 2013 May 2. PubMed PMID: 23690725; PubMed Central PMCID: PMC3655312.
76. Wichmann JL, Hardie AD, Schoepf UJ, Felmly LM, Perry JD, Varga-Szemes A, et al. Single- and dual-energy CT of the abdomen: comparison of radiation dose and image quality of 2nd and 3rd generation dual-source CT. Eur Radiol. 2017;27(2):642–50.
77. Petritsch B, Kosmala A, Gassenmaier T, Weng AM, Veldhoen S, Kunz AS, et al. Diagnosis of pulmonary artery embolism: comparison of single-source CT and 3rd generation dual-source CT using a dual-energy protocol regarding image quality and radiation dose. RoFo: Fortschr Auf Dem Gebiete

Der Rontgenstrahlen Und Der Nuklearmedizin. 2017;189(6):527–36.
78. Pinho DF, Kulkarni NM, Krishnaraj A, Kalva SP, Sahani DV. Initial experience with single-source dual-energy CT abdominal angiography and comparison with single-energy CT angiography: image quality, enhancement, diagnosis and radiation dose. Eur Radiol. 2013;23(2):351–9.
79. Bauer RW, Kramer S, Renker M, Schell B, Larson MC, Beeres M, et al. Dose and image quality at CT pulmonary angiography-comparison of first and second generation dual-energy CT and 64-slice CT. Eur Radiol. 2011;21(10):2139–47.
80. Baxa J, Matouskova T, Krakorova G, Schmidt B, Flohr T, Sedlmair M, et al. Dual-phase dual-energy CT in patients treated with Erlotinib for advanced non-small cell lung cancer: possible benefits of iodine quantification in response assessment. Eur Radiol. 2016;26(8):2828–36.
81. Baxa J, Vondrakova A, Matouskova T, Ruzickova O, Schmidt B, Flohr T, et al. Dual-phase dual-energy CT in patients with lung cancer: assessment of the additional value of iodine quantification in lymph node therapy response. Eur Radiol. 2014;24(8):1981–8.
82. Kim YN, Lee HY, Lee KS, Seo JB, Chung MJ, Ahn MJ, et al. Dual-energy CT in patients treated with anti-angiogenic agents for non-small cell lung cancer: new method of monitoring tumor response? Korean J Radiol. 2012;13(6):702–10.
83. Kalra MK, Singh S, Thrall JH, Mahesh M. Pointers for optimizing radiation dose in abdominal CT protocols. J Am Coll Radiol: JACR. 2011;8(10):731–4.
84. Graser A, Johnson TR, Hecht EM, Becker CR, Leidecker C, Staehler M, et al. Dual-energy CT in patients suspected of having renal masses: can virtual nonenhanced images replace true nonenhanced images? Radiology. 2009;252(2):433–40.
85. De Cecco CN, Darnell A, Macias N, Ayuso JR, Rodriguez S, Rimola J, et al. Virtual unenhanced images of the abdomen with second-generation dual-source dual-energy computed tomography: image quality and liver lesion detection. Investig Radiol. 2013;48(1):1–9.
86. Purysko AS, Primak AN, Baker ME, Obuchowski NA, Remer EM, John B, et al. Comparison of radiation dose and image quality from single-energy and dual-energy CT examinations in the same patients screened for hepatocellular carcinoma. Clin Radiol. 2014;69(12):e538–44.
87. Marin D, Boll DT, Mileto A, Nelson RC. State of the art: dual-energy CT of the abdomen. Radiology. 2014;271(2):327–42.
88. Chen CY, Hsu JS, Jaw TS, Shih MC, Lee LJ, Tsai TH, et al. Split-bolus portal venous phase dual-energy CT urography: protocol design, image quality, and dose reduction. AJR Am J Roentgenol. 2015;205(5):W492–501.
89. Wilhelm K, Schoenthaler M, Hein S, Adams F, Schlager D, Kuehhas FE, et al. Focused dual-energy CT maintains diagnostic and compositional accuracy for urolithiasis using ultralow-dose noncontrast CT. Urology. 2015;86(6):1097–103.
90. Qu M, Yu L, Cardona DG, Liu Y, Duan X, Ai S, et al. Radiation dose reduction in dual-energy CT: does it affect the accuracy of urinary stone characterization? AJR Am J Roentgenol. 2015;205(2):W172–6.
91. Jepperson MA, Cernigliaro JG, el SH I, Morin RL, Haley WE, Thiel DD. In vivo comparison of radiation exposure of dual-energy CT versus low-dose CT versus standard CT for imaging urinary calculi. J Endourol/Endourol Soc. 2015;29(2):141–6.
92. Singh S, Kalra MK, Moore MA, Shailam R, Liu B, Toth TL, et al. Dose reduction and compliance with pediatric CT protocols adapted to patient size, clinical indication, and number of prior studies. Radiology. 2009;252(1):200–8.
93. Singh S, Kalra MK, Thrall JH, Mahesh M. Pointers for optimizing radiation dose in pediatric CT protocols. J Am Coll Radiol JACR. 2012;9(1):77–9.
94. Donnelly LF, Emery KH, Brody AS, Laor T, Gylys-Morin VM, Anton CG, et al. Minimizing radiation dose for pediatric body applications of single-detector helical CT: strategies at a large children's hospital. AJR Am J Roentgenol. 2001;176(2):303–6.
95. Frush DP. Pediatric CT: practical approach to diminish the radiation dose. Pediatr Radiol. 2002;32(10):714–7.. discussion 51-4
96. Kalra MK, Quick P, Singh S, Sandborg M, Persson A. Whole spine CT for evaluation of scoliosis in children: feasibility of sub-milliSievert scanning protocol. Acta Radiol (Stockholm, Sweden: 1987). 2013;54(2):226–30.
97. Rompel O, Glockler M, Janka R, Dittrich S, Cesnjevar R, Lell MM, et al. Third-generation dual-source 70-kVp chest CT angiography with advanced iterative reconstruction in young children: image quality and radiation dose reduction. Pediatr Radiol. 2016;46(4):462–72.
98. Ryu YJ, Kim WS, Choi YH, Cheon JE, Lee SM, Cho HH, et al. Pediatric chest CT: wide-volume and helical scan modes in 320-MDCT. AJR Am J Roentgenol. 2015;205(6):1315–21.
99. Sorantin E, Riccabona M, Stucklschweiger G, Guss H, Fotter R. Experience with volumetric (320 rows) pediatric CT. Eur J Radiol. 2013;82(7):1091–7.
100. Kanal KM, Butler PF, Sengupta D, Bhargavan-Chatfield M, Coombs LP, Morin RL. U.S. diagnostic reference levels and achievable doses for 10 adult CT examinations. Radiology. 2017;284:120.. 161911
101. Verdun FR, Gutierrez D, Vader JP, Aroua A, Alamo-Maestre LT, Bochud F, et al. CT radiation dose in children: a survey to establish age-based diagnostic reference levels in Switzerland. Eur Radiol. 2008;18(9):1980–6.
102. Smans K, Vano E, Sanchez R, Schultz FW, Zoetelief J, Kiljunen T, et al. Results of a European survey on patient doses in paediatric radiology. Radiat Prot Dosim. 2008;129(1–3):204–10.

103. McCollough C, Branham T, Herlihy V, Bhargavan M, Robbins L, Bush K, et al. Diagnostic reference levels from the ACR CT accreditation program. J Ame Coll Radiol JACR. 2011;8(11):795–803.
104. Klosterkemper Y, Appel E, Thomas C, Bethge OT, Aissa J, Kropil P, et al. Tailoring CT dose to patient size: implementation of the updated 2017 ACR size-specific diagnostic reference levels. Acad Radiol. 2018;25:1624.
105. Kim M, Chang K, Hwang J, Nam Y, Han D, Yoon J. Radiation dose for pediatric and young adult Ct: a survey to establish age-based reference levels of 2015-2016 in Korea. Radiat Prot Dosim. 2017;175(2):228–37.
106. European Guidelines on DRLs for Paediatric Imaging 2017. Available from: http://www.eurosafeimaging.org/wp/wp-content/uploads/2014/02/European-Guidelines-on-DRLs-for-Paediatric-Imaging_Revised_18-July-2016_clean.pdf. Accessed on 1st June 2018.
107. Murugan VA, Chatfield MB, Rehani M, Kalra MK. ACR DIR: a User's guide for cardiothoracic radiologists: part 2: how to interpret your DIR report. J Thorac Imaging. 2015;30(6):W69–72.
108. Murugan VA, Bhargavan-Chatfield M, Rehani M, Kalra MK. American college of radiology dose index registry: a user's guide for cardiothoracic radiologists part 1: dose index registry (DIR)-what it means and does for CT? J Thorac Imaging. 2015;30(6):W66–8.
109. Cook TS, Zimmerman SL, Steingall SR, Maidment AD, Kim W, Boonn WW. RADIANCE: an automated, enterprise-wide solution for archiving and reporting CT radiation dose estimates. Radiographics Rev Publ Radiol Soc N Am Inc. 2011;31(7):1833–46.
110. Christianson O, Li X, Frush D, Samei E. Automated size-specific CT dose monitoring program: assessing variability in CT dose. Med Phys. 2012;39(11):7131–9.

CT Practice Monitoring

11

Aiping Ding, Francesco Ria, and Ehsan Samei

Introduction

Computed tomography (CT) is a leading advanced imaging modality today. Over 80 million CT scans are performed every year in the United States [1]. This significant use of CT has raised concerns regarding utilization costs, appropriate applications, and the associated potential radiation risks [2–8]. For example, according to a recent Medicare claim report, hundreds of hospitals across the country needlessly scanned their patients twice even on the same day [7]. Unnecessary repeated scans expose patients to extra radiation resulting in millions of dollars in extra costs on an already overburdened Medicare program [7]. CT alone is responsible for nearly 50% of medical radiation exposures considering all use of ionizing radiation in medicine and for approximately 25% of the US per capita radiation from all radiation resources [1]. CT is also used across all ages, and up to 10% of all CT examinations are performed in children, accounting for about 12% of imaging procedures in the US population [1]. Children have generally higher sensitivity to radiation due to growing tissues, with associated potential cancer risks [9]. Thus, legislative and regulatory organizations, including the US Food and Drug Administration (FDA) [10], the American College of Radiology (ACR) [11], The Joint Commission (TJC) [12], the American Association of Physicists in Medicine (AAPM) [13], and the National Council on Radiation Protection and Measurements (NCRP) [14], have all encouraged and mandated stricter oversight of radiation usage in medical imaging. Accordingly, prevailing considerations have increasingly directed both the scientific and medical communities towards understanding, managing, and mitigating radiation risk or potential risk, especially in younger patients [15, 16].

Risk mitigation is now crucial in radiology and is the core of every optimization action. The aim of the optimization must be to keep radiation exposure reasonably low while ensuring acceptable clinical images. Therefore, evaluation and enhancement of image quality are as critical as radiation risk reduction in the overall CT optimization process. Early approaches to CT optimization focused more on radiation safety: image quality was evaluated only using phantoms or qualitative measures [17]. Such limitations, mostly causing a technological gap in CT performance, didn't allow a comprehensive optimization that simultaneously included radiation dose and image quality. However, recently introduced informatics systems can efficiently and automati-

A. Ding · F. Ria
Clinical Imaging Physics Group, Duke University, Durham, NC, USA
e-mail: aiping.ding@duke.edu; francesco.ria@duke.edu

E. Samei (✉)
Department of Radiology, Duke University, Durham, NC, USA
e-mail: ehsan.samei@duke.edu

© Springer Nature Switzerland AG 2020
E. Samei, N. J. Pelc (eds.), *Computed Tomography*, https://doi.org/10.1007/978-3-030-26957-9_11

cally measure and record important image quality features such as *in vivo* noise magnitude, spatial resolution, and Hounsfield unit (HU) distribution [18–20]. The simultaneous assessment of radiation dose and image quality in CT can enable effective patient-based optimization [21]. This approach is consistent with the last International Commission on Radiological Protection (ICRP) recommendation: "If radiation dose is decreased to a level that results in image quality or diagnostic information inadequate for the medical purpose, either by reducing dose or dose rate excessively or by failing to obtain a sufficient number of images, optimization has not been achieved" [22].

In the context of CT imaging, this calls for a system to comprehensively monitor all aspects of quality and safety in imaging practice including the quality of the equipment, the precision of the applied procedure, the usage of the equipment, the radiation dose to the patient, and the resulting image quality. Monitoring accurate, comprehensive, fast, patient-based metrologies enables effective optimization actions and enhances the benefits for patients, healthcare providers, regulatory agencies, and researchers. Before exploring all the possible benefits, it is important to establish a common nomenclature: Table 11.1 summarizes all the CT exam-related monitoring items. Each item has its own specific quantities that an effective monitoring system should include.

Table 11.1 Summary of CT practice monitoring items

Item	Monitored quantities and parameters
Dose monitoring	CT radiation output (mAs, $CTDI_{vol}$)
	Risk metric surrogates (DLP, SSDE)
	Risk metrics (risk index, effective dose, organ dose)
Scanner parameter monitoring	Scanner model and vendor, kVp, pitch, slice thickness, rotation time, etc.
Patient monitoring	Age, gender, effective diameter (AAPM report No. 204), water equivalent diameter (AAPM report No. 220), weight, BMI, etc.
Image quality monitoring	Noise magnitude, NPS, spatial resolution, Hounsfield units, detectability index (d'), etc.
Operation monitoring	CT protocol, requested procedure, date and time, performing radiographers, performing physician, etc.
Contrast media administration monitoring	Contrast media dose, volume, concentration, brand, pressure, etc.
Performance monitoring	All of the above

Benefits of CT Performance Monitoring: Towards a Value-Based Care

If optimization is paramount for radiology quality improvement, performance monitoring in CT can foster many benefits as briefly discussed below [23].

Regulatory

Recently, many regulations in the United States and Europe have instituted requiring listing of a CT dose estimation in the patient report [24, 25]. Other regulations simply require dose monitoring [26] as well as the comparison with reference levels and the study of the outlier exams [12, 22, 27]. In all these possible scenarios, performance monitoring, and dose monitoring in particular, is a unique and irreplaceable tool providing all the indispensable data to abide by the regulations and international standards.

Healthcare Providers

If regulatory compliance is mandatory, healthcare providers can gain further benefits from CT performance monitoring in multiple ways. First, operation monitoring can positively affect justification and optimization of resource utilization. Second, dose monitoring enables the comparison with national diagnostic reference level (DRL) information while also enabling the development of institutional DRLs and the identification and the analysis of under- and overexposure cases. Third, a comprehensive performance monitoring can impact operational decision-making and analysis through the identification of protocol, equipment, and operator-specific inconsistencies and trends. Lastly, healthcare providers can give important feedback to manufacturers about scanner performance in clinical operation. Manufacturers can use such information to improve scanner design, enabling a quality improvement circle.

Researchers

The incredible amount of data provided by CT performance monitoring systems is a special treat for researchers and can be used towards research goals. For instance, new metrics can be defined to evaluate scanner performance in terms of dose and image quality consistency across patient populations [28]. Furthermore, performance monitoring can provide a quantitative basis for risk assessment in CT in terms of radiation risk (dose) and clinical risk (likelihood of not delivering a proper diagnosis due to poor image quality) [29]. Eventually, performance monitoring provides quantitative data to establish best practices, guidelines, and appropriateness criteria.

Patients

Patients are the ultimate beneficiaries of all quality improvements in medicine. However, there are some specific benefits related to performance monitoring, in particular in terms of increasing awareness. A recent survey across over 700 patients in Europe reported a significant gap in patient awareness about ionizing radiation risk and found that 85% of patients would find it useful to have ionizing radiation dose information in the medical report, in accordance with the latest EU regulation [24, 30]. Furthermore, performance monitoring would provide the opportunity for informed discussion between patients, caregivers, and medical healthcare providers towards a real shared path of care.

In this scenario, it is clear how comprehensive and accurate performance monitoring has become an essential requirement for medical imaging practice, enabling real value-based care. Healthcare institutions that invest in performance monitoring can constantly improve their clinical operations. They can also quantitatively compare the quality of their operations with other institutions in a context of mutual benefit for healthcare providers, regulators, industry, and, of course, patients.

Consistency of Care

In radiology, many scientific articles begin with the pledge to the ALARA principle: *as low as reasonably achievable*. It is related to radiation dose and risk, and it is the principle that regulates optimization and justification of radiological procedures. The key to interpret the acronym is the word *reasonably*: dose as low as possible considering social cost and procedure cost and, most importantly, without threatening the accuracy of the diagnosis.

As a step towards improving consistency across procedures and institutions, the ACR established the CT Dose Index Registry (DIR) [11]. The DIR establishes benchmarks for CT dose indices that can be used for comparisons nationwide. To determine the benchmarks, DIR periodically collects, stores, and statistically analyzes CT dose data from institutions that are enrolled in the program. Initiatives such the DIR represent a leap towards consistency in clinical operations. However, dose reduction and standardization are only "one of the steps in the overall process of optimization" [27]. To really embody the essence of reasonably achievable in the ALARA, the likelihood of obtaining a proper diagnosis should also be considered. The proper diagnosis is strictly related to the quality of the CT images. Therefore, consistency in image quality is paramount in the effort to optimize radiological procedures and to share good practices within a single facility and across multiple institutions.

A recent study investigated the consistency of detectability index (d') across the U.S. facilities that are part of DIR program [31]. The d', calculated in an acrylic phantom, ranged between approximately 60 and 360 across all the protocols, with an interquartile range between 170 and 270. So, even in the facilities that are part of a national program establishing consistency in radiation dose, image quality standardization is far from being achieved. It is important to consider that d' is a metric that incorporates spatial resolution, noise texture, diagnostic task, and viewing conditions. Furthermore, d' is directly correlated to the percentage of correct observer answers in a two-alternative forced-choice model [32]. Therefore, inconsistency in d' results in potential inconsistency in diagnostic performance.

Sources of Variability

To achieve consistency of radiological procedures, the first step is to identify the possible sources of variability. Variabilities can be classified based on their relationships with scanners and operations:

Systematic variabilities are those related to the device and in particular to the automatic adaptation systems, to the detectors, and to the image reconstruction algorithms. For instance, Figure 11.1 shows the distribution of $CTDI_{vol}$

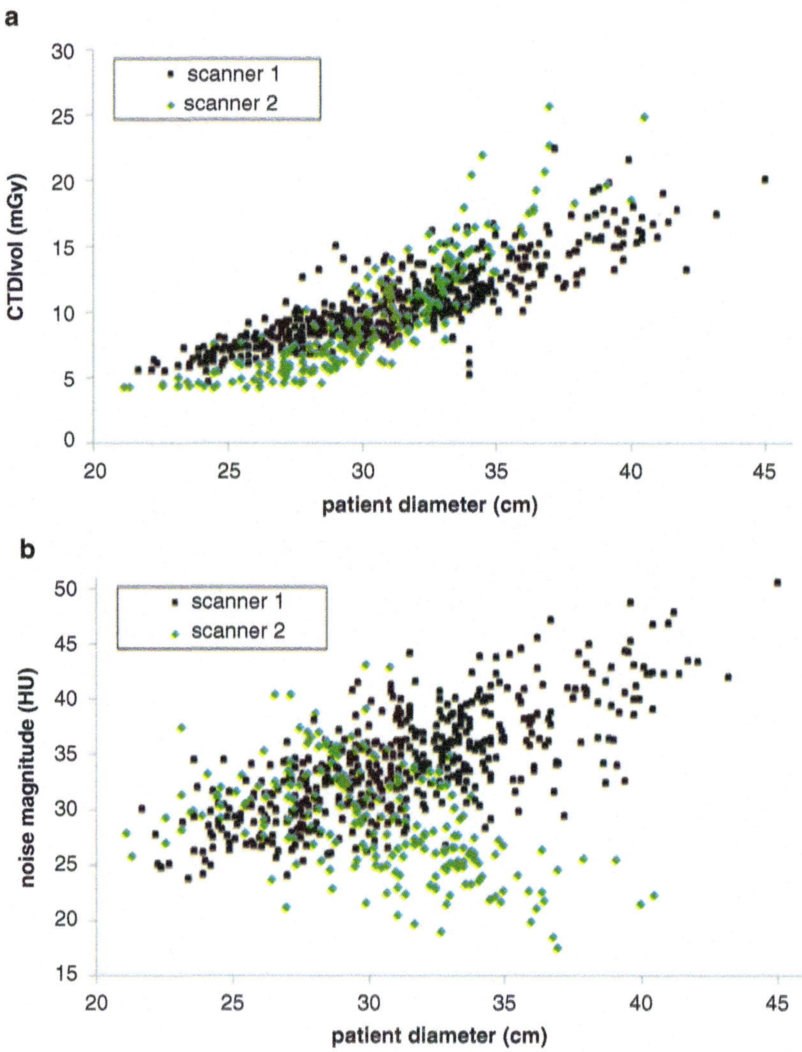

Fig. 11.1 Distribution of $CTDI_{vol}$ (**a**) and noise magnitude (**b**) across different patient diameters for abdominopelvic scans acquired with two scanners from two different vendors. The different automatic adaptation strategies result in different trends both for noise and dose

and noise magnitude across patient diameter for abdominopelvic scans with contrast for two different vendors. The patient images were acquired with similar scanner parameters (kVp, slice thickness, image reconstruction algorithms, and kernels) to avoid other sources of variability. In Figure 11.1a, it is possible to see how, as a result of the tube current adaptation system (ATCM), the dose increases with patient size in both scanners. However, the trends are different, and scanner 1 shows consistently higher doses for small patient sizes (<30 cm) and lower doses for larger patients (>35 cm). So, different ATCM methods introduce an intrinsic variability in terms of radiation dose. Such analysis can be extended, for the same patient population, to the noise magnitude. Figure 11.1b shows different trends of noise across patient size as a consequence of different strategies for ATCM changing the balance between image quality and radiation dose. In particular, scanner 1 allows noise to increase with patient size, whereas scanner 2 shows the opposite behavior [21].

Both variabilities observed in the example above can be determined only with a comprehensive performance monitoring strategy that collects radiation dose and image quality as metrics that can simultaneously describe the actual system output in clinical operation. A limited phantom study, instead, would provide information related to the scanners' performance only in a highly constrained setup without any useful information about scanners' adaptation to different patient sizes in terms of radiation dose and noise magnitude. A possible strategy to reduce the variability in the aforementioned example could be the design of patient size-specific protocols. For instance, the inconsistency can be reduced by designing clinical protocols that allow, in scanner 2, higher dose for patient sizes smaller than 30 cm and lower dose for patient diameters greater than 35 cm and vice versa for scanner 1. The new protocols would also reduce the gap in terms of noise magnitude, dramatically increasing consistency of scanner performances in clinical operation.

Nonsystematic variabilities are those related to users and clinical operations. A typical nonsystematic variability, for example, is related to the use of different scanner parameters in the same protocol and/or population. Figure 11.2a shows the distribution of pitch in a population of patients who underwent a chest without contrast exam with one scanner. About 50% of the studies were performed with a pitch of 3, the rest with variable pitch values. Apparently, there is not a correlation between pitch values and patient habitus. Considering the distribution of $CTDI_{vol}$ across patient diameter for the same patient population (black dots in Fig. 11.2b), it is possible to determine the total variability at a specific reference patient size (i.e., 30 cm). If we consider only the exams performed with pitch = 3 (red dots in Fig. 11.2b), the variability at the same reference size is much smaller, indicating that part of the total variability is related to the use of different pitch values. Therefore, consistency in radiation dose across clinical populations can be improved by targeting consistency in scanner parameters.

Variability can also be induced by the users. In particular, we can consider patient positioning that is critical for automated tube current modulation system performance. A vertical centering offset, for instance, can result in an incorrect magnification of the patient body habitus triggering an over- or underdosage. In the following example, we define the offset as the difference (delta) between the patient geometric center in the axial view and the scanner isocenter: delta X and delta Y are the shifts in horizontal and vertical directions, respectively.

Figure 11.3 shows a set of 37 patients who underwent abdominopelvic with contrast exams with a single scanner. The shifts in both vertical and horizontal axes have been estimated. Considering that radiation dose is exponentially related to the attenuating diameter ($CTDI_{vol} \propto e^{patient\ diameter}$) [33], it is possible to use $ln(CTDI_{vol})$ as a linear descriptor of radiation output as a function of diameter. The linear fit RMSE (root mean square error) can be calculated as a metric of variability across study cases [28]. In the example the RMSE related to the

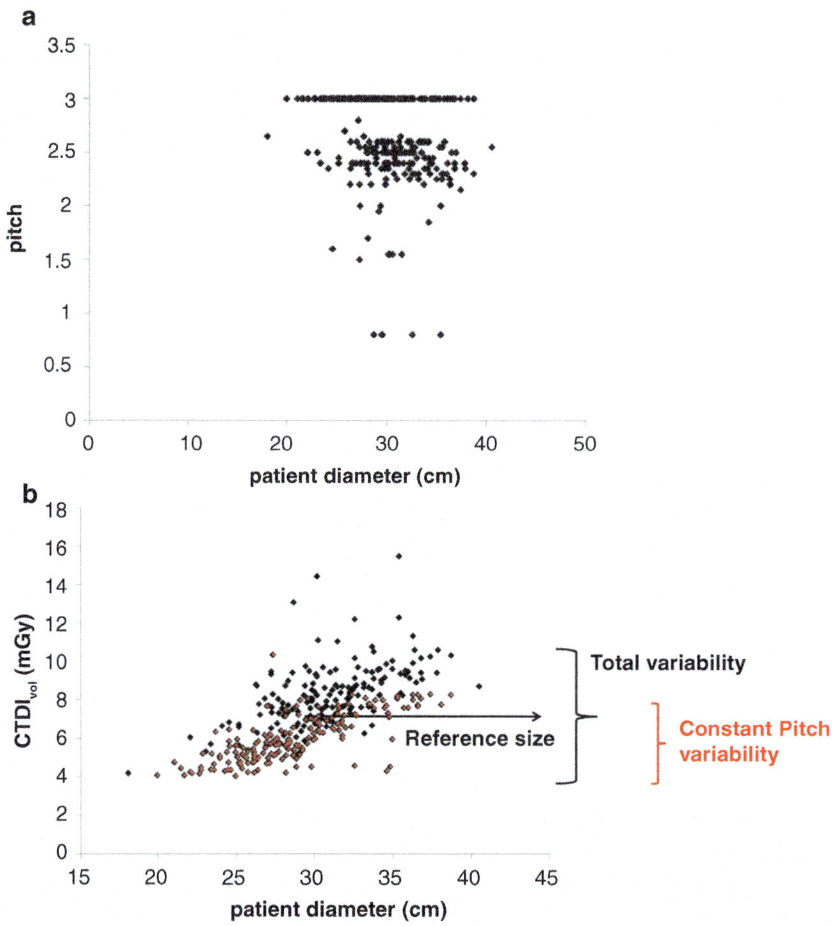

Fig. 11.2 (**a**) Distribution of pitch across patient diameter in a chest scan without contrast population (344 patients, 1 scanner). (**b**) Distribution of CTDI$_{vol}$ across patient diameter for the same population: the black dots are the whole population, whereas the red dots are related only to the patients with pitch = 3. Brackets show the variabilities at a 30 cm reference patient diameter

Fig. 11.3 Vertical and horizontal offset shifts for an abdominopelvic population of 37 patients. The red area includes the patients with horizontal and vertical shift less than ±10 mm and ±20 mm, respectively

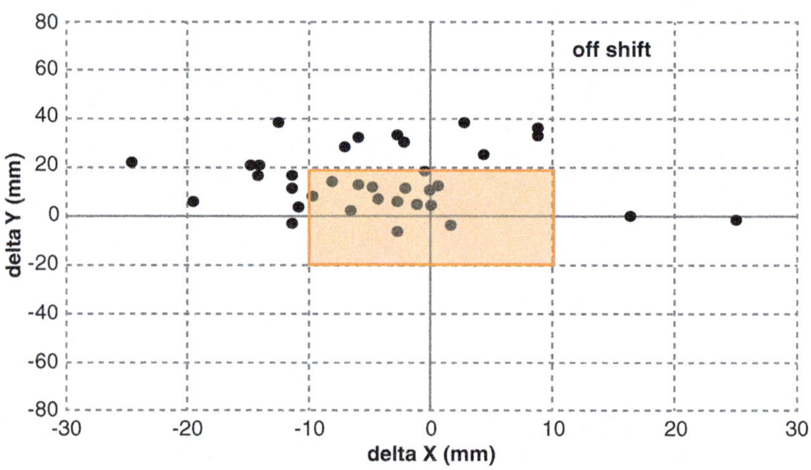

whole population is 0.1350. Instead, considering only the 15 patients with delta X < ±10 mm and delta Y < ±20 mm, the RMSE is 0.1173 (−13%). This example clearly shows how consistency in patient positioning affects the variability of dose in clinical CT populations.

The examples above show how a comprehensive monitoring system can help to highlight inconsistencies in CT performance as well as bad practices. A constant performance monitoring can also identify many other sources of variability (tube voltage, kernels, image reconstructions, etc.). Therefore, a systematic approach in CT practice monitoring can ensure and target consistency of care.

Key Components of an Effective CT Practice Monitoring System

As CT scanning continues to provide patient benefit, it is paramount that we look at dose in a clinical indication paradigm – image quality must inform dose. A poor-quality exam is a disservice to the care of the patient, while an exam with more radiation dose than necessary can reduce its safety. To ensure the benefit of an imaging examination, a proper balance between image quality and radiation safety is essential. Therefore, proper CT imaging requires a combined image-quality and dose monitoring program. There are five key components of an ideal CT imaging practice program [23], as discussed below.

Access: Get Connection and Collection of Exam-Relevant Data

One of the fundamental requirements in CT practice monitoring is to develop an infrastructure capable of acquiring imaging data across equipment and modalities, particularly if the program justifiably extends beyond CT [23]. This requirement is complicated by differences in the data format across different manufactures and models. In practice, image data are usually routed to the monitoring server through the picture archiving and communication system (PACS). An alternative method is to build direct connections with individual imaging systems to collect all exam-relevant data and events comprehensively.

Metrology: Meaningful Quantities to Monitor

A comprehensive CT practice monitoring system integrates metrologies for both dose and image quality and does so in a patient-specific manner. Characterizing dose and quality in terms of patient-specific metrics is a key requirement for effective CT practice monitoring.

The list of quantities needed to assure compliance with national and international regulations is short: $CTDI_{vol}$, DLP; patient diameter or water equivalent diameter, size-specific dose estimate (SSDE); patient accession number, name, gender, and age; exam date and time, scanner name and vendor; and protocol name. To achieve and enhance the benefits of performance monitoring towards a value-based care, a comprehensive monitoring system must track, record, and analyze multiple metrics and parameters that can speak about the actual (as opposed to presumed) output and performance of imaging system. The most relevant metrics to each performance monitoring item are described below.

Dose Monitoring

Over the years, various metrics have been used by the CT community as surrogates for radiation risk. However, some of them only describe the radiation input to the patient and have been treated as risk metrics in the absence of better or more convenient alternatives (i.e., $CTDI_{vol}$ and DLP). Other metrics have been used as a reflection of patient detriment, but they do not account for age and gender which are known to influence the individual risk (i.e., effective dose and organ dose). Currently, the closest surrogate for actual patient risk is the risk index (RI) [32] which includes gender-, age-, and tissue-specific risk coefficients [34].

In this scenario, a recent study explored how 12 different radiation risk metrics characterized radiation burden across clinical CT examination compared to the characterization carried out by Ria *et al* [35]. Metrics that are not strictly related to patient anatomy such as $CTDI_{vol}$ and DLP highly overestimate risk for large patients and underestimate risk for small patients, particularly pediatric exams. Instead, metrics that take into account patient habitus such as SSDE, organ dose, and effective dose characterize risk across clinical populations closer to the RI radiation burden description. Therefore, care should be exercised in drawing risk predictions from unrepresentative risk metrics applied to a population. However, if the purpose of a dose monitoring program is to perform comparisons between institutions or to establish diagnostic reference levels, the International Commission of Radiological Protection "recommends that both $CTDI_{vol}$ and DLP should be assessed in patient surveys performed for the purpose of setting DRL values" [22].

Image Quality Monitoring

The importance of image quality in the overall evaluation of CT performance has already been described. Nowadays, many automatic algorithms have been developed enabling image quality monitoring *in vivo* [18–20]. In this scenario, the challenge is the standardization of the metrics: if radiation dose quantities have their standard definitions and calculation methodologies, the same need exists for image quality-related metrics.

Image quality metrics can actually be used as a surrogate for the benefits carried by the radiological practice. Quantities such as noise magnitude, noise power spectrum, spatial resolution, etc. are a good indicator of the diagnostic image properties. Furthermore, metrics such as d' are directly correlated to the ability of performing an effective diagnosis. Therefore, image quality monitoring is crucial in the overall evaluation of CT performance.

Scanner Parameters, Operations, and Patient Monitoring

Ultimately, radiation dose and image quality are the result of a combination of scanner parameters and settings such as tube voltage, slice thickness, detector configuration, pitch, etc. Therefore, complete CT performance monitoring cannot disregard scanner parameter tracking and analysis. Such analysis is also crucial in the assessment of dose and image quality inconsistency and in the design and implementation of optimization strategies.

Another challenge in the overall CT operations management is the inconsistency in examination and protocol nomenclature. This nomenclature problem is magnified when comparing metrics across institutions. To address this issue, the ACR encourages the use of the RSNA RadLex Playbook which includes a standard set of nomenclature for CT protocols [36].

Lastly, patient information monitoring is also important for multiple reasons. Of course, it's needed to assign the right quantities to the right patient, but it is also needed to retrieve historical dosimetric data of a patient if medical and radiation protection reasons require it. Furthermore, to assess personal and population risks, age and gender information are needed. Finally, anatomical features such as height, weight, body mass index (BMI), effective diameter, water equivalent diameter, and so on enable the calculation of more metrics (e.g., SSDE) as well as more accurate population studies. For instance, the last US DRL survey reports different dose thresholds for different patient size ranges [37].

Contrast Media Administration Monitoring

Achieving image quality that is adequate on a consistent basis is essential for optimizing diagnostic capability. This includes using the optimal contrast media dose and rate as well as the optimal CT scan parameters. When acquiring CT datasets, there are two main determinants of image quality from a diagnostic standpoint. The first determinant of image quality is the set of CT scan parameters: CT parameters such as tube voltage, tube current, pitch, gantry rotation time, image reconstruction algorithm, display field of view, and slice thickness can impact image noise and low-contrast detectability. The second determinant of image quality is the protocol used for intravenous contrast material administration: concentration, volume and rate of contrast media administered intravenously, the timing of the acquisition, and other patient factors such as cardiac output and hydration status may impact the degree of vascular and parenchymal enhancement [38]. Therefore, contrast media administration monitoring is essential in comprehensive CT performance monitoring.

Analytics: From Data to Knowledge

While it is clear that CT practice (dose and quality) monitoring can provide clinically relevant information, it is equally important to know how to best use these data. Collecting data without having a process to convert useful information into knowledge and use that knowledge for improved patient care would be inconsistent with the expectations of stewardship and value-based practices [23]. However, most current CT dose monitoring software solutions limit their data analytics to just display retrospective dose; methods to build models from the data, evaluate them, and deploy them for improved practice have remained largely unanswered [23]. An ideal CT practice monitoring strategy would have the capability to extract useful knowledge from data using comprehensive machine learning-boosted predictive data analytics.

Informatics: Dose and Quality Monitoring as a Secure, Integrated Solution

CT practice monitoring is ultimately an informatics solution [23, 29]. As such, it needs to have all the associated key hardware and software components. A server, whether physical, virtual, or cloud-based, is always needed for data capture, management, analysis, distribution, and display. The data process needs to closely adhere to good informatics practices including data security, encryption, backup, audit trail, and so on. The analyses should be readily accessible and viewable by the users, ideally via a web access with a proper permission management. Therefore, a CT practice monitoring metrology should offer access and analytical solutions to the dose, quality, and device utilization data in an intuitive way with minimal user effort or interactions to access the most pertinent results.

Metis: A New Next-Generation CT Practice Monitoring System

To fulfill the current and future needs of comprehensive CT practice monitoring, Duke University has developed a new "software as a service (SaaS)" CT performance informatics platform, called "Metrology for imaging systems (METIS)," to enable both radiation safety and image quality monitoring, affording prospective and retrospective medical imaging device performance and patient safety assessment.

As the first step, crucial effort was made to build the capability of efficiently and accurately collecting high-quality, comprehensive data from CT clinical practice. As shown in Fig. 11.4, to collect and manage exam-relevant data, the data collection service of METIS was designed in three layers: (1) presentation layer, (2) intermediary business layer, and (3) data source layer. The presentation layer provides a graphical user interface (GUI) where image data is presented to the user and input is taken from the user. The intermediary business layer includes image data access and management, business logic like the integration with the PACS, connection with individual imaging systems, validation of data, querying/retrieving, and data updates. The third layer serves as a database containing all the image data and patient information collected from the PACS, radiology information system (RIS), and individual imaging systems. It provides multiple application program interfaces (APIs) to connect with the database and to perform data insert, update, and deletion, incorporating data based on user's input in the second layer.

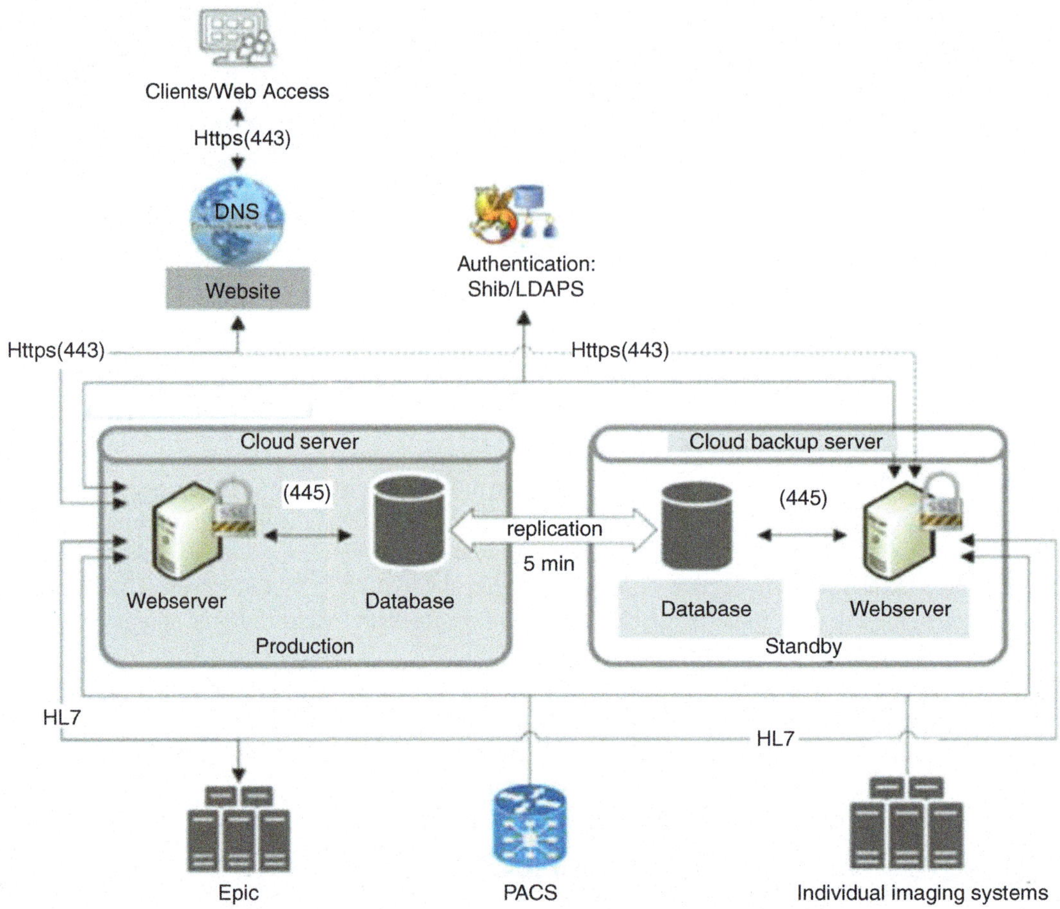

Fig. 11.4 Schema of a multi-infrastructure data connection and collection design in METIS

Patient-Specific Organ Dose Estimation

The $CTDI_{vol}$ and SSDE are currently used in most dose monitoring systems as dose metrics [39, 40]. While they provide a first-order approximation of patient dose, assessing organ dose offers the unique advantage of characterizing radiation exposure in units that are reflective of the dose to the patient independent of the imaging modality. An organ dose database previously generated by Monte Carlo simulations across 100 adult and pediatric human extended cardiac-torso (XCAT) models was incorporated for many CT scan protocols: chest, abdomen, pelvis, abdomen-pelvis, chest-abdomen-pelvis, and head and neck [41]. The organ doses were normalized by the $CTDI_{vol}$ to derive organ dose coefficients independent of the scan parameters. The patient size and scan coverage are used to match the XCAT phantom that has the closest chest height, abdomen height, and abdominopelvic height, respectively. For patients scanned with tube current modulation (TCM), a dose-spread profile was calculated as the dose intensity in the longitudinal (z) direction of a cylindrical volume with sectional diameters from 8 to 50 cm, as illustrated in Fig. 11.5, to represent an average body population. The dose-spread profile was convolved with a TCM profile and fixed tube current, respectively, to derive the accumulated dose distribution. Moreover, METIS combined the knowledge of

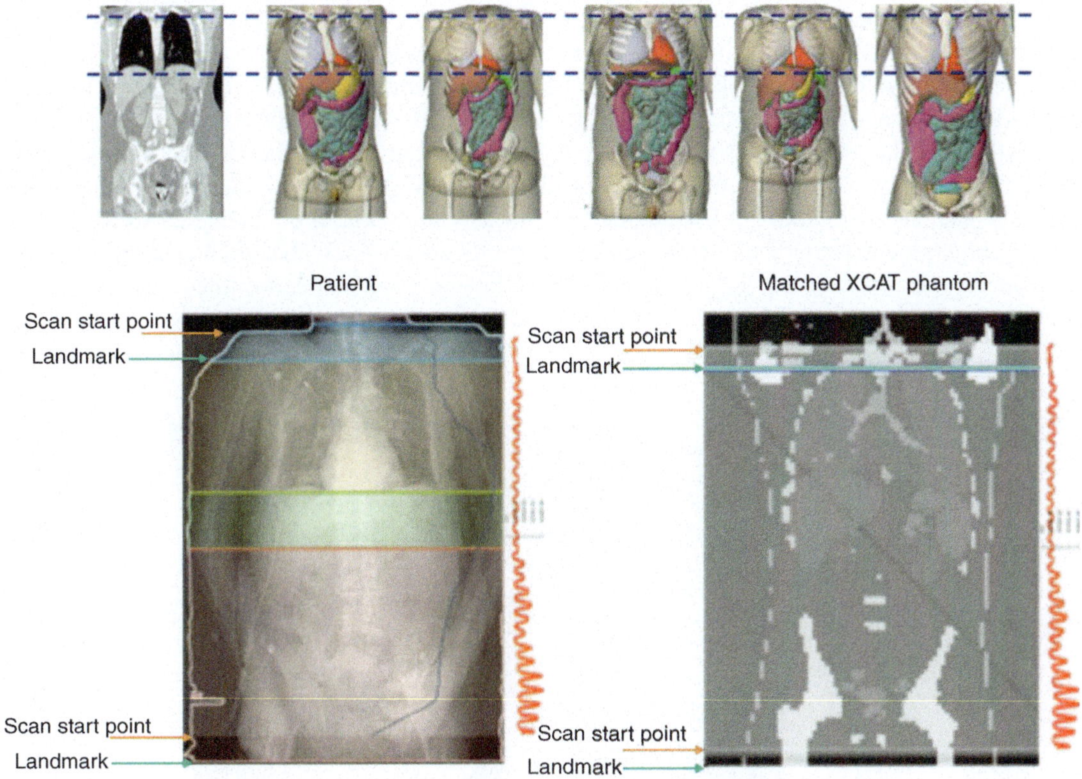

Fig. 11.5 A clinical patient matched to a representative model from an XCAT atlas from which organ doses can be estimated with the knowledge of organ location and radiation field: (top) patient matching to phantom atlas; (down) exposure profile padding from actual patient to the phantom [42]

organ dose with many radiobiological factors that were known relevant to derive an index of risk [41–47]. In this way, METIS provides a comprehensive dose monitoring solution to provide meaningful measures of radiation burden to individual patients by including organ doses and individual risks.

Patient-Specific Image Quality Metric

As previously discussed, the currently available dose monitoring solutions focus primarily on basic metrics of dose that are generic in nature, not reflecting patient risk. Ideally, one wishes to assess patient dose per actual image data and use that to ascertain individualized risk estimates. More importantly, in the current monitoring paradigm, the quality and implied benefit aspects of CT have largely been missing or viewed as peripheral to dose monitoring, creating a potentially detrimental perspective for the optimization of CT dose. Image quality is one primary objective of medical imaging and thus is a necessary attribute to monitor and optimize. Such monitoring enables establishment of target levels based not only on dose but, importantly, based on desired task-based diagnostic performance [23]. The established metrics to quantify image quality are noise, resolution, and contrast. However, these attributes are usually characterized only in static phantoms, while they should ideally be quantified in patient CT images in a patient-specific manner over clinical populations.

To establish patient-specific image quality metrics, the originally collected CT volumetric image data is first anatomically segmented using a pre-trained deep learning model. The model utilizes a deep convolutional neural network (3D-Unet) [46, 47] trained on 200 manually segmented CT images to predict segmentation masks of different organs of a given CT data. The network takes 3D CT volumetric data as input and processes the data with corresponding 3D operations, in particular, 3D convolutions, 3D max pooling, and 3D up-convolutional layers [46, 47]. To avoid bottlenecks in network architecture, METIS adapted batch normalization for faster convergence. The training results show that the method is able to identify the liver with a dice similarity coefficient (DSC) of 0.94 ± 0.02 and other major body organs with DSC > 0.85 (Fig. 11.6). This algorithm streamlines the segmentation process, allowing patient-specific image quality metric to be processed more efficiently.

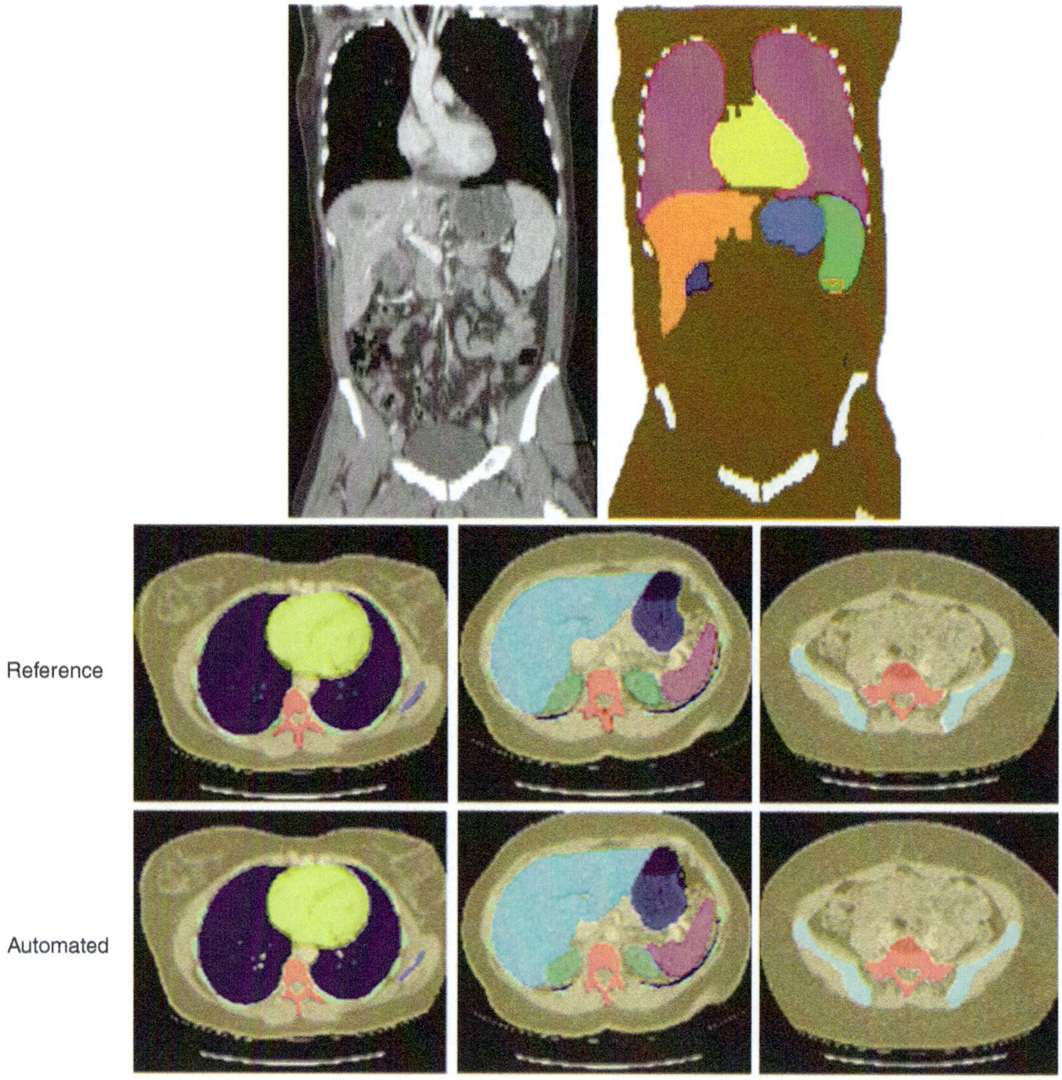

Fig. 11.6 The output of deep learning-powered organ classification (top) and segmentation (bottom) algorithms on CT [46, 47]

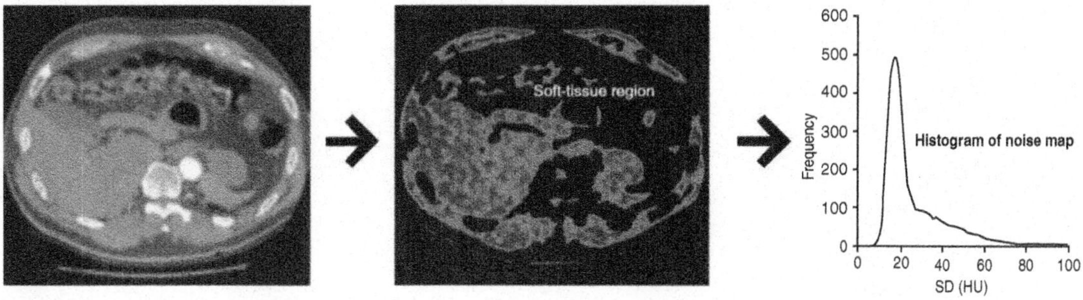

Fig. 11.7 Noise magnitude estimation process. Original CT images (left), noise map showing soft-tissue region (middle), and histogram of noise map for soft-tissue regions (right) [19]

Automated Patient-Specific Noise Estimation

Noise magnitude is a key reflection of image quality directly related to patient dose. It is measured in patient-specific manner from patient CT images using an automated, computationally efficient method previously developed and validated [19]. Since CT noise magnitude is influenced by anatomical variability, it is also characterized in terms of the most frequent noise level in areas of homogeneous tissue with a metric termed "global noise level." The global noise level is calculated in three steps. First, the image is segmented into different tissue types (Fig. 11.7). The tissue types are roughly separated into four categories: aerated tissue (HU< −800), fat (−300 to <0 HU), soft tissue (0 < to 100 HU), and bone (>300 HU). Second, a noise map is generated in which the value at each location corresponds to the noise in an area surrounding that pixel. Third, a histogram is generated for the noise corresponding to the targeted tissue type. The histogram usually comprises two principal categories: homogeneous areas and transitional areas. Transitional areas constitute a surprisingly small portion of the image and are at the boundary of multiple tissue types. Therefore, they exhibit higher and more variable ranges of noise compared with those of homogeneous areas. As a result, the histogram generally has a characteristic high narrow peak corresponding to homogeneous areas and a short broadtail corresponding to transitional areas. The global noise level is determined by identifying the mode of the histogram peak.

Automated Patient-Specific Spatial Resolution Estimation

Resolution is a second important component of image quality. To characterize spatial resolution in CT imaging, the general approach is to measure the CT system's modulation transfer function (MTF) from inserts embedded in uniform phantoms. However, these methods are sufficient only for characterizing system spatial resolution for static, uniformly shaped objects, but not for the spatial resolution of actual clinical images. To better quantify image quality in a patient-specific manner, an automated technique was developed for evaluating the spatial resolution characteristics of clinical CT images *in vivo* [20]. The method is based on automated characterization of the patient's air skin interface. First, the patient is segmented from the image using a thresholding technique. Next, a mesh of the patient is constructed from the segmented dataset. Third, edge-spread function (ESF) measurements are made across the patient's skin and are binned by their radial distance from the isocenter to construct oversampled ESF measurements. The oversampled ESF measurements are binned by a fraction of the in-plane pixel size and differentiated to obtain the line-spread function (LSF). Finally, the Fourier

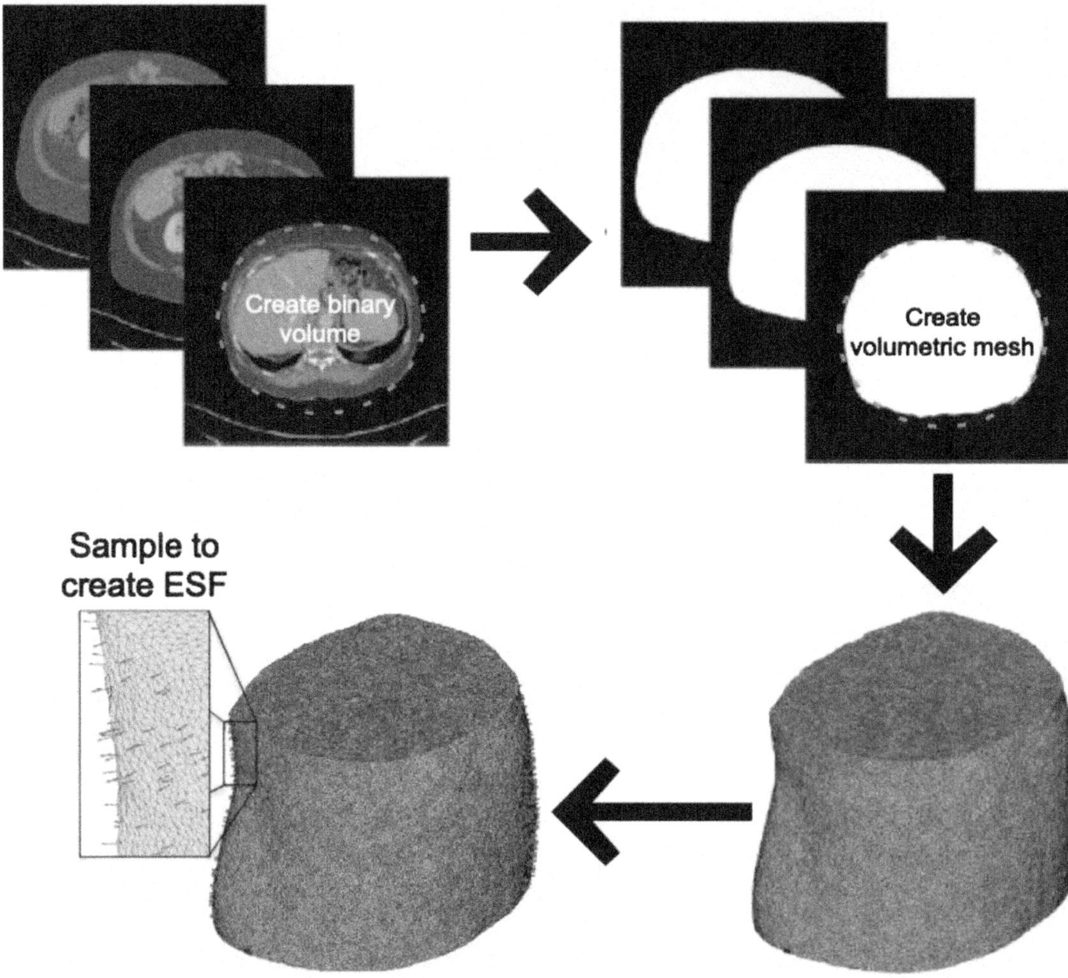

Fig. 11.8 Steps of the resolution measurements made on clinical CT datasets [20]

transform of the LSF is calculated and normalized by the value at zero frequency to obtain a CT spatial resolution index (RI) analogous to the MTF, as shown in Fig. 11.8 [20]. The technology is deployed as a provision to assess and monitor resolution across clinical cases on a patient-specific basis. The measured variability in image quality among clinical images is being used to optimize clinical protocols in an effort to make image quality consistent throughout all scanners in the clinic.

Automated Patient-Specific HU Contrast Estimation

Image contrast is the third important component of image quality. This is particularly important in CT as about 60% of CT imaging is done with the administration of contrast agents for additional opacification, which can vary significantly from case to case. Operating on a clinical CT dataset, the patient's body is segmented into key organs, the lung, liver, aorta, and spine (Fig. 11.9). An algorithm automatically samples

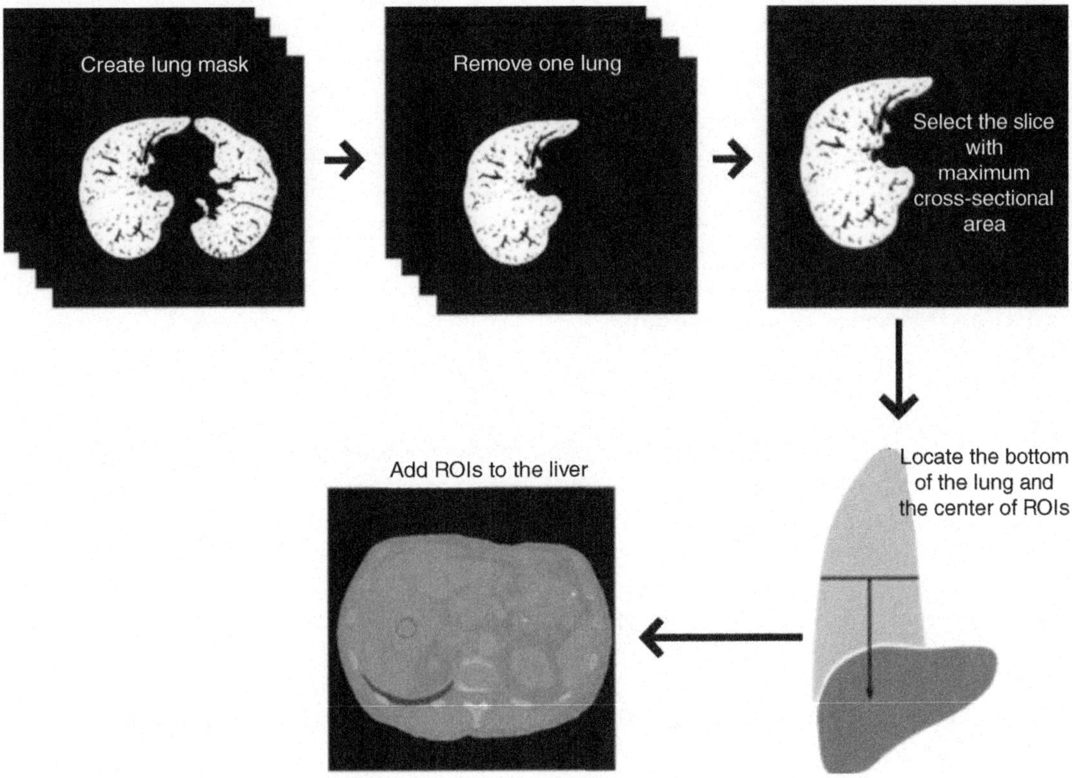

Fig. 11.9 Process for determining the ideal location to position a cylindrical ROI inside a patient's liver [18]

these organs to measure histograms of the HUs. This automated technique has been validated against manual segmentation of the organs in 15 (8 male, 7 female) non-contrast-enhanced and 15 (8 male and 7 female) contrast-enhanced datasets (administrated with 75–150 mL of 300–370 mgI/mL of iodine (Isovue, Bracco Diagnostics, Inc., Princeton, NJ) acquired on 2 CT scanners (Discovery CT750 HD, LightSpeed VCT, General Electric Medical Systems, Milwaukee, WI) [18].

Results show HU histograms from the automated technique closely match those of a manual technique. The histograms exhibit the expected Gaussian distribution for both the automated and manual techniques. These histograms demonstrate qualitative agreement between the automated and manual techniques. Overall, the algorithm successfully measured the histograms of the four organs in both contrast-enhanced and non-contrast-enhanced CT exams for all of the cases examined. This technology is implemented in METIS to enable automated estimations of HU and contrast in patient CT images.

Predictive Analytic Models on Captured Dose, Image Quality, and Associated CT Examination Data

Dose and image quality monitoring is expected to be used to extract meaningful knowledge towards quality and clinical patient care improvement. In METIS, a number of analytical techniques have been deployed towards that end, which includes trends and variations within patient cohorts, inconsistencies across systems, operators, and patients of different sizes, and identifying outliers towards optimization of CT practice. Keeping track of corrective actions, METIS offers continuous improvement of analyses and corrective actions over time.

Ascertain Protocol- and Size-Specific Radiation Dose and Quality Reference Levels

DRLs in medical imaging were developed as guidance for performance evaluation based on ionizing radiation dose estimations but only by inference of diagnostic quality. Following that philosophy, the dose and quality monitoring data can be used to define appropriate reference dose and quality levels so that the protocols that deliver excessive dose can be easily identified. Towards that goal, the use of universal alerts based on dose alone, as adopted in most current dose monitoring systems, may be of limited clinical utility. That is due to the fact that different protocols have different dose requirements because of the differences in anatomical regions, patient sizes, and imaging tasks. Additionally, the radiation dose necessary to generate a diagnostic image quality depends strongly on the amount of attenuation. Therefore, both protocol- and patient size-specific monitoring should be used to define the dose and quality reference alert levels to establish the most meaningful references and alert levels as a function of protocol and patient size [21].

Figure 11.10 shows an example of how such protocol-specific reference levels can be established. The results are used in the protocol definitions to serve as guidelines for technologists to improve examination consistency across the operation. It also demonstrates an alert that ignores patient size is ill-informed: a level that is appropriate for smaller (and perhaps younger) patients leads to excessive false alarms for large patients. Aiming to avoid that, the level can be set to a higher level, but that would obscure overdose cases for small patients. Our analytics address this inadequacy

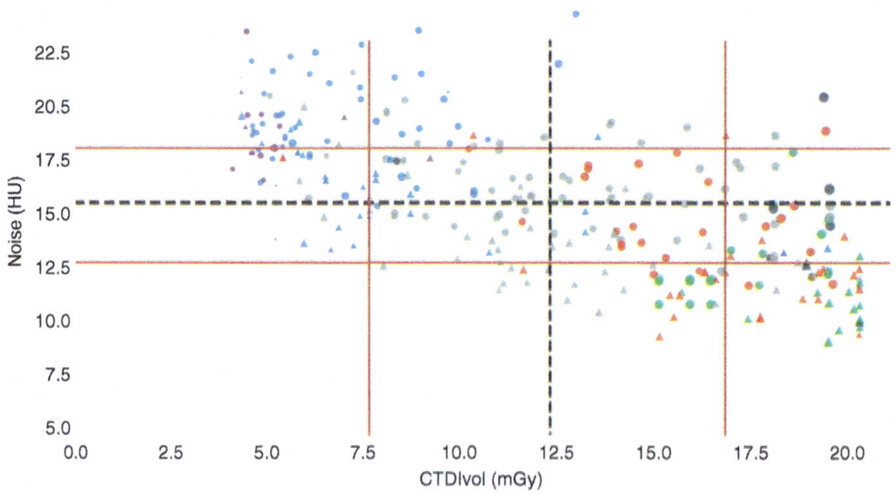

Fig. 11.10 Plots of protocol- and size-specific reference noise levels. Lines are 25th, 50th, and 75th percentile. Points are color-coded based on patient BMI, with shape indicating reconstruction algorithm and size representing the patient diameter

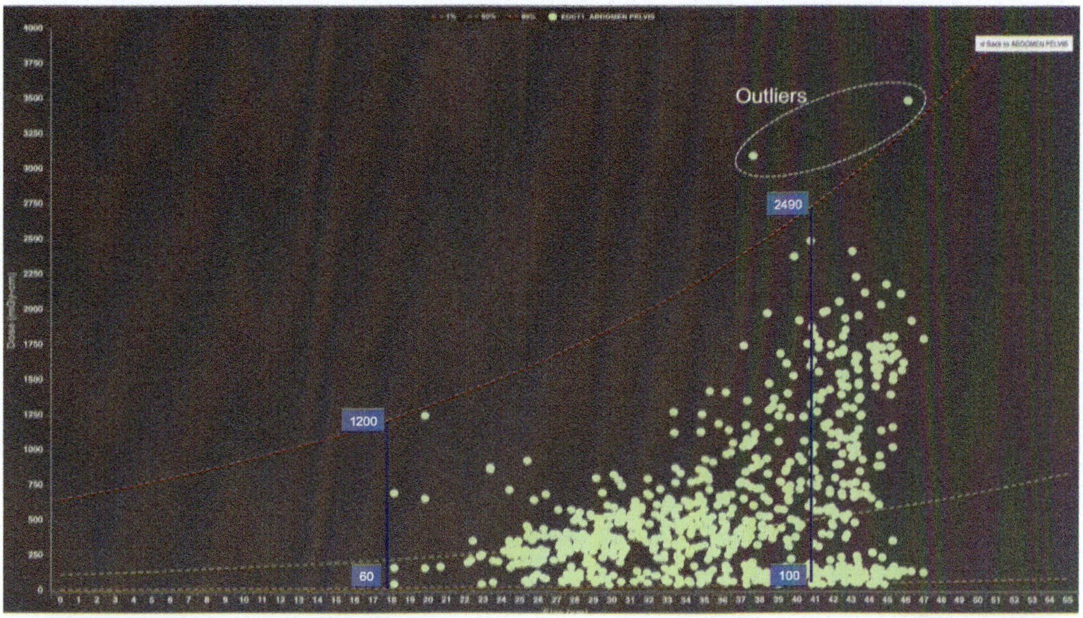

Fig. 11.11 Plots of protocol- and size-specific reference dose levels. Each point represents a patient undergoing abdomen-pelvis CT. The red, yellow, and amber dash lines represent the 99th, 50th, and 1st percentile fitting lines. The points circled in the white elliptical shapes are overexposured cases

Identify and Investigate Over- and Underexposure Cases

With the establishment of protocol- and size-specific dose and noise reference levels, it would be easy to rapidly identify the true outliers. Those would include both over- and underexposure conditions. This will help educate CT technologists to be aware of this problem and to verify that the correct scanning settings are used. By efficiently identifying and understanding potential outliers, METIS enables continuous assurance of the exam quality (Fig. 11.11).

Ascertain Intra- and Intersystem Variability

At large medical institutions, it is very common that multiple CT systems of different vendors and models are used. The imaging protocols across those systems are not necessarily the same or applied consistently. When imaging patients, there is an underlying assumption that images should be more about the patients themselves and less about the conditions under which the images are acquired. Therefore, there is a need to standardize dose and image quality across systems. Figure 11.12 illustrates dose variation between different CT scanners and protocols. Ascertaining these trends enables one to adjust the protocol parameters associated with different systems so that the patient dose and imaging quality could meet certain target requirements, in effect making patient care (quality and safety) more consistent and less system-dependent.

Web-Based Graphical User Interface

METIS is designed based on the service-oriented architecture (SOA) approach by

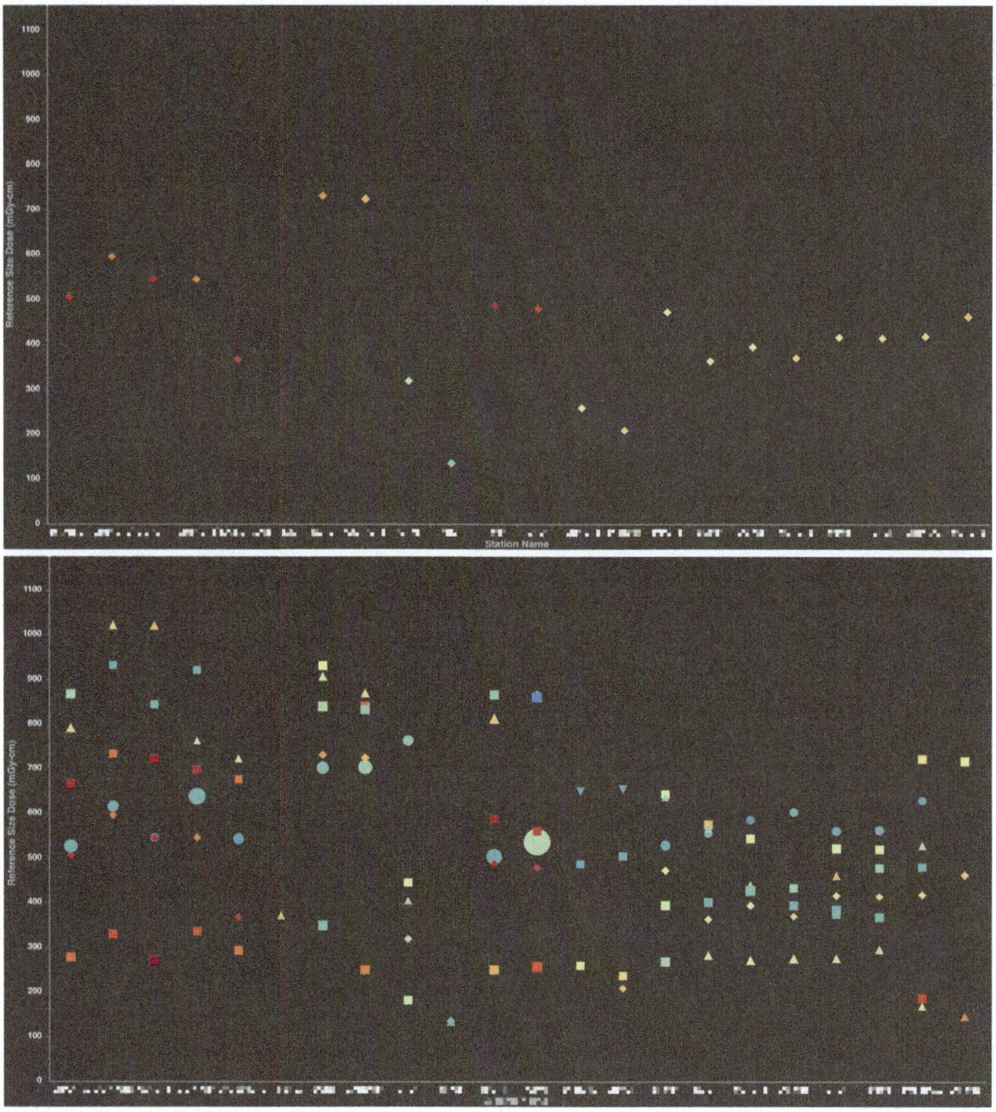

Fig. 11.12 Plots of dose variances between different CT scanners for a given protocol (top) and across some protocols (bottom). Each point on this plot represents the performance of one protocol for the entire period studied. The shape of the marker represents the protocol name. The color of the marker represents the slope of the aforementioned trend line. The size of the marker represents the variability of the data [48]

grouping all the dose and quality assessment algorithms together as interposable services. We will develop a web-based graphical user interface (GUI) including the clinical DICOM image management, web-based DICOM display, and data visualization dashboard. Some of the possible visualizations are demonstrated in Fig. 11.13. The web-based DICOM viewer is developed using hypertext markup language (HTML) and an open-source DICOM server package. The data dashboard is developed using the MongoDB, Express.js, AngularJS, and NodeJS (MEAN) stack. Related dose and image quality data are stored together in a database that provides fast query access for a high-performance user interface. Data analysis and data visualization methods are integrated into the data dashboard.

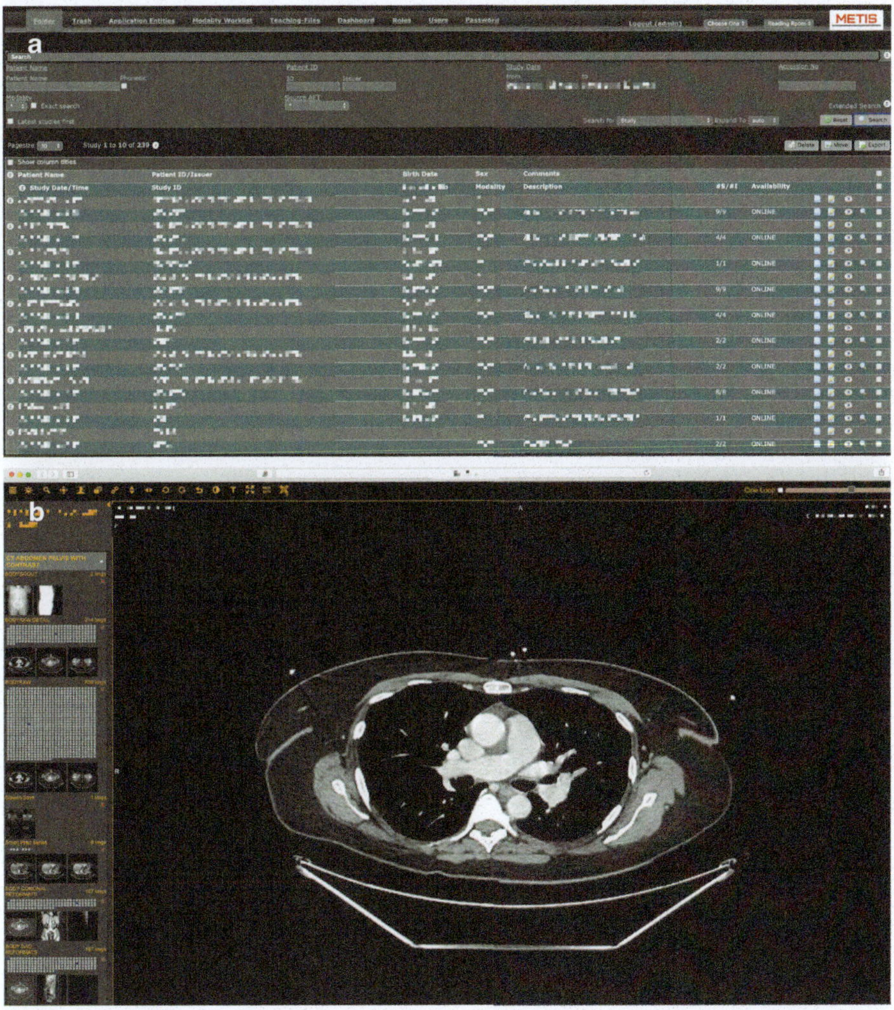

Fig. 11.13 Some preliminary web-based GUIs and dashboard visualizations for METIS: (**a**) DICOM image data management interface; (**b**) web-based DICOM viewer; (**c**) plot of scanner usage; (**d**) plot of protocol usage

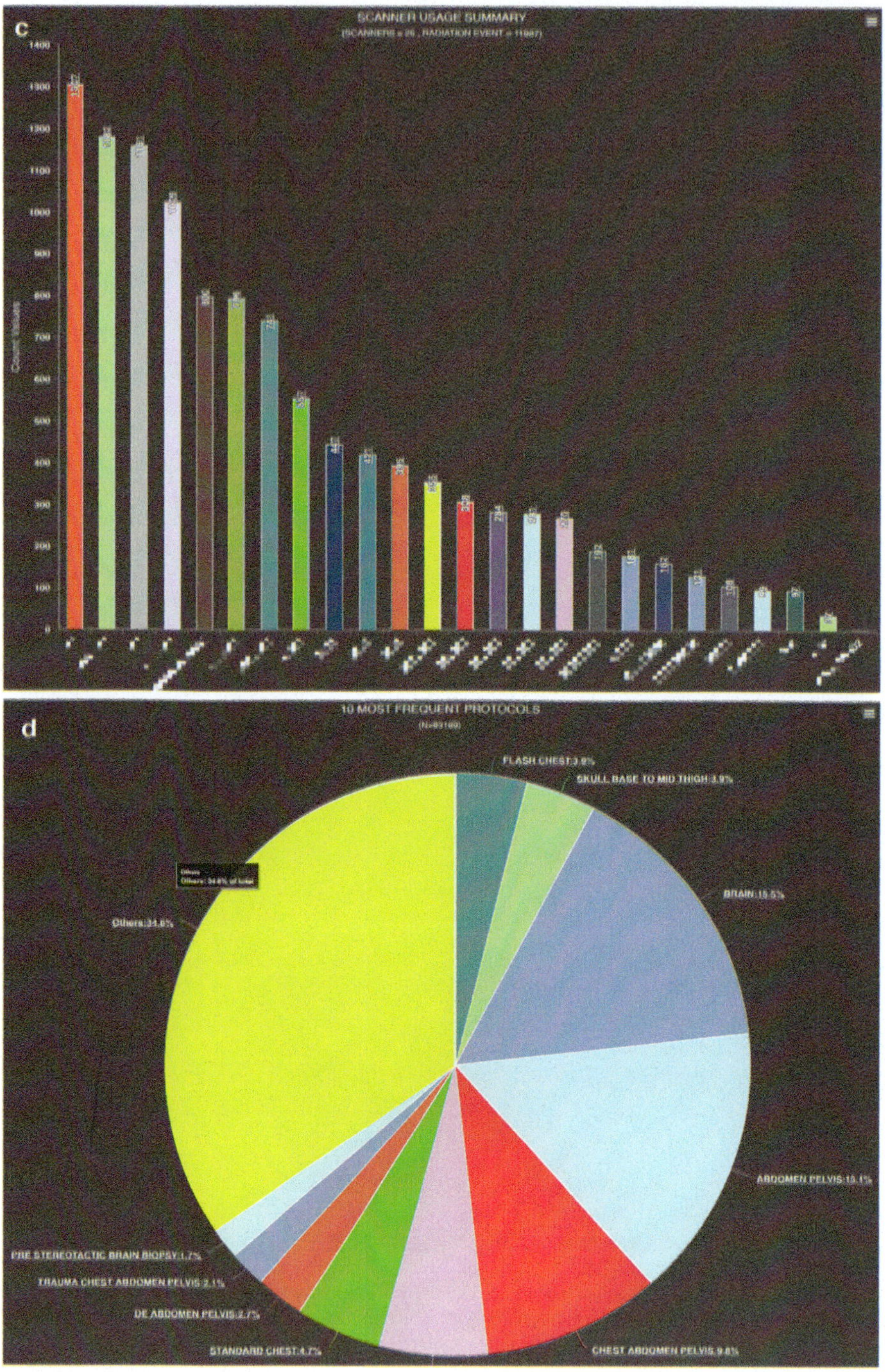

Fig. 11.13 (continued)

Conclusion

CT practice monitoring is a crucial tool for guiding imaging interpreters and operators in optimizing imaging radiation dose and quality-level matching expected values to ensure consistent device usage and apply best practices in medical imaging for improved patient care. Programmatic radiation dose-reporting software has emerged to understand, manage, and mitigate radiation exposure towards proper imaging. However, proper imaging implies not only radiation risk but also clinical value in caring for illness and injury across all ages. Ensuring the benefit of CT examination requires a combined image-quality and dose monitoring program. Such a program is a required element of value-based practice in CT imaging, providing opportunities for improved individual decision-making as well as for assessing and addressing the aggregate aspects of CT imaging practice.

METIS offers the first ever strategy for combined dose and image quality monitoring. Adding quality-dose metrics and advanced prospective and retrospective data analysis, METIS provides opportunities for improved patient care and for assessing and addressing the aggregate aspects of clinical imaging practice to ensure rigorous patient safety and consistent imaging quality. This in turn paves the way towards consistent and high-quality imaging care across the healthcare enterprise.

References

1. Brenner DJ. Should we be concerned about the rapid increase in CT usage? Rev Environ Health. 2010;25(1):63–8.
2. Sodickson A, Beayens PF, Andriole KP, Prevedello LM, Nawfel RD, Hanson R, et al. Recurrent CT, cumulative radiation exposure, and associated radiation-induced cancer risks from CT of adults. Radiology. 2009;251(1):175–84.
3. Pearce MS, Salotti JA, Little MP, McHugh K, Lee C, Pyo Kim K, et al. Radiation exposure from CT scans in childhood and subsequent risk of leukaemia and brain tumours: a retrospective cohort study. Lancet. 2012;380(9840):499–505.
4. Boone JM, Hendee WR, McNitt-Gray MF, Seltzer SE. Radiation exposure from CT scans: how to close our knowledge gaps, monitor and safeguard exposure--proceedings and recommendations of the radiation dose summit, sponsored by NIBIB, February 24–25, 2011. Radiology. 2012;265(2):544–54.
5. Brenner DJ. Radiation risks potentially associated with low-dose CT screening of adult smokers for lung cancer. Radiology. 2004;231(2):440–5.
6. Meeson S, Patel R, Golding S. Clinical expansion of CT and radiation dose. In: Tack D, Kalra MK, Gevenois PA, editors. Radiation dose from multidetector CT. 2nd ed. Berlin: Springer-Verlag; 2012. p. 21–32.
7. Bogdanich W, McGinty JC. Medicare claims show overuse for CT scanning. The New York Times [internet]. 17th June 2011. Available from http://www.nytimes.com/2011/06/18/health/18radiation.html.
8. United Nations Scientific Committee on the Effects of Atomic Radiation. Sources and effects of ionizing radiation. UNSCEAR 2008 report to the general assembly with scientific annexes. New York: United Nations; 2010.
9. Brenner DJ. Estimating cancer risks from pediatric CT: going from the qualitative to the quantitative. Pediatr Radiol. 2002;32(4):228–31.
10. US Food and Drug Administration. White paper: initiative to reduce unnecessary radiation exposure from medical imaging. 2010. http://www.fda.gov/Radiation-EmittingProducts/RadiationSafety/RadiationDoseReduction/ucm199994.htm.
11. Morin RL, Coombs LP, Chatfield MB. ACR dose index registry. J Am Coll Radiol. 2011;8(4):288–91.
12. The Joint Commission. Radiation risks of diagnostic imaging. The joint commission: sentinel event alert. 2011;47:1–4.. http://www.jointcommission.org/assets/1/18/sea_471.pdf
13. Boone S, Cody D, Mc Collough C, McNitt-Gray M, Toth T. Size specific dose estimates (SSDE) in pediatric and adult body CT examinations. AAPM report no. 204. College Park: American Association of Physicists in Medicine; 2011.
14. NCRP 2009 Ionizing radiation exposure of the population of the United States NCRP Report no. 160. National Council on Radiation Protection and Measurements, 2009.
15. Li X, Samei E, Segars WP, Sturgeon GM, Colsher JG, Frush DP. Patient-specific radiation dose and cancer risk for pediatric chest CT. Radiology. 2011;259(3):862–74.
16. Samei E, Tian X, Segars WP, Frush DP. Radiation risk index for pediatric CT: a patient-derived metric. Pediatr Radiol. 2017;47(13):1737–174.
17. Dougeni E, Faulkner K, Panayiotakis G. A review of patient dose and optimization methods in adult and paediatric CT scanning. Eur J Radiol. 2012;81:e665–83.
18. Abadi E, Sanders J, Samei E. Patient-specific quantification of image quality: an automated technique for measuring the distribution of organ Hounsfield units in clinical chest CT images. Med Phys. 2017;44(9):4736–46.
19. Christianson O, Winslow J, Frush DP, Samei E. Automated technique to measure noise in clinical CT examinations. AJR. 2015;205:W93–9.

20. Sanders J, Hurwitz L, Samei E. Patient-specific quantification of image quality: an automated method for measuring spatial resolution in clinical CT images. Med Phys. 2016;43(10):5330–8.
21. Ria F, Davis JT, Solomon JB, Wilson JM, Smith TB, Frush DP, et al. Expanding the Concept of Diagnostic Reference Levels to Noise and Dose Reference Levels in CT. AJR Am J Roentgenol. 2019;213:1–6.
22. ICRP. Diagnostic reference levels in medical imaging, ICRP Publication 135. Ann ICRP. 2017;46(1).
23. Frush DP, Samei E. CT radiation dose monitoring: current state and new prospects CME. Medscape [internet]. 19th March 2015. Available from http://www.medscape.org/viewarticle/839485.
24. Council Directive 2013/59/Euratom http://eurlex.europa.eu/LexUriServ/LexUriServ.do?uri=OJ:L:2014:013:0001:0073:IT:PDF
25. Radiation Control: Health Facilities and Clinics, SB1237, 19 February 2010. http://www.leginfo.ca.gov/pub/09-10/bill/sen/sb_1201-1250/sb_1237_bill_20100929_chaptered.html.
26. Texas Department of State Health Services. Computed Tomography (CT): Radiation Control Program. Updated 29 Dec 2011. https://www.dshs.state.tx.us/radiation/x-ray/laws-rules.aspx#medical-x-ray.
27. International Atomic Energy Agency, Radiation Protection of Patients (RPOP) – Diagnostic Reference Levels (DRLs). IAEA; 2017. https://www.iaea.org/resources/rpop/health-professionals/radiology/diagnostic-reference-levels.
28. Ria F, Wilson JM, Zhang Y, Samei E. Image noise and dose performance across a clinical population: patient size adaptation as a metric of CT performance. Med Phys. 2017;44(6):2141–7.
29. Samei E, Järvinen H, Kortesniemi M, Simantirakis G, Goh C, Wallace A, et al. Medical imaging dose optimization from ground up: expert opinion of an international summit. J Radiol Prot. 2018;38:967–89.
30. Ria F, Bergantin A, Vai A, Bonfanti P, Martinotti AS, Redaelli I, et al. Awareness of medical radiation exposure among patients: a patient survey as a first step for effective communication of ionizing radiation risks. Phys Med. 2017;43:57–62.
31. Zhang Y, Samei E, Nair S, Coombs LP, Jackson EF, Sullivan DC. Quantitative performance for ACR CT accreditation images across different vendors, protocols, and institutions: initial report of an ACR-RSNA collaboration. 102th RSNA conference, Nov 27th–Dec 2nd 2016, Chicago.
32. Christianson O, Chen JS, Yang Z, et al. An improved index of image quality for task-based performance of CT iterative reconstruction across three commercial implementations. Radiology. 2015;275(3):725–34.
33. Christianson O, Li X, Frush DP, Samei E. Automated size-specific CT dose monitoring program: assessing variability in CT dose. Med Phys. 2012;39(11):7131–9.
34. National Research Council. Health risks from exposure to low levels of ionizing radiation: BEIR VII phase 2. 2006.
35. Ria F, Fu W, Hoye J, Segars WP, Kapadia A, Samei E. Characterization of radiation risk across a clinical CT patient population: comparison across 12 risks metrics. 104th RSNA conference. Nov 25th–30th 2018, Chicago, IL.
36. Mabotuwana T, Lee MC, Cohen-Solal EV, Chang P. Mapping institution-specific study descriptions to RadLex playbook entries. J Digit Imaging. 2014;27:321–30.
37. Kanal KM, Butler PF, Sengupta D, Bhargavan-Chatfield M, Coombs LP, Morin RLUS. Diagnostic reference levels and achievable doses for 10 adult CT examinations. Radiology. 2017;284:120–34.
38. Bae KT. Intravenous contrast medium administration and scan timing at CT: considerations and approaches. Radiology. 2010;256:32–61.
39. American Association of Physicists in Medicine. Use of water equivalent diameter for calculating patient size and size-specific dose estimates (SSDE) in CT, Report no. 220. Report of the AAPM task group 220. College Park: AAPM; 2014.
40. McCollough CH, Leng S, Yu L, Cody DD, Boon JM, McNitt-Gray MF. CT dose index and patient dose: they are not the same thing. Radiology. 2011;259(2):311–6.
41. Tian X, Li X, Segars WP, Frush DP, Paulson EK, Samei E. Dose coefficients in pediatric and adult abdominopelvic CT based on 100 patient models. Phys Med Biol. 2013;58(24):8755–68.
42. Tian X, Li X, Segars WP, Frush DP, Samei E. Prospective estimation of organ dose in CT under tube current modulation. Med Phys. 2015;42(4):1575–85.
43. Tian X, Samei E. Accurate assessment and prediction of noise in clinical CT images. Med Phys. 2015;43(1):475–82.
44. Li X, Samei E, Segars WP, Sturgeon GM, Colsher JG, Toncheva G, et al. Patient-specific radiation dose and cancer risk estimation in CT: part I. development and validation of a Monte Carlo program. Med Phys. 2011;38(1):397–407.
45. Li X, Samei E, Segars WP, Sturgeon GM, Colsher JG, Toncheva G, et al. Patient-specific radiation dose and cancer risk estimation in CT: part II. Application to patients. Med Phys. 2011;38(1):408–19.
46. Fu W, Sturgeon GM, Agasthya G, Segars WP, Kapadia AJ, Samei E. Breast dose reduction with organ-based, wide-angle tube current modulated CT. J Med Imaging. 2017;4(3):031208.
47. Fu W, Sharma S, Smith TB, Hou R, Abadi E, Vignesh S, et al. Multi-organ segmentation in clinical-computed tomography for patient-specific image quality and dose metrology. Proceedings Volume 10948, Medical Imaging 2019: Physical of Medical Imaging. 2019:1094829.
48. Ding A, Wilson J, Solomon J, Zhang Y, Mann S, Nelson J, Wells J, Samei E. METIS: next-generation performance informatics platform for value-based clinical imaging practice, 104th RSNA conference, 25th–30th Nov 2018, Chicago.

Part IV

Spectral CT

12 Methods for Spectral CT Imaging

Cynthia H. McCollough

Introduction

Clinical Motivation

Because CT numbers depend on X-ray attenuation, they are impacted by the mass density and effective atomic number of the imaged materials. Therefore, different materials can have the same CT number if the effective atomic number differences are offset by appropriate differences in the mass density. Spectral CT imaging acquires data at two or more energies, allowing mathematical methods to separately determine the mass density and effective atomic number. Clinically, this has been implemented using two spectral measurements and is referred to as dual-energy CT. Currently under research and development, energy-resolving photon-counting-detector (PCD) CT technology will allow acquisition of more than two spectral measurements. This is often referred to as multi-energy CT. However, because there are only two fundamental determinants of X-ray attenuation, namely, photoelectric effect and Compton scattering, the acquisition of more than two spectral measurements does not necessarily allow the discrimination of more than two material types. Materials with K edges in the diagnostic energy range can be separately measured with energy-resolving PCD techniques if spectral data are acquired below and above the K edge. Otherwise, three-material decomposition requires some a priori information, such as the assumption of mass or volume conservation [1]. Figure 12.1 gives an example of the clinical utility of dual-energy CT data.

History of Dual-Energy CT

The concept of dual-energy CT is not necessarily a new one, even though its use in clinical practice began in earnest in only 2006. In Hounsfield's 1973 paper, he noted "Two pictures are taken of the same slice, one at 100 kV and the other at 140 kV… so that areas of high atomic numbers can be enhanced. Tests carried out to date have shown that iodine ($z = 53$) can be readily differentiated from calcium ($z = 20$)" [2]. The technique was explored further in the 1970s and adopted for a short period in the mid-1980s by one commercial CT manufacturer (Siemens Healthcare) [3]; however, limitations in CT scanner technology at that time limited the clinical utility of the technique, which disappeared from commercial systems until 2006.

C. H. McCollough (✉)
Department of Radiology, Mayo Clinic,
Rochester, MN, USA
e-mail: mccollough.cynthia@mayo.edu

© Springer Nature Switzerland AG 2020

E. Samei, N. J. Pelc (eds.), *Computed Tomography*, https://doi.org/10.1007/978-3-030-26957-9_12

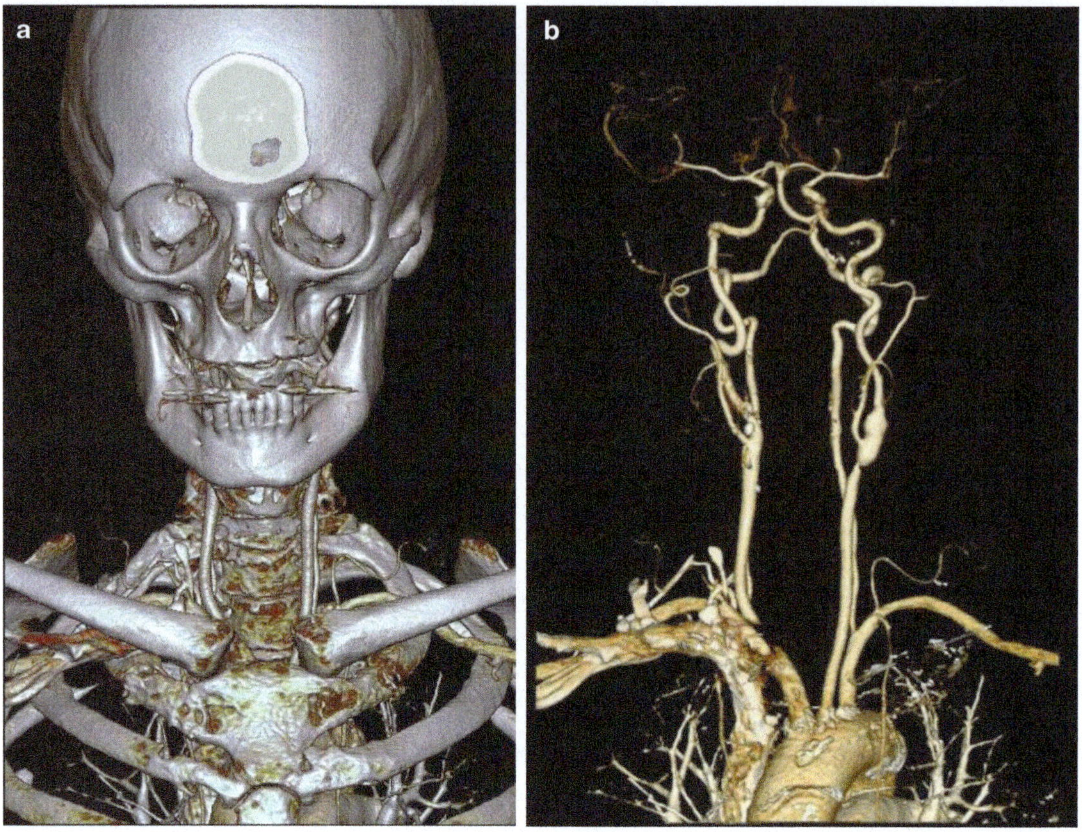

Fig. 12.1 3D volume rendered image of a dual-energy CT angiogram of the head and neck. Because dual-energy CT processing can classify a voxel as containing either iodine or calcium, an image with bone overlapping the vascular anatomy (**a**) can be turned into an image containing only vascular anatomy (**b**) with a single click of a button. This eliminates the need for manual or semiautomated bone removal

Importance of Spectral Separation

Because of the material-specific, energy-dependent behavior of X-ray absorption coefficients, measurements taken at two different effective energies can be used to identify two materials, as shown in Fig. 12.2. As the effective energy of the beam changes from about 75 keV to about 55 keV, the difference in X-ray absorption for iodine is much greater than that for bone, allowing the two materials to be separated, as demonstrated in Fig. 12.1. The greater the difference between the effective energies of the spectra, i.e., the amount of spectral overlap is lower, the more different these material-specific signatures will be, making the job of separating them easier. Kelcz et al. demonstrated that as spectral separation increases, the noise in the material-specific images decreases dramatically [4]. Therefore, in considering the technology used to acquire data having different energy spectra, it is important to consider the amount of resulting spectral overlap [5, 6]. In the following section, the various approaches to acquiring CT data with different energy spectra will be reviewed.

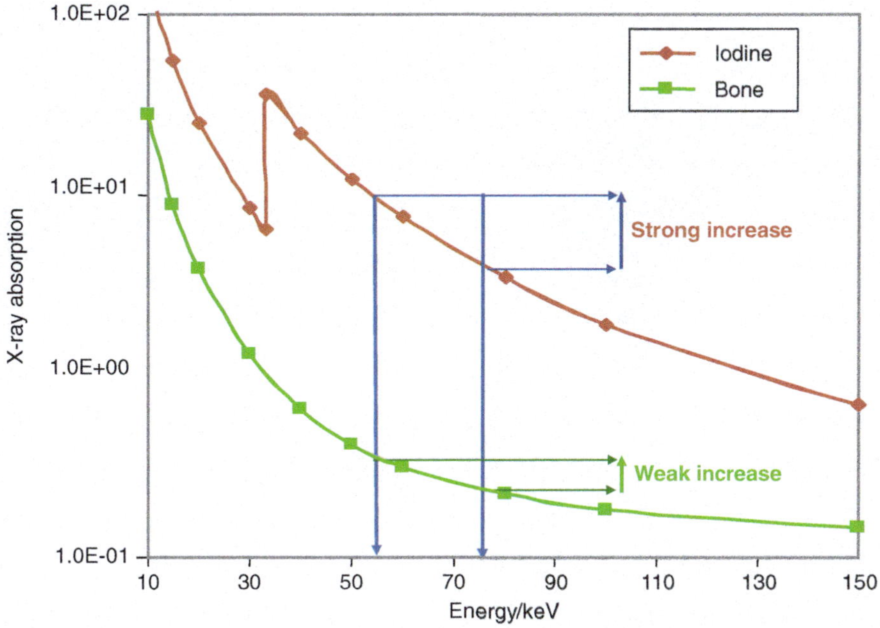

Fig. 12.2 The X-ray absorption of a material is dependent on the material composition (e.g., bone or iodine) and on the photon energy. Therefore, for measurements taken at two different energies, e.g., 75 and 55 keV, the increase in absorption as the energy is decreased is greater for iodine than it is for bone. This energy-dependent and material-dependent behavior is what allows dual-energy CT to differentiate between bone and iodine

Multi-energy CT Data Acquisition Methods

Split-Beam Filtration

Using a single X-ray source and single X-ray tube potential, dual-energy CT data can be acquired by placing a filter composed of two different materials in front of the X-ray beam [7]. For example, one of the materials might be tin, which shifts the energy spectrum to the right, increasing the effective energy of the spectrum. The other material might be gold, which has a K edge of approximately 80 keV. Because the attenuation is dramatically increased above the K edge, this preferentially absorbs higher-energy photons, above 80 keV, shifting the effective energy of the spectra to the left to lower energies. Figure 12.3 illustrates the concept of this split-beam filtration approach, and Fig. 12.4 shows how the two energy spectra are altered by the two filters. For this technique to be successful, data must be acquired using a spiral technique. In this manner, the spectral data acquired are spatially offset from one another. During the spiral interpolation process, the data can be appropriately aligned and used for reconstruction and dual-energy processing.

Dual-Layer Detectors

Another manner in which dual-energy data can be acquired using a single X-ray tube and a single X-ray tube potential is to differentiate the low- and high-energy spectra at the detector. This can be accomplished using a detector having two absorption and readout layers (Fig. 12.5). Lower-energy photons are stopped in the more superficial detector, closest to the patient, and higher-energy photons are preferentially absorbed

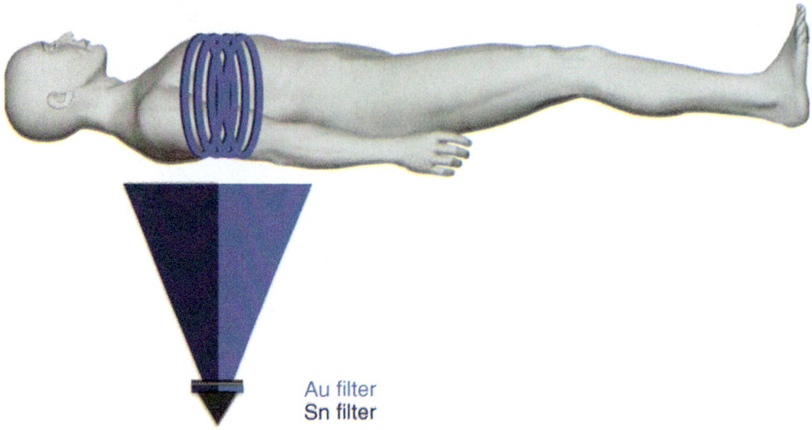

Fig. 12.3 Illustration of the split-beam approach for acquiring dual-energy CT data. The gold (Au) filter reduces the effective energy of a 120 kV spectrum, while the tin (Sn) filter increases the effective energy. During a spiral acquisition, low- and high-energy spectral data are using a single X-ray source, a single tube potential setting, and a conventional single-layer detector

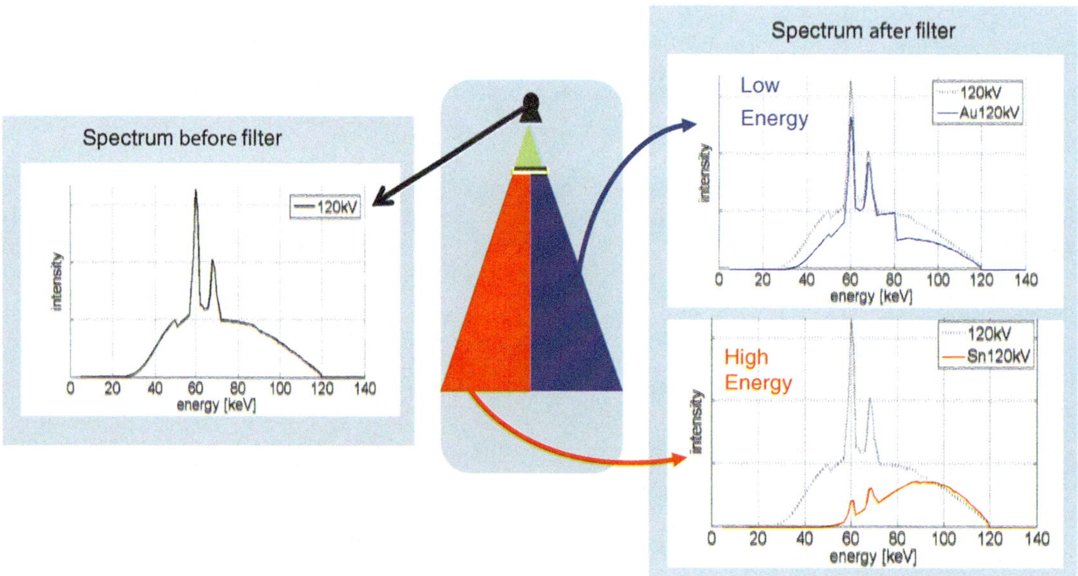

Fig. 12.4 Illustration of the beam softening that occurs with the Au filter and the beam hardening that occurs with the Sn filter

in the deeper detector layer, farther from the patient. The two sets of measured data can be added together to create a conventional, single-energy data set, or the two sets of data can be processed separately to create dual-energy images. In this manner, dual-energy data are collected at all times and can be used in spiral or axial acquisition modes. The data are perfectly registered both temporally and spatially [8]. In Fig. 12.6, the spectral separation that results is shown [9].

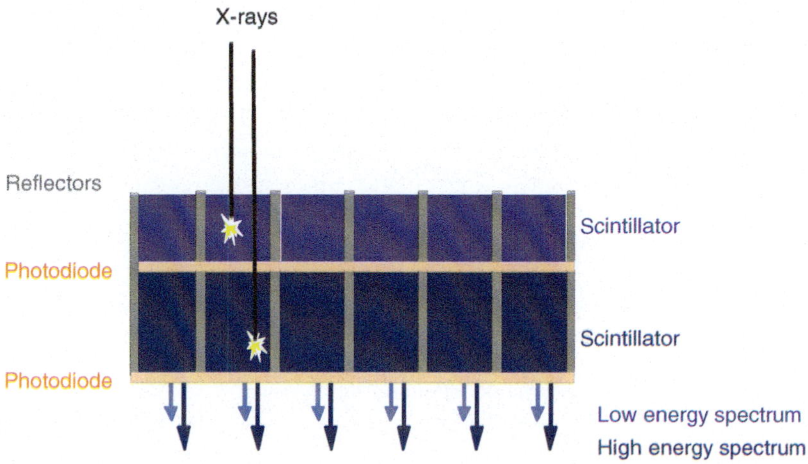

Fig. 12.5 Illustration of a dual-layer detector. Lower-energy photons are more likely to be stopped in the front layer (closest to the patient) to collect data of a relatively low-energy spectrum. Higher-energy photons are more likely to pass through the front layer and be absorbed in the back layer, resulting in a relatively higher-energy spectrum

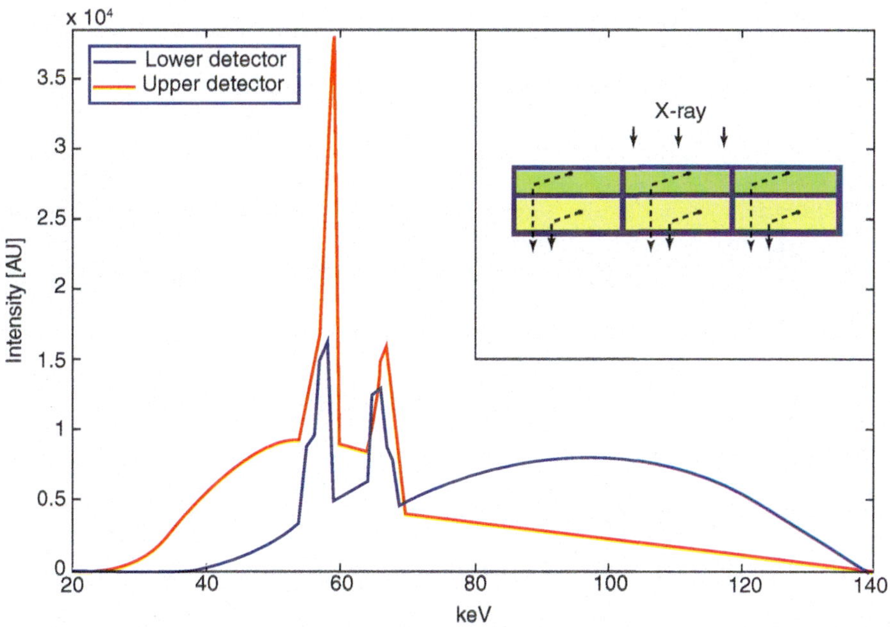

Fig. 12.6 Spectral separation resulting from a dual-layer detector is shown in this plot (Reprinted with permission from Carmi et al. [9])

Photon-Counting Detectors (PCDs)

An emerging technology, which is currently only in research use, is to use energy-resolving PCD technology, a single X-ray tube, and a single tube potential to simultaneously acquire data that are binned according to the energy level of the detected photon [10–14]. See also Chap. 14. To accomplish this, the detector must directly convert the detected X-ray energy to charge, as shown in Fig. 12.7. This is done using a semiconductor detector technology, such as cadmium zinc telluride (CZT) or CdTe. The spectral separation for a detector allowing two energy thresholds is shown in Fig. 12.8.

Slow Tube Potential Switching

The most straightforward way to acquire two data sets, each with a different energy spectrum, is simply to perform two separate acquisitions at two different tube potential settings. This can be

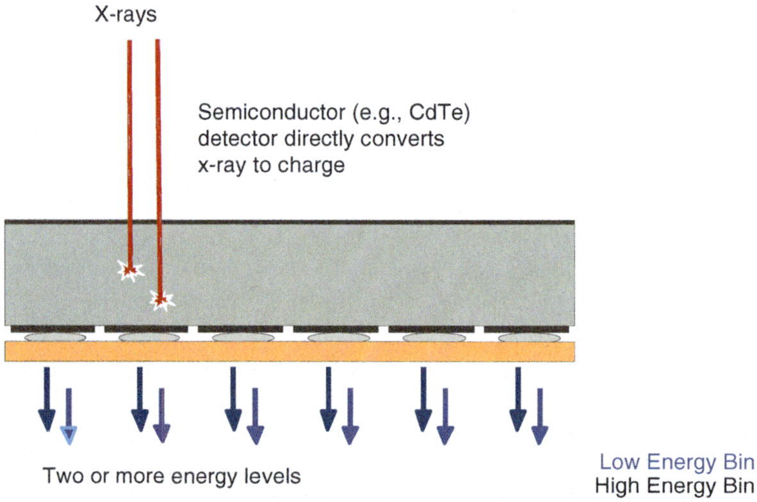

Fig. 12.7 Energy-resolving, photon-counting detectors involve a direct conversion of X-rays into electrons, unlike conventional CT detectors, which first convert X-rays into visible light and then visible light into electrons. The single-step process is associated with several desirable features, including the ability to exclude electronic noise from the measured data and the ability to categorize measured events according to the incoming photon energy. This latter property allows for binning of the data according to energy, which yields multiple energy bins of simultaneously acquired data for use in multi-energy CT data processing

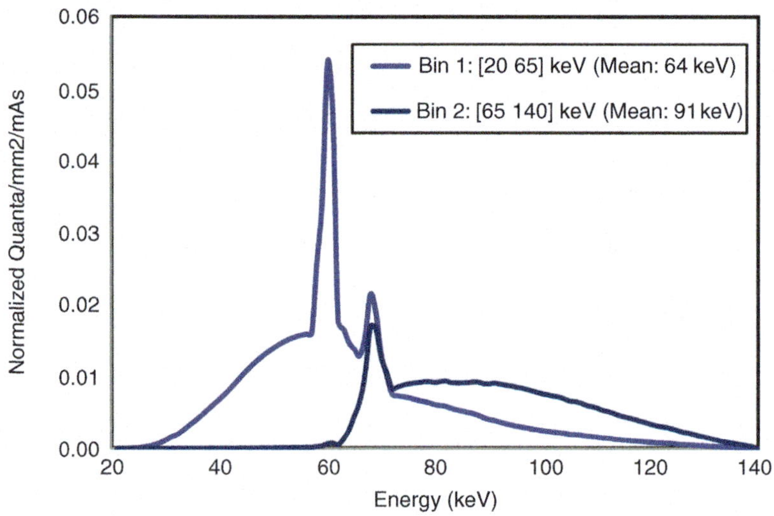

Fig. 12.8 Energy spectra resulting from the two-bin mode of the photon-counting detector used in a research photon-counting-detector system

done in either axial or spiral acquisition mode. However, the interscan delay, which is the scan time plus the time to move the table (if necessary) and initiate a new scan, can pose serious motion misregistration challenges, particularly for imaging of dynamic processes such as contrast enhancement. For scanners that can acquire data over a large scan volume in a single rotation, this may be an acceptable approach (Fig. 12.9) [15]. For most scanners, 80 kV and 140 kV represent the lowest and highest tube potential settings, respectively. Figure 12.10 gives an example of these two energy spectra. The low-energy (low tube potential) spectrum is fully encompassed within the high-energy (high tube potential) spectrum, resulting in relatively poor energy separation.

Rapid Tube Potential Switching

Instead of acquiring two consecutive scans, each at a different tube potential setting, the tube potential can be quickly switched between successive views as the tube rotates about the patient (Fig. 12.11) [16]. This switching must be very rapid, as approximately 2000 separate views must be acquired within 1 gantry rotation period, which can be less than 0.5 second. It is technically challenging to change the tube potential at

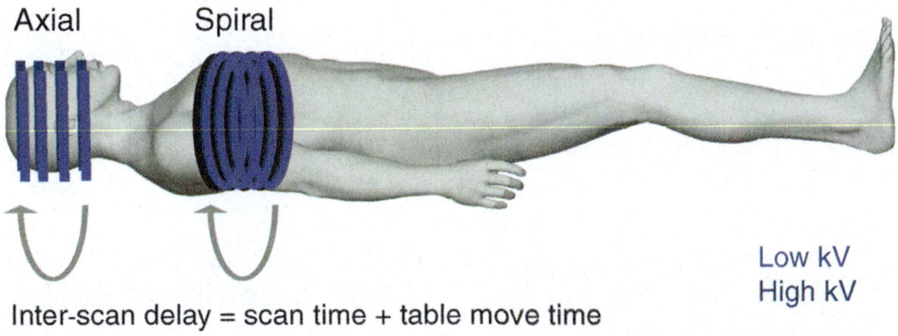

Fig. 12.9 In slow tube potential switching dual-energy CT data acquisitions, the entire volume of interest is scanned first at one tube potential, the tube potential is switched to the alternate setting, and the volume is rescanned. The interscan time delay may result in unacceptable motion artifacts due to misregistration of the anatomy or changes in the contrast enhancement. For large-coverage CT systems, however, the time delay may be acceptable for some applications (Reprinted with permission from [15])

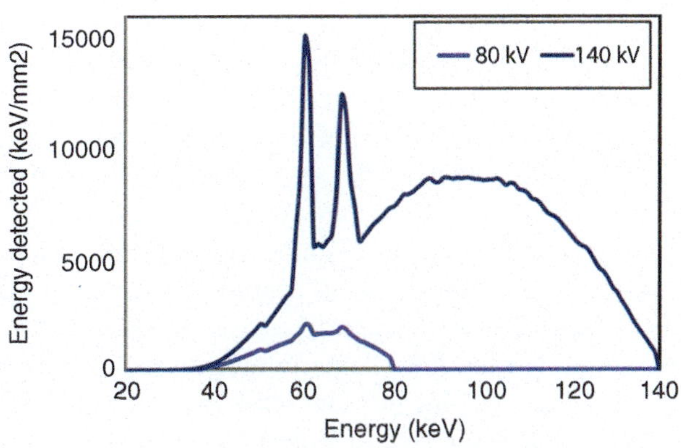

Fig. 12.10 Typical 80 and 140 kV spectra are shown. These are the typical settings for slow tube potential switching, as they maximize the spectral separation. Because the low-energy spectrum is fully encompassed by the high-energy spectrum, there is relatively poor spectral separation

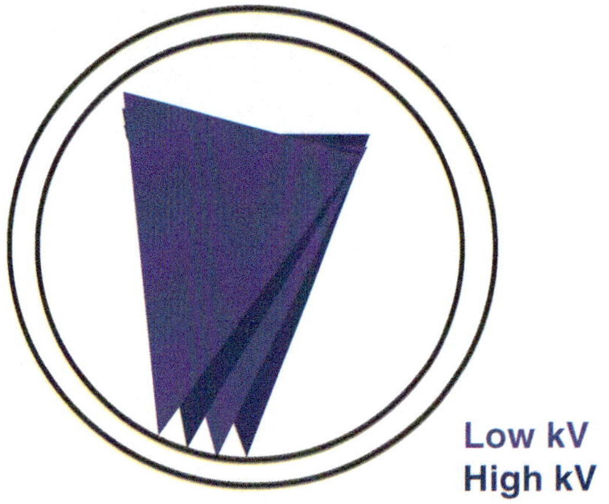

Fig. 12.11 In fast tube potential switching dual-energy CT data acquisitions, the tube potential is switched for every different projection, minimizing the misregistration between the low- and high-energy data sets. (Reprinted with permission from [15]). Assuming the tube potentials are 80 and 140 kV, the spectra will have overlap similar to that for slow tube potential switching (Fig. 12.10)

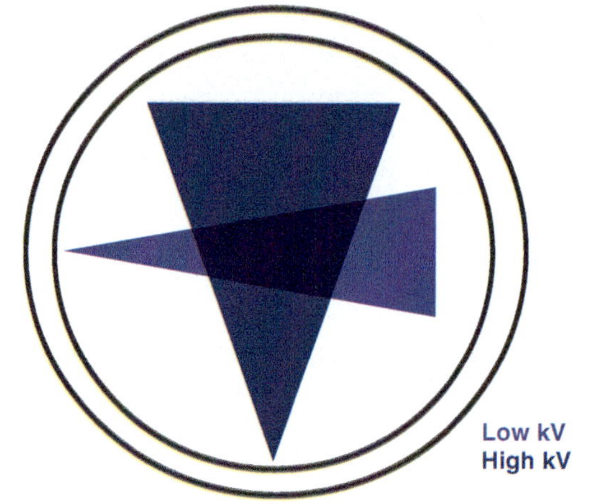

Fig. 12.12 A dual-source CT system uses two different tube-detector pairs, located about 90° apart from one another on the same slip-ring gantry (Reprinted with permission from [15])

such a rapid rate; thus, instead of a square-wave type of wave form, the tube potential is varying quickly but continuously from the maximum to minimum values. Assuming the tube potentials are 80 and 140 kV, the spectra will have overlap similar to that for slow tube potential switching (Fig. 12.10). Because the switching is not instantaneous, there is likely to be more blending of the two spectra, which would be expected to further degrade energy separation.

Dual-Source Geometry

In dual-source geometry, two X-ray tubes and two detector arrays are located on the same slip-ring gantry, with the two tube-detector pairs offset from one another by approximately 90° (Fig. 12.12) [17, 18]. Data are collected simultaneously with both beams in either axial or spiral mode, but because of the 90-degree offset, the dual-energy data are not exactly registered. Dual-energy processing must be performed on reconstructed images due to the 90-degree offset between the low- and high-energy projection data. Because each X-ray spectrum is created by its own tube, the beam filtration for each tube can be tailored to maximize spectra separation, as shown in Fig. 12.13 [5, 6, 19].

Image Rendition Methods

The data acquired in a dual- or multi-energy CT acquisition can be processed and displayed in a number of different ways. In the following sections, each of the different methods and its optimal usage will be described. Examples will also be provided.

Low- or High-Energy Source Images

Some systems reconstruct and provide to the users both the images from the low-energy spectrum and the high-energy spectrum. These could be from low and high tube potentials (e.g., from dual-source CT or tube potential switching), low- and high-energy bin data (e.g., from PCD CT), or low- and high-energy spectral data from the front and back layers of a dual-layer detector. These images are the source data from which subsequent dual-

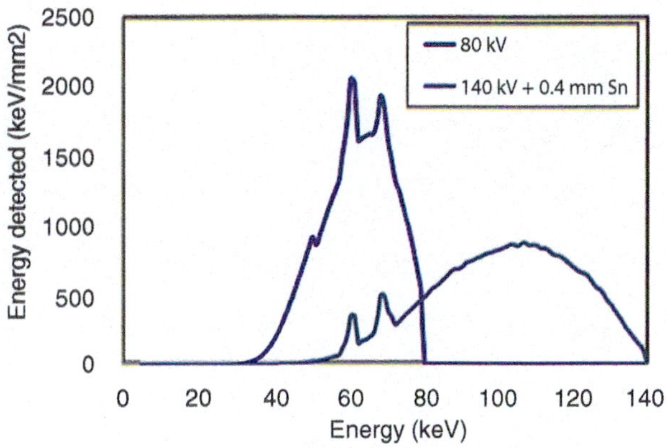

Fig. 12.13 The tube current and beam filtration can be set differently for each tube-detector pair of a dual-source CT scanner, resulting in very good spectral separation

energy processing is performed. These images are not typically viewed by a radiologist but can be used if questions arise about the processed images. It is helpful to archive these source data for future reprocessing if new algorithms become available or new parameter settings are desired.

Mixed or Blended Images

The source images referred to in the previous section have the disadvantage that neither are formed using all photons exiting the patient. Thus, the low- and high-energy images are often combined, either linearly or nonlinearly, to form what are referred to as mixed or blended images (Fig. 12.14). The weighting between the two energy spectrum images can be varied depending on the specific diagnostic task; however, an image is often presented that approximates a conventional 120 kV image [20]. These mixed images are the "routine" images that are used for primary interpretation by radiologists and clinicians. These provide a single set of images that utilize all delivered photons, and therefore, they should always be archived.

Material-Selective Images

In order to create images, sometimes referred to as maps, of a single material (e.g., an iodine image, a water image, or a bone image), the low- and high-energy spectrum data must be decomposed into these basis (or base) materials. This process can be performed using projection [3, 21–24] or image data [1, 25]. For research purposes, it can be difficult for algorithm developers to obtain access to projection data, and hence, image-based approaches can be easier to implement for the research community. This also poses no problem with regard to requiring spatial and temporal registration between views in projection data. In theory, projection-based techniques can provide an exact correction for beam hardening, but in practice, some can remain due to calibration issues. That said, while beam hardening cannot be totally removed with image-based decomposition, in practice it is reasonably well corrected for.

The decomposition process creates pairs of images with complementary properties. This could be a photoelectric effect and Compton scattering pair of images, an effective atomic number and mass density pair of images, or any two materials that behave relatively differently in their energy dependence, such as iodine and water image pairs or iodine and calcium image pairs. With the use of volume or mass conservation, the equations can be solved for a third material, and with energy-resolving PCD CT, additional materials having K edges above approximately 50 keV can also be determined.

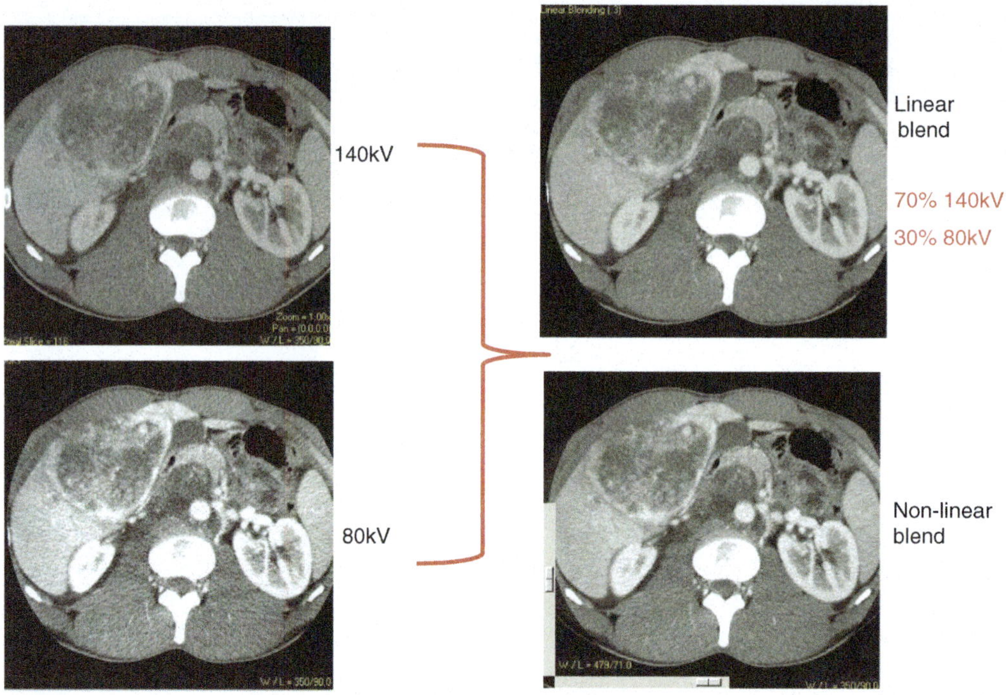

Fig. 12.14 Low- and high-energy images can be mixed (or blended) to create a new image series that uses all detected photons. In linearly mixed images, the same ratios of low- and high-energy images are used for all voxels and images. The result are images with lower noise than either source image or an iodine signal that is somewhere between that of the two source images. In nonlinear blending, a different ratio is applied to each voxel [26]. For bright voxels, which presumably contain a lot of iodine or calcium, more of the low-energy image is used to maintain the higher brightness. For low-brightness voxels, which are presumably soft tissue, more of the high-energy image is used because it has a lower noise level. While this is visually quite pleasing and may allow better qualitative visualization of anatomic structures and pathology, these images cannot be used for quantitative assessments due to the extreme nonlinearity of the data on a voxel by voxel basis

Classification vs. Quantification

After decomposition, the resultant data can be used to either classify a material (e.g., is it iodine or bone) or to quantify the material (e.g., the concentration of iodine is 7.4 mg/ml). Table 12.1 lists some examples of dual-energy CT clinical applications and whether the application classifies material type or quantifies material density.

Material Classification

Material classification can be used to answer common clinical questions, such as whether or not a kidney stone is made of uric acid or non-uric-acid minerals, whether a voxel contains bone or iodine, or whether a voxel contains gout or pseudo-gout crystals. The diagram in Fig. 12.15 helps to explain how this is accomplished. In a diagram that plots the CT number in the low-energy image against the CT number of the high-energy image, materials of different effective atomic numbers will be represented as lines having different slopes. The slope of the line, sometimes referred to as the CT number ratio or dual-energy ratio, is a function of effective atomic number. By definition, water is at the origin of such a plot. A line is drawn that bisects the triangle formed between water, material 1 and mate-

Table 12.1 The clinical applications listed here can be classified as either a material classifiction task or a material quantification task

Material classification	Material quantification
Kidney stone characterization	Blood pool imaging (perfused blood volume)
Gout detection and quantification	Virtual non-contrast (iodine removal/iodine image)
Silicone breast implant leakage	Virtual non-calcium (bone removal/bone image)
Automated bone removal in CT angiography	
Plaque removal	

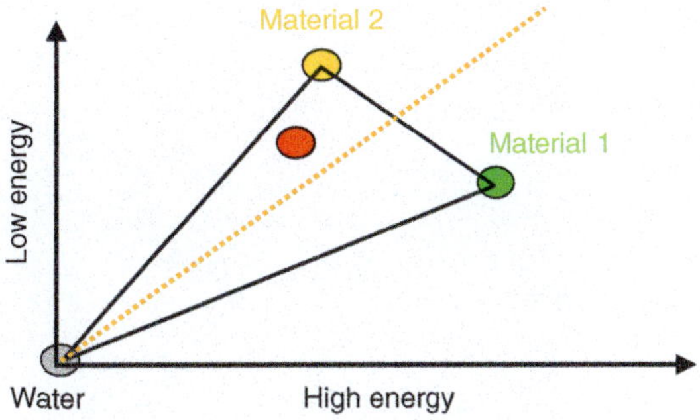

Fig. 12.15 Dual-energy CT data can be used to classify material type into one of two choices. Pictorially, this can be represented as a triangle in a plot of low-energy CT number to high-energy CT number. The slope of the lower and upper sides of the triangle is determined by the material composition. To determine whether an unknown voxel is material 1 or material 2, the voxel is mapped onto this plot and compared to a line that bisects the triangle between the lines connecting to material 1 and material 2. For the example shown, the unknown voxel (in red) lies above the bisecting line and is thus labeled as material 2

rial 2, and any voxels above the line, in this case, closer to material 2, are classified as material 2. Numerous publications have demonstrated the success of material classification for a number of applications [27–47].

With classification of iodine vs. bone, it becomes very easy to quickly "remove the bone" in a CT angiogram, allowing clear visualization of vascular structures. This avoids manual or semiautomated bone removal, which can be labor intensive and/or operator dependent. Figure 12.16 provides an example of a dual-energy CT angiogram of the abdominal aorta and lower extremities.

Material Quantitation

A quantitative application of dual-energy CT is the assessment of the iodine concentration within tissue. This provides an image of the amount of iodinated blood in tissue or a vessel and is sometimes referred to as perfused blood volume, which should not be confused with direct perfusion measurements, which require temporally distinct measurements. However, quantitative assessment of perfused blood volume has been shown to serve as surrogate markers for ischemia and infarct and to correlate with direct measures of blood perfusion [48–50] and flow [51, 52]. Figure 12.17 shows a large perfusion deficit in a dual-energy CT pulmonary embolus examination.

Virtual Non-contrast Images

A large number of CT exams are performed after injection of iodine-containing contrast media or after ingestion of iodine- or barium-containing contrast agents. To reduce unnecessary radiation exposure and to improve workflow, scans are not typically performed prior to injection or ingestion of contrast media. However, some situations require the use of an unenhanced image in order to quantify the increase in enhancement. For example, the unexpected finding of a modestly enhancing renal mass may be uninterpretable without a non-contrast scan to determine the amount of enhancement that occurs from baseline to differentiate between cystic lesions and enhancing masses [53–56].

By being able to quantify the concentration of iodine in each voxel, the signal associated with the iodine can be "subtracted" to create virtual non-contrast images. This can be helpful in differentiating between hemorrhages or extravasated iodine in the brain (Fig. 12.18) [57–59]. Similarly, the amount of calcium in a voxel can be determined quantitatively and

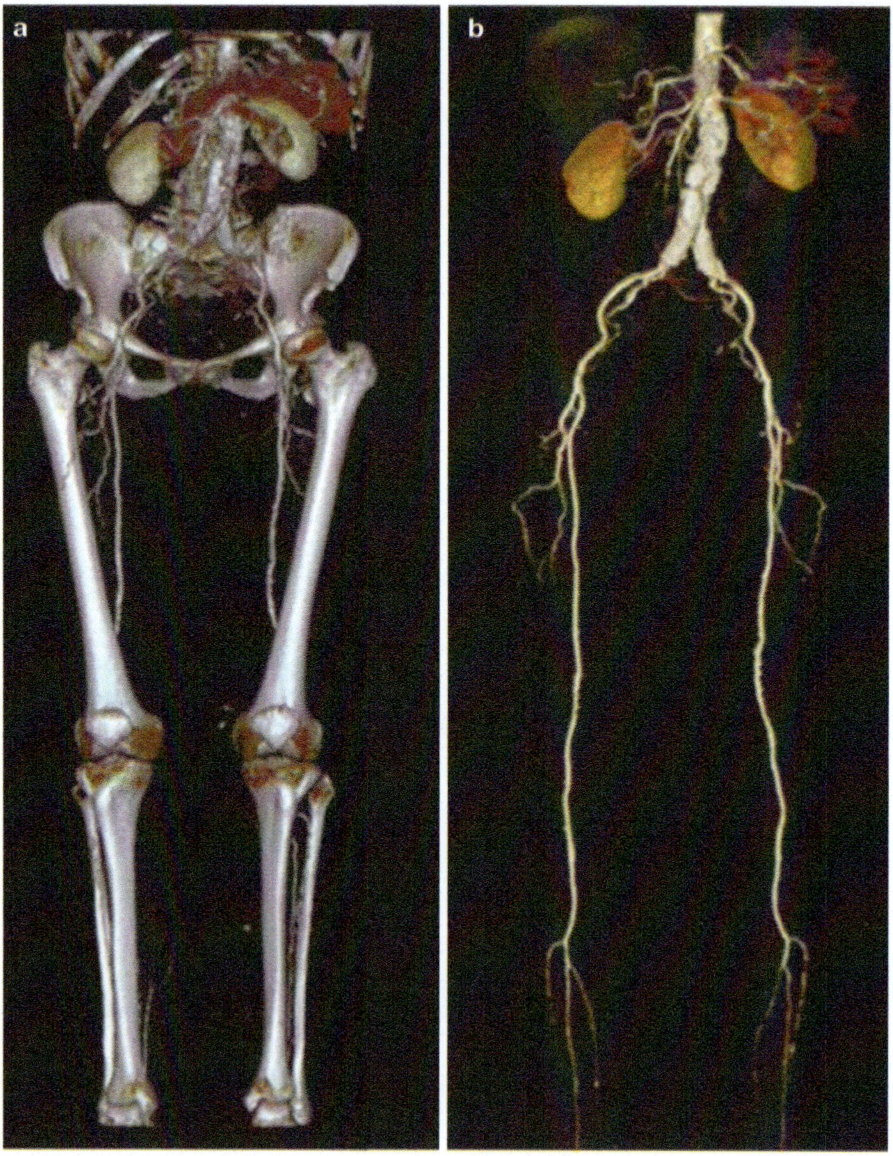

Fig. 12.16 3D volume rendered image of a dual-energy CT angiogram of the abdomen, pelvis, and lower extremities. Because dual-energy CT processing can classify a voxel as containing either iodine or calcium, an image with bone overlapping the vascular anatomy (**a**) can be turned into an image containing only vascular anatomy or iodine-containing soft tissue (**b**) (Reprinted with permission from [15])

subtracted to created virtual non-calcium images [60–62]. The removal of the bright calcium signal allows edematous bone lesions or bone bruising to be visualized, something that was previously only able to be appreciated with MRI (Fig. 12.19).

Energy-Selective Images

After decomposition into basis material maps (or effective atomic number and density maps), images can be synthesized that emulate the appearance of an image acquired with a monoenergetic

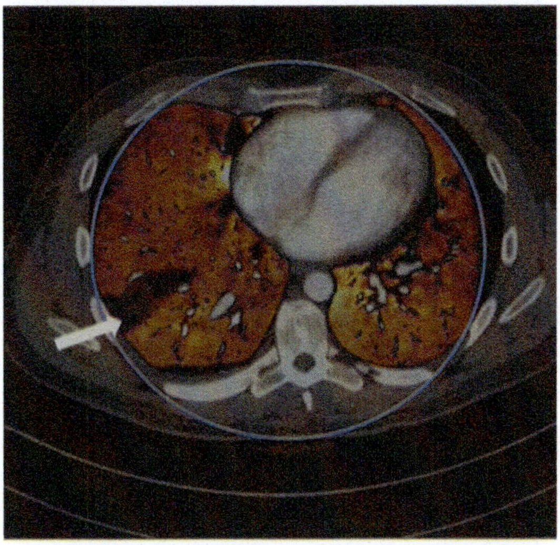

Fig. 12.17 Axial image of a patient with a pulmonary embolism and large perfusion deficit (arrow). In this image, the iodine signal is colored between red and yellow, with yellow denoting higher iodine concentrations. The absolute value of iodine concentration can be measured using provided tools. This image is from a dual-source CT system, which has a smaller field of view for the second tube-detector pair. Beyond that field of view (blue circle), only single-energy information is shown (Reprinted with permission from [15])

X-ray source (virtual monoenergetic images). This is accomplished by looking up and applying the mass attenuation coefficients for each identified material at the photon energy value of interest. The linear attenuation coefficient can then be calculated from knowledge of the material density and converted into CT numbers. This process is demonstrated in Fig. 12.20 [63]. As shown in Fig. 12.21, iodine signal is very bright in the low-keV images and becomes increasingly darker as the target photon energy is increased [64]. However, because lower-energy photons are more readily attenuated, these images are considerably noisier. The use of energy-domain noise reduction techniques can result in acceptable noise levels, even at 40, 50, or 60 keV (Fig. 12.22) [65].

Virtual monoenergetic imaging can be used to increase iodine signal, which can increase conspicuity of subtle lesions, compensate for poor venous access that results in slow injection rates, or allow the use of lower volumes of contrast media (Fig. 12.23) [66–71]. Conversely, using high keV values reduces the attenuation of

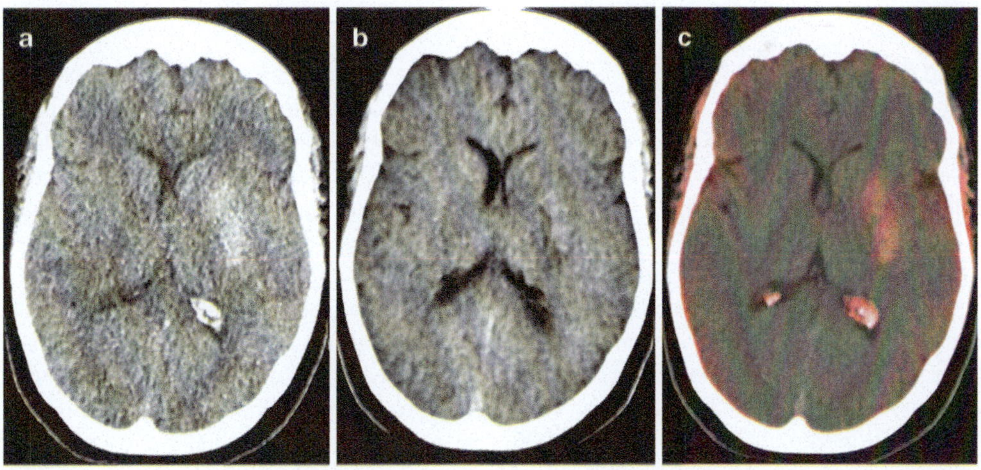

Fig. 12.18 (**a**) Mixed image demonstrating an enhancing portion of the brain subsequent to a neurologic interventional procedure. This image is indeterminate for hemorrhage vs. retention of extravasated iodinated contrast media. (**b**) Virtual non-contrast image demonstrated minimal enhancement in the region of interest, indicating that hemorrhage is unlikely. (**c**) Iodine map (in red) overlaid on top of the mixed image demonstrated bright iodinated signal in the region of interest, demonstrating a high likelihood that the enhancement seen in (**a**) is due to retained contrast material

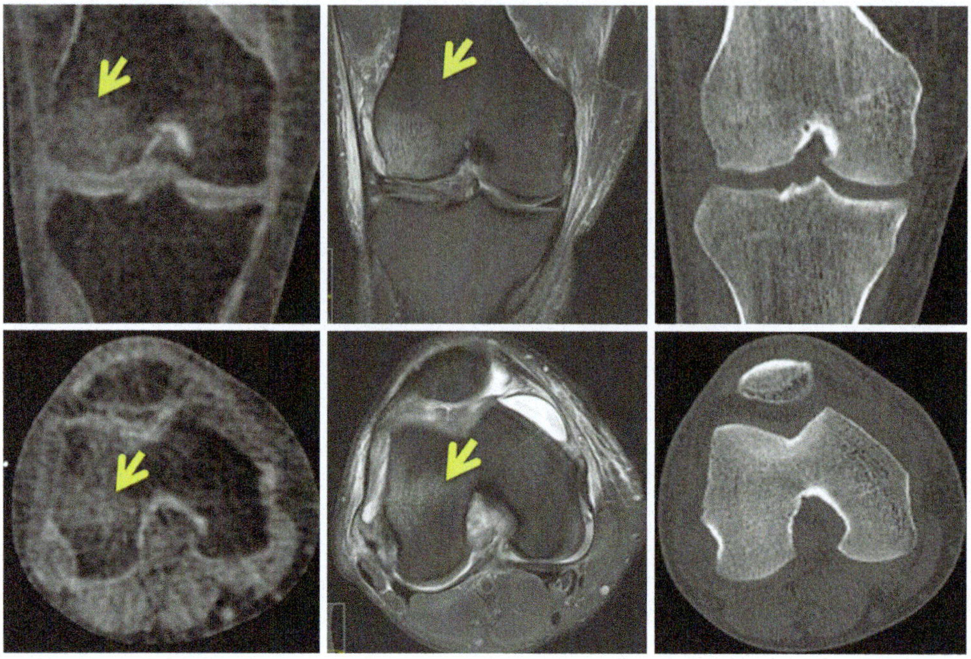

Fig. 12.19 Coronal (top row) and axial (bottom row) images of a patient's knee subsequent to a traumatic injury to his knee. The MRI images (center column) demonstrate signal within the bone marrow (arrows), which corresponds to bone edema secondary to trauma. The conventional CT images (right column) do not demonstrate any pathology; the calcium signal overwhelms the small signal due to the bone marrow edema. The virtual non-calcium dual-energy CT images (left column) demonstrate that after removal of the bright calcium signal, the bone marrow edema (arrows) can be visualized and matches the MRI images extremely well (Reprinted with permission from [15])

metal and can reduce metal artifacts (Fig. 12.24) [72–76].

Discussion and Conclusion

In summary, spectral CT images can be acquired using a variety of techniques and geometries and can be processed and displayed in a number of different ways. The clinical utilization of dual-energy CT has continued to increase since its reintroduction into clinical practice in 2006, with thousands of peer-reviewed publications in the literature in 2019 since then related to dual-energy CT. The nonmaterial-specific types of images, such as the low- and high-energy spectrum source images, the mixed images, or the virtual monoenergetic images, can be used in a variety of ways. Mixed or monoenergetic images can be used for routine examination interpretation, and monoenergetic images can reduce metal artifacts or improve iodine contrast-to-noise ratio. This latter property can be used to decrease radiation dose or contrast media dose.

Material-specific images, which can be a pair of basis materials, a photoelectric and Compton pair of images, or even k-edge material maps, are being used to add new clinical applications to CT imaging. These include applications that classify materials, such as in kidney stone applications, or that quantify materials, allowing the suppression of the amount of signal contributed from a given material (e.g., virtual non-calcium or non-contrast images).

When discussing dual- or multi-energy CT, either for clinical purposes or in research environments, it is in general very important that both

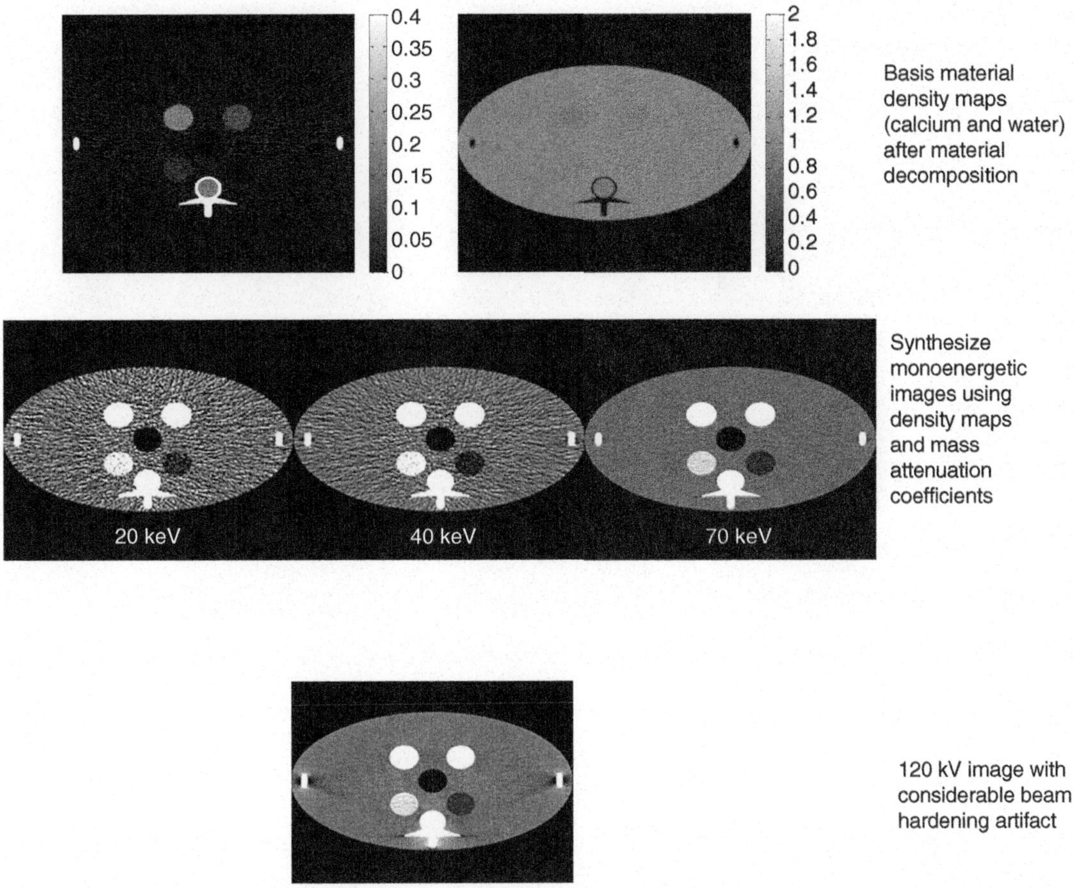

Fig. 12.20 Numerical simulations using a test phantom demonstrate the potential benefit of virtual monoenergetic images. The top row shows basis material density maps (calcium at left, water at right) after material decomposition. The center row shows the monoenergetic images created from the measured density maps and the mass attenuation coefficients for calcium and water, at the specific energy of interest (20, 40, or 70 keV). Because materials are much more attenuating at lower X-ray energies, fewer photons are detected in the simulation process, and hence the 20 keV image is much noisier than the 70 keV image. The bottom row shows the considerable beam-hardening artifacts produced for a conventional 120 kV image

the acquisition technology responsible for data collection and the image rendition methods be specified. For example, each of the different acquisition methods described has the ability to produce dual-energy data sets. The degree of spectral separation, however, can differ substantially, potentially impacting the accuracy and precision of material decomposition applications. With respect to image processing and display, window and level values for "routine image review" need to be adjusted according to the type of image being evaluated. Thus even "hanging protocols" need to be informed of the type of "dual-energy image" under review.

In conclusion, the different types of images that can be formed, and the different clinical applications that have arisen (and that are likely to continue to be developed), make spectral CT a very rich addition to the capabilities of CT. The use of dual- and multi-energy CT is anticipated to continue to increase as the technology continues to advance and as spectral CT-capable scanners continue to be installed around the world. Hounsfield was correct in his prediction of the ability to sepa-

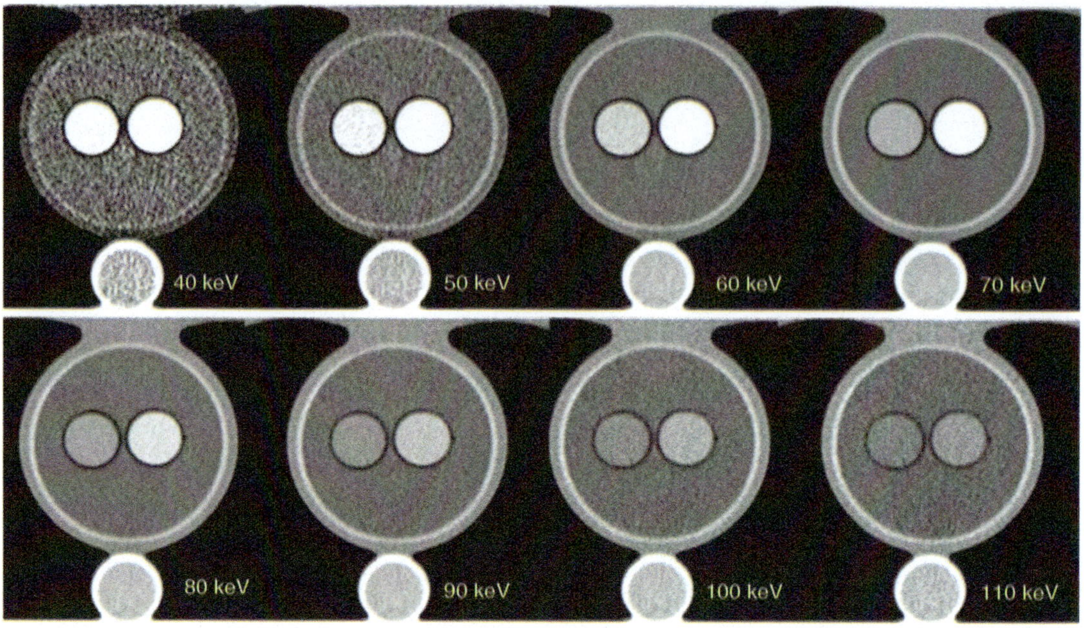

Fig. 12.21 In a test phantom containing two vials, each filled with a different concentration of iodine, the change in the appearance of iodine as the energy of the virtual monoenergetic image is varied and can be appreciated. The same window and level settings are used for all images. At 40 keV, the iodine is very bright, saturating the image in those regions. As the photon energy is increased, the iodine signal is decreased, allowing differentiation of the two iodine concentrations. At 110 keV, the iodine signal is very faint, approaching the brightness of the water background (Reprinted with permission from [64])

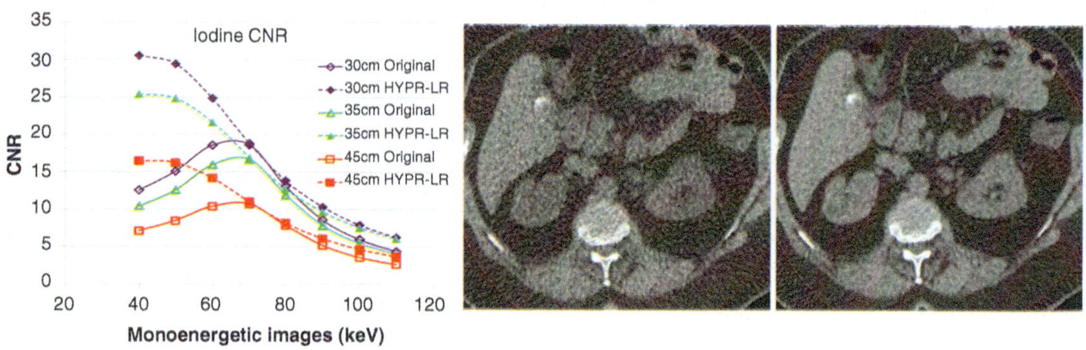

Fig. 12.22 The plot at left demonstrates the value of energy-domain noise reduction in the context of virtual monoenergetic imaging. Although the iodine brightness continues to increase as the photon energy is decreased, the iodine contrast-to-noise ratio (CNR) falls due to the rapidly increasing noise level as the photon energy is decreased (solid curves). With the use of energy-domain noise reduction, the increase in noise at decreased photon energy can be avoided, allowing an increased iodine CNR for energies as low as 40 keV. The magnitude of the effect varies according to patient size. In this example, water-filled torso-shaped phantoms of 30, 35, and 45 cm lateral width were evaluated. (Reprinted with permission from [65])

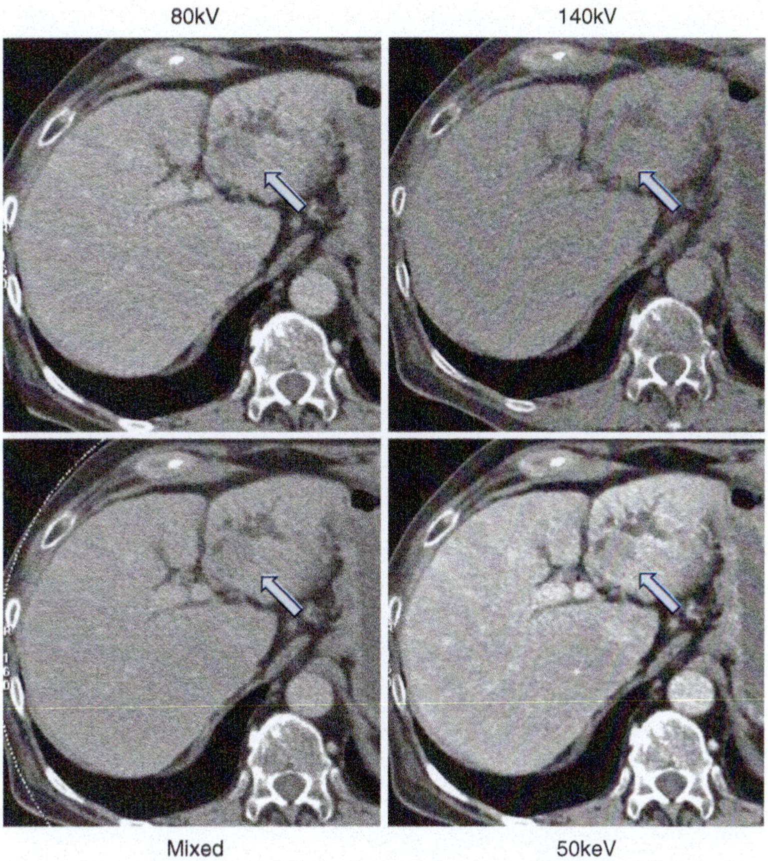

Fig. 12.23 The hypoattenuating liver lesion (arrows) has more contrast relative to the enhancing liver parenchyma at 80 kV compared to at 140 kV, albeit the 80 kV image is somewhat noisy. The mixed image uses all measured photons and thus has lower image noise but similar contrast to the 80 kV image. The 50 keV virtual monoenergetic image, however, has substantially increased contrast between the contrast-enhanced liver (which has become much brighter) and the lesion of interest

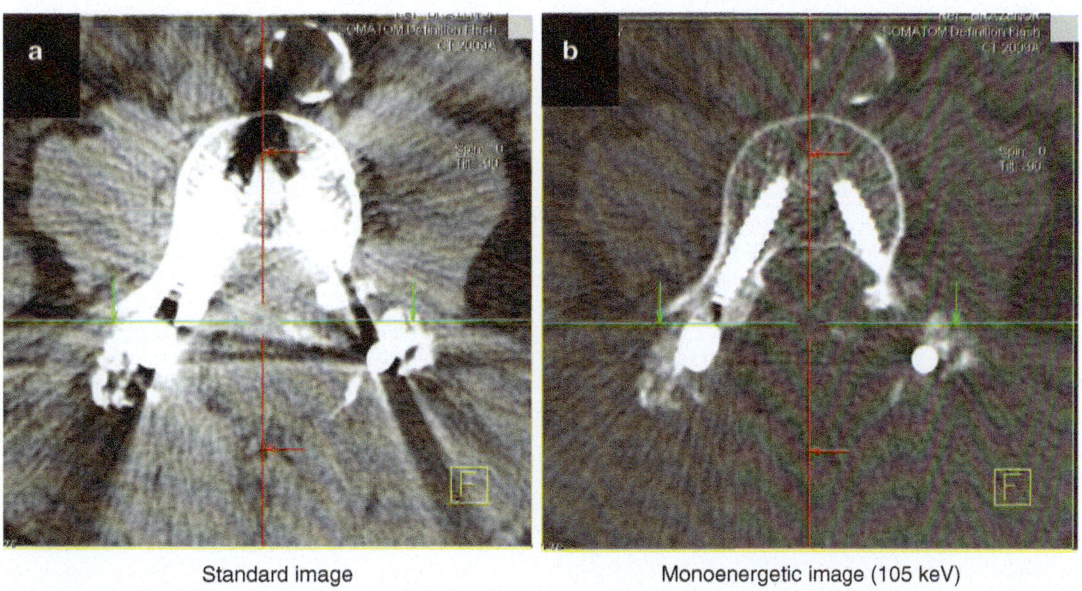

Fig. 12.24 The virtual monoenergetic image (**b**) created with a high photon energy (105 keV) demonstrates decreased attenuation of metal and hence decreased metal artifacts, relative to a conventional CT acquired using 120 kV

rate iodine from calcium, and he would likely be pleased to see this capability of CT finally brought into, and utilized, in the clinical arena.

Acknowledgments The author would like to thank colleagues from the Mayo Clinic for their collaboration on dual- and multi-energy CT over the course of many years, including Drs. J.G. Fletcher, Lifeng Yu, Shuai Leng, Amy Kotsenas, Terri Vrtiska, Katie Glazebrook, and Liqiang Ren. She would also like to thank Drs. Thomas Flohr and Bernhard Schmidt, for their collaboration on this topic, and Ms. Kris Nunez, for her expert assistance in manuscript and figure preparation.

Disclosure Dr. McCollough is the principal investigator of a research grant to the Mayo Clinic from Siemens Healthineers.

References

1. Liu X, Yu L, Primak AN, McCollough CH. Quantitative imaging of element composition and mass fraction using dual-energy CT: three-material decomposition. Med Phys. 2009;36:1602–9.
2. Hounsfield GN. Computerized transverse axial scanning (tomography). 1. Description of system. Br J Radiol. 1973;46:1016–22.
3. Kalender WA, Perman WH, Vetter JR, Klotz E. Evaluation of a prototype dual-energy computed tomographic apparatus. I. Phantom studies. Med Phys. 1986;13:334–9.
4. Kelcz F, Joseph PM, Hilal SK. Noise considerations in dual energy CT scanning. Med Phys. 1979;6:418–25.
5. Krauss B, Grant KL, Schmidt BT, Flohr TG. The importance of spectral separation: an assessment of dual-energy spectral separation for quantitative ability and dose efficiency. Investig Radiol. 2015;50:114–8.
6. Primak AN, Ramirez Giraldo JC, Liu X, Yu L, McCollough CH. Improved dual-energy material discrimination for dual-source CT by means of additional spectral filtration. Med Phys. 2009;36:1359–69.
7. Rutt B, Fenster A. Split-filter computed tomography: a simple technique for dual energy scanning. J Comput Assist Tomogr. 1980;4:501–9.
8. Ozguner O, Dhanantwari A, Halliburton S, Wen G, Utrup S, Jordan D. Objective image characterization of a spectral CT scanner with dual-layer detector. Phys Med Biol. 2018;63:025027.
9. Carmi R, Naveh G, Altman A. Material separation with dual-layer CT. IEEE Nucl Sci Symp. 2005;4:1876–8.
10. Gutjahr R, Halaweish AF, Yu Z, et al. Human imaging with photon counting-based computed tomography at clinical dose levels: contrast-to-noise ratio and cadaver studies. Investig Radiol. 2016;51:421–9.
11. Kappler S, Hannemann T, Kraft E, et al. First results from a hybrid prototype CT scanner for exploring benefits of quantum-counting in clinical CT. Proc SPIE. 2012;8313:83130X.
12. Roessl E, Proksa R. K-edge imaging in x-ray computed tomography using multi-bin photon counting detectors. Phys Med Biol. 2007;52:4679–96.
13. Taguchi K, Iwanczyk JS. Vision 20/20: single photon counting x-ray detectors in medical imaging. Med Phys. 2013;40:100901.
14. Yu Z, Leng S, Kappler S, et al. Noise performance of low-dose CT: comparison between an energy integrating detector and a photon counting detector using a whole-body research photon counting CT scanner. J Med Imaging (Bellingham). 2016;3:043503.
15. McCollough C, Leng S, Yu L, Fletcher JG. Dual- and multi-energy computed tomography: principles, technical approaches and clinical applications. Radiology. 2015;273:637–53.
16. Wu X, Langan DA, Xu D, et al. Monochromatic CT image representation via fast switching dual kVp. Proc SPIE. 2009;7258:725845.
17. Flohr TG, McCollough CH, Bruder H, et al. First performance evaluation of a dual-source CT (DSCT) system. Eur Radiol. 2006;16:256–68.
18. Johnson TR, Krauss B, Sedlmair M, et al. Material differentiation by dual energy CT: initial experience. Eur Radiol. 2007;17:1510–7.
19. Primak AN, Giraldo JC, Eusemann CD, et al. Dual-source dual-energy CT with additional tin filtration: dose and image quality evaluation in phantoms and in vivo. AJR Am J Roentgenol. 2010;195:1164–74.
20. Yu L, Primak AN, Liu X, McCollough CH. Image quality optimization and evaluation of linearly mixed images in dual-source, dual-energy CT. Med Phys. 2009;36:1019–24.
21. Alvarez RE, Macovski A. Energy-selective reconstructions in X-ray computerized tomography. Phys Med Biol. 1976;21:733–44.
22. Lehmann LA, Alvarez RE, Macovski A, et al. Generalized image combinations in dual KVP digital radiography. Med Phys. 1981;8:659–67.
23. Macovski A, Alvarez RE, Chan JL, Stonestrom JP, Zatz LM. Energy dependent reconstruction in X-ray computerized tomography. Comput Biol Med. 1976;6:325–36.
24. Marshall WH Jr, Alvarez RE, Macovski A. Initial results with prereconstruction dual-energy computed tomography (PREDECT). Radiology. 1981;140:421–30.
25. Heismann B, Leppert J, Stierstorfer K. Density and atomic number measurements with spectral x-ray attenuation method. J Appl Phys. 2003;94:2073–9.
26. Eusemann, Christian, David R. Holmes III, Bernhard Schmidt, Thomas G. Flohr, Richard Robb, Cynthia McCollough, David M. Hough et al. "Dual energy CT: How to best blend both energies in one fused image?." In Medical imaging 2008: visualization, image-guided procedures, and modeling, vol. 6918, p. 691803. International Society for Optics and Photonics, 2008.

27. Bongartz T, Glazebrook KN, Kavros SJ, et al. Dual-energy CT for the diagnosis of gout: an accuracy and diagnostic yield study. Ann Rheum Dis. 2015;74:1072–7.
28. Brockmann C, Jochum S, Sadick M, et al. Dual-energy CT angiography in peripheral arterial occlusive disease. Cardiovasc Intervent Radiol. 2009;32:630–7.
29. Buerke B, Wittkamp G, Seifarth H, Heindel W, Kloska SP. Dual-energy CTA with bone removal for transcranial arteries: intraindividual comparison with standard CTA without bone removal and TOF-MRA. Acad Radiol. 2009;16:1348–55.
30. Choi HK, Burns LC, Shojania K, et al. Dual energy CT in gout: a prospective validation study. Ann Rheum Dis. 2012;71:1466–71.
31. Eiber M, Holzapfel K, Frimberger M, et al. Targeted dual-energy single-source CT for characterisation of urinary calculi: experimental and clinical experience. Eur Radiol. 2012;22:251–8.
32. Glazebrook KN, Leng S, Jacobson SR, McCollough CM. Dual-energy CT for evaluation of intra- and extracapsular silicone implant rupture. Case Rep Radiol. 2016;2016:6323709.
33. Huppertz A, Hermann KG, Diekhoff T, Wagner M, Hamm B, Schmidt WA. Systemic staging for urate crystal deposits with dual-energy CT and ultrasound in patients with suspected gout. Rheumatol Int. 2014;34:763–71.
34. Johnson TR, Himsl I, Hellerhoff K, et al. Dual-energy CT for the evaluation of silicone breast implants. Eur Radiol. 2013;23:991–6.
35. Kaza RK, Ananthakrishnan L, Kambadakone A, Platt JF. Update of dual-energy CT applications in the genitourinary tract. AJR Am J Roentgenol. 2017;208:1185–92.
36. Kiefer T, Diekhoff T, Hermann S, et al. Single source dual-energy computed tomography in the diagnosis of gout: diagnostic reliability in comparison to digital radiography and conventional computed tomography of the feet. Eur J Radiol. 2016;85:1829–34.
37. Kulkarni NM, Eisner BH, Pinho DF, Joshi MC, Kambadakone AR, Sahani DV. Determination of renal stone composition in phantom and patients using single-source dual-energy computed tomography. J Comput Assist Tomogr. 2013;37:37–45.
38. Lee YH, Song GG. Diagnostic accuracy of dual-energy computed tomography in patients with gout: a meta-analysis. Semin Arthritis Rheum. 2017;47:95–101.
39. Leng S, Huang A, Cardona JM, Duan X, Williams JC, McCollough CH. Dual-energy CT for quantification of urinary stone composition in mixed stones: a phantom study. AJR Am J Roentgenol. 2016;207:321–9.
40. Morhard D, Fink C, Graser A, Reiser MF, Becker C, Johnson TR. Cervical and cranial computed tomographic angiography with automated bone removal: dual energy computed tomography versus standard computed tomography. Investig Radiol. 2009;44:293–7.
41. Primak AN, Fletcher JG, Vrtiska TJ, et al. Noninvasive differentiation of uric acid versus non-uric acid kidney stones using dual-energy CT. Acad Radiol. 2007;14:1441–7.
42. Qu M, Ramirez-Giraldo JC, Leng S, et al. Dual-energy dual-source CT with additional spectral filtration can improve the differentiation of non-uric acid renal stones: an ex vivo phantom study. AJR Am J Roentgenol. 2011;196:1279–87.
43. Schulz B, Kuehling K, Kromen W, et al. Automatic bone removal technique in whole-body dual-energy CT angiography: performance and image quality. AJR Am J Roentgenol. 2012;199:W646–50.
44. Shi D, Xu JX, Wu HX, Wang Y, Zhou QJ, Yu RS. Methods of assessment of tophus and bone erosions in gout using dual-energy CT: reproducibility analysis. Clin Rheumatol. 2015;34:755–65.
45. Sommer WH, Johnson TR, Becker CR, et al. The value of dual-energy bone removal in maximum intensity projections of lower extremity computed tomography angiography. Investig Radiol. 2009;44:285–92.
46. Sun Y, Chen H, Zhang Z, et al. Dual-energy computed tomography for monitoring the effect of urate-lowering therapy in gouty arthritis. Int J Rheum Dis. 2015;18:880–5.
47. Zhang LJ, Wu SY, Poon CS, et al. Automatic bone removal dual-energy CT angiography for the evaluation of intracranial aneurysms. J Comput Assist Tomogr. 2010;34:816–24.
48. Okada M, Kunihiro Y, Nakashima Y, et al. Added value of lung perfused blood volume images using dual-energy CT for assessment of acute pulmonary embolism. Eur J Radiol. 2015;84:172–7.
49. Miura S, Ohno Y, Kimura H, Kichikawa K. Quantitative lung perfused blood volume imaging on dual-energy CT: capability for quantitative assessment of disease severity in patients with acute pulmonary thromboembolism. Acta Radiol. 2015;56:284–93.
50. Sakamoto A, Sakamoto I, Nagayama H, Koike H, Sueyoshi E, Uetani M. Quantification of lung perfusion blood volume with dual-energy CT: assessment of the severity of acute pulmonary thromboembolism. AJR Am J Roentgenol. 2014;203:287–91.
51. Mileto A, Marin D, Alfaro-Cordoba M, et al. Iodine quantification to distinguish clear cell from papillary renal cell carcinoma at dual-energy multidetector CT: a multireader diagnostic performance study. Radiology. 2014;273:813–20.
52. Zarzour JG, Milner D, Valentin R, et al. Quantitative iodine content threshold for discrimination of renal cell carcinomas using rapid kV-switching dual-energy CT. Abdom Radiol (NY). 2017;42:727–34.
53. Wortman JR, Bunch PM, Fulwadhva UP, Bonci GA, Sodickson AD. Dual-energy CT of incidental findings in the abdomen: can we reduce the need for follow-up imaging? Am J Roentgenol. 2016;207:W58–W68.
54. Graser A, Johnson TR, Chandarana H, Macari M. Dual energy CT: preliminary observations and potential clinical applications in the abdomen. Eur Radiol. 2009;19:13–23.

55. Graser A, Johnson TR, Hecht EM, et al. Dual-energy CT in patients suspected of having renal masses: can virtual nonenhanced images replace true nonenhanced images? Radiology. 2009;252:433–40.
56. Arndt N, Staehler M, Siegert S, Reiser MF, Graser A. Dual energy CT in patients with polycystic kidney disease. Eur Radiol. 2012;22:2125–9.
57. Gupta R, Phan CM, Leidecker C, et al. Evaluation of dual-energy CT for differentiating intracerebral hemorrhage from iodinated contrast material staining. Radiology. 2010;257:205–11.
58. Phan CM, Yoo AJ, Hirsch JA, Nogueira RG, Gupta R. Differentiation of hemorrhage from iodinated contrast in different intracranial compartments using dual-energy head CT. AJNR Am J Neuroradiol. 2012;33:1088–94.
59. Kim SJ, Lim HK, Lee HY, et al. Dual-energy CT in the evaluation of intracerebral hemorrhage of unknown origin: differentiation between tumor bleeding and pure hemorrhage. AJNR Am J Neuroradiol. 2012;33:865–72.
60. Ai S, Qu M, Glazebrook KN, et al. Use of dual-energy CT and virtual non-calcium techniques to evaluate post-traumatic bone bruises in knees in the subacute setting. Skelet Radiol. 2014;43:1289–95.
61. Pache G, Krauss B, Strohm P, et al. Dual-energy CT virtual noncalcium technique: detecting posttraumatic bone marrow lesions – feasibility study. Radiology. 2010;256:617–24.
62. Wang CK, Tsai JM, Chuang MT, Wang MT, Huang KY, Lin RM. Bone marrow edema in vertebral compression fractures: detection with dual-energy CT. Radiology. 2013;269:525–33.
63. Yu L, Leng S, McCollough CH. Dual-energy CT-based monochromatic imaging. AJR Am J Roentgenol. 2012;199:S9–S15.
64. Yu L, Christner JA, Leng S, Wang J, Fletcher JG, McCollough CH. Virtual monochromatic imaging in dual-source dual-energy CT: radiation dose and image quality. Med Phys. 2011;38:6371–9.
65. Leng S, Yu L, Fletcher JG, McCollough C. Maximizing iodine contrast-to-noise ratios in abdominal CT imaging through use of energy domain noise reduction and virtual monoenergetic dual-energy CT. Radiology. 2015;276:562–70.
66. Carrascosa P, Leipsic JA, Capunay C, et al. Monochromatic image reconstruction by dual energy imaging allows half iodine load computed tomography coronary angiography. Eur J Radiol. 2015;84:1915–20.
67. Nagayama Y, Nakaura T, Oda S, et al. Dual-layer DECT for multiphasic hepatic CT with 50 percent iodine load: a matched-pair comparison with a 120 kVp protocol. Eur Radiol. 2018;28:1719–30.
68. Pomerantz SR, Kamalian S, Zhang D, et al. Virtual monochromatic reconstruction of dual-energy unenhanced head CT at 65-75 keV maximizes image quality compared with conventional polychromatic CT. Radiology. 2013;266:318–25.
69. Schneider D, Apfaltrer P, Sudarski S, et al. Optimization of kiloelectron volt settings in cerebral and cervical dual-energy CT angiography determined with virtual monoenergetic imaging. Acad Radiol. 2014;21:431–6.
70. Tsang DS, Merchant TE, Merchant SE, Smith H, Yagil Y, Hua CH. Quantifying potential reduction in contrast dose with monoenergetic images synthesized from dual-layer detector spectral CT. Br J Radiol. 2017;90:20170290.
71. Wichmann JL, Noske EM, Kraft J, et al. Virtual monoenergetic dual-energy computed tomography: optimization of kiloelectron volt settings in head and neck cancer. Investig Radiol. 2014;49:735–41.
72. Bamberg F, Dierks A, Nikolaou K, Reiser MF, Becker CR, Johnson TR. Metal artifact reduction by dual energy computed tomography using monoenergetic extrapolation. Eur Radiol. 2011;21:1424–9.
73. Cha J, Kim HJ, Kim ST, Kim YK, Kim HY, Park GM. Dual-energy CT with virtual monochromatic images and metal artifact reduction software for reducing metallic dental artifacts. Acta Radiol. 2017;58:1312–9.
74. Dunet V, Bernasconi M, Hajdu SD, Meuli RA, Daniel RT, Zerlauth JB. Impact of metal artifact reduction software on image quality of gemstone spectral imaging dual-energy cerebral CT angiography after intracranial aneurysm clipping. Neuroradiology. 2017;59:845–52.
75. Filograna L, Magarelli N, Leone A, et al. Value of monoenergetic dual-energy CT (DECT) for artefact reduction from metallic orthopedic implants in post-mortem studies. Skelet Radiol. 2015;44:1287–94.
76. Stolzmann P, Winklhofer S, Schwendener N, Alkadhi H, Thali MJ, Ruder TD. Monoenergetic computed tomography reconstructions reduce beam hardening artifacts from dental restorations. Forensic Sci Med Pathol. 2013;9:327–32.

Clinical Applications of Spectral CT 13

André Euler and Sebastian T. Schindera

Neuroradiology

Stroke Imaging

DECT has proven its impact on patient treatment and outcome in brain imaging after endovascular stroke treatment. The detection of a post-interventional intracerebral hemorrhage (ICH) is crucial in the planning of posttreatment anti-aggregation therapy. Commonly, non-contrast single-energy CT (SECT) is performed to rule out post-interventional ICH. However, this modality does not allow for the differentiation of hyperdense ICH from periprocedural extravasation of contrast material. Several studies have shown that DECT can reliably distinguish between hemorrhage and iodine [1–3] and thus affect accurate diagnosis and patient management. Material decomposition algorithms enable the post-processing of iodine maps and production of virtual non-contrast (VNC) images which are used to identify both entities (Fig. 13.1). In a clinical study, VNC images demonstrated good agreement in the diagnosis of subarachnoid hemorrhage compared to true non-contrast (TNC) images [4]. The advantage of the utilization of VNC images is the perfect registration with the iodine maps and potential for radiation dose reduction by eliminating an additional non-contrast CT scan. A disadvantage of the VNC images, however, is an increase in image noise and therefore a decrease in image quality [4].

Another advantage of VNC images is the improved detection of areas of acute ischemia or infarction after endovascular stroke treatment [5]. The brain-blood barrier (BBB) is often affected during an infarction. If contrast material is applied during endovascular stroke treatment, it can diffuse through the BBB into the adjacent brain tissue. Consequently, the affected area can appear hyperdense on conventional non-contrast CT images and therefore mask underlying hypodense infarctions. VNC images improve the detection of these infarctions by removing the contrast material staining in brain tissue.

Recent research has focused on the investigation of so-called X-maps or Edema maps (EM) which use a modified three-material decomposition algorithm to create modified VNC images. These maps are able to visualize ischemic areas by detecting edema as an increase in water content of brain parenchyma. X- and EM-maps have been demonstrated to detect edema and to measure core infarct volume more accurately than TNC and VNC images (Fig. 13.2) [6, 7]. Furthermore, one study found comparable

A. Euler (✉)
Institute of Diagnostic and Interventional Radiology, University Hospital Zurich, Zurich, Switzerland

S. T. Schindera
Institute of Radiology, Cantonal Hospital Aarau, Aarau, Switzerland
e-mail: sebastian.schindera@ksa.ch

© Springer Nature Switzerland AG 2020

E. Samei, N. J. Pelc (eds.), *Computed Tomography*, https://doi.org/10.1007/978-3-030-26957-9_13

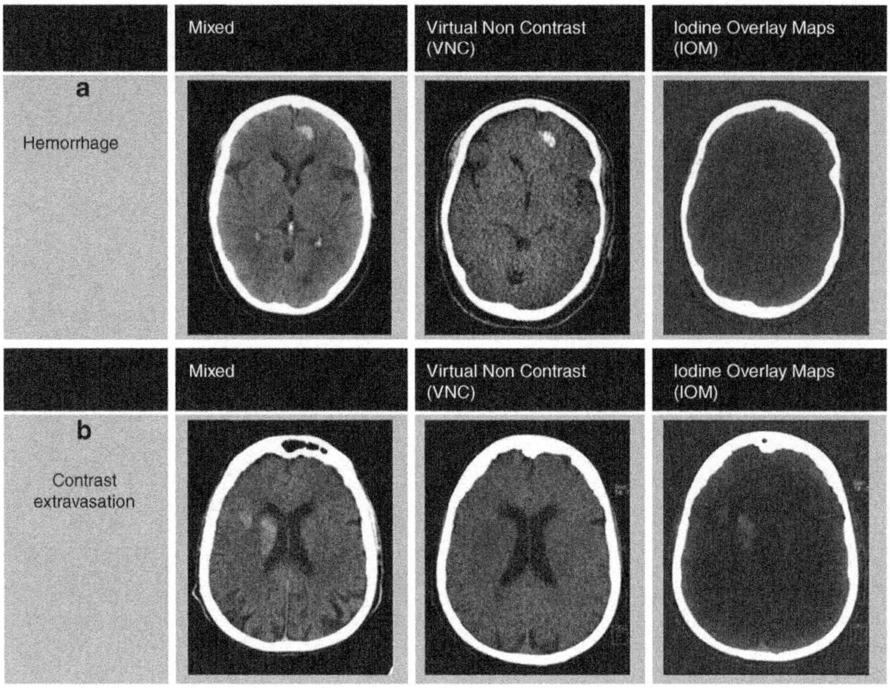

Fig. 13.1 DECT offers the reconstruction of virtual non-contrast images (VNC) and iodine maps which allow the differentiation of intracerebral hemorrhage from contrast extravasation. Both entities demonstrate as a hyperdensity on conventional mixed images. In hemorrhage, this hyperdensity remains in VNC images while being subtracted from the iodine map (**a**). In the case of a contrast extravasation, the hyperdensity is subtracted from VNC images while it remains on the iodine map (**b**) (© With permission of Springer: Tijssen et al. [3])

delineation of acute ischemia on X-maps compared to diffusion-weighted MRI images [8].

Emergency Imaging

Material decomposition algorithms have been proven to be useful in emergency settings due to their ability to detect calcium. This enables the reconstruction of calcium and virtual non-calcium images. These image sets can be used to differentiate acute hemorrhage from parenchymal calcifications. This potentially impacts clinical workflow because the detection of calcifications can eliminate additional follow-up CT studies in cases where prior imaging examinations are not available. One study demonstrated an accuracy of 99% of calcium images to differentiate between calcification and hemorrhage in emergency patients [9]. An important pitfall of three-material imaging with two-material decomposition, however, is that iodine appears bright on calcium images and vice versa. Therefore, both materials cannot be differentiated in the presence of soft tissue on material density maps only. Material density maps must always be interpreted in conjunction with their corresponding VNC images to avoid misinterpretation.

Further Applications

Virtual monochromatic or monoenergetic imaging (VMI) can be used to improve the gray matter to white matter contrast-to-noise ratio (GM-WM CNR) and to reduce artifacts in the posterior fossa. Pomerantz et al. compared VMI to conventional polychromatic imaging at 120 kV in non-contrast CT [10]. The study

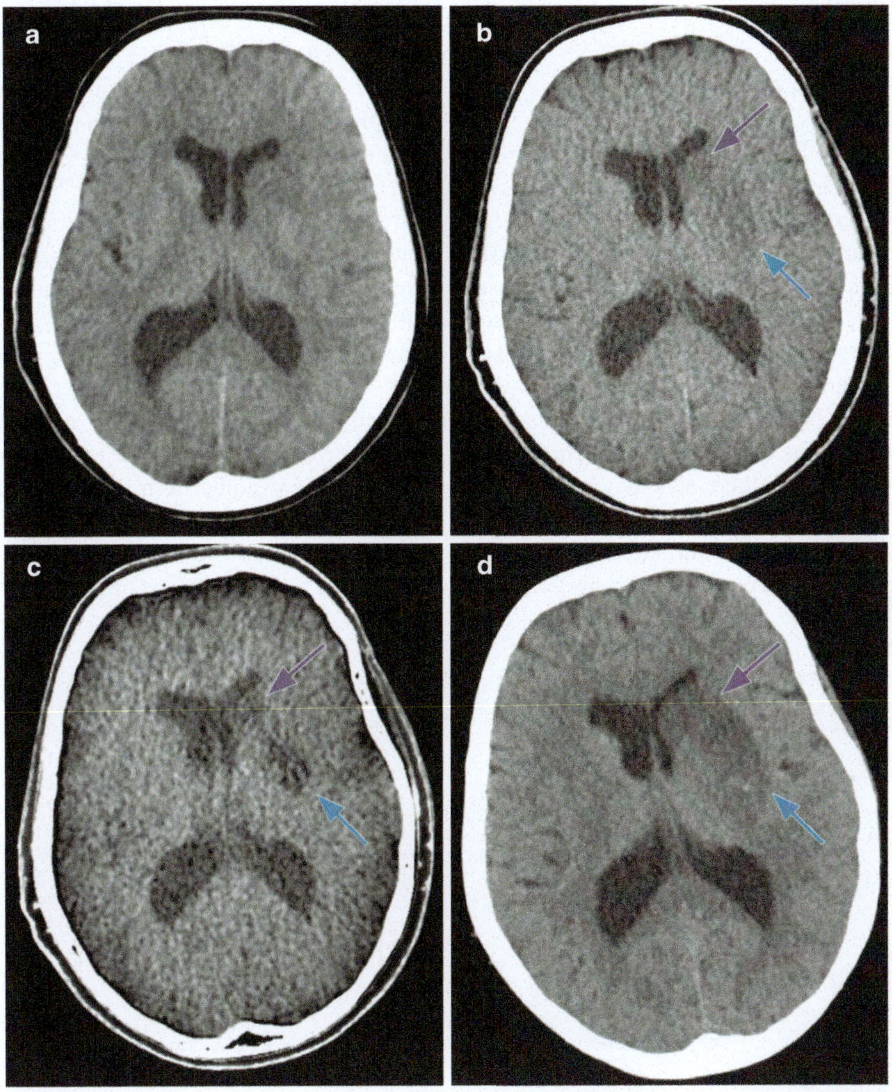

Fig. 13.2 DECT-based edema maps can be used to improve the visualization of ischemic lesions. In this patient, ischemic areas in the caudate nucleus (violet arrow) and putamen (blue arrow) are identified on the edema map (**c**) but are less visible in the brain window (**a**) and VNC images (**b**). Follow-up CT confirmed area of infarction (© With permission of Springer: Grams et al. [7])

demonstrated that a maximum GM-WM CNR was achieved at 65 keV for the supratentorial brain. Minimal artifacts were observed in VMI at 75 keV. In addition, VMI can be used to reduce metal artifacts by using VMI at high energy levels [11]. Artifacts are reduced by a reduction of the beam-hardening effect caused by metallic material [12]. Unfortunately, high-energy VMIs will decrease the CT attenuation of iodinated structures which can be disadvantageous if vessels are assessed in CT angiography.

On the other hand, VMI at low energy levels can be used to increase the CT attenuation of cerebral and cervical vessels. One study found that VMI at 60 keV improved the vessel attenuation and CNR compared to conventional polychromatic images at 120 kV in cerebral and cervical CT angiography for dual-source DECT [13].

Thoracic Imaging

Lung Perfusion and Pulmonary Embolism

DECT pulmonary angiography is a reliable tool to generate lung parenchyma iodine perfusion maps and to quantify pulmonary perfused blood volume (PBV). These maps can be used to volumetrically measure lung perfusion defects (PD_{vol}) after pulmonary thromboembolic events (Fig. 13.3). Previous studies have shown positive agreement between DECT-based pulmonary perfusion assessment and perfusion scintigraphy [14] as well as even higher accuracy in the detection of perfusion defects compared to a combination of SPECT/CT and ventilation scintigraphy [15]. The scoring of perfusion defects has been shown to correlate with the severity of acute pulmonary embolism (PE) [16]. However, controversy exists about the benefit of PD_{vol} assessment as a predictive parameter for all-cause mortality. Traditionally, the quantitative CT assessment of right ventricular dysfunction, defined as an increased ratio between right ventricular and left ventricular axial diameter, has been used as a strong predictor for the clinical outcome of patient with acute pulmonary embolism [17]. Takx et al. reported that PD_{vol} was superior to traditionally used ventricular diameter ratio as a significant predictor for 6-month mortality in patients without thromboembolic clot in CT pulmonary angiography [18]. Another retrospective study by Im et al., however, observed no significant added benefit of PD_{vol} compared to ventricular diameter ratio alone when 30-day mortality was assessed

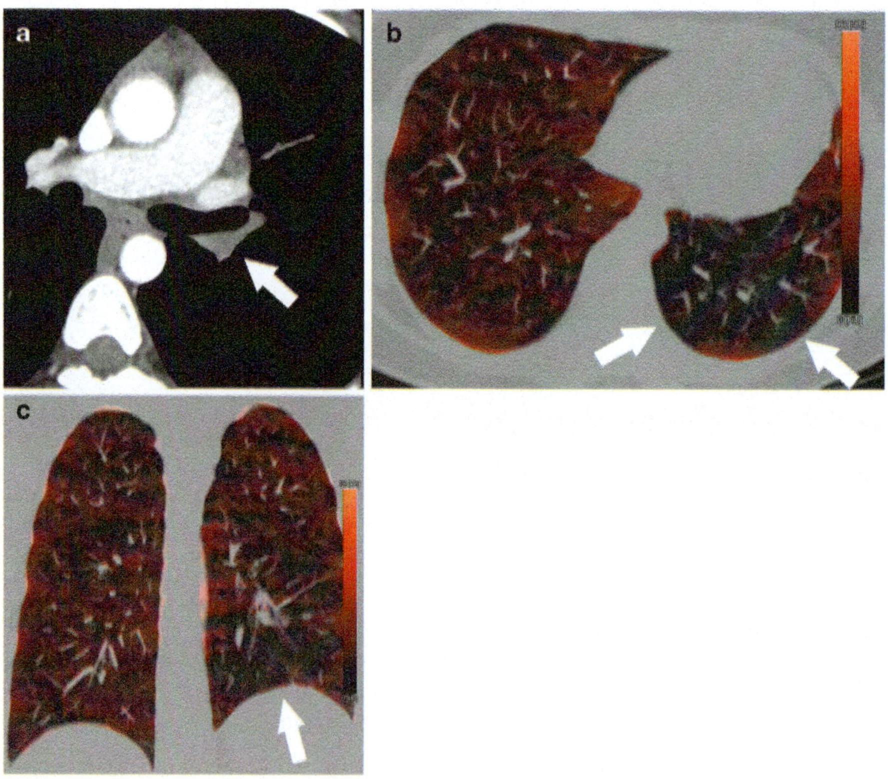

Fig. 13.3 Lung perfusion iodine maps reconstructed from DECT pulmonary angiography enable the quantification and visualization of parenchymal perfusion defects. On conventional linearly blended images, chronic thromboembolism is present as a contrast medium filling defect in a segmental pulmonary artery of the left lower lobe (white arrow in **a**). Axial and coronal iodine maps demonstrate the corresponding perfusion defect in the posterior segment of the left lower lobe (white arrows in **b** and **c**)

among patient with acute pulmonary embolism [19]. Prospective, multicenter studies are needed to further assess the impact of PD_{vol} on disease prediction, prognosis, and patient treatment.

DECT can be further used to reconstruct color-coded vessel maps, demonstrating the iodine content in pulmonary arteries. One study observed significantly improved detection of subsegmental PE with the use of these vessel maps in combination with conventional gray scale images in arterial phase DECT of oncologic patients [20].

A few studies have investigated the capability of DECT to differentiate acute from chronic PE. In chronic PE, vascular remodeling occurs in which the lung tissue distal of the obstruction is collateralized by bronchial arteries. Therefore, chronic PE is more often associated with dilated bronchial arteries compared to acute PE. Hong et al. investigated the utility of two-phase DECT with scans at pulmonary arterial and delayed phases [21]. The authors observed significantly increased iodine attenuation of the obstructed lung segments in the delayed phase images in chronic PE compared to acute PE, demonstrating the increased perfusion by bronchial collaterals in chronic PE. Another study by Kim et al. showed that the ratio of iodine concentration between the pulmonary thrombus and the main pulmonary artery can be used to successfully differentiate between acute and chronic PE [22].

Virtual monoenergetic images (VMIs) can be used to improve the CT attenuation and CNR of pulmonary arteries, thus increasing the detection of incidentally discovered thromboembolism in portal-venous phase [23] and salvaging nondiagnostic scans (Fig. 13.4). The use of VMIs allowed for a reduction of contrast medium in CT pulmonary angiography of up to 84% in patients with acute or chronic renal failure (from 32 to 5.4 g iodine) [24]. The recommendation for the optimal keV level of VMIs varies in the literature and also depends on the dual-energy approach and the algorithm used to produce the images. Newer algorithms enable a noise-optimized reconstruction of low-keV VMIs, e.g., 40 keV images. A study using a first-generation monoenergetic algorithm on a dual-source DECT reported that VMIs at 70 keV significantly increased quantitative image quality parameters [25]. In contrast, using a second-generation monoenergetic reconstruction algorithm, VMIs at 40–50 keV have been shown to optimize quantitative and qualitative image quality parameters [26]. Two studies reported that suboptimal PE exams can be salvaged if low-energy VMIs are used for dual-layer detector-based DECT [27, 28]. Suboptimal exams are usually caused by reduced cardiac output or inadequate bolus timing. Care has to be taken, however, to optimize the window settings for displaying low-energy VMIs for image interpretation as standard window settings may result in inferior image perception [29].

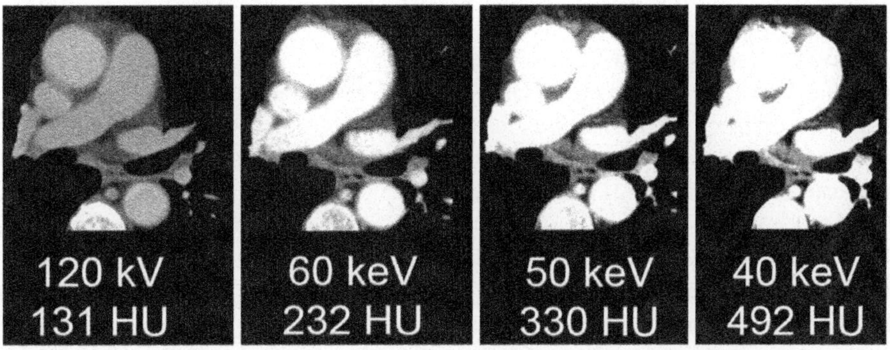

Fig. 13.4 Example of the use of VMI to improve the CT attenuation of the pulmonary arteries: Axial CT images of a single-source split-filter DECT pulmonary angiography at the level of the pulmonary trunk. CT attenuation increases significantly with decreasing energy level of VMI. CT attenuation of 40 keV images is almost fourfold compared to conventional linearly blended images simulating 120 kV. Care has to be taken, however, to adjust the window settings in low-energy VMI

Cardiovascular Imaging

Cardiac Imaging

Recent studies have investigated the utility of cardiac DECT in the characterization and differentiation of myocardial disease. In routine clinical practice CT-angiography of the heart is commonly used to assess the extent of coronary artery disease. However, many patients with chronic heart failure are additionally referred to MRI with late gadolinium-enhanced (LGE) imaging to obtain further information about the myocardium. LGE can be used to differentiate myocardial infarction from non-ischemic dilated cardiomyopathy. Nevertheless, this approach is time-consuming and cost-intensive. Ideally, CT angiography of the heart could be combined with DECT to assess coronary and myocardial function in a "one-stop shop" approach. A recent study by Ohta et al. prospectively compared late contrast enhancement DECT with late gadolinium-enhanced MRI in patients with ischemic and non-ischemic myocardial disease in 44 patients [30]. The authors reported high concordance between areas of late gadolinium enhancement and DECT delayed enhancement using iodine maps and low-energy VMIs with reported accuracies of 95.5% and 93.3%, respectively [30]. They concluded that delayed enhancement DECT of the myocardium enables accurate detection of scars in patients with heart failure. High diagnostic accuracy for the detection of myocardial infarction has been reported when combining DECT iodine maps with CT angiography in patients with suspected myocardial infarction [31]. Furthermore, DECT demonstrated non-inferiority to MRI in the quantification of infarct volumes in patients with chronic myocardial infarction [32]. A potential future clinical tool could be automatic volumetric infarct segmentation, which has been successfully applied in an experimental animal study [33].

DECT-derived iodine maps can be used in perfusion imaging of the heart because the quantification of myocardial iodine uptake has been shown to be a useful surrogate for myocardial perfusion. Typically, DECT perfusion is performed at rest and under pharmacological stress [34, 35]. Here, reversible ischemia is represented by hypoattenuating myocardium only in the stress phase, while myocardial infarction is depicted as a perfusion defect at both rest and stress phases. In one study, DECT-derived iodine quantification demonstrated high concordance with stress-rest single-photon emission computed tomography (SPECT) perfusion imaging [36]. However, another study by Meinel et al., comparing rest-stress DECT perfusion to SPECT perfusion revealed that almost half of reversible myocardial defects at SPECT were classified as fixed defects using DECT perfusion [35].

VMIs at low energy levels are another option to improve myocardial evaluation. VMIs at low-keV levels have shown improved detection of perfusion defects in stress DECT compared to high-keV levels [37]. Chang et al. reported improved assessment of late enhancement using 70 keV images in patients with cardiomyopathy compared to conventional linearly blended images simulating 120 kV [38].

Another benefit of DECT is the possibility to reconstruct virtual non-contrast images (VNC). VNCs can be used to assess the calcium score of coronary vessels. Calcium scoring is a viable tool in the risk stratification of low- to intermediate-risk patients for coronary artery disease. Typically, calcium scoring is performed on true non-contrast CT scans. VNCs can be used to replace these additional non-contrast scans in patients who need a post-contrast study and consequently decrease the radiation burden to the patient [39]. Caution has to be taken, however, that VNCs tend to reduce calcium signal and slightly underestimate the burden of calcified plaques.

Another potential role of DECT in cardiac imaging lies in the diagnosis of cardiac amyloidosis. One study utilized the quantification of the myocardial iodine concentration in late phase DECT scans 5 min after contrast medium injection to differentiate patients with amyloidosis from patients with non-amyloid hypertrophic cardiomyopathy and control patients [40]. Here, significantly higher myocardial iodine concentrations were measured in amyloidosis.

Vascular Imaging

VMIs at low energy levels offer a promising tool for vascular imaging, due to their ability to increase the CT signal of iodinated structures, improve the CNR, and reduce beam-hardening artifacts when compared to conventional CT images at 120 kV. Furthermore, low-keV VMI can be used to decrease the amount of contrast medium and consequently the iodine dose to the patient, which improves patient safety and examination costs [41–43]. Shuman et al. demonstrated that VMI at 50 keV can be used in CT angiography of the aorta to reduce the iodine dose by 70% (from 50 to 15 g iodine) compared to a single-energy protocol at 120 kV without impairment in CNR and SNR [44]. VMIs at energy levels of 40–60 keV have been shown to provide the best compromise between improved CNR and slightly impaired subjective image quality for reduced-iodine CT angiography studies.

One main clinical application of DECT in vascular imaging is the assessment of endoleaks after endovascular repair. Typically, endoleaks are diagnosed using multiphasic CT scans (non-contrast, arterial, and venous phase). Using DECT, however, Javor et al. recently demonstrated the feasibility of a single-acquisition split-bolus DECT protocol as a one-stop shop approach in the evaluation of endoleaks [45]. Here, VNC were used to replace the true non-contrast scan [46–48]. The authors reported a radiation dose reduction of 42% compared to a biphasic acquisition [45]. Furthermore, VMIs at 40 keV have been shown to improve the detection of endoleaks compared to conventional linearly blended images at 120 kV [49].

Abdominal Imaging

Radiation Dose Reduction with Virtual Non-contrast Imaging

VNC images reconstructed from contrast-enhanced DECT scans enable the elimination of a true non-contrast scan. Multiple studies have suggested replacing the TNC scan by VNC images in order to reduce the radiation dose to the patient [50–53]. To date, most of these studies have been limited to dual-source (DS) DECT scanners. A radiation dose reduction between 21% and 33% has been reported using VNC images for liver mass evaluation by reducing a 3-phase to a 2-phase scan protocol [50–53]. Graser et al. demonstrated a radiation dose saving potential of 35–49% by omitting the TNC scan in patients under investigation for renal masses [54, 55]. A dose reduction of 26% was reported for imaging of the pancreas [56] and 30% for imaging of gastrointestinal bleeding [57]. In single-source fast kV-switching DECT, radiation dose reductions of 25% and 30% were observed for multiphase exams assessing liver masses and gastric masses, respectively [58, 59].

VNC imaging has been described as a potential diagnostic imaging strategy in the management of incidental adrenal and hepatic findings by the American College of Radiology [60, 61]. A consensus statement by radiologists of nine academic institutions in the USA recommended that VNC images reconstructed from the arterial phase could replace TNC images for dual-phase liver and pancreatic exams [62]. However, certain pitfalls have to be taken into account when applying VNC images in routine clinical practice. These will be highlighted in the last section of this chapter.

Characterization of Incidental Adrenal Nodules

Adrenal nodules are an extremely common incidental finding in abdominal CT, with an incidence of approximately 5% [63]. Traditionally, true non-contrast CT, multiphase contrast-enhanced CT washout technique, and chemical-shift MRI have been used to diagnose adrenal adenomas. In non-contrast CT, an attenuation of <10 HU has been shown to be highly specific for lipid-rich adrenal adenomas [64]. In clinical routine, however, adrenal nodules are often incidentally detected on single-energy single-phase contrast-enhanced CT scans for which their CT attenuation will overlap between benign adenomas and malignant entities (e.g., metastases). In this case, either additional multiphase CT imaging or MRI has to be performed for further lesion characterization. This dilemma can potentially be solved by the implementation of DECT as the default single-phase contrast-enhanced protocol. DECT offers the ability to generate virtual non-contrast (VNC) images from single-phase contrast-enhanced DECT scans. These VNC images can be used to replace TNC scans and consequently reduce the cumulative radiation dose.

Several studies have compared the accuracy of VNC images to TNC images in the diagnosis of adrenal adenoma [65–68]. For dual-source DECT, a meta-analysis reported comparable sensitivity between VNC images (54%) and conventional TNC images (57%) [69]. However, the pooled sensitivity was rather low, and a pooled specificity could not be calculated. Furthermore, a high heterogeneity for the sensitivity of VNC images was identified, which may have been caused by different timing of the application of intravenous contrast medium among the studies [69]. Interestingly, for single-source DECT, only a small number of studies on differentiation of adrenal nodules have been done. These studies reported high sensitivity and specificity to differentiate between adenomas and non-adenomas when using material density analysis [70] or between adenomas and metastases when using VMI [71]. Further prospective multicenter studies are needed to validate the accuracy of VNC images to diagnose adrenal adenomas.

Martin et al. demonstrated that DECT-based iodine and fat quantification could be used as another tool to distinguish adrenal adenomas from metastases and normal adrenal parenchyma [72]. Here, adrenal adenomas showed lower iodine concentration and higher fat fraction values compared to adrenal metastases. Furthermore, iodine maps help to differentiate adrenal hemorrhage from other disease entities (Fig. 13.5).

Characterization of Urinary Stones

The characterization of urinary stones is a prime example of an application of DECT that potentially impacts patient treatment. There are different treatment options for urinary stones dependent on the stone composition. Stones are classified based on their etiology, e.g., noninfectious stones (calcium oxalate, calcium phosphate including brushite and carbonate apatite, uric acid), infectious stones (magnesium ammonium phosphate, calcium apatite, ammonium urate), and genetic stones (cystine, xanthine, 2, 8-dihydroxyadenine) [73]. The majority of stones are composed of calcium oxalate and these are usually treated with invasive procedures like ureterorenoscopy, extracorporeal shock wave lithotripsy, and percutaneous nephrolithotomy. On the other hand, uric acid stones can be treated by pharmacotherapy (oral chemolysis). This treatment involves alkalization of the urine to achieve a pH of 6.5–7.2 [74] and monitoring of urine pH by the patient multiple times a day [73]. Stone characterization can be

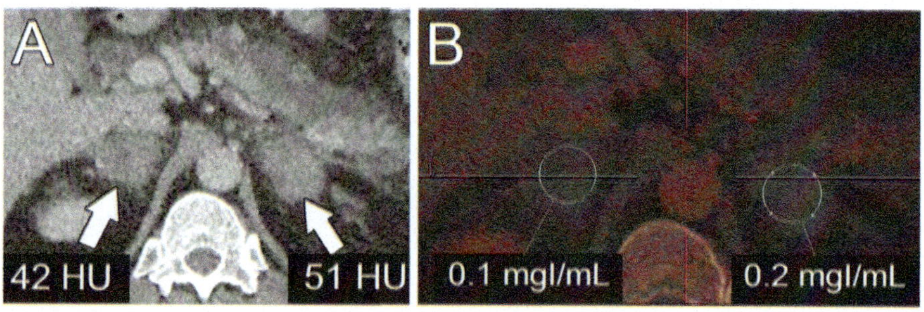

Fig. 13.5 (**a**) Contrast-enhanced DECT of the adrenal glands in a patient in septic shock. Both lesions are hyperdense with CT attenuation values of about 50 HU. (**b**) Reconstructed iodine maps showed no relevant iodine uptake of both lesions. VNC images (not shown) demonstrated hyperdensity of the lesions. Findings indicated stress-induced adrenal hemorrhages

used to guide patient treatment. In a prospective clinical trial, Nestler et al. demonstrated a positive predictive value of 100% and a negative predictive value of 98.5% for the characterization of uric acid stones [75]. Therefore, DECT has the potential to reduce invasive procedures and their associated risks by identifying patients suitable for oral chemolysis (Fig. 13.6) [76].

The analysis of stone composition is limited when using conventional polychromatic single-energy CT because of an overlap in the CT attenuation of different types of stones. Some DECT approaches use a threshold-based assessment of the dual-energy ratio (DE ratio) to characterize stone composition. The DE ratio is defined as the ratio of the CT attenuation of the stone at the low-energy spectrum compared to the high-energy spectrum. DE ratios have been shown to be greater than 1.24 for calcium oxalate and calcium phosphate stones, between 1.13 and 1.24 for cystine stones, and less than 1.1 for uric acid stones [77]. Other options include the assessment of attenuation values of VMI [78] or to calculate

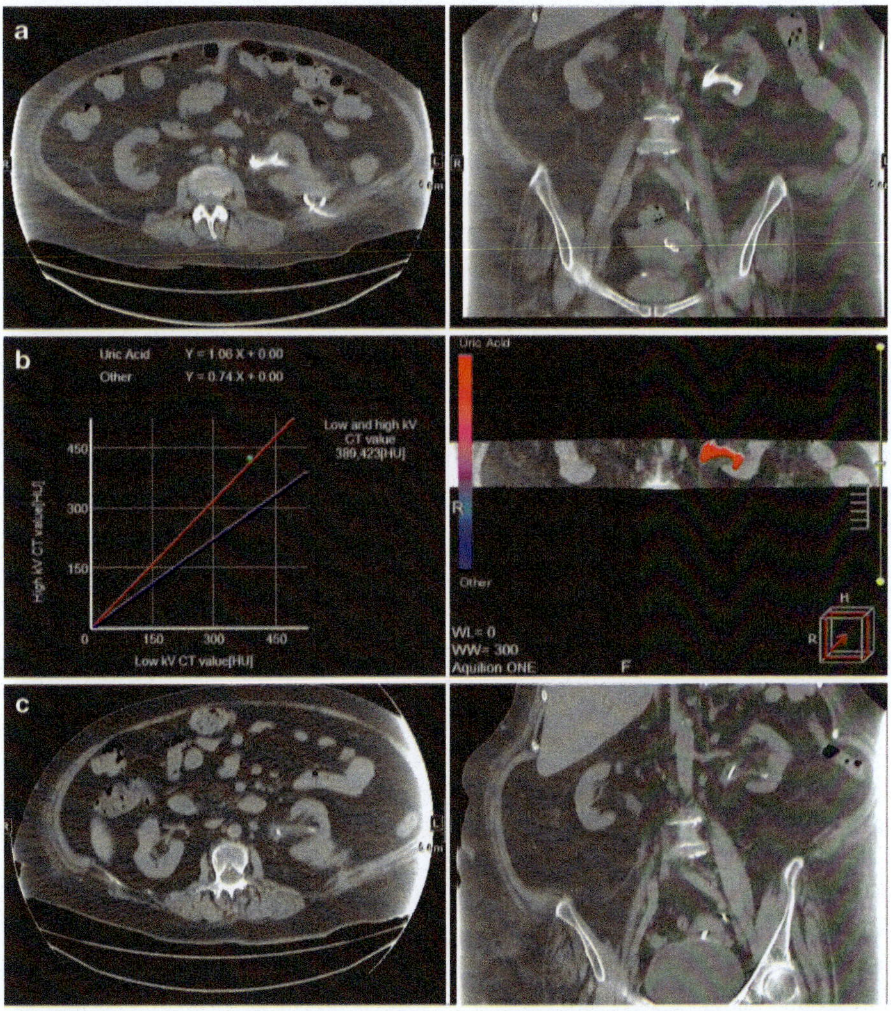

Fig. 13.6 Urinary stone characterization with material decomposition algorithms. (**a**) Axial on coronal CT images showing a large stone in the left renal pelvis in an obese patient with left flank pain. (**b**) DECT-stone analysis classified the stone as a uric acid stone based on a dual-energy ratio of 1.06 (color-coded in red). Chemolysis by alkalinization of the urine was performed. (**c**) After treatment the stone was almost completely dissolved

and compare the effective atomic number (Z_{eff}) of the investigated stone compared to the Z_{eff} of stones of known composition. Most vendors use color-coded maps to visualize stone composition. DECT demonstrated high accuracy to differentiate uric acid from non-uric acid stones or different subtypes of non-uric acid stones [79–81]. A meta-analysis reported a pooled sensitivity of 95.5% and a pooled specificity of 98.5% to differentiate uric acid and non-uric acid stones [82].

The main limitation of DECT in the characterization of urinary stones is the decreased accuracy in stones smaller than 3 mm [83]. This may, however, have little impact on patient treatment as it is estimated that 95% of stones up to 4 mm are non-obstructing and pass within 40 days [73]. Furthermore, another limitation of DECT is non-characterization of a large proportion of stones <5 mm [84] at a reduced radiation dose, pointing out that a certain minimum radiation dose level is needed to successfully characterize stone composition. A possible solution to overcome the limitations of DECT in the characterization of small stones is the use of photon-counting detector CT (PCD-CT). A phantom study reported an improved accuracy for the characterization of stones <3 mm using PCD-CT compared to traditional DECT [83].

Evaluation of Bowel Disease

The utility of DECT, including multi-material decomposition (MMD) and VMI imaging, has been demonstrated for neoplastic, vascular, and inflammatory diseases of the bowel. Focal or segmental hyper- or hypoenhancement of the bowel wall in contrast-enhanced CT scans is a key finding in the majority of bowel diseases. Iodine maps and VMI at low-keV levels can improve the visualization of enhancement differences between affected and normal bowel wall and therefore improve the conspicuity of pathologic conditions. Boellaard et al. demonstrated an increased accuracy for the detection of colorectal cancer in contrast-enhanced DECT if iodine maps were used in addition to conventional mixed images at 120 kV (96.7% vs. 90%) [85]. Interestingly, results were sufficient even without bowel preparation or insufflation prior to the DECT scan. Moreover, VNC and iodine maps have been shown to be useful in the differentiation between malignant neoplastic and benign neoplastic findings in suspected colorectal cancer [86]. First steps have been taken to assess the potential of quantitative DECT parameters to assess tumor differentiation [87, 88].

Another potential application of DECT in bowel disease is the improvement of the detection of bowel ischemia. In an animal study, DECT with iodine maps and VMIs significantly improved the conspicuity of ischemic small bowel compared with conventional CT [89]. In a retrospective clinical study of patients with small bowel obstruction, VMI at 70 keV improved CNR and diagnostic confidence in the assessment of mural bowel wall enhancement [90]. Lourenco et al. demonstrated a substantial increase in sensitivity for the detection of acute bowel ischemia (from 63.6% to 81.8%) if iodine maps and VMI at 40 keV were added to the assessment of conventional images [91].

Not only do quantitative DECT parameters (e.g., iodine quantification) allow for improved visualization of hypoenhancing bowel wall in ischemia, they also enable the differentiation of normal bowel wall from hyperenhancing wall in inflammatory diseases [92, 93]. In Crohn's disease, the wall of inflamed bowel segments showed significantly higher iodine concentrations compared to normal segments. Nevertheless, a limitation of iodine quantification of the bowel wall is the difficulty to define an appropriate region of interest in thin bowel walls. Lee et al. proposed the use of VMI at 40 keV in addition to conventional polychromatic images at 120 kV to improve diagnostic accuracy for active Crohn's disease [94]. However, considering the low number of scientific publications to date, further prospective clinical studies are needed to validate the diagnostic accuracy of quantitative DECT parameters in bowel disease.

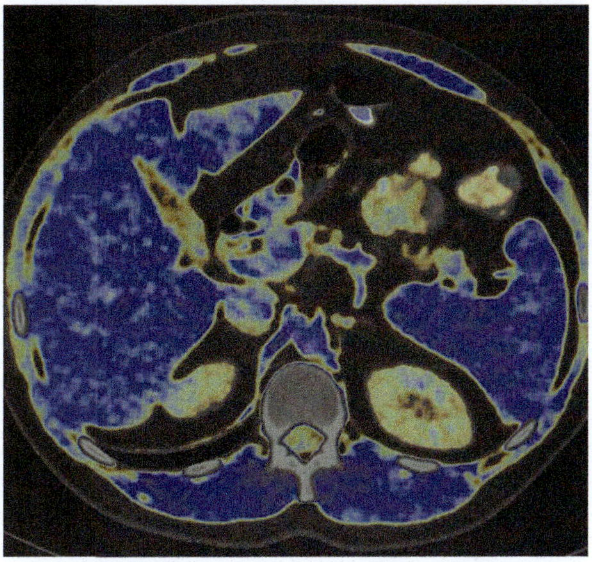

Fig. 13.7 Example of a fat map reconstructed from DECT. Increased fat content is color-coded in yellow to red. In this case, the liver parenchyma demonstrated normal fat distribution indicated by the blue/violet color

Quantification of Liver Fat

Multi-material decomposition algorithms of contrast-enhanced DECT scans offer the ability to generate hepatic fat volume fraction (FVF) images (Fig. 13.7). The reconstruction of FVF is a rather recent technology with only a few references in the literature [95, 96]. In a prospective study, these images showed accurate and reproducible quantification of hepatic fat compared to MR spectroscopy with liver biopsy as the reference standard [95]. Moreover, Cao et al. demonstrated the potential of multi-material imaging and VMI to assess the heterogeneity of fat deposition in the liver in an animal study [96]. Further clinical studies are needed to validate DECT as a reliable tool in the quantification of liver fat.

Oncologic Imaging

Tumor Detection and Characterization

DECT offers some promising quantification tools that can be beneficial in the detection and characterization of benign and malignant lesions in oncologic imaging.

DECT-based iodine quantification (DECT-IQ) and VMI are the two main applications that have been shown to improve lesion detection and conspicuity in different areas of the body. The combined use of iodine material density images and VMI images at low energy levels (i.e., 52 keV) has been successfully demonstrated to improve lesion contrast and reader confidence of hypoattenuating pancreatic adenocarcinomas [97, 98] as well as to improve the detection of hypervascular pancreatic neoplasms [99]. Moreover, iodine material density images have shown promising results as an addition to conventional scans for the assessment of local recurrence in surgically treated pancreatic adenocarcinoma [100]. Improved conspicuity has also been reported using VMI at low energy levels in the assessment of liver lesions [101] (Figs. 13.8 and 13.9). Moreover, DECT-IQ has been used to diagnose tumor thrombus in the portal vein in hepatocellular carcinoma [102]. Marin et al. demonstrated improved specificity for the characterization of small renal lesions using DECT-IQ over traditional CT attenuation measurements [103]. The authors reported a threshold of 1.9 mg iodine per mL (mgI/mL) to differentiate between benign (simple cyst, hemorrhagic cyst, oncocytoma, fat-poor angiomyolipoma) and malignant renal lesions (clear cell, papillary, and

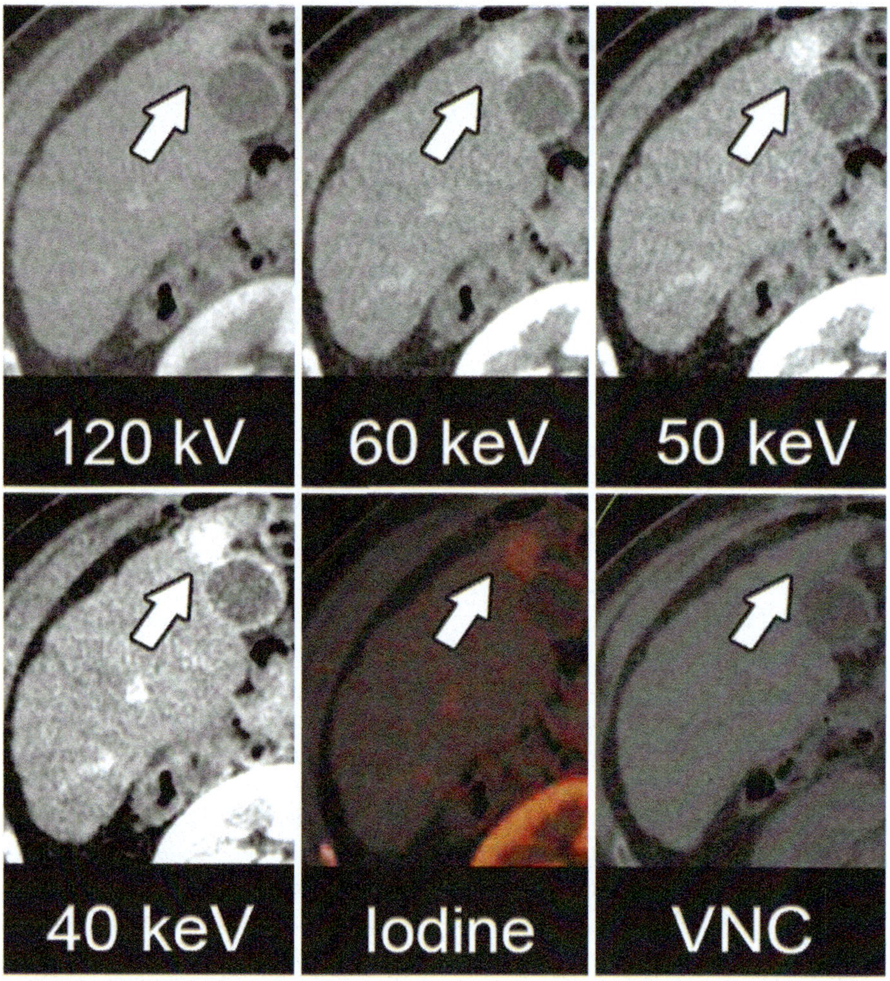

Fig. 13.8 Example of the benefit of DECT to improve the detection and conspicuity of a hyperenhancing liver lesion (LI-RADS 4). Images show (from left to right): a linearly blended DECT image simulating 120 kV, VMI images from 60 to 40 keV, iodine map, and VNC image. Note the increased CT attenuation of the lesion at low-keV VMI. The lesion is bright on the iodine map but disappears on VNC images indicating a strong iodine uptake (Courtesy of Fides R. Schwartz, Duke University, USA)

chromophobe renal cell carcinoma) with a high specificity of 93% [103]. In that study malignant lesions demonstrated iodine concentrations above this threshold (Fig. 13.10).

In thoracic imaging, DECT-IQ and spectral attenuation curves can be used to distinguish pulmonary cancer from inflammatory masses [104]. In a small clinical study, pulmonary sarcomas were successfully differentiated from pulmonary thromboembolism [105]. Additionally, DECT-IQ has been reported to distinguish benign from malignant mediastinal lesions [106]. Furthermore, DECT-IQ can be used to discriminate between metastatic and nonmetastatic lymph nodes in lung and gynecological malignancies [107, 108] (Fig. 13.11).

Treatment Response Assessment

DECT-IQ demonstrated promising results as a predictive biomarker in oncologic imaging. This is of high importance in the assessment of tumor treatment response. Iodine quantification

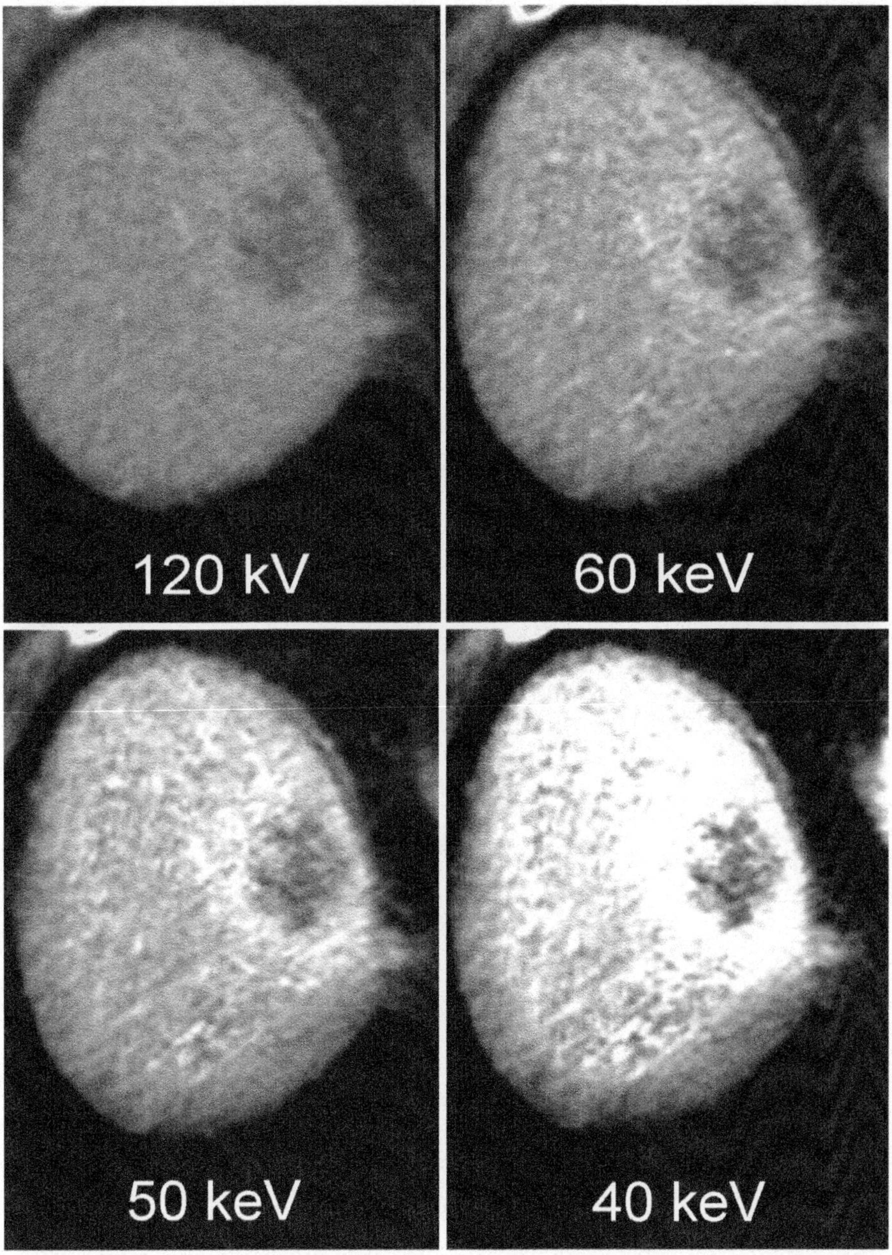

Fig. 13.9 Improvement of CNR and conspicuity of a hypoattenuating liver metastasis in the liver dome using low-energy virtual monoenergetic images compared to conventional linearly blended images simulating 120 kV. CT attenuation of the rim enhancement increases with decreasing energy level of VMI. This improvement is so high in the 40 keV image that the window settings would have to be adjusted during clinical image evaluation to compensate for the overly bright hyperattenuation. As a trade-off, image noise is increased at low-energy VMIs. Images were acquired using a second-generation VMI algorithm on a single-source split-filter DECT

was demonstrated to be helpful in the prediction of outcome for cervical cancer treated with radiochemotherapy [109]. In lung cancers treated with traditional radio- or chemoradiotherapy, DECT-IQ showed comparable response evaluation compared to metabolism-based param-

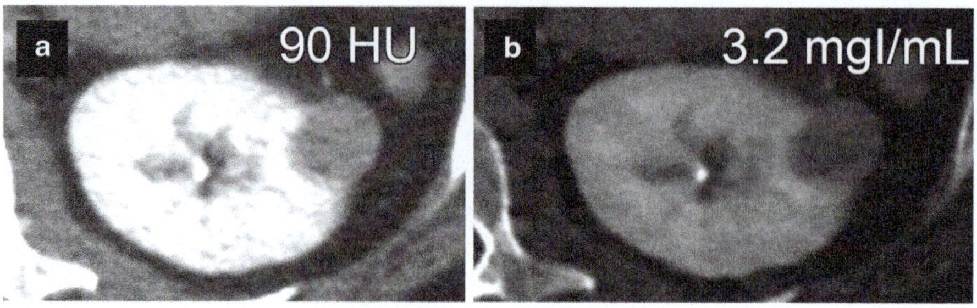

Fig. 13.10 Example of an incidental renal lesion with increased CT attenuation in contrast-enhanced portal-venous phase DECT (**a**). In SECT, further imaging would be required to differentiate between a hemorrhagic cyst and a malignant lesion. Iodine material density images demonstrated moderate iodine uptake of the lesion (**b**). The lesion was resected and proved to be a renal cell carcinoma

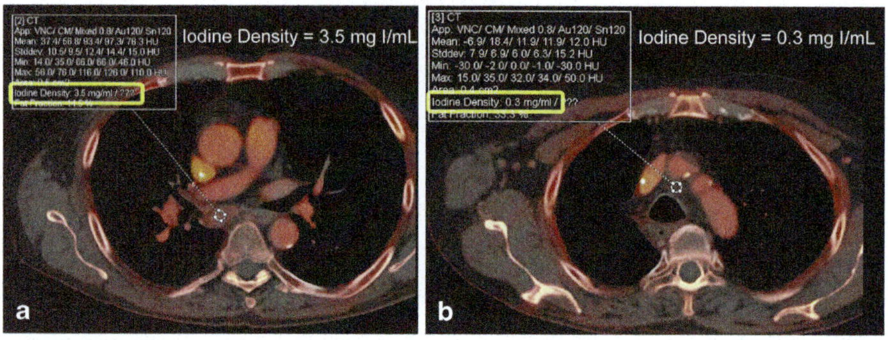

Fig. 13.11 Mediastinal lymph node metastasis in a patient with adenosquamous lung cancer. Quantification of iodine concentration on iodine density maps can be helpful to differentiate metastatic (**a**) from benign (**b**) lymph node. In this example, the metastatic lymph node shows substantially higher iodine concentration compared to a benign lymph node

eters in fluorine-18 fluorodeoxyglucose (FDG) positron emission tomography (PET) [110]. Moreover, iodine concentration in the arterial phase has been reported as a predictive biomarker for recurrence of lung cancer after stereotactic radiotherapy [111]. Lung cancers with low iodine concentrations demonstrated higher recurrence rates. It is postulated that these lower concentrations represent hypoxic cell populations that are more resistant to radiotherapy.

DECT-IQ was also shown to be useful in the response assessments of tumors that are treated with antiangiogenic therapy. This oncologic therapy attacks tumor neovascularization and therefore alters its iodine uptake which can be assessed by a volumetric quantification of the iodine concentration. Promising results have been reported in clinical studies for advanced non-small cell lung cancer (NSCLC) [112, 113] and metastatic renal cell carcinoma [114]. Moreover, DECT achieved improved prediction of tumor treatment response in advanced gastrointestinal stromal tumors treated with antiangiogenic therapy compared to established response criteria (RECIST and CHOI) [115].

Iodine Quantification as a Predictive Biomarker

Recent research investigated if DECT-IQ can reliably predict the invasiveness and potential of tumors to metastasize. One study successfully developed DECT-IQ-based nomograms to preoperatively predict lymph node metastases in gastric cancer [116]. Moreover, Shimamoto et al. reported that iodine volume measured using a VOI-tool on iodine maps was significantly associated with the differentiation grade of non-small cell lung cancers [117]. Here, well-differentiated tumors showed higher iodine-related attenuation compared to poorly differentiated tumors. Low iodine volume also correlated with greater invasiveness. A potential correlation of DECT-IQ and gene expression has been shown for the expression of vascular endothelial growth factor (VEGF), a biomarker for neo-angiogenesis [118]. Li et al. demonstrated that iodine concentration, spectral HU curves, and CT attenuation at 40 keV monoenergetic images correlate significantly with VEGF expression in NSCLC.

Musculoskeletal Imaging

Detection of Bone Marrow Edema

MDCT serves as a primary tool in the assessment of acute bone fractures in trauma patients, especially of the spine. However, single-energy CT has lacked the ability to assess the existence of bone marrow edema (BME) which serves as a major criterion to determine the acuity of a fracture. This is especially important in the estimation of the age of compression fractures in osteoporotic patients. The detection of BME, traditionally performed with MRI, is an important step to initiate patient treatment, e.g., balloon kyphoplasty, which has been used in the treatment of acute compression fractures. Recent studies have shown that DECT can be used to detect BME in various body regions and has the potential to serve as a reasonable alternative if MRI is not immediately available or is contraindicated [119–121] (Fig. 13.12). A three-material decomposition algorithm is applied to create so-called virtual non-calcium images. In contrast to the calculation of virtual non-contrast images, the algorithm uses calcium instead of iodine as the third material (alongside fat and water). Virtual non-calcium images can therefore be used to visualize increased water content which is present in BME. These images can be used for qualitative and quantitative assessment.

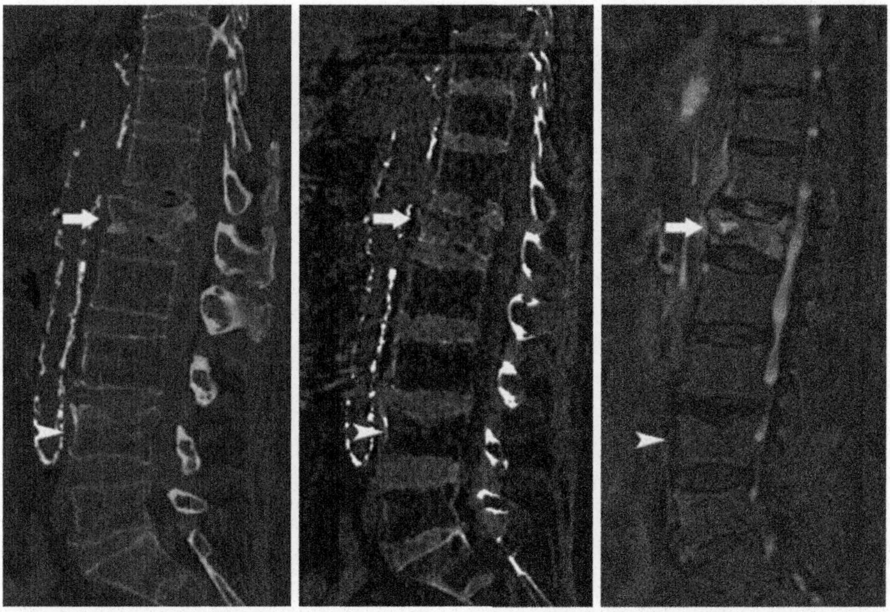

Fig. 13.12 Eighty-three-year-old-patient with suspected traumatic compression fractures. Sagittal reformatted CT images: Unenhanced CT (left), virtual non-calcium image (middle), and sagittal STIR MR image (right). L1 and L4 demonstrated morphological changes suggestive of compression fractures. However, acute bone marrow edema was only confirmed in L1 (as hyperdensity on the virtual non-calcium image and hyperintensity on the STIR MR image). L4 did not show bone marrow edema, indicating an old compression fracture (© With permission from Springer: Bierry et al. [121])

A recent meta-analysis reported a pooled sensitivity of 85% and specificity of 97% of DECT for the detection of BME in the spine and appendicular skeleton [122]. The meta-analysis also revealed that qualitative (visual) assessment was superior to quantitative assessment. However, another recent prospective study reported only a sensitivity of 73% and specificity of 70% for the detection of BME in osteoporotic compression fractures [123]. The authors also observed that a certain level of experience was needed for the correct interpretation of virtual non-calcium images [123]. This limitation was confirmed by the variation among readers reported by Kaup et al. [124]. Another limitation is a decreased detection of edema in subcortical regions due to misregistration with the adjacent cortex [119].

Detection of Gout

Gout is the most prevalent crystal arthropathy. In gout, monosodium urate crystal depositions are found in and around joints, especially in periarticular soft tissues. The gold standard for monosodium urate detection is joint aspiration and the utilization of polarization microscopy. However, this method is rather invasive and can fail in up to 25% of cases [125]. DECT has proven to be a noninvasive alternative in the early diagnosis and treatment monitoring of gout (Fig. 13.13) [126, 127]. DECT can reliably distinguish between urate deposition and calcification. A meta-analysis reported a pooled sensitivity of 88% and specificity of 90% for the diagnostic accuracy of DECT in gout [128]. Furthermore, intra- and interobserver reproducibility was shown to be excellent for DECT [129]. However, radiologists have to be aware of the typical artifacts seen in color-coded urate maps. Typically, signal of urate exists artificially in the nails, nail bed, skin calluses, arteries, and areas affected by degraded image quality due to motion or noise [130]. Therefore, color-coded urate maps should always be interpreted together with the conventional polychromatic reconstruction.

Reduction of Metal Artifacts

Metal implants are known to cause relevant image artifacts due to beam hardening and photon starvation in conventional single-energy polychromatic CT. Beam-hardening artifacts occur if low-energy photons are absorbed by metal, which leads to higher energies of the beam penetrating the implant. This leads to a shift of the x-ray spectrum toward higher energies. A reduced tissue x-ray absorption of this "hardened" beam consequently results in dark streaks adjacent to the implant. Photon starvation artifacts occur if a large portion of photons are absorbed by the metal leading to very low signal at the detector. This results in fine dark and bright streaks. DECT offers the possibility to generate virtual monochromatic images (VMI) at energy levels between 40 and 200 keV by combining weighted low- and high-energy image information. VMI at high energy levels is particularly suitable to suppress beam-hardening artifacts while so-called projection-based metal artifact reduction algorithms (MARs) are primarily able to compensate for photon starvation. Photon starvation is more prevalent in larger metallic implants or implants with high atomic numbers (in which case MARs prove to be superior over VMIs) [131]. In patients with total hip replacements, MARs demonstrated improved assessment of adjacent soft tissues and VMIs improved assessment of the bone structure [132] (Fig. 13.14).

The application of DECT-based metal artifact reduction has been investigated for several metals used in different regions of the body. Optimal energy levels to reduce artifacts from metallic implants have been found between 95 and 150 keV [133–135]. However, a recent investigation of dental implants on a spectral detector CT reported optimal artifact reduction at higher energy levels of 130–160 keV [136]. The downside of VMI at high energy levels is reduced tissue contrast of the adjacent tissue, especially in contrast-enhanced scans [137, 138]. This points out that the energy level of monochromatic images has to be adjusted individually depending

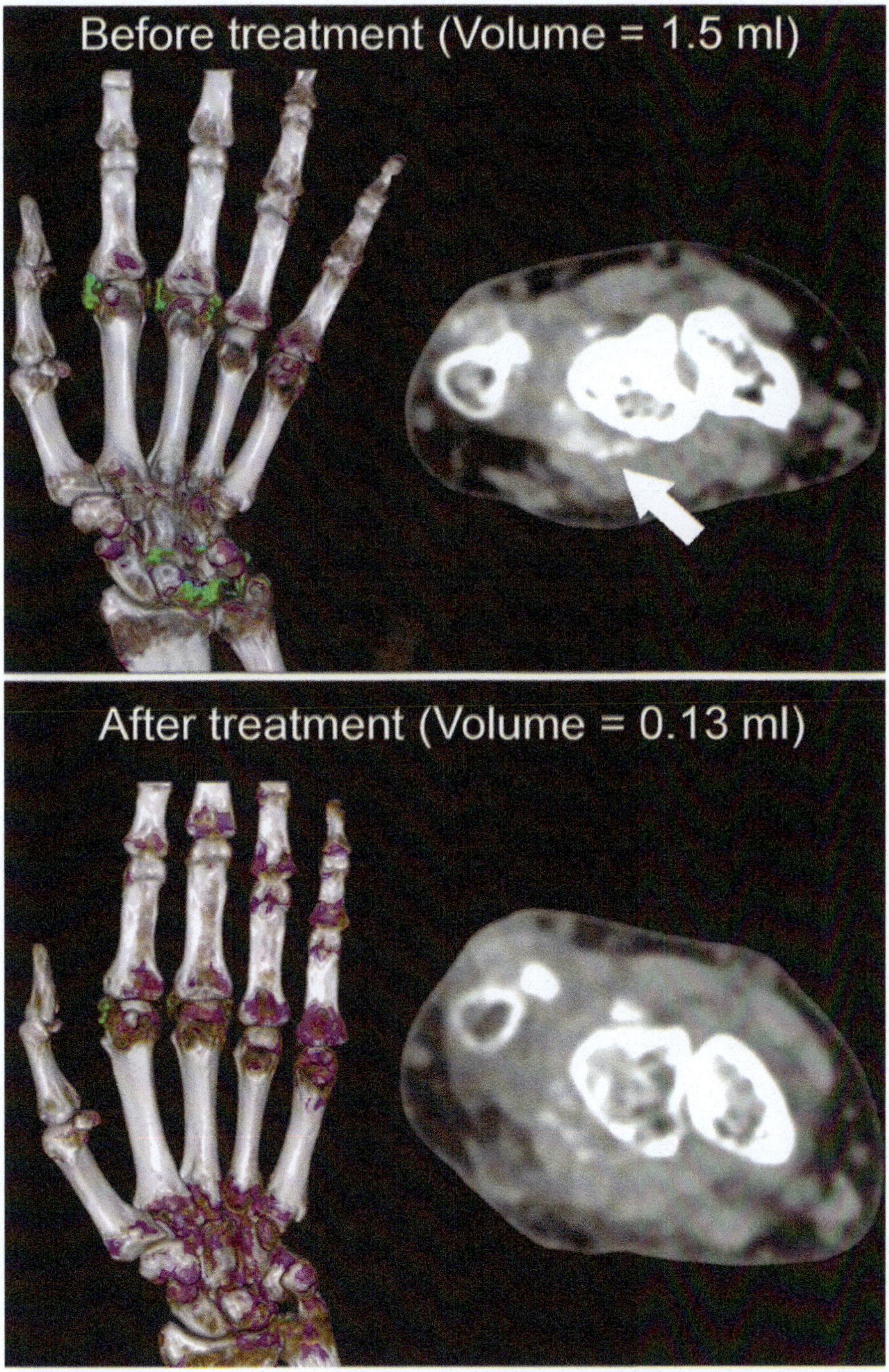

Fig. 13.13 DECT in the detection and quantification of gout. Upper image shows a volumetric rendering (VRT) and axial linearly blended image of the right hand in a patient with symptomatic gout before treatment. Gout deposits (arrow) are color-coded in green on the VRT. DECT enables quantification of the volume of gout deposits and the assessment of treatment response: after treatment most of the gout deposits disappeared

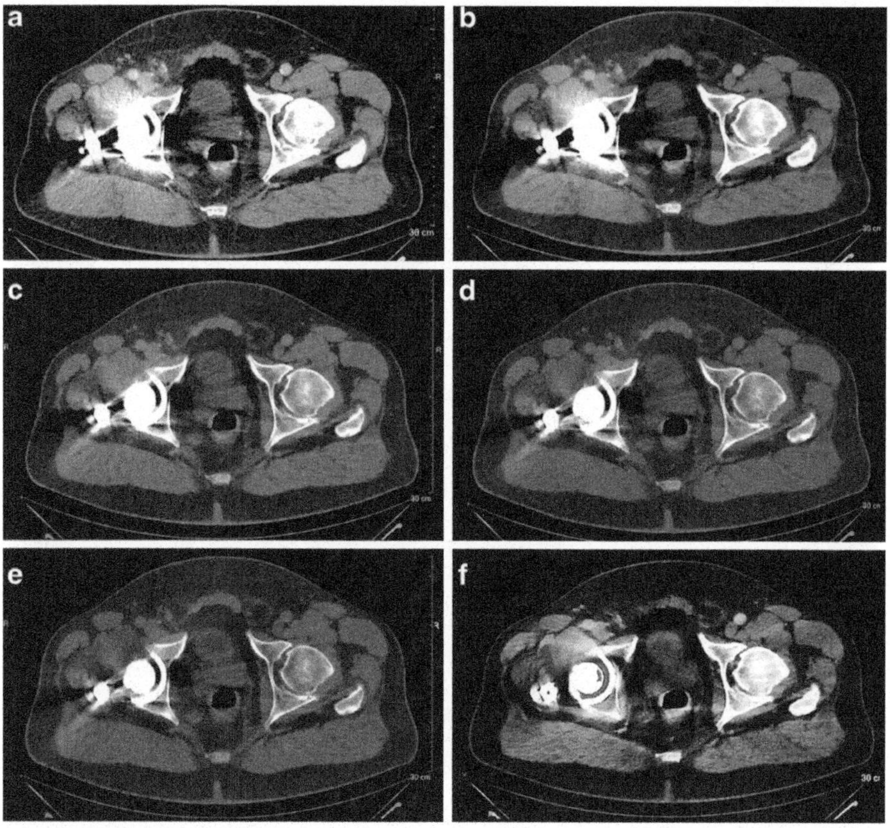

Fig. 13.14 Seventy-nine-year-old patient with a total hip replacement on the right. Axial CT image of (**a**) conventional CT image, (**b–e**) VMIs at 70, 110, 150, and 200 keV, and (**f**) MAR. VMIs and MAR demonstrate strong artifact reduction (© With permission from Springer: Laukamp et al. [132])

on the type of metal. Furthermore, VMIs can be combined with iterative metal artifact reduction algorithms (iMARs) to further improve image quality [139–141].

Pitfalls in Dual-Energy Imaging

Accuracy of Virtual Non-contrast Imaging

Radiologists have to be aware of the potential pitfalls and inaccuracies of DECT imaging to avoid misinterpretation of results in routine clinical practice. Controversy exists in the literature in regards to the ability of VNC images to accurately reflect CT attenuation values measured on TNC scans. Several studies reported differences between CT attenuation values measured on VNC and TNC (these were not statistically significant for the liver) [50, 53, 54]. Borhani et al., however, observed a considerable percentage of cases in which the CT attenuation difference of various abdominal organs was >10 HU between VNC and TNC images in the same patient [142]. In addition, Durieux et al. concluded that VNC should still not replace TNC on a third-generation DS-DECT based on their finding of substantial differences in the CT attenuation for fluid, fat, and renal tissue [143].

Reliability and Reproducibility of DECT Parameters

Recently, investigation of the reliability and reproducibility of DECT-based quantitative parameters has been of major interest for the research community. Multiple studies have revealed major differences in quantitative imaging parameters within (intra-conditional) and among different DECT approaches (inter-conditional). Obmann et al. demonstrated in a clinical study that the CT attenuation values of virtual non-contrast images (VNC) varied significantly between dual-source DECT and split-filter DECT [144]. Furthermore, the authors reported increased intrascanner variability for split-filter DECT compared to dual-source DECT. In a phantom study, Jacobsen et al. compared the accuracy of iodine quantification and virtual monoenergetic imaging among five different DECT approaches [145]. The authors concluded that both parameters vary among DECT systems with dual-source and fast kV-switching DECT providing the most accurate results in a large phantom. Another phantom study reported that the minimum detectable difference in iodine concentration among different generations of single-source and dual-source DECT ranged from 0.4 to 1.5 mg iodine/mL [146]. This is of major concern if a patient is imaged repeatedly on different DECT scanners or with different scan parameters at the same or different radiologic departments during an oncologic follow-up.

Artifacts in VNC and Iodine Imaging

Pitfalls occur particularly when imaging the lungs and the genitourinary system. Focal artificial iodine defects that can mimic perfusion defects were reported for color-coded iodine perfusion maps of the lung [147]. Beam-hardening artifacts caused by contrast medium in the superior vena cava, cardiac motion, and diaphragmatic motion are the most common causes for these artificial iodine defects. Another pitfall is that calcium appears hyperdense/bright on color-coded iodine maps that are based on three-material decomposition algorithms [148]. This can lead to misinterpretation of iodine enhancement if a calcification is present in, e.g., a renal mass. Therefore, it is crucial to review these iodine maps in conjunction with the corresponding VNC images to differentiate calcium (hyperdense on VNC) from iodine (not apparent on VNC). Based on the same principle that calcium is hyperdense on both iodine maps and VNC images, small urinary stones can be falsely subtracted and disappear from VNC images that are reconstructed from post-contrast DECT urography scans [149]. Very small (<3 mm) and less dense stones (<400 HU) are affected [150]. If VNC images are used to replace true non-contrast scans in DECT urography, it is recommend to reconstruct these images from the nephrographic phase instead of the excretory phase [149, 151].

References

1. Gupta R, Phan CM, Leidecker C, Brady TJ, Hirsch JA, Nogueira RG, et al. Evaluation of dual-energy CT for differentiating intracerebral hemorrhage from iodinated contrast material staining. Radiology. 2010;257(1):205–11.
2. Phan CM, Yoo AJ, Hirsch JA, Nogueira RG, Gupta R. Differentiation of hemorrhage from iodinated contrast in different intracranial compartments using dual-energy head CT. AJNR Am J Neuroradiol. 2012;33(6):1088–94.
3. Tijssen MP, Hofman PA, Stadler AA, van Zwam W, de Graaf R, van Oostenbrugge RJ, et al. The role of dual energy CT in differentiating between brain haemorrhage and contrast medium after mechanical revascularisation in acute ischaemic stroke. Eur Radiol. 2014;24(4):834–40.
4. Jiang XY, Zhang SH, Xie QZ, Yin ZJ, Liu QY, Zhao MD, et al. Evaluation of virtual noncontrast images obtained from dual-energy CTA for diagnosing subarachnoid hemorrhage. AJNR Am J Neuroradiol. 2015;36(5):855–60.
5. Gariani J, Cuvinciuc V, Courvoisier D, Krauss B, Mendes Pereira V, Sztajzel R, et al. Diagnosis of acute ischemia using dual energy CT after mechanical thrombectomy. J Neurointerv Surg. 2016;8(10):996–1000.
6. Mohammed MF, Marais O, Min A, Ferguson D, Jalal S, Khosa F, et al. Unenhanced dual-energy computed tomography: visualization of brain edema. Investig Radiol. 2018;53(2):63–9.
7. Grams AE, Djurdjevic T, Rehwald R, Schiestl T, Dazinger F, Steiger R, et al. Improved visualisation of early cerebral infarctions after endovascular stroke therapy using dual-energy computed tomography oedema maps. Eur Radiol. 2018;28:4534–41.
8. Noguchi K, Itoh T, Naruto N, Takashima S, Tanaka K, Kuroda S. A novel imaging technique (X-map) to identify acute ischemic lesions using noncontrast dual-energy computed tomography. J Stroke Cerebrovasc Dis. 2017;26(1):34–41.

9. Hu R, Daftari Besheli L, Young J, Wu M, Pomerantz S, Lev MH, et al. Dual-energy head CT enables accurate distinction of intraparenchymal hemorrhage from calcification in emergency department patients. Radiology. 2016;280(1):177–83.
10. Pomerantz SR, Kamalian S, Zhang D, Gupta R, Rapalino O, Sahani DV, et al. Virtual monochromatic reconstruction of dual-energy unenhanced head CT at 65–75 keV maximizes image quality compared with conventional polychromatic CT. Radiology. 2013;266(1):318–25.
11. Jia Y, Zhang J, Fan J, Li C, Sun Y, Li D, et al. Gemstone spectral imaging reduced artefacts from metal coils or clips after treatment of cerebral aneurysms: a retrospective study of 35 patients. Br J Radiol. 2015;88(1055):20150222.
12. Yu L, Leng S, McCollough CH. Dual-energy CT-based monochromatic imaging. AJR Am J Roentgenol. 2012;199(5 Suppl):S9–S15.
13. Schneider D, Apfaltrer P, Sudarski S, Nance JW Jr, Haubenreisser H, Fink C, et al. Optimization of kiloelectron volt settings in cerebral and cervical dual-energy CT angiography determined with virtual monoenergetic imaging. Acad Radiol. 2014;21(4):431–6.
14. Thieme SF, Becker CR, Hacker M, Nikolaou K, Reiser MF, Johnson TR. Dual energy CT for the assessment of lung perfusion – correlation to scintigraphy. Eur J Radiol. 2008;68(3):369–74.
15. Thieme SF, Graute V, Nikolaou K, Maxien D, Reiser MF, Hacker M, et al. Dual energy CT lung perfusion imaging – correlation with SPECT/CT. Eur J Radiol. 2012;81(2):360–5.
16. Chae EJ, Seo JB, Jang YM, Krauss B, Lee CW, Lee HJ, et al. Dual-energy CT for assessment of the severity of acute pulmonary embolism: pulmonary perfusion defect score compared with CT angiographic obstruction score and right ventricular/left ventricular diameter ratio. AJR Am J Roentgenol. 2010;194(3):604–10.
17. Meinel FG, Nance JW Jr, Schoepf UJ, Hoffmann VS, Thierfelder KM, Costello P, et al. Predictive value of computed tomography in acute pulmonary embolism: systematic review and meta-analysis. Am J Med. 2015;128(7):747–59 e2.
18. Takx RAP, Henzler T, Schoepf UJ, Germann T, Schoenberg SO, Shirinova A, et al. Predictive value of perfusion defects on dual energy CTA in the absence of thromboembolic clots. J Cardiovasc Comput Tomogr. 2017;11(3):183–7.
19. Im DJ, Hur J, Han KH, Lee HJ, Kim YJ, Kwon W, et al. Acute pulmonary embolism: retrospective cohort study of the predictive value of perfusion defect volume measured with dual-energy CT. AJR Am J Roentgenol. 2017;209(5):1015–22.
20. Uhrig M, Simons D, Schlemmer HP. Incidental pulmonary emboli in stage IV melanoma patients: prevalence in CT staging examinations and improved detection with vessel reconstructions based on dual energy CT. PLoS One. 2018;13(7):e0199458.
21. Hong YJ, Kim JY, Choe KO, Hur J, Lee HJ, Choi BW, et al. Different perfusion pattern between acute and chronic pulmonary thromboembolism: evaluation with two-phase dual-energy perfusion CT. AJR Am J Roentgenol. 2013;200(4):812–7.
22. Kim SS, Hur J, Kim YJ, Lee HJ, Hong YJ, Choi BW. Dual-energy CT for differentiating acute and chronic pulmonary thromboembolism: an initial experience. Int J Card Imaging. 2014;30(Suppl 2):113–20.
23. Weiss J, Notohamiprodjo M, Bongers M, Schabel C, Mangold S, Nikolaou K, et al. Effect of noise-optimized monoenergetic postprocessing on diagnostic accuracy for detecting incidental pulmonary embolism in portal-venous phase dual-energy computed tomography. Investig Radiol. 2017;52(3):142–7.
24. Meyer M, Haubenreisser H, Schabel C, Leidecker C, Schmidt B, Schoenberg SO, et al. CT pulmonary angiography in patients with acute or chronic renal insufficiency: evaluation of a low dose contrast material protocol. Sci Rep. 2018;8(1):1995.
25. Apfaltrer P, Sudarski S, Schneider D, Nance JW Jr, Haubenreisser H, Fink C, et al. Value of monoenergetic low-kV dual energy CT datasets for improved image quality of CT pulmonary angiography. Eur J Radiol. 2014;83(2):322–8.
26. Dane B, Patel H, O'Donnell T, Girvin F, Brusca-Augello G, Alpert JB, et al. Image quality on dual-energy CTPA virtual monoenergetic images: quantitative and qualitative assessment. Acad Radiol. 2018;25(8):1075–86.
27. Ghandour A, Sher A, Rassouli N, Dhanantwari A, Rajiah P. Evaluation of virtual monoenergetic images on pulmonary vasculature using the dual-layer detector-based spectral computed tomography. J Comput Assist Tomogr. 2018;42:858–65.
28. Bae K, Jeon KN, Cho SB, Park SE, Moon JI, Baek HJ, et al. Improved opacification of a suboptimally enhanced pulmonary artery in chest CT: experience using a dual-layer detector spectral CT. AJR Am J Roentgenol. 2018;210(4):734–41.
29. D'Angelo T, Bucher AM, Lenga L, Arendt CT, Peterke JL, Caruso D, et al. Optimisation of window settings for traditional and noise-optimised virtual monoenergetic imaging in dual-energy computed tomography pulmonary angiography. Eur Radiol. 2018;28(4):1393–401.
30. Ohta Y, Kitao S, Yunaga H, Fujii S, Mukai N, Yamamoto K, et al. Myocardial delayed enhancement CT for the evaluation of heart failure: comparison to MRI. Radiology. 2018;288(3):682–91.
31. Han R, Sun K, Lu B, Zhao R, Li K, Yang X. Diagnostic accuracy of coronary CT angiography combined with dual-energy myocardial perfusion imaging for detection of myocardial infarction. Exp Ther Med. 2017;14(1):207–13.
32. Ha SJ, Jang Y, Lee BK, Cho IJ, Shim CY, Hong GR, et al. Assessment of myocardial viability based on dual-energy computed tomography in patients

with chronic myocardial infarction: comparison with magnetic resonance imaging. Clin Imaging. 2017;46:8–13.
33. Sandfort V, Kwan AC, Elumogo C, Vigneault DM, Symons R, Pourmorteza A, et al. Automatic high-resolution infarct detection using volumetric multiphase dual-energy CT. J Cardiovasc Comput Tomogr. 2017;11(4):288–94.
34. Weininger M, Schoepf UJ, Ramachandra A, Fink C, Rowe GW, Costello P, et al. Adenosine-stress dynamic real-time myocardial perfusion CT and adenosine-stress first-pass dual-energy myocardial perfusion CT for the assessment of acute chest pain: initial results. Eur J Radiol. 2012;81(12):3703–10.
35. Meinel FG, De Cecco CN, Schoepf UJ, Nance JW Jr, Silverman JR, Flowers BA, et al. First-arterial-pass dual-energy CT for assessment of myocardial blood supply: do we need rest, stress, and delayed acquisition? Comparison with SPECT. Radiology. 2014;270(3):708–16.
36. Nakahara T, Toyama T, Jinzaki M, Seki R, Saito Y, Higuchi T, et al. Quantitative analysis of iodine image of dual-energy computed tomography at rest: comparison with 99mTc-tetrofosmin stress-rest single-photon emission computed tomography myocardial perfusion imaging as the reference standard. J Thorac Imaging. 2018;33(2):97–104.
37. Carrascosa P, Deviggiano A, de Zan M, Capunay C, Campisi R, Rodriguez-Granillo GA. Improved discrimination of myocardial perfusion defects at low energy levels using virtual monochromatic imaging. J Comput Assist Tomogr. 2017;41(4):661–7.
38. Chang S, Han K, Youn JC, Im DJ, Kim JY, Suh YJ, et al. Utility of dual-energy CT-based monochromatic imaging in the assessment of myocardial delayed enhancement in patients with cardiomyopathy. Radiology. 2018;287(2):442–51.
39. Yamada Y, Jinzaki M, Okamura T, Yamada M, Tanami Y, Abe T, et al. Feasibility of coronary artery calcium scoring on virtual unenhanced images derived from single-source fast kVp-switching dual-energy coronary CT angiography. J Cardiovasc Comput Tomogr. 2014;8(5):391–400.
40. Chevance V, Damy T, Tacher V, Legou F, Ridouani F, Luciani A, et al. Myocardial iodine concentration measurement using dual-energy computed tomography for the diagnosis of cardiac amyloidosis: a pilot study. Eur Radiol. 2018;28(2):816–23.
41. Agrawal MD, Oliveira GR, Kalva SP, Pinho DF, Arellano RS, Sahani DV. Prospective comparison of reduced-iodine-dose virtual monochromatic imaging dataset from dual-energy CT angiography with standard-iodine-dose single-energy CT angiography for abdominal aortic aneurysm. AJR Am J Roentgenol. 2016;207(6):W125–W32.
42. Shuman WP, Chan KT, Busey JM, Mitsumori LM, Koprowicz KM. Dual-energy CT aortography with 50% reduced iodine dose versus single-energy CT aortography with standard iodine dose. Acad Radiol. 2016;23(5):611–8.
43. Tsang DS, Merchant TE, Merchant SE, Smith H, Yagil Y, Hua CH. Quantifying potential reduction in contrast dose with monoenergetic images synthesized from dual-layer detector spectral CT. Br J Radiol. 2017;90(1078):20170290.
44. Shuman WP, O'Malley RB, Busey JM, Ramos MM, Koprowicz KM. Prospective comparison of dual-energy CT aortography using 70% reduced iodine dose versus single-energy CT aortography using standard iodine dose in the same patient. Abdom Radiol (NY). 2017;42(3):759–65.
45. Javor D, Wressnegger A, Unterhumer S, Kollndorfer K, Nolz R, Beitzke D, et al. Endoleak detection using single-acquisition split-bolus dual-energy computer tomography (DECT). Eur Radiol. 2017;27(4):1622–30.
46. Stolzmann P, Frauenfelder T, Pfammatter T, Peter N, Scheffel H, Lachat M, et al. Endoleaks after endovascular abdominal aortic aneurysm repair: detection with dual-energy dual-source CT. Radiology. 2008;249(2):682–91.
47. Maturen KE, Kleaveland PA, Kaza RK, Liu PS, Quint LE, Khalatbari SH, et al. Aortic endograft surveillance: use of fast-switch kVp dual-energy computed tomography with virtual noncontrast imaging. J Comput Assist Tomogr. 2011;35(6):742–6.
48. Flors L, Leiva-Salinas C, Norton PT, Patrie JT, Hagspiel KD. Imaging follow-up of endovascular repair of type B aortic dissection with dual-source, dual-energy CT and late delayed-phase scans. J Vasc Interv Radiol. 2014;25(3):435–42.
49. Martin SS, Wichmann JL, Weyer H, Scholtz JE, Leithner D, Spandorfer A, et al. Endoleaks after endovascular aortic aneurysm repair: improved detection with noise-optimized virtual monoenergetic dual-energy CT. Eur J Radiol. 2017;94:125–32.
50. Zhang LJ, Peng J, Wu SY, Wang ZJ, Wu XS, Zhou CS, et al. Liver virtual non-enhanced CT with dual-source, dual-energy CT: a preliminary study. Eur Radiol. 2010;20(9):2257–64.
51. De Cecco CN, Buffa V, Fedeli S, Luzietti M, Vallone A, Ruopoli R, et al. Dual energy CT (DECT) of the liver: conventional versus virtual unenhanced images. Eur Radiol. 2010;20(12):2870–5.
52. De Cecco CN, Darnell A, Macias N, Ayuso JR, Rodriguez S, Rimola J, et al. Virtual unenhanced images of the abdomen with second-generation dual-source dual-energy computed tomography: image quality and liver lesion detection. Investig Radiol. 2013;48(1):1–9.
53. De Cecco CN, Muscogiuri G, Schoepf UJ, Caruso D, Wichmann JL, Cannao PM, et al. Virtual unenhanced imaging of the liver with third-generation dual-source dual-energy CT and advanced modeled iterative reconstruction. Eur J Radiol. 2016;85(7):1257–64.
54. Graser A, Johnson TR, Hecht EM, Becker CR, Leidecker C, Staehler M, et al. Dual-energy CT in patients suspected of having renal masses: can vir-

tual nonenhanced images replace true nonenhanced images? Radiology. 2009;252(2):433–40.
55. Graser A, Becker CR, Staehler M, Clevert DA, Macari M, Arndt N, et al. Single-phase dual-energy CT allows for characterization of renal masses as benign or malignant. Investig Radiol. 2010;45(7):399–405.
56. Mileto A, Mazziotti S, Gaeta M, Bottari A, Zimbaro F, Giardina C, et al. Pancreatic dual-source dual-energy CT: is it time to discard unenhanced imaging? Clin Radiol. 2012;67(4):334–9.
57. Sun H, Xue HD, Wang YN, Qian JM, Yu JC, Zhu F, et al. Dual-source dual-energy computed tomography angiography for active gastrointestinal bleeding: a preliminary study. Clin Radiol. 2013;68(2):139–47.
58. Chai Y, Xing J, Gao J, Lv P, Liang P, Liu J, et al. Feasibility of virtual nonenhanced images derived from single-source fast kVp-switching dual-energy CT in evaluating gastric tumors. Eur J Radiol. 2016;85(2):366–72.
59. Li Y, Li Y, Jackson A, Li X, Huang N, Guo C, et al. Comparison of virtual unenhanced CT images of the abdomen under different iodine flow rates. Abdom Radiol (NY). 2017;42(1):312–21.
60. Mayo-Smith WW, Song JH, Boland GL, Francis IR, Israel GM, Mazzaglia PJ, et al. Management of incidental adrenal masses: a white paper of the ACR incidental findings committee. J Am Coll Radiol. 2017;14(8):1038–44.
61. Gore RM, Pickhardt PJ, Mortele KJ, Fishman EK, Horowitz JM, Fimmel CJ, et al. Management of incidental liver lesions on CT: a white paper of the ACR incidental findings committee. J Am Coll Radiol. 2017;14(11):1429–37.
62. Patel BN, Alexander L, Allen B, Berland L, Borhani A, Mileto A, et al. Dual-energy CT workflow: multi-institutional consensus on standardization of abdominopelvic MDCT protocols. Abdom Radiol (NY). 2017;42(3):676–87.
63. Song JH, Chaudhry FS, Mayo-Smith WW. The incidental adrenal mass on CT: prevalence of adrenal disease in 1,049 consecutive adrenal masses in patients with no known malignancy. AJR Am J Roentgenol. 2008;190(5):1163–8.
64. Boland GW, Lee MJ, Gazelle GS, Halpern EF, McNicholas MM, Mueller PR. Characterization of adrenal masses using unenhanced CT: an analysis of the CT literature. AJR Am J Roentgenol. 1998;171(1):201–4.
65. Ho LM, Marin D, Neville AM, Barnhart HX, Gupta RT, Paulson EK, et al. Characterization of adrenal nodules with dual-energy CT: can virtual unenhanced attenuation values replace true unenhanced attenuation values? AJR Am J Roentgenol. 2012;198(4):840–5.
66. Gnannt R, Fischer M, Goetti R, Karlo C, Leschka S, Alkadhi H. Dual-energy CT for characterization of the incidental adrenal mass: preliminary observations. AJR Am J Roentgenol. 2012;198(1):138–44.
67. Botsikas D, Triponez F, Boudabbous S, Hansen C, Becker CD, Montet X. Incidental adrenal lesions detected on enhanced abdominal dual-energy CT: can the diagnostic workup be shortened by the implementation of virtual unenhanced images? Eur J Radiol. 2014;83(10):1746–51.
68. Helck A, Hummel N, Meinel FG, Johnson T, Nikolaou K, Graser A. Can single-phase dual-energy CT reliably identify adrenal adenomas? Eur Radiol. 2014;24(7):1636–42.
69. Connolly MJ, McInnes MDF, El-Khodary M, McGrath TA, Schieda N. Diagnostic accuracy of virtual non-contrast enhanced dual-energy CT for diagnosis of adrenal adenoma: a systematic review and meta-analysis. Eur Radiol. 2017;27(10):4324–35.
70. Mileto A, Nelson RC, Marin D, Roy Choudhury K, Ho LM. Dual-energy multidetector CT for the characterization of incidental adrenal nodules: diagnostic performance of contrast-enhanced material density analysis. Radiology. 2015;274(2):445–54.
71. Ju Y, Liu A, Dong Y, Liu Y, Wang H, Sun M, et al. The value of nonenhanced single-source dual-energy CT for differentiating metastases from adenoma in adrenal glands. Acad Radiol. 2015;22(7):834–9.
72. Martin SS, Weidinger S, Czwikla R, Kaltenbach B, Albrecht MH, Lenga L, et al. Iodine and fat quantification for differentiation of adrenal gland adenomas from metastases using third-generation dual-source dual-energy computed tomography. Investig Radiol. 2018;53(3):173–8.
73. Turk C, Petrik A, Sarica K, Seitz C, Skolarikos A, Straub M, et al. EAU guidelines on diagnosis and conservative management of urolithiasis. Eur Urol. 2016;69(3):468–74.
74. Ma Q, Fang L, Su R, Ma L, Xie G, Cheng Y. Uric acid stones, clinical manifestations and therapeutic considerations. Postgrad Med J. 2018;94(1114):458–62.
75. Nestler T, Nestler K, Neisius A, Isbarn H, Netsch C, Waldeck S, et al. Diagnostic accuracy of third-generation dual-source dual-energy CT: a prospective trial and protocol for clinical implementation. World J Urol. 2019;37(4):735–41.
76. Habashy D, Xia R, Ridley W, Chan L, Ridley L. Impact of dual energy characterization of urinary calculus on management. J Med Imaging Radiat Oncol. 2016;60(5):624–31.
77. Hidas G, Eliahou R, Duvdevani M, Coulon P, Lemaitre L, Gofrit ON, et al. Determination of renal stone composition with dual-energy CT: in vivo analysis and comparison with x-ray diffraction. Radiology. 2010;257(2):394–401.
78. Lombardo F, Bonatti M, Zamboni GA, Avesani G, Oberhofer N, Bonelli M, et al. Uric acid versus non-uric acid renal stones: in vivo differentiation with spectral CT. Clin Radiol. 2017;72(6):490–6.
79. Stolzmann P, Kozomara M, Chuck N, Muntener M, Leschka S, Scheffel H, et al. In vivo identification of uric acid stones with dual-energy CT: diagnostic performance evaluation in patients. Abdom Imaging. 2010;35(5):629–35.

80. Qu M, Ramirez-Giraldo JC, Leng S, Williams JC, Vrtiska TJ, Lieske JC, et al. Dual-energy dual-source CT with additional spectral filtration can improve the differentiation of non-uric acid renal stones: an ex vivo phantom study. AJR Am J Roentgenol. 2011;196(6):1279–87.
81. Leng S, Shiung M, Ai S, Qu M, Vrtiska TJ, Grant KL, et al. Feasibility of discriminating uric acid from non-uric acid renal stones using consecutive spatially registered low- and high-energy scans obtained on a conventional CT scanner. AJR Am J Roentgenol. 2015;204(1):92–7.
82. Zheng X, Liu Y, Li M, Wang Q, Song B. Dual-energy computed tomography for characterizing urinary calcified calculi and uric acid calculi: a meta-analysis. Eur J Radiol. 2016;85(10):1843–8.
83. Marcus RP, Fletcher JG, Ferrero A, Leng S, Halaweish AF, Gutjahr R, et al. Detection and characterization of renal stones by using photon-counting-based CT. Radiology. 2018;289: 436–42:180126
84. Franken A, Gevenois PA, Muylem AV, Howarth N, Keyzer C. In vivo differentiation of uric acid versus non-uric acid urinary calculi with third-generation dual-source dual-energy CT at reduced radiation dose. AJR Am J Roentgenol. 2018;210(2):358–63.
85. Boellaard TN, Henneman OD, Streekstra GJ, Venema HW, Nio CY, van Dorth-Rombouts MC, et al. The feasibility of colorectal cancer detection using dual-energy computed tomography with iodine mapping. Clin Radiol. 2013;68(8):799–806.
86. Schaeffer B, Johnson TR, Mang T, Kreis ME, Reiser MF, Graser A. Dual-energy CT colonography for preoperative "one-stop" staging in patients with colonic neoplasia. Acad Radiol. 2014;21(12):1567–72.
87. Gong HX, Zhang KB, Wu LM, Baigorri BF, Yin Y, Geng XC, et al. Dual energy spectral CT imaging for colorectal cancer grading: a preliminary study. PLoS One. 2016;11(2):e0147756.
88. Chuang-Bo Y, Tai-Ping H, Hai-Feng D, Yong-Jun J, Xi-Rong Z, Guang-Ming M, et al. Quantitative assessment of the degree of differentiation in colon cancer with dual-energy spectral CT. Abdom Radiol (NY). 2017;42(11):2591–6.
89. Potretzke TA, Brace CL, Lubner MG, Sampson LA, Willey BJ, Lee FT Jr. Early small-bowel ischemia: dual-energy CT improves conspicuity compared with conventional CT in a swine model. Radiology. 2015;275(1):119–26.
90. Darras KE, McLaughlin PD, Kang H, Black B, Walshe T, Chang SD, et al. Virtual monoenergetic reconstruction of contrast-enhanced dual energy CT at 70keV maximizes mural enhancement in acute small bowel obstruction. Eur J Radiol. 2016;85(5):950–6.
91. Lourenco PDM, Rawski R, Mohammed MF, Khosa F, Nicolaou S, McLaughlin P. Dual-energy CT iodine mapping and 40-keV monoenergetic applications in the diagnosis of acute bowel ischemia. AJR Am J Roentgenol. 2018;211(3):564–70.
92. Villanueva Campos AM, Tardaguila de la Fuente G, Utrera Perez E, Jurado Basildo C, Mera Fernandez D, Martinez Rodriguez C. Value of dual-energy CT enterography in the analysis of pathological bowel segments in patients with Crohn's disease. Radiologia. 2018;60(3):223–9.
93. De Kock I, Delrue L, Lecluyse C, Hindryckx P, De Vos M, Villeirs G. Feasibility study using iodine quantification on dual-energy CT enterography to distinguish normal small bowel from active inflammatory Crohn's disease. Acta Radiol. 2019;60(6):679–86.
94. Lee SM, Kim SH, Ahn SJ, Kang HJ, Kang JH, Han JK. Virtual monoenergetic dual-layer, dual-energy CT enterography: optimization of keV settings and its added value for Crohn's disease. Eur Radiol. 2018;28(6):2525–34.
95. Hyodo T, Hori M, Lamb P, Sasaki K, Wakayama T, Chiba Y, et al. Multimaterial decomposition algorithm for the quantification of liver fat content by using fast-kilovolt-peak switching dual-energy CT: experimental validation. Radiology. 2017;282(2):381–9.
96. Cao Q, Shang S, Han X, Cao D, Zhao L. Evaluation on heterogeneity of fatty liver in rats: a multiparameter quantitative analysis by dual energy CT. Acad Radiol. 2019;26(5):e47–e55.
97. McNamara MM, Little MD, Alexander LF, Carroll LV, Beasley TM, Morgan DE. Multireader evaluation of lesion conspicuity in small pancreatic adenocarcinomas: complimentary value of iodine material density and low keV simulated monoenergetic images using multiphasic rapid kVp-switching dual energy CT. Abdom Imaging. 2015;40(5):1230–40.
98. Patel BN, Thomas JV, Lockhart ME, Berland LL, Morgan DE. Single-source dual-energy spectral multidetector CT of pancreatic adenocarcinoma: optimization of energy level viewing significantly increases lesion contrast. Clin Radiol. 2013;68(2):148–54.
99. Lin XZ, Wu ZY, Tao R, Guo Y, Li JY, Zhang J, et al. Dual energy spectral CT imaging of insulinoma-value in preoperative diagnosis compared with conventional multi-detector CT. Eur J Radiol. 2012;81(10):2487–94.
100. Parakh A, Patino M, Muenzel D, Kambadakone A, Sahani DV. Role of rapid kV-switching dual-energy CT in assessment of post-surgical local recurrence of pancreatic adenocarcinoma. Abdom Radiol (NY). 2018;43(2):497–504.
101. Shuman WP, Green DE, Busey JM, Mitsumori LM, Choi E, Koprowicz KM, et al. Dual-energy liver CT: effect of monochromatic imaging on lesion detection, conspicuity, and contrast-to-noise ratio of hypervascular lesions on late arterial phase. AJR Am J Roentgenol. 2014;203(3):601–6.
102. Ascenti G, Sofia C, Mazziotti S, Silipigni S, D'Angelo T, Pergolizzi S, et al. Dual-energy CT with iodine quantification in distinguishing between bland and neoplastic portal vein thrombosis in

patients with hepatocellular carcinoma. Clin Radiol. 2016;71(9):938 e1–9.

103. Marin D, Davis D, Roy Choudhury K, Patel B, Gupta RT, Mileto A, et al. Characterization of small focal renal lesions: diagnostic accuracy with single-phase contrast-enhanced dual-energy CT with material attenuation analysis compared with conventional attenuation measurements. Radiology. 2017;284(3):737–47.
104. Hou WS, Wu HW, Yin Y, Cheng JJ, Zhang Q, Xu JR. Differentiation of lung cancers from inflammatory masses with dual-energy spectral CT imaging. Acad Radiol. 2015;22(3):337–44.
105. Chang S, Hur J, Im DJ, Suh YJ, Hong YJ, Lee HJ, et al. Dual-energy CT-based iodine quantification for differentiating pulmonary artery sarcoma from pulmonary thromboembolism: a pilot study. Eur Radiol. 2016;26(9):3162–70.
106. Lee SH, Hur J, Kim YJ, Lee HJ, Hong YJ, Choi BW. Additional value of dual-energy CT to differentiate between benign and malignant mediastinal tumors: an initial experience. Eur J Radiol. 2013;82(11):2043–9.
107. Li X, Meng X, Ye Z. Iodine quantification to characterize primary lesions, metastatic and non-metastatic lymph nodes in lung cancers by dual energy computed tomography: an initial experience. Eur J Radiol. 2016;85(6):1219–23.
108. Rizzo S, Radice D, Femia M, De Marco P, Origgi D, Preda L, et al. Metastatic and non-metastatic lymph nodes: quantification and different distribution of iodine uptake assessed by dual-energy CT. Eur Radiol. 2018;28(2):760–9.
109. Jiang C, Yang P, Lei J, Li J, Yan K, Li F, et al. The application of iodine quantitative information obtained by dual-source dual-energy computed tomography on chemoradiotherapy effect monitoring for cervical cancer: a preliminary study. J Comput Assist Tomogr. 2017;41(5):737–45.
110. Ren Y, Jiao Y, Ge W, Zhang L, Hua Y, Li C, et al. Dual-energy computed tomography-based iodine quantitation for response evaluation of lung cancers to chemoradiotherapy/radiotherapy: a comparison with fluorine-18 fluorodeoxyglucose positron emission tomography/computed tomography-based positron emission tomography/computed tomography response evaluation criterion in solid tumors. J Comput Assist Tomogr. 2018;42(4):614–22.
111. Aoki M, Hirose K, Sato M, Akimoto H, Kawaguchi H, Hatayama Y, et al. Prognostic impact of average iodine density assessed by dual-energy spectral imaging for predicting lung tumor recurrence after stereotactic body radiotherapy. J Radiat Res. 2016;57(4):381–6.
112. Kim YN, Lee HY, Lee KS, Seo JB, Chung MJ, Ahn MJ, et al. Dual-energy CT in patients treated with anti-angiogenic agents for non-small cell lung cancer: new method of monitoring tumor response? Korean J Radiol. 2012;13(6):702–10.
113. Baxa J, Matouskova T, Krakorova G, Schmidt B, Flohr T, Sedlmair M, et al. Dual-phase dual-energy CT in patients treated with erlotinib for advanced non-small cell lung cancer: possible benefits of iodine quantification in response assessment. Eur Radiol. 2016;26(8):2828–36.
114. Hellbach K, Sterzik A, Sommer W, Karpitschka M, Hummel N, Casuscelli J, et al. Dual energy CT allows for improved characterization of response to antiangiogenic treatment in patients with metastatic renal cell cancer. Eur Radiol. 2017;27(6):2532–7.
115. Meyer M, Hohenberger P, Apfaltrer P, Henzler T, Dinter DJ, Schoenberg SO, et al. CT-based response assessment of advanced gastrointestinal stromal tumor: dual energy CT provides a more predictive imaging biomarker of clinical benefit than RECIST or Choi criteria. Eur J Radiol. 2013;82(6):923–8.
116. Li J, Fang M, Wang R, Dong D, Tian J, Liang P, et al. Diagnostic accuracy of dual-energy CT-based nomograms to predict lymph node metastasis in gastric cancer. Eur Radiol. 2018;28:5241–9.
117. Shimamoto H, Iwano S, Umakoshi H, Kawaguchi K, Naganawa S. Evaluation of locoregional invasiveness of small-sized non-small cell lung cancers by enhanced dual-energy computed tomography. Cancer Imaging. 2016;16(1):18.
118. Li GJ, Gao J, Wang GL, Zhang CQ, Shi H, Deng K. Correlation between vascular endothelial growth factor and quantitative dual-energy spectral CT in non-small-cell lung cancer. Clin Radiol. 2016;71(4):363–8.
119. Pache G, Krauss B, Strohm P, Saueressig U, Blanke P, Bulla S, et al. Dual-energy CT virtual noncalcium technique: detecting posttraumatic bone marrow lesions – feasibility study. Radiology. 2010;256(2):617–24.
120. Guggenberger R, Gnannt R, Hodler J, Krauss B, Wanner GA, Csuka E, et al. Diagnostic performance of dual-energy CT for the detection of traumatic bone marrow lesions in the ankle: comparison with MR imaging. Radiology. 2012;264(1):164–73.
121. Bierry G, Venkatasamy A, Kremer S, Dosch JC, Dietemann JL. Dual-energy CT in vertebral compression fractures: performance of visual and quantitative analysis for bone marrow edema demonstration with comparison to MRI. Skelet Radiol. 2014;43(4):485–92.
122. Suh CH, Yun SJ, Jin W, Lee SH, Park SY, Ryu CW. Diagnostic performance of dual-energy CT for the detection of bone marrow oedema: a systematic review and meta-analysis. Eur Radiol. 2018;28:4182–94.
123. Diekhoff T, Engelhard N, Fuchs M, Pumberger M, Putzier M, Mews J, et al. Single-source dual-energy computed tomography for the assessment of bone marrow oedema in vertebral compression fractures: a prospective diagnostic accuracy study. Eur Radiol. 2019;29(1):31–9.
124. Kaup M, Wichmann JL, Scholtz JE, Beeres M, Kromen W, Albrecht MH, et al. Dual-energy

CT-based display of bone marrow edema in osteoporotic vertebral compression fractures: impact on diagnostic accuracy of radiologists with varying levels of experience in correlation to MR imaging. Radiology. 2016;280(2):510–9.
125. Mallinson PI, Coupal TM, McLaughlin PD, Nicolaou S, Munk PL, Ouellette HA. Dual-energy CT for the musculoskeletal system. Radiology. 2016;281(3):690–707.
126. Glazebrook KN, Guimaraes LS, Murthy NS, Black DF, Bongartz T, Manek NJ, et al. Identification of intraarticular and periarticular uric acid crystals with dual-energy CT: initial evaluation. Radiology. 2011;261(2):516–24.
127. Bongartz T, Glazebrook KN, Kavros SJ, Murthy NS, Merry SP, Franz WB 3rd, et al. Dual-energy CT for the diagnosis of gout: an accuracy and diagnostic yield study. Ann Rheum Dis. 2015;74(6):1072–7.
128. Yu Z, Mao T, Xu Y, Li T, Wang Y, Gao F, et al. Diagnostic accuracy of dual-energy CT in gout: a systematic review and meta-analysis. Skelet Radiol. 2018;47:1587–93.
129. Ramon A, Bohm-Sigrand A, Pottecher P, Richette P, Maillefert JF, Devilliers H, et al. Role of dual-energy CT in the diagnosis and follow-up of gout: systematic analysis of the literature. Clin Rheumatol. 2018;37(3):587–95.
130. Mallinson PI, Coupal T, Reisinger C, Chou H, Munk PL, Nicolaou S, et al. Artifacts in dual-energy CT gout protocol: a review of 50 suspected cases with an artifact identification guide. AJR Am J Roentgenol. 2014;203(1):W103–9.
131. Pagniez J, Legrand L, Khung S, Faivre JB, Duhamel A, Krauss A, et al. Metal artifact reduction on chest computed tomography examinations: comparison of the iterative metallic artefact reduction algorithm and the monoenergetic approach. J Comput Assist Tomogr. 2017;41(3):446–54.
132. Laukamp KR, Lennartz S, Neuhaus VF, Grosse Hokamp N, Rau R, Le Blanc M, et al. CT metal artifacts in patients with total hip replacements: for artifact reduction monoenergetic reconstructions and post-processing algorithms are both efficient but not similar. Eur Radiol. 2018;28:4524–33.
133. Wang Y, Qian B, Li B, Qin G, Zhou Z, Qiu Y, et al. Metal artifacts reduction using monochromatic images from spectral CT: evaluation of pedicle screws in patients with scoliosis. Eur J Radiol. 2013;82(8):e360–6.
134. Guggenberger R, Winklhofer S, Osterhoff G, Wanner GA, Fortunati M, Andreisek G, et al. Metallic artefact reduction with monoenergetic dual-energy CT: systematic ex vivo evaluation of posterior spinal fusion implants from various vendors and different spine levels. Eur Radiol. 2012;22(11):2357–64.
135. Bamberg F, Dierks A, Nikolaou K, Reiser MF, Becker CR, Johnson TR. Metal artifact reduction by dual energy computed tomography using monoenergetic extrapolation. Eur Radiol. 2011;21(7):1424–9.
136. Grosse Hokamp N, Laukamp KR, Lennartz S, Zopfs D, Abdullayev N, Neuhaus VF, et al. Artifact reduction from dental implants using virtual monoenergetic reconstructions from novel spectral detector CT. Eur J Radiol. 2018;104:136–42.
137. Kuchenbecker S, Faby S, Sawall S, Lell M, Kachelriess M. Dual energy CT: how well can pseudo-monochromatic imaging reduce metal artifacts? Med Phys. 2015;42(2):1023–36.
138. Kidoh M, Utsunomiya D, Oda S, Nakaura T, Funama Y, Yuki H, et al. CT venography after knee replacement surgery: comparison of dual-energy CT-based monochromatic imaging and single-energy metal artifact reduction techniques on a 320-row CT scanner. Acta Radiol Open. 2017;6(2):2058460117693463.
139. Cha J, Kim HJ, Kim ST, Kim YK, Kim HY, Park GM. Dual-energy CT with virtual monochromatic images and metal artifact reduction software for reducing metallic dental artifacts. Acta Radiol. 2017;58(11):1312–9.
140. Winklhofer S, Hinzpeter R, Stocker D, Baltsavias G, Michels L, Burkhardt JK, et al. Combining monoenergetic extrapolations from dual-energy CT with iterative reconstructions: reduction of coil and clip artifacts from intracranial aneurysm therapy. Neuroradiology. 2018;60(3):281–91.
141. Yue D, Fan Rong C, Ning C, Liang H, Ai Lian L, Ru Xin W, et al. Reduction of metal artifacts from unilateral hip arthroplasty on dual-energy CT with metal artifact reduction software. Acta Radiol. 2018;59(7):853–60.
142. Borhani AA, Kulzer M, Iranpour N, Ghodadra A, Sparrow M, Furlan A, et al. Comparison of true unenhanced and virtual unenhanced (VUE) attenuation values in abdominopelvic single-source rapid kilovoltage-switching spectral CT. Abdom Radiol (NY). 2017;42(3):710–7.
143. Durieux P, Gevenois PA, Muylem AV, Howarth N, Keyzer C. Abdominal attenuation values on virtual and true unenhanced images obtained with third-generation dual-source dual-energy CT. AJR Am J Roentgenol. 2018;210(5):1042–58.
144. Obmann MM, Kelsch V, Cosentino A, Hofmann V, Boll DT, Benz MR. Interscanner and intrascanner comparison of virtual unenhanced attenuation values derived from twin beam dual-energy and dual-source, dual-energy computed tomography. Invest Radiol. 2019;54(1):1–6.
145. Jacobsen MC, Schellingerhout D, Wood CA, Tamm EP, Godoy MC, Sun J, et al. Intermanufacturer comparison of dual-energy CT iodine quantification and monochromatic attenuation: a phantom study. Radiology. 2018;287(1):224–34.
146. Euler A, Solomon J, Mazurowski MA, Samei E, Nelson RC. How accurate and precise are CT based measurements of iodine concentration? A comparison of the minimum detectable concentration difference among single source and dual source dual energy CT in a phantom study. Eur Radiol. 2019;29(4):2069–78.

147. Kang MJ, Park CM, Lee CH, Goo JM, Lee HJ. Focal iodine defects on color-coded iodine perfusion maps of dual-energy pulmonary CT angiography images: a potential diagnostic pitfall. AJR Am J Roentgenol. 2010;195(5):W325–30.
148. Wortman JR, Sodickson AD. Pearls, pitfalls, and problems in dual-energy computed tomography imaging of the body. Radiol Clin N Am. 2018;56(4):625–40.
149. Moon JW, Park BK, Kim CK, Park SY. Evaluation of virtual unenhanced CT obtained from dual-energy CT urography for detecting urinary stones. Br J Radiol. 2012;85(1014):e176–81.
150. Mangold S, Thomas C, Fenchel M, Vuust M, Krauss B, Ketelsen D, et al. Virtual nonenhanced dual-energy CT urography with tin-filter technology: determinants of detection of urinary calculi in the renal collecting system. Radiology. 2012;264(1):119–25.
151. Sahni VA, Shinagare AB, Silverman SG. Virtual unenhanced CT images acquired from dual-energy CT urography: accuracy of attenuation values and variation with contrast material phase. Clin Radiol. 2013;68(3):264–71.

14 Future Prospects of Spectral CT: Photon Counting

Taly Gilat Schmidt

How Photon-Counting Detectors Differ from Conventional CT Detectors

Conventional CT Detectors: Indirect Conversion and Energy Integration

The basic functionality of a conventional CT detector and a photon-counting detector is illustrated in Fig. 14.1. Conventional CT detectors detect photons by a two-step process known as an indirect conversion process. Photons are absorbed in a high-attenuating, scintillating material that converts X-ray photons to light photons. Light photons disperse throughout the scintillator and are randomly reflected until they are absorbed by the photodiode, where they are converted to an electrical voltage. Each photon creates a signal whose amplitude is theoretically proportional to its energy. However, there are many statistical uncertainties and inefficiencies in the conversion from X-ray to light photons and from light photons to electrical signal. These inefficiencies and uncertainties introduce variations in the detected signal for a given photon energy, causing indirect-conversion detectors to have poor energy resolution [1]. The readout electronics in a conventional CT detector integrate the signal generated by the photodiode during the readout time, thereby combining the signals from the millions of photons detected during a measurement period. Conventional CT detectors are thus referred to as energy-integrating detectors. Information about the energy deposited by each detected photon is lost during this integration process. Pixels in conventional CT detectors are separated by reflecting material to prevent the light from spreading between pixels. This reflective material constitutes dead space on the detector, causing a loss of dose efficiency.

T. G. Schmidt (✉)
Department of Biomedical Engineering, Marquette University and Medical College of Wisconsin, Milwaukee, WI, USA
e-mail: tal.gilat-schmidt@marquette.edu

Photon-Counting CT (PCCT): Direct Conversion and Pulse-Height Analysis

Photon-counting detectors are made from a semiconductor material that converts the absorbed photon energy to electrical charge, known as direct-conversion detection. [1] A high-voltage bias is applied between electrodes across the semiconductor. The resulting electric field causes the charge carriers to be collected at the electrodes. The readout electronics consist of an amplifier, pulse shaper, and a series of comparator channels with digital counters. Ideally, the readout electronics generate a pulse for each absorbed photon, with pulse height proportional to the absorbed photon energy. The readout

© Springer Nature Switzerland AG 2020

E. Samei, N. J. Pelc (eds.), *Computed Tomography*, https://doi.org/10.1007/978-3-030-26957-9_14

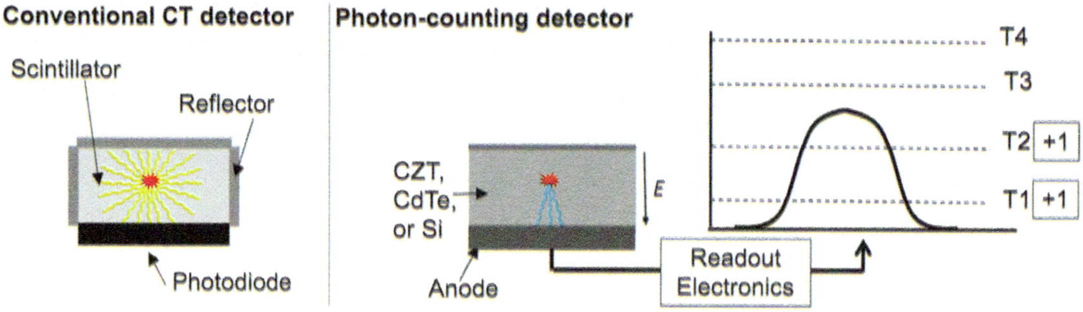

Fig. 14.1 (Left) Illustration of the operation of a conventional CT detector, where the absorbed photon energy is converted to light by the scintillator. Some of the light photons travel toward the photodiode, where they are converted to electrical charge. (Right) Illustration of the operation of a photon-counting detector, where the absorbed photon energy is converted to charge carriers, which are steered toward the anode by the applied electric field. The readout electronics generate a pulse that is proportional to the deposited energy. The readout electronics contain a series of comparator channels, each with a set threshold level. Each channel increments a counter if the pulse height is above the channel threshold level

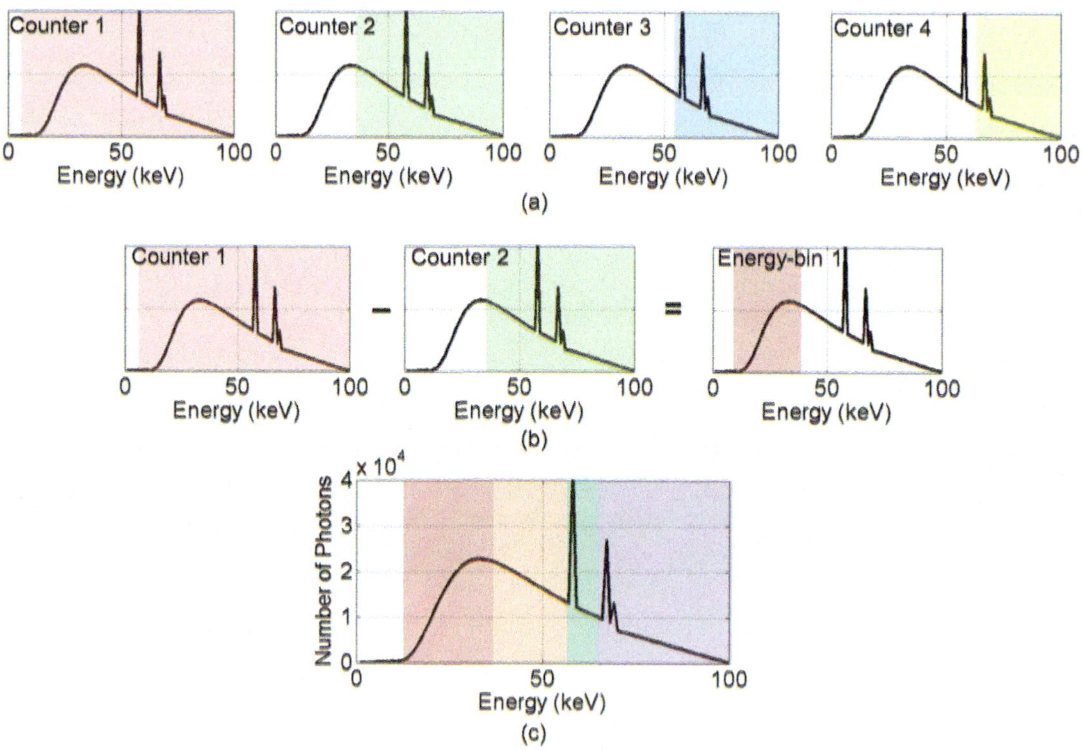

Fig. 14.2 Illustration of the spectral acquisition performed by photon-counting detectors. (**a**) The portion of the spectra acquired by each channel, where each channel measures the number of photons counted above the channel's set energy threshold level. (**b**) The counts measured by consecutive channels can be subtracted to calculate the number of photons counted with energy between the threshold levels of the two channels, forming an "energy-bin" measurement. (**c**) The four spectral measurements acquired by an ideal photon-counting detector with four comparator channels

electronics of each pixel contain a set of comparator circuits each with a set threshold level. Each comparator channel increments a counter if the height of the pulse is above the set threshold. At the end of the readout time, each channel measurement is the number of photons detected with energy above the set threshold level, as illustrated in Fig. 14.2.

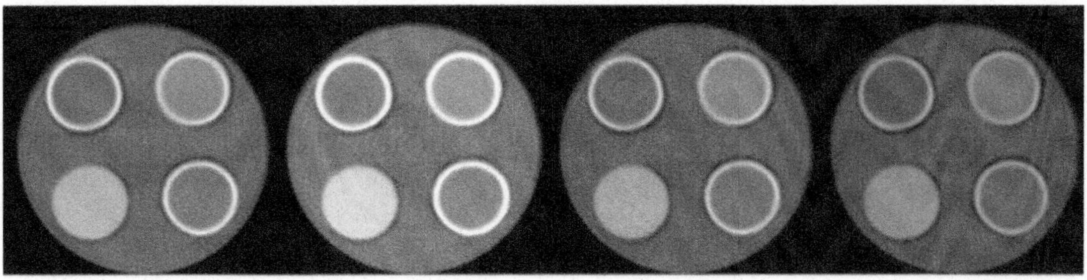

Fig. 14.3 Images of a phantom reconstructed from a benchtop PCCT system with three comparator channels, displayed at the same window/level settings. The photon-counting image on the left is the result of reconstructing all counts detected above the lowest energy threshold, which is similar to a conventional CT image. The images reconstructed from each of the three energy bins are also displayed, demonstrating higher CT numbers and higher contrast in the lower energy bins

The number of photons detected between two energy thresholds, referred to as an energy bin in this chapter, can be calculated by subtracting the counts detected in consecutive channels, as illustrated in Fig. 14.2. In this way, photon-counting detectors can simultaneously acquire multiple spectral measurements that ideally correspond to separated energy bins. The number of energy-bin measurements acquired simultaneously is equal to the number of comparator channels per pixel. Because the photons are converted to charge directly, reflectors are not needed between pixels. Direct-conversion semiconductor detectors produce more signal carriers (electron-hole pairs) per photon than the signal carriers produced by indirect-conversion scintillating detectors [1]. The larger number of signal carriers reduces the variation in the pulse height generated for each detected photon, thus providing improved energy resolution compared to indirect-conversion detectors.

Cadmium zinc telluride (CZT) and cadmium telluride (CdTe) are examples of semiconductors with high atomic number used for PCCT [2–4]. The high atomic number provides high photon stopping power, so that small thicknesses of the sensor can be used (2–3 mm). Silicon photon-counting detectors have also been developed for X-ray and CT imaging [5]. Silicon has low photon stopping power due to its low atomic number; therefore the pixel must have large depth (e.g., 3 cm).

The number of counts detected above the lowest threshold setting can be reconstructed to form a nonspectral CT image that is very similar to a conventional CT image, as shown in Fig. 14.3. Throughout this chapter, this nonspectral image is referred to as the photon-counting image. The counts data acquired in each energy bin can be reconstructed separately to create energy-bin images, as shown in Fig. 14.3. Figure 14.3 demonstrates the higher contrast in the lower-energy-bin images. The energy-bin data can be combined before or after reconstruction to create an improved nonspectral CT image or to perform material decomposition.

Advantages of Photon-Counting CT Compared to Conventional Spectral CT Approaches

Photon-counting detectors provide several potential advantages for both conventional (non-spectral) CT acquisition and for spectral CT acquisition.

Reduction of electronic noise Electronic noise, which is additive Gaussian noise introduced by the detector electronics, occurs in every X-ray detector measurement in addition to photon noise. Figure 14.4 demonstrates an example of the analog signal measured by a detector, with and without electronic noise (Fig. 14.4). In a conventional CT detector, all electronic noise contributes to the final measurement because the signal is integrated across the readout time. When the overall detected flux is low, for example, in low-dose acquisitions, acquisitions of large patients, or with very small pixels, the impact of electronic noise on the final CT image can be significant [6]. Photon-counting detectors can

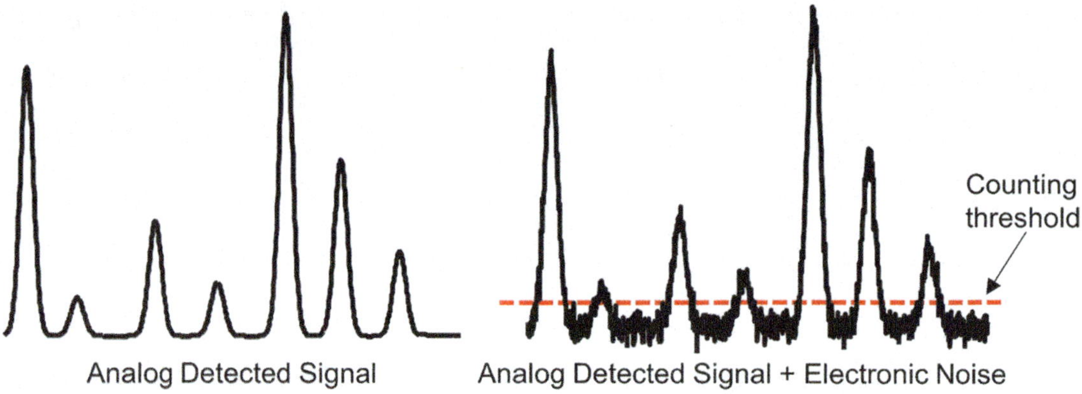

Fig. 14.4 Generated signal (left) without and (right) with electronic noise, where each pulse corresponds to the energy deposited by a photon absorption event. Photon-counting detectors can reject most of the electronic noise by setting the lowest energy threshold above the expected electronic noise signal, as demonstrated by the red dashed line

reject much of the electronic noise by setting the lowest threshold level higher than the majority of electronic noise signal [7], as shown in Fig. 14.4. However, this low threshold also reduces the detector efficiency by rejecting real photon events that register below the threshold, either due to low photon energy or due to low-energy tailing effects to be described in section "Flux-Independent Spectral Degradations". Electronic noise detected above the lowest photon-counting threshold causes uncertainty in the pulse height generated by the photon, thereby impacting the energy resolution of the photon-counting detector.

Improved spatial resolution If pixel sizes are reduced to improve spatial resolution in conventional CT detectors, the proportion of dead space due to reflectors increases, thus reducing the detective quantum efficiency (DQE). Since photon-counting detectors do not have dead space due to reflectors, the pixel size can be decreased without this dose efficiency penalty. The electronic noise reduction property of photon-counting detectors further enables detectors with smaller pixels.

Improved detective quantum efficiency (DQE) The lack of dead space in photon-counting detectors is one reason for increased DQE compared to conventional CT detectors. Reduced noise aliasing due to smaller pixel sizes provides an additional DQE improvement [8]. Improved weighting of the signal carried by the photons also increases DQE [9]. Conventional CT detectors integrate the energy of absorbed photons, thereby giving more weight to the higher-energy photons with less contrast information and resulting in reduced DQE. Photon-counting detectors improve the DQE, as photons at all energies are weighted equally. Ideally, each photon would be weighted based on its information content, for example, giving more weight to the lower-energy photons [9], as illustrated in Fig. 14.5. Optimal methods for weighting the energy-bin data in PCCT have been developed and demonstrated to improve the contrast-to-noise ratio [9–11].

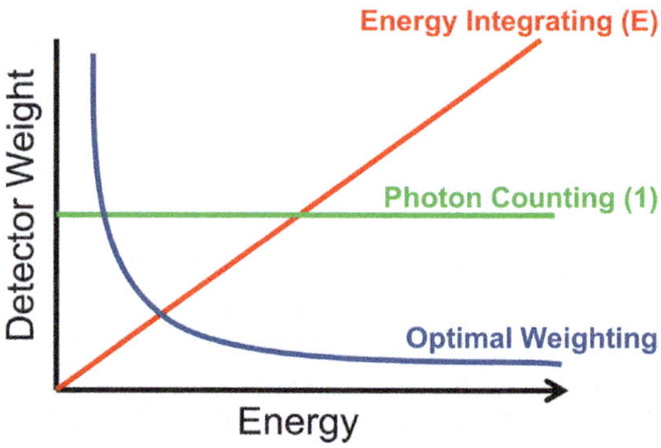

Fig. 14.5 Illustration of how photons of different energies are weighted during detection. By integrating the detected signal, conventional CT detectors weight each photon by its energy. By counting all photons, photon-counting detectors weight photons at all energies equally. Optimal weighting of the photons gives the highest weight to the lower-energy photons, thereby improving DQE [9]

Perfect spatial registration of spectral measurements In a photon-counting detector, the multiple spectral measurements for each ray are acquired at the same time and thus are perfectly registered. This advantage is also true for multilayer detector spectral CT systems, but is not true for dual-kV systems.

Spectral information acquired as part of conventional CT protocol Photon-counting detectors acquire the spectral energy-bin data while also acquiring a nonspectral CT image from the total number of counted photons. Because the energy bins are always acquired, the decision to use the spectral information can be determined after acquisition. This advantage is also true for multilayer detector spectral CT.

Acquisition of more than two spectral measurements Photon-counting detectors can acquire more than two spectral measurements simultaneously, as compared to clinical spectral CT systems that use two tube voltage settings or a dual-layer spectral detector. The number of spectral measurements depends on the number of comparator channels per pixel. Some photon-counting detector designs acquire more spectral measurements than comparator channels by varying the thresholds across subpixels (e.g., checkerboard detectors [12]); however this incurs a substantial noise penalty [13].

Theoretically improved spectral separation The two spectra acquired by dual-kV or dual-layer spectral CT systems overlap in energy, although beam filtration has been used in dual-source spectral CT systems to reduce overlap [14]. Photon-counting detectors ideally acquire spectral measurements in separated energy bins, as illustrated in Fig. 14.2. Since spectral overlap between measurements reduces the dose efficiency of spectral CT systems [14], photon-counting detectors have the potential to improve dose efficiency. In practice, the pulse height generated by a photon-counting detector does not always correctly represent the true photon energy, thus introducing overlap between energy-bin spectra and limiting this potential benefit of PCCT, as will be discussed in section "Challenges and Limitations of Photon-Counting CT".

Figure 14.6 demonstrates how improved spectral separation and an increased number of spectral

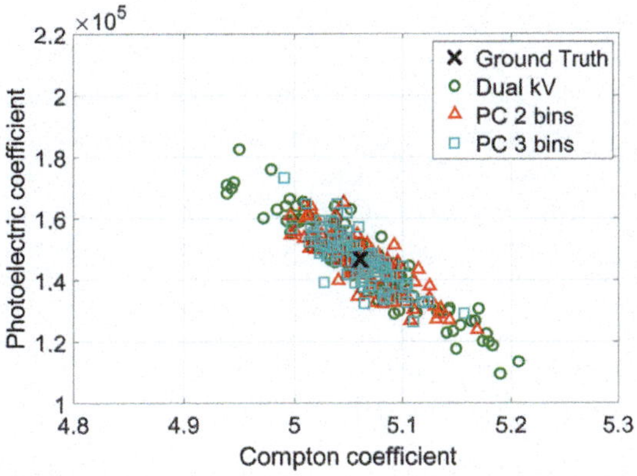

Fig. 14.6 Material decomposition coefficients for 30-cm thickness of water estimated from simulated dual-kV measurements (80 kV and 140 kV without extra filtration), ideal photon-counting measurements with two energy bins ([20–56], [56–120] keV), and ideal photon-counting measurements with three energy bins ([20–50], [50–66], [66–120] keV) all at equal dose. Each marker represents the basis coefficients estimated from one simulated trial. The photon-counting measurements estimate the same mean coefficients as dual-kV but with reduced noise

measurements can improve the dose efficiency of PCCT material decomposition compared to dual-energy CT. The transmission of X-rays through 30 cm of water was simulated for a dual-energy acquisition and an ideal photon-counting acquisition with two energy bins and three energy bins. Material decomposition into photoelectric and Compton basis functions was performed using a maximum likelihood estimator [15]. As seen in Fig. 14.6, the dual-kV and ideal photon-counting methods accurately estimate the mean material decomposition estimates. The ideal photon-counting acquisition with two energy bins reduced the noise in the material decomposition estimates by 40% compared to the dual-kV acquisition, due to improved spectral separation. Noise was reduced by an additional 10–15% when using three photon-counting spectral measurements.

Overall, the benefits of photon-counting detectors can potentially improve the quality of conventional (nonspectral) CT images, by providing images with reduced noise and/or dose, improved contrast-to-noise ratio, and improved spatial resolution. PCCT can potentially provide material decomposition images with higher dose efficiency (less noise and/or less dose) than conventional spectral CT. By acquiring more than two spectral measurements, PCCT can perform material decomposition to identify and quantify K-edge contrast agents, including differentiating multiple contrast agents. The potential and demonstrated impact of PCCT on clinical applications will be described in more detail and with examples in section "Overcoming the Challenges of PCCT".

Challenges and Limitations of Photon-Counting CT

Photon-counting detectors acquire spectral measurements in separated energy bins only if the pulse height of each detected photon represents the true photon energy and only if the pulses generated by different photons can be resolved in time. In practice, there are many nonideal effects that cause photons to be detected at incorrect energies or to not be detected at all. These nonideal effects can be categorized as spectral degradations that are independent of the flux and spectral degradations that are flux dependent.

Flux-Independent Spectral Degradations

The detector spectral response functions can be represented as the probability of a photon with energy E being detected at energy E'. For an ideal detector, the response functions look like impulse functions (Fig. 14.7), because the probability of a photon being detected at its true energy is 1. Figure 14.7 illustrates the spectral response functions of an example photon-counting detector with 0.38 × 1.6 mm pixels and 3-mm sensor thickness [2] and an example photon-counting detector with 1.0 × 1.4 mm pixels with 1-mm sensor thickness [16], where a photon has a relatively high probability of being detected as having incorrect energy.

When a photon is absorbed in the semiconductor material, the number of generated charge carriers is stochastic. This effect, along with electronic noise, causes the spectral response functions to have a Gaussian shape around the true photon energy as illustrated in Fig. 14.7.

If the photon absorption event occurs near the edge of a pixel, the charge cloud may spread across multiple pixels, as illustrated in Fig. 14.8. When charge sharing occurs, the photon is detected as multiple pulses in the true and neighboring pixels, with each detected pulse having lower energy than the true photon absorption event [17]. Charge sharing causes many photons to be erroneously detected in low energy bins, resulting in the low-energy tail in the spectral response functions (Fig. 14.7), while also introducing noise correlations and blurring across pixels. Charge sharing effects increase as pixel size decreases and as sensor thickness increases, which is demonstrated by the higher contribution of low-energy tails in Fig. 14.7b compared to Fig. 14.7c.

In photon-counting detectors made of semiconductors with high atomic number, such as cadmium and telluride, photons are absorbed primarily by the photoelectric effect. The secondary fluorescent

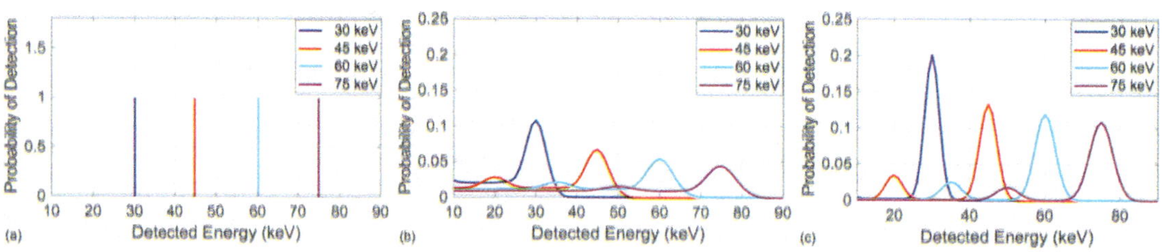

Fig. 14.7 Spectral response functions representing the probability of a photon being detected at different energies, plotted for photons with true energies of 30 keV, 45 keV, 60 keV, and 75 keV. Response functions are plotted for (**a**) an ideal photon-counting detector, where each photon has a probability of one of being detected at its true energy, (**b**) an example photon-counting detector [2] with 0.38 × 1.6 mm pixels and 3-mm sensor thickness, and (**c**) an example photon-counting detector [16] with 1.0 × 1.4 mm pixels and 1-mm sensor thickness. Plots (**b**, **c**) demonstrate that in realistic photon-counting detectors, photons have a non-zero probability of being detected at an incorrect energy and that the low-energy tail due to charge sharing is greater for smaller pixels, as shown in (**b**)

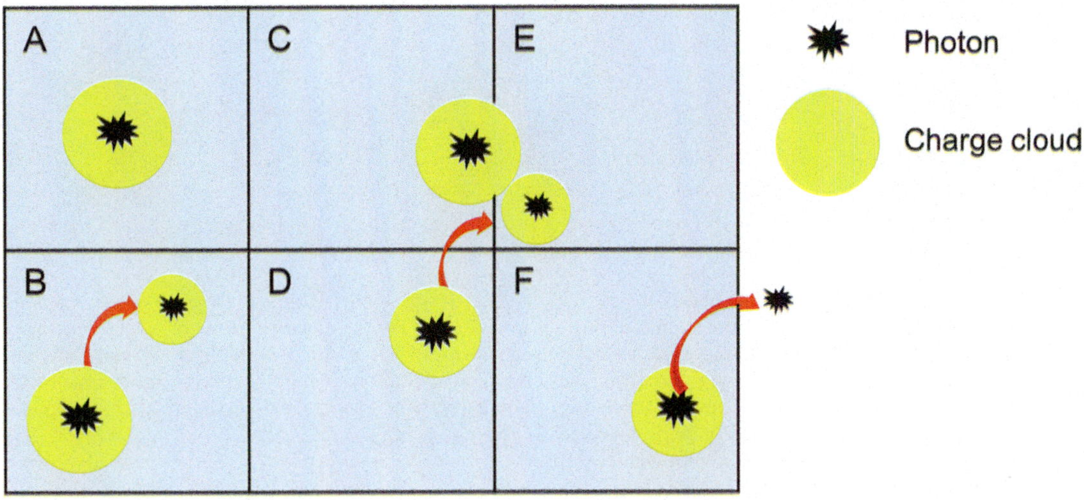

Fig. 14.8 Illustration of the flux-independent effects that degrade the spectral response of photon-counting detectors. Pixel A detects the correct photon energy, as the charge cloud is contained in the pixel. Pixel B detects the correct photon energy because the secondary photon (characteristic K-escape photon for CdTe/CZT or Compton scattered photon for silicon) is reabsorbed in the pixel. Pixel C detects the photon at an erroneously low energy because the charge cloud spreads to pixel E. Pixel D detects the primary photon at an erroneously low energy because the secondary or scattered photon travels to Pixel E. Pixel E erroneously counts photons due to charge sharing from Pixel C and absorption of a secondary or scattered photon emitted from Pixel D. Pixel F detects the photon at an erroneously low energy, because the emitted secondary or scattered photon leaves the detector

X-rays emitted during photoelectric absorption have sufficient energy to escape the pixel volume [18]. For silicon detectors, scattered photons produced by Compton interactions have sufficient energy to escape the pixel volume. Possible detection scenarios are illustrated in Fig. 14.8. Both fluorescent and scattered photons may be reabsorbed in the correct pixel, in which case the photon energy is correctly detected. If fluorescent or scattered photons travel outside of the pixel, the original photon is detected as having an erroneously low energy. If the fluorescent or scattered photon is absorbed in a neighboring pixel, the neighboring pixel detects an erroneous count and has increased correlation to the neighboring pixel.

The net effect of the flux-independent spectral degradations is that photons are detected in the incorrect energy bins, typically with high-energy photons detected at lower energy bins. As shown in Fig. 14.9, the nonideal spectral response functions cause overlap between the spectra contributing to each energy bins, thus reducing dose efficiency.

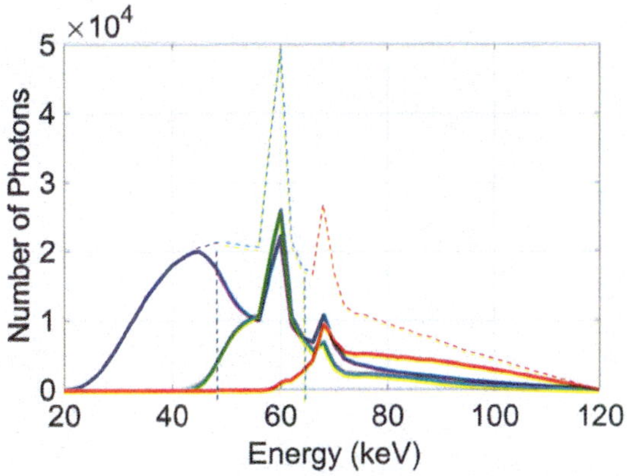

Fig. 14.9 The spectra of photons detected in a low (blue), medium (green), and high (red) energy bin of an ideal photon-counting detector (dashed lines) and for a photon-counting detector with example spectral response functions shown in Fig. 14.7b (solid lines)

Figure 14.10 demonstrates the effects of flux-independent spectral degradations on material decomposition estimates for the simulated example first presented in Fig. 14.6. The nonideal photon-counting detector spectral response introduces a large bias in the material decomposition estimates if the spectral response is not accounted for during material decomposition. Figure 14.10 also shows that accurate modeling of the detector spectral response removes the

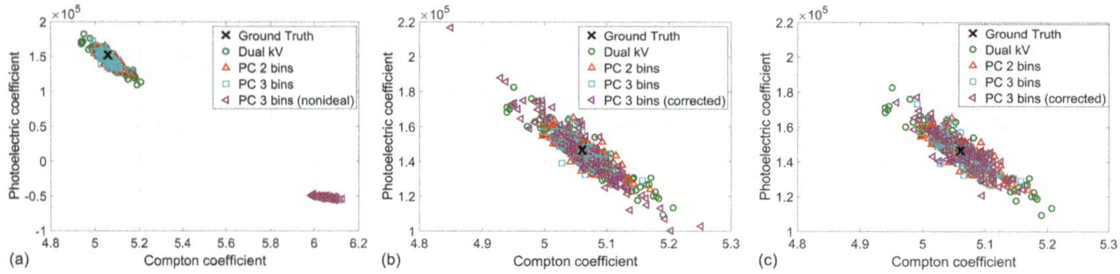

Fig. 14.10 Material decomposition coefficients for 30-cm thickness of water estimated from simulated dual-kV measurements and photon-counting measurements assuming an ideal and an example spectral response. The nonideal spectral response was not accounted for during material decomposition in (**a**) but was properly modeled in (**b**). Nonideal spectral response can (**a**) introduce bias if not accurately modeled and (**b**) increase noise compared to an ideal photon-counting detector when accurately modeled. Plots (**a**, **b**) assumed the example photon-counting spectral response functions shown in Fig. 14.7b, while plot (**c**) assumed the example spectral response functions of Fig. 14.7c

bias in the material decomposition estimates. However, the spectral overlap caused by nonideal spectral response increases the noise compared to an ideal photon-counting detector. Figure 14.10b assumed a photon-counting detector with spectral responses of Fig. 14.7b (smaller detector pixels), demonstrating slightly increased material decomposition noise compared to the dual-energy simulation. Figure 14.10c assumed the spectral responses of Fig. 14.7c (larger detector pixels), demonstrating decreased material decomposition noise compared to the dual-energy simulation.

In summary, flux-independent spectral degradations cause overlap between the spectra of the energy bins, limiting the potential of photon-counting detectors to improve dose efficiency compared to dual-energy systems. Flux-independent degradations increase as the pixel size decreases.

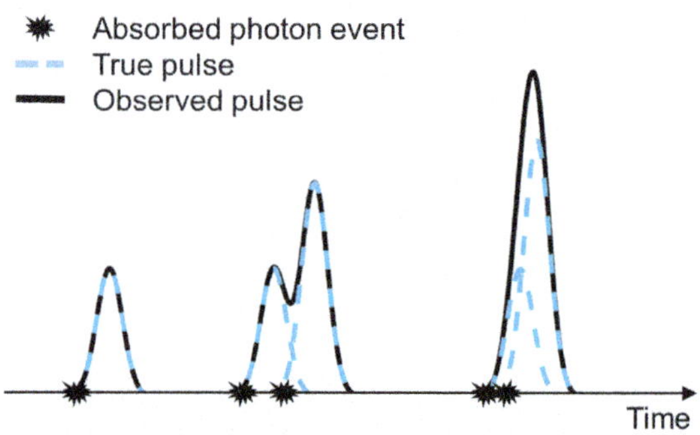

Fig. 14.11 When photons hit the detector within a short time window, the pulses overlap, causing pulse pileup. Photon A is detected correctly. Photons B and C arrive within the detector dead time and thus are detected as a single event with erroneously high energy. Photons D and E may be detected as two separate events, depending on the detector dead time, but photon E would be detected at an erroneously high energy, because of the overlap with the tail of the pulse generated for photon D

Flux-Dependent Spectral Degradations (Pulse Pileup)

The detector dead time is defined as the minimum time between two photon absorption events for which the detector will register the events as two separate photons. If two or more photons are absorbed in a pixel within this dead time, their pulses will combine, causing the multiple pulses to be detected as one event with energy represented by the total pulse height, as illustrated in Fig. 14.11. If the pulse of one photon overlaps with the tail of a pulse from a previous photon, both pulses may be detected as separate events but with errors in the height of the second pulse (Fig. 14.11). Pulse-pileup effects depend on the detector operating mode, detector dead time, detector pixel size, and the photon flux reaching the detector [19]. When operating in non-paralyzable mode, the detector returns to its active counting state after the dead time, regardless of how many photons are detected during the dead time. In paralyzable mode, an additional dead time occurs for each detected photon. Pulse pileup causes a loss in the overall number of counted photons, also known as dead time loss, which reduces DQE and increases noise [20]. Dead time losses

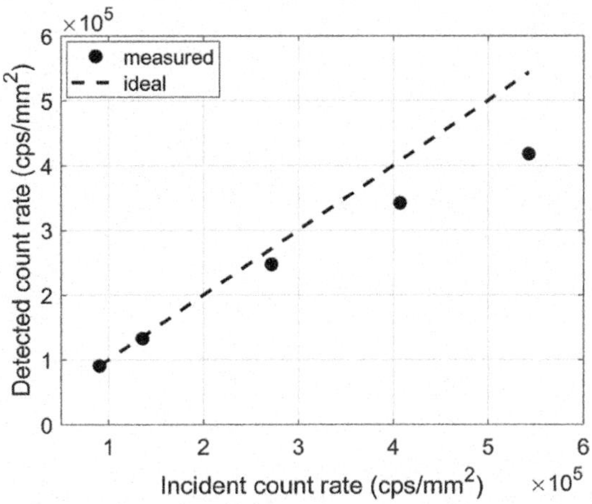

Fig. 14.12 Detected count rate plotted against the count-rate incident on the detector, as measured on a benchtop PCCT system with maximum count rate of 1 million counts per second per mm^2, demonstrating dead time losses at higher flux

depend on the count-rate incident on the detector (Fig. 14.12). Since pileup varies with object attenuation, pileup can also introduce artifacts if dead time losses are not corrected. Pulse pileup decreases with decreasing pixel size. A shorter pulse shaping time can also reduce pileup effects; however the minimum shaping time is limited by the time needed to collect the charges generated by a photon absorption event [21].

Overcoming the Challenges of PCCT

Numerous approaches have been developed and are under development to address the spectral limitations of photon-counting detectors, a selection of which is highlighted in this section.

Detector Hardware Solutions: Charge Summing and Layered Detectors

Larger pixels reduce charge sharing but at the expense of pileup and spatial resolution. Charge summing circuitry is one example of an electronic solution to reduce the effects of charge sharing across pixels while maintaining spatial resolution [22]. Charges are summed in adjacent 2×2 pixels so that the pulse height more accurately represents the true photon energy. Coincidence logic assigns the photon to the pixel with the highest deposited charge. Charge summing improves the spectral response of small pixels but requires lower count rates than reading out the small pixels individually [22, 23].

A hardware solution to reduce pulse pileup is to divide the detector into multiple layers in the depth direction, with each layer having its own anode and readout electronics, as has been implemented for silicon detectors [24]. Since detected photons are distributed across depth, the count-rate incident on each layer is reduced compared to the total count-rate incident on the pixel.

CT System Solutions: Improved Beam-Shaping Filters and Interior PCCT Imaging

The count rate reaching the detector in a CT acquisition has a wide dynamic range [21]. Pulse-pileup effects will be greatest in regions where the beam attenuation is small, such as at toward the edge of the patient or when traveling through the lungs.

Dynamic, patient-specific beam-shaping filters are under development to improve the optimization of flux across the range of patient anatomies [25, 26]. While the primary purpose of these dynamic beam filters is to reduce patient dose, successful implementation would also reduce pileup effects for photon-counting detectors in regions of low patient attenuation [27].

Since pulse-pileup effects are greater toward the periphery of patients, another approach is to acquire photon-counting data only in a central region of interest, by either using hybrid counting/integrating systems [28–30] or by using interior reconstruction algorithms [31].

Algorithmic Solutions: Detector Modeling and Empirical Decomposition

When considering the reconstruction of nonspectral PCCT images, the loss of photons due to nonideal effects reduces dose efficiency and increases noise and may cause artifacts due to the dependence of photon losses on object attenuation The deterministic effects of the losses can be corrected [32–34], but not the noise penalty [20].

The spectral distortion due nonideal detector effects can have a large impact on material decomposition (Fig. 14.10). Bias can be reduced by accurately modeling the nonideal detector effects during material decomposition. Numerous spectral models have been developed or are under development, including models based on synchrotron or isotope measurements [2], Monte Carlo models [35], analytical models [19, 36], or models of effective energy-bin spectra [37].

An alternative approach is to create an empirical model of the relationship between the counts data and the basis material pathlengths, based on calibration methods rather than explicit modeling of detector effects. The relationship between the energy-bin data and basis material pathlengths has been modeled using polynomials [38, 39], a linearized maximum likelihood estimator with correction table [40], and neural networks [41].

Overall, algorithmic methods to model and compensate the nonideal spectral responses of photon-counting detectors can effectively reduce the bias introduced by the spectral distortion. However, these compensation methods cannot recover dose efficiency due to lost counts and spectral overlap.

The Demonstrated and Future Impact of Photon-Counting CT

This section provides examples demonstrating the benefit of PCCT for conventional (nonspectral) CT imaging and for material decomposition applications. Gantry-based PCCT prototypes that are under commercial development are summarized in Table 14.1.

Improved Conventional (Nonspectral) CT Images

Conventional (nonspectral) PCCT images can be reconstructed from all counts detected above the lowest threshold, by generating virtual monoenergetic images after material decomposition (as in dual-energy CT) or by optimally weighting the energy-bin images. Conventional PCCT images have improved image quality compared to images from conventional CT scanners, due to improved dose efficiency, higher spatial resolution, and improved energy weighting.

Figure 14.13 demonstrates the improved spatial resolution of a full-body PCCT prototype scanner (Prismatic). Figure 14.14 demonstrates the improved spatial resolution and noise performance of a full-body PCCT prototype (Siemens Healthineers) [44]. Improved DQE and reduced electronic noise are two benefits of PCCT that reduce noise. A study using a full-body PCCT prototype demonstrated ~33% reduction in noise for a PCCT acquisition at 120 effective mAs compared to a conventional CT system and a ~40% reduction at 30 effective mAs, where electronic noise has a larger contribution, as shown in Fig. 14.15 [7]. Optimal energy weighting has demonstrated CNR improvements ranging from 10% to 35% [18, 45], as well as reduced beam-hardening artifacts [11].

Table 14.1 Summary of gantry-based PCCT prototypes under development. Detector sizes are the physical detector sizes, not scaled to isocenter. The preclinical MARS Bioimaging system includes charge summing mode

Manufacturer	Detector material	Pixel size	Detector size	Energy bins
Siemens Healthineers [3]	CdTe	0.225 × 0.225 mm subpixels that can be grouped into high-resolution mode (0.45 × 0.45 mm) or macro mode (0.9 × 0.9 mm)	43.2 × 2.88 cm	2 per subpixel
Philips Medical Systems [4]	CZT	0.5 × 0.5 mm	30 × 0.45 cm (preclinical) 92.4 × 3.2 cm (planned clinical)	5
Prismatic Sensors [42]	Silicon	0.5 × 0.4 mm	90.0 × 0.1 cm	8
MARS Bioimaging [43]	CdTe	0.11 × 0.11 mm	1.408 × 1.408 (can be translated)	4

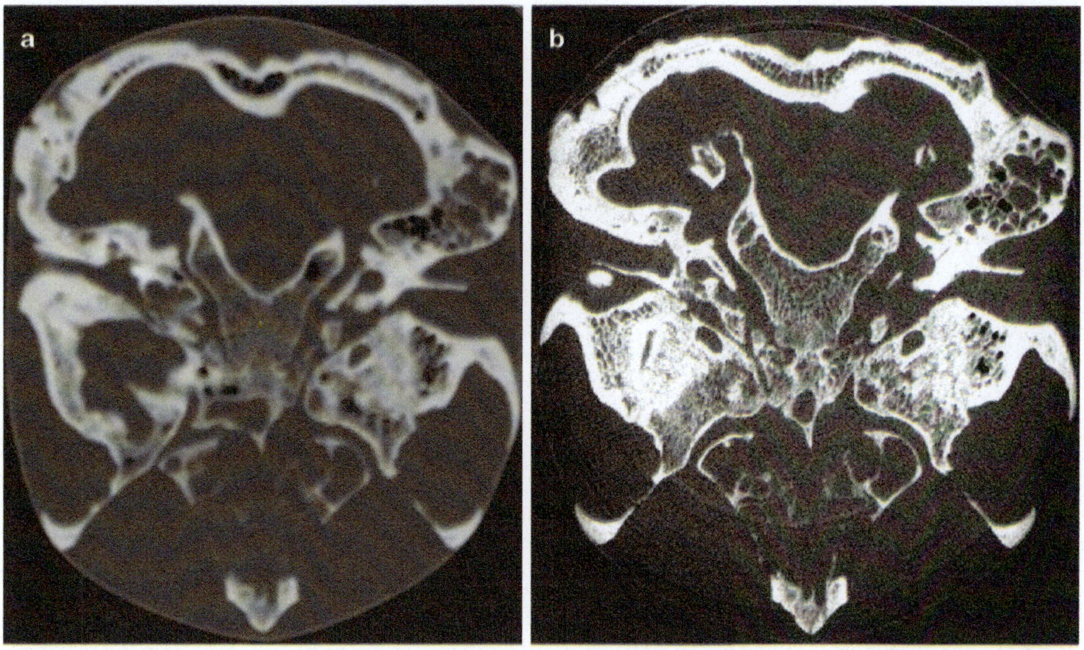

Fig. 14.13 Images of a skull phantom acquired by (**a**) conventional dual-energy CT scanner and (**b**) a full-body PCCT prototype (Prismatic Sensors), demonstrating the higher spatial resolution of the PCCT image. (Images courtesy of Mats Danielsson, KTH Royal Institute of Technology and Prismatic Sensors)

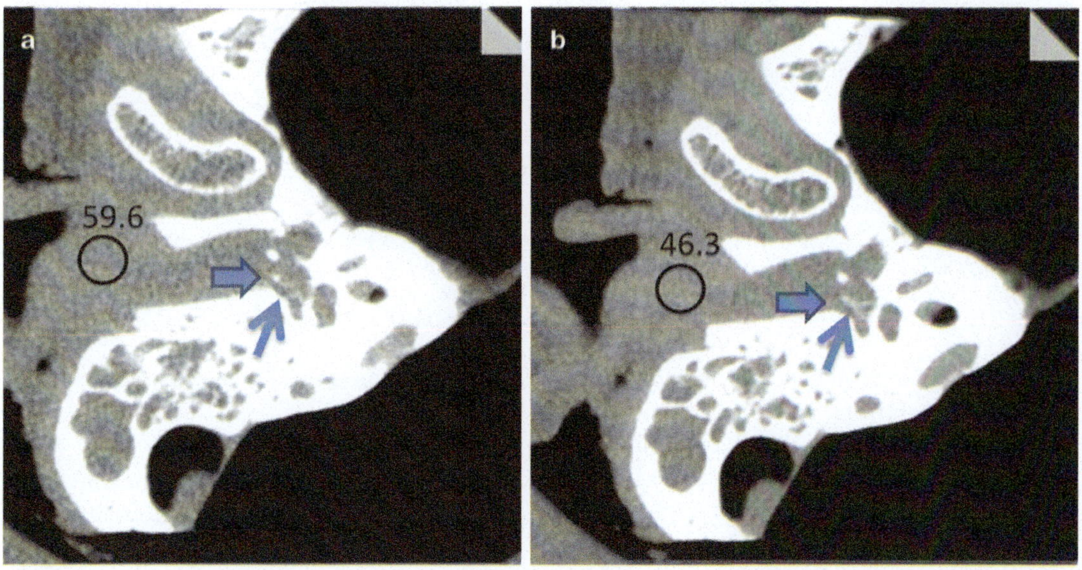

Fig. 14.14 Images of a temporal bone specimen acquired by (**a**) clinical CT scanner (SOMATOM Definition FLASH, Siemens Healthineers) and (**b**) a full-body PCCT prototype (Siemens Healthineers) at equal dose. Higher spatial resolution can be seen in the PCCT image, including improved depiction of the stapes superstructure. Noise standard deviation in the marked ROI is also shown, demonstrating reduced noise standard deviation for the PCCT in addition to the higher spatial resolution and thinner slices. (Images reprinted with permission from [44])

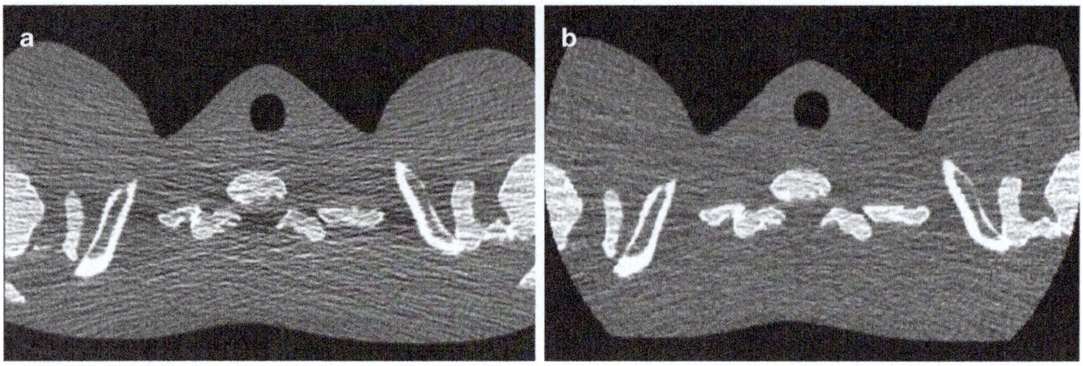

Fig. 14.15 Images of a shoulder phantom acquired by (**a**) clinical dual-source CT scanner (SOMATOM Definition FLASH, Siemens Healthineers) and (**b**) a full-body PCCT prototype (Siemens Healthineers) at an effective 30 mAs, demonstrating reduced noise in the PCCT images due to increased DQE and reduced electronic noise. (Images reprinted with permission from [7])

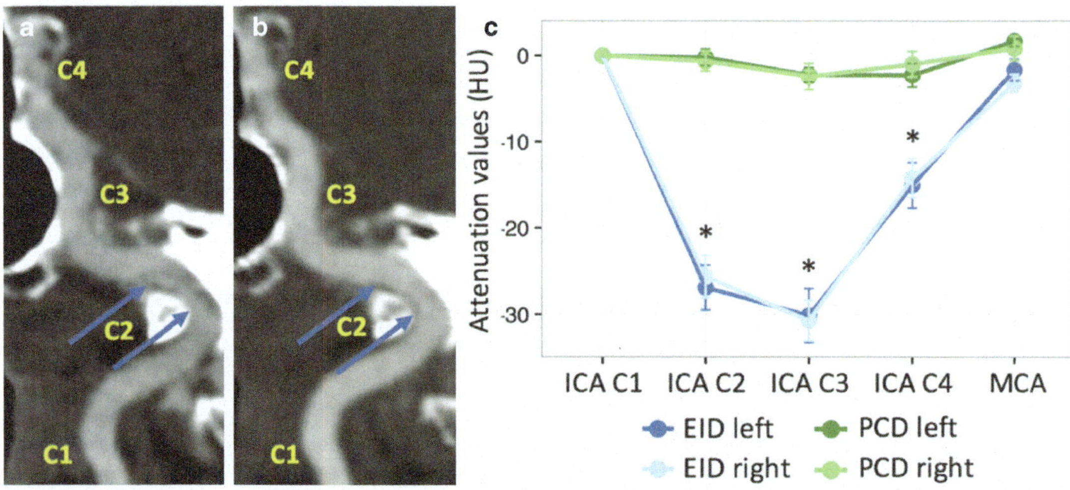

Fig. 14.16 Curved multiplanar reconstructions of the carotid artery acquired by (**a**) CT scanner (SOMATOM Definition FLASH, Siemens Healthineers) and (**b**) a full-body PCCT prototype (Siemens Healthineers). The CT numbers in different segments of the artery are plotted in **c**. The PCCT images demonstrated reduced beam-hardening artifacts and more consistent CT numbers across segments. (Reprinted with permission from [47])

Clinical studies using full-body CT prototypes have further quantified the image quality improvement of PCCT for brain [46], head/neck [47], lung [48], and abdominal [49] applications. These studies have demonstrated equal or higher subjective image quality scores, reduced noise, and improved CNR for the nonspectral PCCT images compared to conventional CT images. For example, Fig. 14.16 demonstrates that PCCT increased iodine CNR and reduced beam hardening in the carotid artery compared to conventional CT [47].

Improved Material Decomposition Imaging

Despite the additional spectral measurements provided by photon-counting detectors, PCCT cannot decompose more materials than dual-energy systems unless there is a contrast agent with detectable K-edge. The limitation of two basis materials (or three basis materials with prior information) occurs because there are two energy-dependent processes that dominate photon attenuation in the CT energy range. The examples presented in Figs. 14.6 and 14.10 dem-

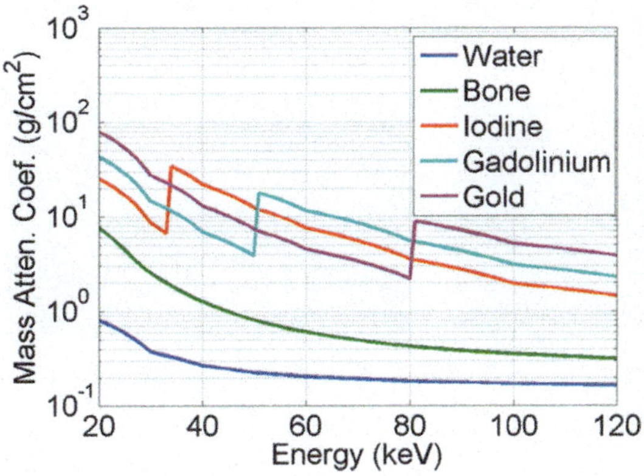

Fig. 14.17 X-ray mass attenuation coefficients of water, bone, and three materials with K-absorption edges in the CT energy range

onstrate that PCCT can provide the same material decomposition information as dual-energy CT, with the potential for reduced noise or dose.

Contrast agents, such as iodine, barium, and gadolinium, have K-absorption edges within CT energy range, as plotted in Fig. 14.17. These K-edges provide material-specific spectral signatures that enable decomposing additional basis functions if there are more than two spectral measurements [2, 15]. Typically, K-edge material decomposition is performed by estimating two-basis material images that represent tissues and by estimating an additional basis image for each K-edge contrast agent [2]. The number of spectral measurements should be at least equal to the number of basis images to be estimated. Unlike dual-energy methods, the resulting K-edge basis material image depicts only the contrast agent without contamination from tissues. Another advantage of K-edge material decomposition is that the reconstructed basis image values are in units of concentration, providing direct quantitative information.

PCCT also has the capability of decomposing more than one contrast agent simultaneously, for example, an intravenous agent and a targeted agent, or different contrast agents for different phases of enhancement.

There are several challenges to K-edge material decomposition. The noise in the material decomposition estimates, and therefore the noise in the basis images, increases with the number of estimated basis coefficients [50]. The K-edges of iodine (33 keV) and barium (37 keV) occur

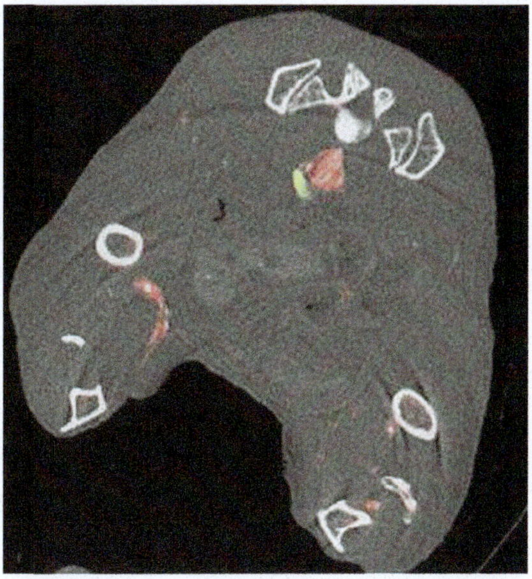

Fig. 14.18 In vivo image of mouse model of atherosclerosis reconstructed from a preclinical PCCT prototype. The gold overlay represents the distribution of targeted gold lipoprotein nanoparticles (gold basis map). The red overlay represents the distribution of the iodine blood contrast agent (iodine basis map). (Reprinted with permission from [51]

at relatively low energies, such that the K-edge signature for these contrast agents may be lost due to severe attenuation of low-energy photons when scanning humans.

Nanoparticle K-edge contrast agents, both targeted and intravenous agents, have been explored for PCCT applications. For example, gold nanoparticles targeted to atherosclerosis (Au-HDL) have been imaged simultaneously with an iodine blood-pool contrast agent in small animals, as shown in Fig. 14.18 [51]. Studies have demonstrated the feasibility of PCCT imaging of clots using bismuth and ytterbium nanoparticle contrast agents targeted to fibrin [52, 53]. Compared to other molecular imaging modalities, PCCT has the advantage of high spatial resolution, high temporal resolution, and direct quantification of concentration. However, PCCT is challenged by its very low sensitivity, which is several orders of magnitude lower than other molecular imaging modalities [54].

Another potential dual-contrast agent application enabled by PCCT is multiphase imaging at a single time point. An in vivo animal study with

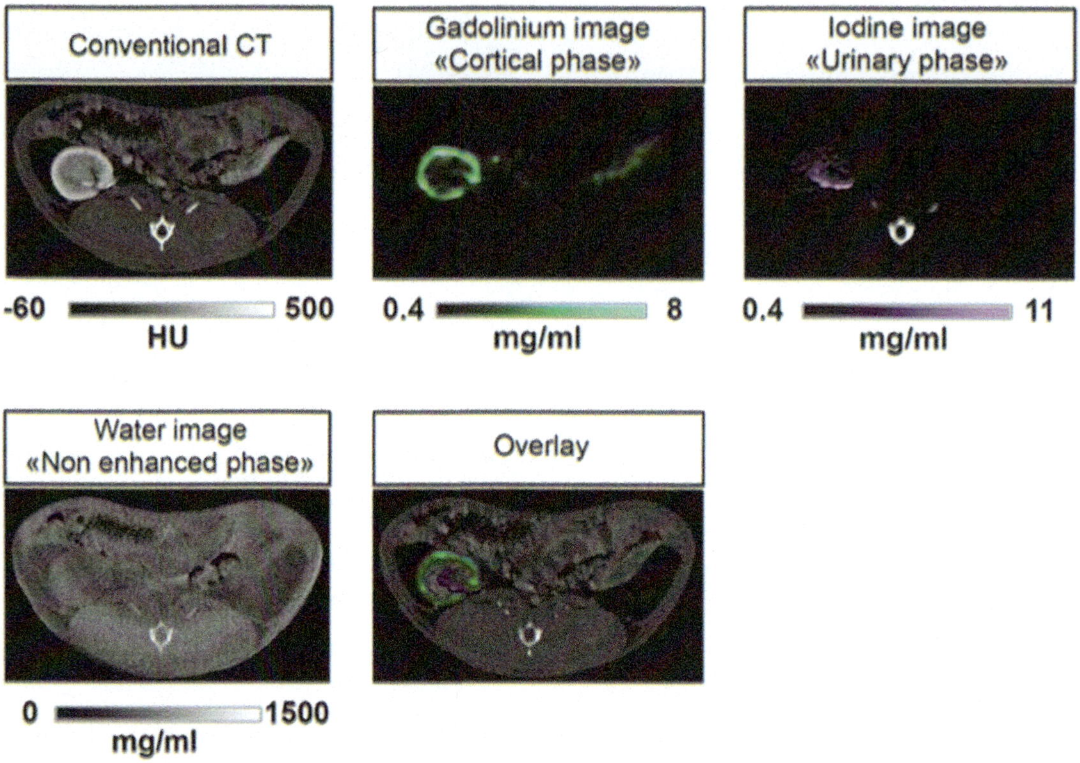

Fig. 14.19 Example of dual-contrast multiphase kidney imaging at a single time point, acquired by a preclinical PCCT prototype (Philips Healthcare) as part of an in vivo animal study. CT acquisition was performed at a single time point 20 s after injection of a gadolinium contrast agent and 60 s after injection of an iodine contrast agent. The conventional CT image cannot discriminate the two contrast agents. The gadolinium basis image depicts the cortical phase, and the iodine basis image depicts the urinary phase. Material decomposition also produces a water basis image, corresponding to a virtual non-enhanced scan, onto which the cortical and urinary enhancement can be visualized with a color overlay. (Images courtesy of Philips Healthcare and Salim Si-Mohamed, Hospices Civils de Lyon)

a preclinical PCCT prototype demonstrated multiphase imaging of the kidney at a single time point, 20 s after injection of a gadolinium contrast agent and 60 s after injection of an iodine contrast agent. Material decomposition was performed into iodine, gadolinium, and water basis images. The gadolinium basis image depicts enhancement of the cortical phase, while the iodine map represents the urinary phase as seen in Fig. 14.19.

An in vivo animal study demonstrated a protocol of injecting a gadolinium contrast agent followed by an iodinated contrast agent [55]. Cardiac PCCT imaging was performed at single time point, followed by material decomposition to create iodine, gadolinium, and non-contrast images. The iodine images represent the first-pass enhancement, while the gadolinium images represent the late myocardial enhancement, demonstrating dual-phase imaging from a single CT acquisition as shown in Fig. 14.20.

The potential benefits of these dual-contrast protocols include reduced dose, because imaging is performed at only one time point, and the coregistration of the phases. A comparison of dose and image quality of dual-contrast agent/single time point PCCT protocols to conventional single contrast agent/multi-time point protocol is required to quantify the improvement made possible by PCCT. Also, the medical and logistical issues of injecting two contrast agents require further study.

An in vivo animal study demonstrated dynamic imaging of a gold nanoparticle contrast agent with long blood residence time and an iodinated contrast agent with rapid excretion [56]. PCCT imaging was performed at multiple time points, with material decomposition into gold, iodine, and water basis images, enabling quantification of the dynamic enhancement of each contrast agent, as shown in Fig. 14.21.

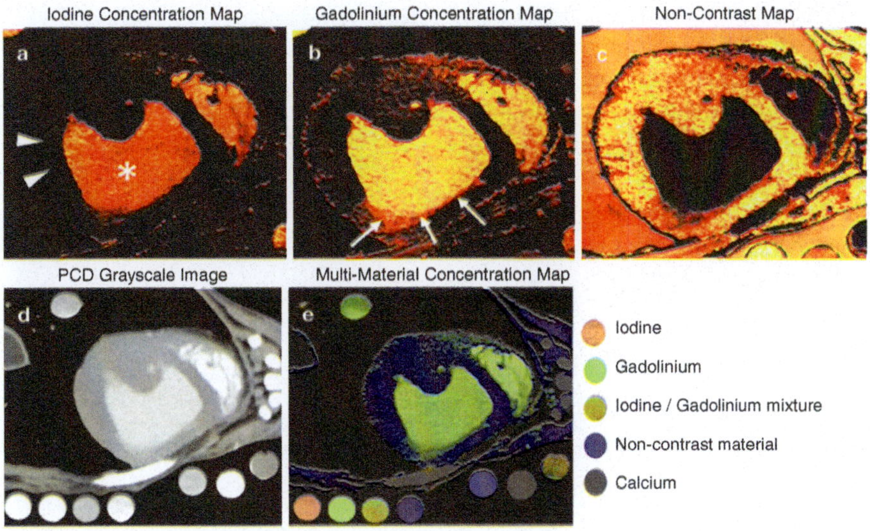

Fig. 14.20 Example of dual-contrast multiphase cardiac imaging at a single time point, acquired by a full-body PCCT prototype (Siemens Healthineers) as part of an in vivo animal study. Acquisition was performed 10 min after injection of a gadolinium blood-pool agent and immediately after injection of an iodine blood-pool agent. Material decomposition of the spectral PCCT data produced (**a**) gadolinium, (**b**) iodine, and (**c**) non-contrast basis images. The gadolinium image shows late enhancement of the subendocardial scar (arrows in (**b**)), while the iodine image shows first-pass enhancement of the blood pool (asterisk in (**a**)). The (**d**) nonspectral PCCT image is compared to (**e**) a multicolor combination of the basis images. (Reprinted with permission from [55])

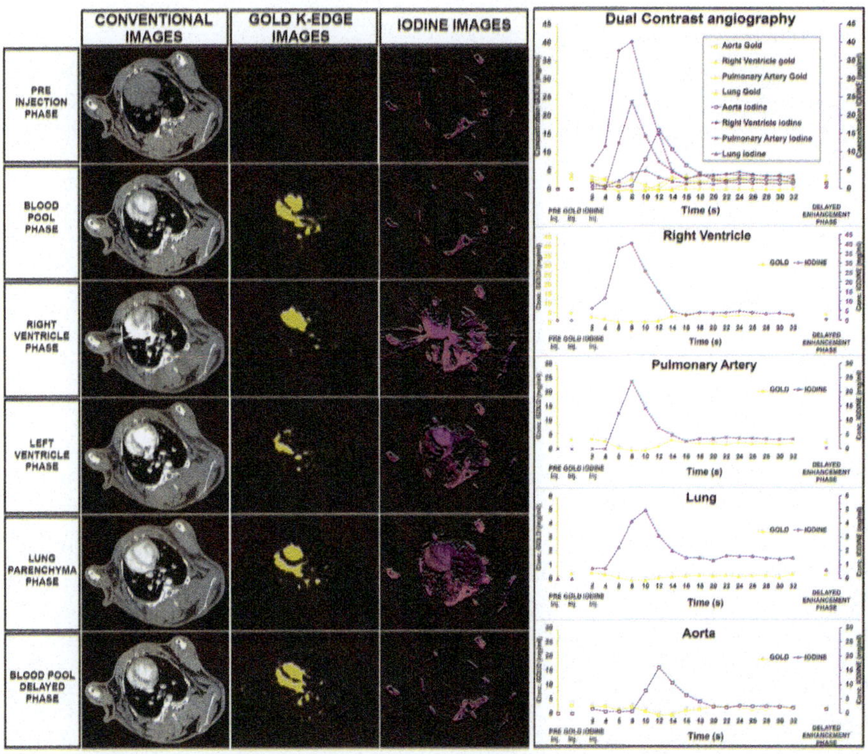

Fig. 14.21 Example of dual-contrast dynamic cardiac images, acquired by a preclinical PCCT prototype (Philips Healthcare) as part of an in vivo animal study. The non-spectral (conventional), gold, and iodine images are shown on the left. Quantification of the gold and iodine concentrations at different time points and locations is displayed on the right. (Reprinted from [56] with permission from https://creativecommons.org/licenses/by/4.0/)

Another potential application of dual-contrast CT imaging is using different K-edge materials for oral and intravenous contrast. A phantom study on a preclinical PCCT prototype proposed using an iodine oral contrast for fecal tagging and gadolinium as the blood-pool agent [57]. Material decomposition of iodine and gadolinium images enabled visualization of the polyps from the feces.

Summary

Photon-counting detectors use direct-conversion semiconductors, combined with pulse-height analysis electronics, to sort detected photons into energy bins. Photon-counting detectors can acquire more than two spectral measurements simultaneously, while also acquiring a nonspectral CT image. In addition to the spectral acquisition capabilities, photon-counting detectors have the additional benefits of higher resolution imaging with higher dose efficiency, compared to conventional CT detectors. However, photon-counting detectors are challenged by numerous effects in the detector that degrade the spectral information and cause photons to be detected in the incorrect energy bins. Numerous efforts are underway to minimize and compensate for these nonideal effects, including detector hardware, system, and algorithmic approaches.

Overall, photon-counting detectors have potential to (1) produce nonspectral CT images with increased contrast, improved spatial resolution, reduced beam-hardening artifacts, and reduced noise and/or dose, (2) improve the dose efficiency of two-material decomposition, and (3) quantify K-edge contrast agents, including multi-contrast studies. Whole-body clinical PCCT prototypes have been developed, with animal and clinical studies underway to evaluate the benefits and new applications made possible by PCCT.

Acknowledgments The author thanks David Cormode (University of Pennsylvania), Mats Danielsson (KTH Royal Institute of Technology and Prismatic Sensors), Cynthia McCollough (Mayo Clinic), Salim Si-Mohamed (Hospices Civils de Lyon), and Yoad Yagil (Philips Healthcare) for sharing images and information for this chapter.

References

1. Knoll GF. Radiation detection and measurement. 3rd ed. New York: Wiley; 2000.
2. Schlomka JP, et al. Experimental feasibility of multi-energy photon-counting K-edge imaging in pre-clinical computed tomography. Phys Med Biol. 2008;53(15):4031–47.
3. Yu Z, et al. Evaluation of conventional imaging performance in a research whole-body CT system with a photon-counting detector array. Phys Med Biol. 2016;61(4):1572.
4. Si-Mohamed S, et al. Review of an initial experience with an experimental spectral photon-counting computed tomography system. Nucl Inst Methods Phys Res Sect A Accel Spectrometers Detect Assoc Equip. 2017;873:27–35.
5. Bornefalk H, Danielsson M. Photon-counting spectral computed tomography using silicon strip detectors: a feasibility study. Phys Med Biol. 2010;55(7):1999–2022.
6. Duan X et al. Electronic noise in CT detectors: impact on image noise and artifacts. 2013. https://doi.org/10.2214/AJR.12.10234.
7. Yu Z, et al. Noise performance of low-dose CT: comparison between an energy integrating detector and a photon counting detector using a whole-body research photon counting CT scanner. J Med Imaging. 2016;3(4):043503.
8. Baek J, Pineda AR, Pelc NJ. To bin or not to bin? The effect of CT system limiting resolution on noise and detectability. Phys Med Biol. 2013;58(5):1433.
9. Tapiovaara MJ, Wagner RF. SNR and DQE analysis of broad spectrum X-ray imaging. Phys Med Biol. 1985;30(6):519–29.
10. Giersch J, Niederlöhner D, Anton G. The influence of energy weighting on X-ray imaging quality. Nucl Inst Methods Phys Res Sect A Accel Spectrometers, Detect Assoc Equip. 2004;531(1–2):68–74.
11. Schmidt TG. Optimal 'image-based' weighting for energy-resolved CT. Med Phys. 2009;36(7):3018–27.
12. Kappler S, et al. Multi-energy performance of a research prototype CT scanner with small-pixel counting detector. Proc SPIE. 2013;8668:86680O–86680O-8.
13. Schmidt TG, Zimmerman KC, Sidky EY. The effects of extending the spectral information acquired by a photon-counting detector for spectral CT. Phys Med Biol. 2015;60(4):1583–600.
14. Krauss B, Grant KL, Schmidt BT, Flohr TG. The importance of spectral separation. Investig Radiol. 2015;50(2):114–8.
15. Roessl E, Proksa R. K-edge imaging in x-ray computed tomography using multi-bin photon counting detectors. Phys Med Biol. 2007;52(15):4679–96.
16. Touch M, Clark DP, Barber W, Badea CT. A neural network-based method for spectral distortion correction in photon counting x-ray CT. Phys Med Biol. 2016;61(16):6132–53.

17. Xu C, Danielsson M, Bornefalk H. Evaluation of energy loss and charge sharing in cadmium telluride detectors for photon-counting computed tomography. IEEE Trans Nucl Sci. 2011;58(3):614–25.
18. Shikhaliev PM, Fritz SG, Chapman JW. Photon counting multienergy x-ray imaging: effect of the characteristic x rays on detector performance. Med Phys. 2009;36(11):5107–19.
19. Taguchi K, Frey EC, Wang X, Iwanczyk JS, Barber WC. An analytical model of the effects of pulse pileup on the energy spectrum recorded by energy resolved photon counting x-ray detectors. Med Phys. 2010;37:3957.
20. Wang AS, Harrison D, Lobastov V, Tkaczyk JE. Pulse pileup statistics for energy discriminating photon counting x-ray detectors. Med Phys. 2011;38(7):4265–75.
21. Taguchi K, Iwanczyk JS. Vision 20/20: single photon counting x-ray detectors in medical imaging. Med Phys. 2013;40(10):100901.
22. Koenig T, et al. Charge summing in spectroscopic X-ray detectors with high-Z sensors. IEEE Trans Nucl Sci. 2013;60(6):4713–8.
23. Koenig T, et al. How spectroscopic x-ray imaging benefits from inter-pixel communication. Phys Med Biol. 2014;59(20):6195–213.
24. Liu X, Grönberg F, Sjölin M, Karlsson S, Danielsson M. Count rate performance of a silicon-strip detector for photon-counting spectral CT. Nucl Inst Methods Phys Res Sect A Accel Spectrometers, Detect Assoc Equip. 2016;827:102–6.
25. Hsieh SS, Fleischmann D, Pelc NJ. Dose reduction using a dynamic, piecewise-linear attenuator. Med Phys. 2014;41(2):021910.
26. Szczykutowicz TP, Mistretta CA. Design of a digital beam attenuation system for computed tomography: part I. System design and simulation framework. Med Phys. 2013;40(2):021905.
27. Hsieh SS, Pelc NJ. The piecewise-linear dynamic attenuator reduces the impact of count rate loss with photon-counting detectors. Phys Med Biol. 2014;59(11):2829–47.
28. Schmidt TG, Pektas F. Region-of-interest material decomposition from truncated energy-resolved CT. Med Phys. 2011;38(10):5657–66.
29. Xu Q, et al. Image reconstruction for hybrid true-color micro-CT. IEEE Trans Biomed Eng. 2012;59(6):1711–9.
30. Yu Z, et al. How low can we go in radiation dose for the data-completion scan on a research whole-body photon-counting computed tomography system. J Comput Assist Tomogr. 2016;40:663–70.
31. Taguchi K, Xu J, Srivastava S, Tsui BMW, Cammin J, Tang Q. Interior region-of-interest reconstruction using a small, nearly piecewise constant subregion. Med Phys. 2011;38:1307.
32. Johns PC, Yaffe MJ. Correction of pulse-height spectra for peak pileup effects using periodic and random pulse generators. Nucl Inst Methods Phys Res Sect A Accel Spectrometers, Detect Assoc Equip. 1987;255(3):559–81.
33. Gardner RP, Wielopolski L. A generalized method for correcting pulse-height spectra for the peak pile-up effect due to double sum pulses: part I. Predicting spectral distortion for arbitrary pulse shapes. Nucl Inst Methods. 1977;140(2):289–96.
34. Roessl E, Daerr H, Proksa R. A Fourier approach to pulse pile-up in photon-counting x-ray detectors. Med Phys. 2016;43(3):1295.
35. Liu X, et al. Spectral response model for a multi-bin photon-counting spectral computed tomography detector and its applications. J Med Imaging. 2015;2(3):033502.
36. Cammin J, Xu J, Barber WC, Iwanczyk JS, Hartsough NE, Taguchi K. A cascaded model of spectral distortions due to spectral response effects and pulse pileup effects in a photon-counting x-ray detector for CT. Med Phys. 2014;41(4):041905.
37. Schmidt TG, Barber RF, Sidky EY. A spectral CT method to directly estimate basis material maps from experimental photon-counting data. IEEE Trans Med Imaging. 2017;36(9):1808–19.
38. Alvarez RE, Macovski A. Energy-selective reconstructions in X-ray computerised tomography. Phys Med Biol. 1976;21(5):733–44.
39. Wu D, Zhang L, Zhu X, Xu X, Wang S. A weighted polynomial based material decomposition method for spectral x-ray CT imaging. Phys Med Biol. 2016;61(10):3749–83.
40. Alvarez RE. Estimator for photon counting energy selective x-ray imaging with multibin pulse height analysis. Med Phys. 2011;38:2324.
41. Zimmerman KC, Schmidt TG. Experimental comparison of empirical material decomposition methods for spectral CT. Phys Med Biol. 2015;60(8):3175–91.
42. Persson M, et al. Energy-resolved CT imaging with a photon-counting silicon-strip detector. Phys Med Biol. 2014;59(22):6709–27.
43. Panta RK, et al. Element-specific spectral imaging of multiple contrast agents: a phantom study. J Instrum. 2018;13(02):T02001–T02001.
44. Leng S, et al. Dose-efficient ultrahigh-resolution scan mode using a photon counting detector computed tomography system. J Med Imaging. 2016;3(4):043504.
45. Le HQ, Ducote JL, Molloi S. Radiation dose reduction using a CdZnTe-based computed tomography system: comparison to flat-panel detectors. Med Phys. 2010;37(3):1225–36.
46. Pourmorteza A, et al. Photon-counting CT of the brain: in vivo human results and image-quality assessment. AJNR Am J Neuroradiol. 2017;38(12):2257–63.
47. Symons R, et al. Photon-counting computed tomography for vascular imaging of the head and neck. Investig Radiol. 2018;53(3):135–42.
48. Symons R, et al. Feasibility of dose-reduced chest CT with photon-counting detectors: initial results in humans. Radiology. 2017;285(3):980–9.

49. Pourmorteza A, et al. Abdominal imaging with contrast-enhanced photon-counting CT: first human experience. Radiology. 2016;279(1):239–45.
50. Roessl E, Herrmann C. Cram{é}r--Rao lower bound of basis image noise in multiple-energy x-ray imaging. Phys Med Biol. 2009;54(5):1307.
51. Roessl E et al. Preclinical spectral computed tomography of gold nano-particles. Nuclear Instruments and Methods in Physics Research Section A: Accelerators, Spectrometers, Detectors and Associated Equipment. 2011;648:S259–S264.
52. Pan D, et al. Computed tomography in color: nanoK-enhanced spectral CT molecular imaging. Angew Chem Int Ed. 2010;49(50):9635–9.
53. Pan D, et al. An early investigation of ytterbium nanocolloids for selective and quantitative 'multicolor' spectral CT imaging. ACS Nano. 2012;6(4):3364–70.
54. Roessl E, Brendel B, Engel K, Schlomka J, Thran A, Proksa R. Sensitivity of photon-counting based K-edge imaging in X-ray computed tomography. IEEE Trans Med Imaging. 2011;30:1678–90.
55. Symons R, et al. Dual-contrast agent photon-counting computed tomography of the heart: initial experience. Int J Cardiovasc Imaging. 2017;33(8):1253–61.
56. Cormode DP, et al. Multicolor spectral photon-counting computed tomography: in vivo dual contrast imaging with a high count rate scanner. Sci Rep. 2017;7(1):4784.
57. Muenzel D, et al. Spectral photon-counting CT: initial experience with dual–contrast agent K-edge colonography. Radiology. 2017;283(3):723–8.

Part V

Quantitative CT

CT-Based Quantification

15

Ehsan Samei and Jocelyn Hoye

Introduction

Quantitative imaging refers to the science, the technology, and the process of extracting quantitative values from medical images. The Radiological Society of North America defines quantitative imaging as "the extraction of quantifiable features from medical images for the assessment of normal or the severity, degree of change, or status of a disease, injury, or chronic condition relative to normal" [1]. The key aspect of quantitative imaging is that it is not only the extraction of quantitative numbers – it is also using those numbers to assess the patient. Examples of quantities that might be extracted from medical images include measured image intensity values in a region of interest, measured diameters and volumes of different structures, and mathematical descriptions of texture to quantify internal anatomical heterogeneity for regions of interest. These quantifications might be used, for example, to decide if a lung nodule is responding to a therapy, to determine if there is stenosis in a cardiac vessel and the degree of severity of a stenosis, or to determine the likelihood of malignancy of a liver lesion. With first applications in oncology, cardiology, pulmonology, orthopedics, and neurology, quantitative imaging is a goal shared by many physicians and scientists across medical specialties with the end goal of improving patient care.

Historically, medical imaging was developed to allow physicians to see a visual representation of the internal structures of the human body. Medical images were valued for their ability to provide a noninvasive representation of internal anatomy that would allow for improved diagnosis and treatment of patients. For many years, medical images were used qualitatively by radiologists and physicians who would describe their findings based on what they were able to see in the images. However, scientists and physicians have realized that images have the potential to provide also a wealth of quantitative information toward the diagnosis and the treatment of the patient.

One goal of using medical images for quantification is to improve patient care by making patient assessment and treatment decisions less susceptible to intra- and interobserver differences. The use of quantitative imaging can make patient

E. Samei (✉)
Department of Radiology, Duke University, Durham, NC, USA
e-mail: ehsan.samei@duke.edu

J. Hoye
Carl E. Ravin Advanced Imaging Laboratories (RAI Labs) and Medical Physics Graduate Program, Department of Radiology, Duke University, Durham, NC, USA
e-mail: jocelyn.hoye@duke.edu

© Springer Nature Switzerland AG 2020

E. Samei, N. J. Pelc (eds.), *Computed Tomography*, https://doi.org/10.1007/978-3-030-26957-9_15

care more consistent by extracting numbers from patient images, with the idea being the numbers are less subjective and more consistent from one interpreter to another and for the same interpreter over time. Quantitative imaging also allows for the understanding of the degree of severity of a change in condition. For example, qualitative imaging allows a physician to see that a lung nodule increased in size between the first scan 6 months ago and the scan of the patient today. However, quantitative imaging, in theory, allows the physician to say that the lung nodule increased in size by 30%, for example. Quantitative information can help healthcare professionals ensure consistent care is delivered across patients and facilitates evidence-based decisions based on the significance of the findings.

Each imaging modality has its own unique image quantification applications and technical challenges, with some modalities having more quantification potential. Computed Tomography (CT) offers such a potential as the intensity values in the image correspond with the fundamental physical properties of the tissues. Even though the final image displayed is not in units of linear attenuation coefficient, the final image can be, to some extent, considered a normalized linear attenuation coefficient scaled with water set to a value of 0 Hounsfield Units (HU) and air set to −1000 HU. Generally, physicians know the expected HU for a given tissue at a given kV and can therefore use an average HU measurement to understand the extent of disease. In addition to HU measurements, iodine concentration can be quantified using dual energy CT to create iodine material decomposition images. Iodine quantification can be used to infer the iodine contrast uptake in tissue. Other quantitative measurements in CT include measurements of distances, areas, and volumes of interest for differentiation of image features. Recently, an emerging field of radiomics has offered expanded quantitative measurements including intensity enhancement reflecting temporal properties of perfusion and diffusion in tissue, texture reflecting internal heterogeneity of tissue, and morphology reflecting the shape and geometry of a region of interest [2–4].

In CT, there are several challenges to quantification. While the fundamental measure of CT is linear attenuation coefficient, there are many factors that alter the final CT image properties. Quantitative measures from CT are likely susceptible to the many "knobs" that can be manipulated in image acquisition and reconstruction, including kV, mAs, pitch, reconstructed slice thickness, reconstruction type, and reconstruction kernel. An example of an image "knob" which can impact quantification is the combination of kV, mAs, pitch, and average patient size which interact to determine the noise magnitude in the image. Images with greater noise magnitude may result in highly variable quantification of specific patient attributes. Further, manufacturers deploy different reconstruction kernels in the process of creating CT images which are not necessarily designed for quantitation. A CT image may be reconstructed using a reconstruction kernel that makes the images more appealing to be viewed by a radiologist; however, that does not necessarily make the image better for quantitation. Different kernels may alter the size and shape of an object and the gray levels of the final CT image. The processes of beam-hardening and scatter correction further impact the quantitative capability of the scanner. In CT, most manufacturers keep the details of reconstruction and correction methods as proprietary information, making it difficult to undo the effects. The precision of quantification in CT must be addressed if one is to ensure that evidence-based decision-making is relevant to the patient and not simply a reflection of the imaging acquisition and reconstruction settings.

In principle, any imaging quantification, including that in CT, needs to meet four requirements to be most effective (Table 15.1). Those include:

1. Clinical and biological relevance (ensuring the attribute of an image is worth quantifying)
2. Objectivity (ensuring the quantification measures what we believe to be the truth of the object being measured)
3. Robust quantification (ensuring the imprecision in the quantification is understood and mitigated)

Table 15.1 Definitions of the four main aspects of quantitative metrics to ensure high-quality quantification in CT

Quantification requirement	Definition	Determination
Relevance	Quantification that is associated with a useful biological or clinical outcome of a patient	Ascertaining the correlation of metrics with clinical outcomes or intermediary clinical outcomes (e.g., progression)
Objectivity	Quantification that is associated with accurate and representative of the underlying truth of the patient or the disease	Ascertaining the bias or accuracy of metrics in comparison to known property of the tissue or object (i.e., gold standard)
Robustness	Quantification that is associated with metrics which can be measured precisely	Ascertaining the variability of metrics in repeated measurements
Implementation	Quantification that is associated with metrics which can be effectively implemented clinically	Ascertaining the needed tools and their usability in clinical settings

4. Clinical implementability (ensuring the quantification is possible to implement clinically in a way that is usable by medical professionals)

The following sections of this chapter will give an in-depth description of the four main aspects of quantification and describe the requirements and challenges associated with each.

Relevance

It is fundamental to CT-based quantitative imaging that the quantification of an attribute has clinical and biological relevance to the patient. Relevance is ascribed to a quantification metric which can successfully quantify the usable biological or clinical outcome of a patient. A relevant metric would be correlated with an observable biological phenomenon. Relevance is the overall end goal of quantitative imaging; however, it is so integral and important to quantification that it must be addressed at the beginning. The end goal of quantification in CT, or in any other imaging modality, is to be able to make an assessment or decision about patient disease status. If a quantification does not give information about a patient disease status, related to the biological truth of the patient, then the quantification is not relevant, and physicians and scientists should not continue to investigate the quantification. In another word, all quantifications must be relevant by being grounded in some clinical or biological understanding of the disease or disease process. Example biological and clinical phenomena in CT which have been quantified include tumor/lesion size, tumor/lesion spiculation, and extent of cardiac stenosis, each of which is relevant attributes of a disease independent of imaging.

Tumor/lesion size is a known indicator of patient outcome, with the general trend that patients with larger tumors and lesions tend to have worse survival than patients with smaller lesions [5]. Tumor size is also used as an endpoint for clinical trials to indicate whether a patient is responding to a therapy [6]. Since this phenomenon has been observed and understood biologically, any quantification that seeks to measure tumor size and is successfully able to do so would be considered a relevant quantification. In-plane diameter, area, and volume are all metrics which seek to quantify tumor size. While there may be debate about which of these metrics can be measured robustly and accurately in a clinical scenario (which we tackle as a third requirement below), all these metrics are considered relevant because they quantify the size of the tumor/lesion which has also been known to correlate with patient outcome.

Degree of coronary artery stenosis is another example of an observable biological phenomenon which is predictive of patient outcome. A stenosis is defined as the narrowing of a blood vessel. When blood vessels are narrowed, the flow of blood through the region is restricted. Therefore, patients whose vessels have more stenosis are more likely to have worse outcomes. The degree of stenosis might also indicate to a physician that a more extensive intervention may be needed for the patient. Since the degree of coronary artery stenosis is understood clinically and biologically, any metric that successfully quantifies the extent of stenosis is a relevant quantification. Coronary artery stenosis can be measured as a percentage of the normal size by measuring the area of the normal vessel and the area of the stenosed region and relating the two measurements in a ratio. While this quantification may not be robust and accurate across all cardiac CTs and all patient heart rates, the quantification is relevant because it seeks to quantify an observable trait which correlates with a clinical outcome.

A final example of a biological and clinical disease process which has been quantified is lesion spiculation. In general, lesions which are more spiculated at the edges, rather than having well-defined smooth boarders, are more likely to be malignant [7]. Researchers in the field of radiomics have developed several metrics which seek to quantify the extent of spiculation of a lesion by calculating the variability of the distance from the perimeter to the center of the lesion [8]. Others have quantified spiculation by measuring the average gradient of the edge of the lesion to quantify the level of definition in the lesion margins [9]. Metrics that seek to quantify lesion spiculation are examples of biologically and clinically relevant metrics.

It is essential that quantification be grounded in patient outcomes and biology to ensure that the metrics are worth implementing clinically. Ensuring biological and clinical relevance will also give an understanding of the expected trends against which to check that the metrics are giving the results we expect. For example, a new metric to quantify lesion spiculation can be tested against images of lesions with a range of known spiculations. If the metric is found not to be correlated with observable changes in spiculation level of lesions, the quantification is not relevant to the biological phenomenon aimed to be quantified. Ultimately, if quantitative metrics extracted from patient images are not biologically relevant, then the metrics will not be useful for improving patient care.

While it may seem obvious that quantitative metrics should be metrics which are relevant to biological and clinical outcomes, it can be easy to get caught up in quantification for quantification sake and lose sight of the overall goal and purpose of image quantification. Along these lines, statistically, it is easy to find a quantification metric which seems relevant if enough candidate metrics are tested. For example, let's say we have CT images of 200 patients, and we know how long the patients survived after being diagnosed with lung cancer, and we wanted to find a quantification which correlates with patient survival. If we decide to skip the assessment of biological relevance and simply test many quantification metrics, we may find a metric correlated with survival simply due to chance. If we do not take the time to (1) account for multiple hypothesis testing by either correcting for it or acquiring more patient cases or (2) determine scientifically how the mathematics of the quantification might relate to what we are able to see in the patient images, then we cannot be sure that the quantifications are relevant to clinical outcomes and patient biology, rather than simply being due to random chance [10].

When the precise underlying biological processes are unknown, the expertise of expert clinicians can be harnessed to identify and create clinically meaningful quantifications. For example, when radiologists read and interpret patient images containing lesions, they often subjectively deploy image signatures associated with malignancy, such as qualities associated with borders or necrosis. Those attribute can be made into quantitative biomarkers. This method of creating quantitative features can create disease-targeted quantitation that takes advantage of radiologist expert information. Needless to say, having biomarkers founded on biological or clinical foundations, it would still be necessary to follow appropriate statistical methodology to ensure that any newly developed metric is statistically predictive of patient outcomes.

In summary, quantitative metrics extracted from patient CT images must be biologically and clinically relevant. For metrics to be relevant, they must be correlated with observable changes in patient anatomy and disease which are reflective of changes in biology and anatomy of the underlying ground truth of the patient. Examples of metrics which are based in biological relevance are quantification of lesion size, cardiac plaque stenosis, and lesion spiculation. While not all metrics developed to quantify biological phenomena can be measured with adequate accuracy and precision, metrics which are relevant to biological and clinical ground truth are the only metrics worth studying for the improvement of patient care. Even if a metric were developed which could be measured accurately and precisely for every patient, if the metric did not give information to clinicians about the disease state and did not aid the clinicians in their decision-making process about patient care, then the metric would not be relevant.

Objectivity

Objective quantification metrics are ones which accurately assign a number to the observable expected phenotypic variation for normal patient anatomy and disease. In other words, objective quantifications are quantifications which are accurate and representative of the underlying *ground truth* of the patient. Objective quantifications are ones which are accurate and not biased depending on how the quantity is measured. An easy way to understand objective measurements is with the example of height. When a person asks how tall you are, you can give an objective measurement of your height if you used a tape measure. You know that your measurement is accurate because there is a reference standard object which represents 1 m against which all other methods were evaluated. The development of the reference standard meter stick allowed the measurements of distances to be objective and standardized.

In CT, objectivity is sometimes difficult to achieve because there is variation in the ways that CT images are presented depending on which settings were chosen to both acquire and reconstruct the CT images. This is partially because CT was largely developed to obtain a qualitative image of internal anatomy rather than to obtain quantitative data points. As such, the many different settings can lead to different quantifications depending on how the images were acquired and reconstructed. As a result, quantitative metrics measured from CT scans are not necessarily objective. As an example, if one seeks to quantify tumor volume, the objectivity is compromised if the value is dependent on the CT machine – such as if volume on one CT scanner is 500 mm^3 and on another is 550 mm^3.

While CT is not an inherently objective way to acquire data, the challenge of objectivity can be overcome if you can account for differences between CT scanners and methods. By accounting for any systematic bias, then we can make the quantification objective. If we return to the height example, a biased tape measure would be one that you know underestimates your height by 5 in. Since you know that the tape measure underestimates by 5 in, you can correct for the bias by adding 5 in to your height as measured using that specific tool. Similarly, if you can determine that with scanner model A, all volumes are underestimated by 20%, then you can add 20% to whatever measure of volume you get from scanner model A. Underlying this discussion is the need to have a gold standard reference object which can be used to compare different CT scanner acquisition and reconstruction settings. To assess the objectivity of a quantification, it is necessary to have such a gold standard reference to ensure that the quantification is an objective measure of the ground truth of a patient, rather than an effect of the scanning or analysis process.

In CT, a gold standard can be supplied by a known object, which can be physical or computational. The object should be made with material and morphological realism. The object either can then be physically scanned by a CT scanner or can be virtually scanned by a simulated CT scanner through so-called the virtual clinical trial process [11]. The CT scanned versions of the object can be visually and quantitatively compared to the ground truth. The quantitative features from both the ground truth and the CT image can be compared to calculate any bias which was introduced by the specific CT scanning acquisition and reconstruction settings. This process can be repeated for multiple acquisition and reconstruction settings to determine the exact bias in any specific imaging settings. For example, a study was performed to calculate the bias in morphology features of lung lesions across different protocols [12]. The results can be displayed in a heatmap with different protocols along one axis and different morphology features along another axis and the feature bias displayed in color as shown in Fig. 15.1.

The process of creating ground truth objects to be scanned by CT scanners to verify quantitative accuracy has been done for several applications. For example, ground truth objects which have internal heterogeneity have been developed to allow verification that texture features measured from CT scans are truly indicative of the ground truth of the object and are not merely unintended quantification of image noise or some other image feature [13, 14]. Figure 15.2 shows the process of computationally creating 3D printed texture lesion models. Another example is coronary artery stenosis. When physicians measure percent stenosis from CT scans, they want to be sure that their measurement is reflective of the ground truth stenosis in the patient. Using a ground truth phantom with a known stenosis, the effects of different CT imaging acquisition settings and different motion profiles of the moving vessels in the heart were tested [15]. A final example is related to metal artifacts in images. If a physician wants to measure the contrast of the aorta to determine the enhancement curve over

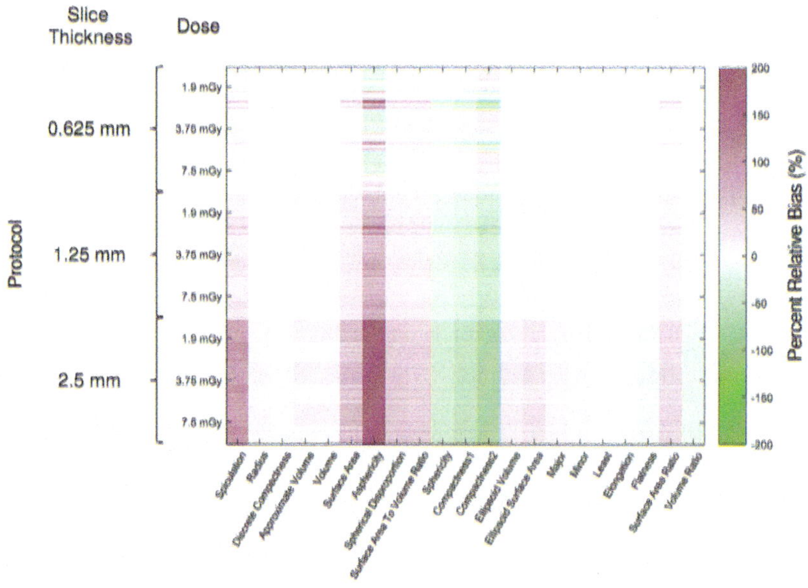

Fig. 15.1 The percent relative bias of morphology features is shown for lung nodules imaged by different imaging protocols from multiple vendors using different kernels, doses, and slice thicknesses. The positive bias (overestimation) is shown in pink, and the negative bias (underestimation) is shown in green

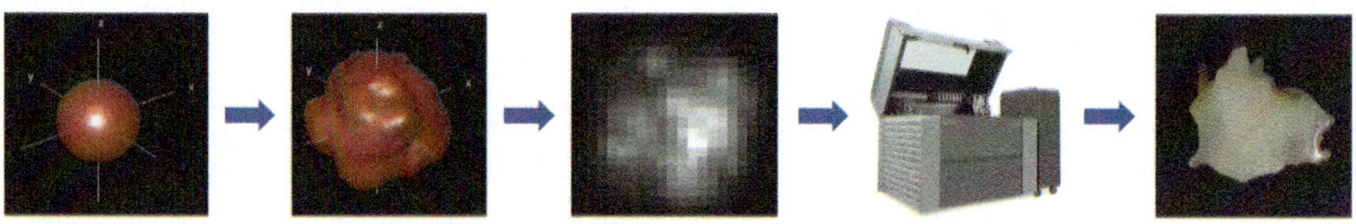

Fig. 15.2 3D printed textured lesion models were created by starting with a simple geometrical sphere. The sphere was updated to have anatomically informed morphology, and texture before it was sent to the 3D printer to create a physical model

time after administering IV contrast, and the aorta is affected by a metal artifact, it would be necessary to quantify the extent that the metal artifact impacts the objectivity of the measurement. This was previously studied by creating an exact replica of a metal object using a nonmetal material [16]. Both the metal object and nonmetal replica were separately inserted into models of the aorta and imaged with a CT scanner. The difference in contrast was calculated for the metal and nonmetal cases for a variety of imaging acquisitions or reconstruction settings.

While it may sound simple to determine the objectivity of quantification, sometimes it can be quite difficult to determine if a metric is correlated with underlying biological truth. To ensure independence of CT system influence, it is necessary to have ground truth biological models which are (1) representative of patient anatomy and disease and (2) are made of materials which are anatomically realistic when imaged by CT. For simulated CT scans, biological material properties of the model need to be known so that the attenuation through the model can be simulated. In terms of ground truth realism, it may be possible that the ground truth objects used to test imaging acquisition settings are not similar enough to the underlying ground truth anatomy of patients, and therefore the results would not give objective information about the patients.

Generation of realistic anatomic and disease models is challenging because it is incredibly difficult to ever know the ground truth anatomy of the patient, and therefore it is difficult to ensure that models are representative of patient anatomy and disease. Ground truth of the patient cannot be determined directly from CT scans because the patient anatomy as displayed by CT scans has already been affected by the imaging system. Ground truth anatomy cannot always be determined even by surgical means because the surgery itself changes the morphological and anatomical appearance of the area of interest. For example, lung tissue that has been removed from a patient and scanned by a micro-CT scanner does not retain its shape and morphology outside of the living and breathing patient. Several solutions to the problem of creating anatomical models include (1) iteratively generating ground truth models which are blurred by the system MTF and injected with noise according to the system NPS and are then updated based on comparison with a CT representation of the anatomy [17, 18] and (2) using biomechanical and physiological theoretical models to create models grounded in biology [19, 20]. Example anatomical models with realism have included morphological lung and liver lesion models [21], internal heterogeneity liver models [17], internal heterogeneity lesion models (Fig. 15.3) [13], and cardiac plaque models [15].

Another challenging aspect of ascertaining objectivity is ensuring the fidelity of the ground

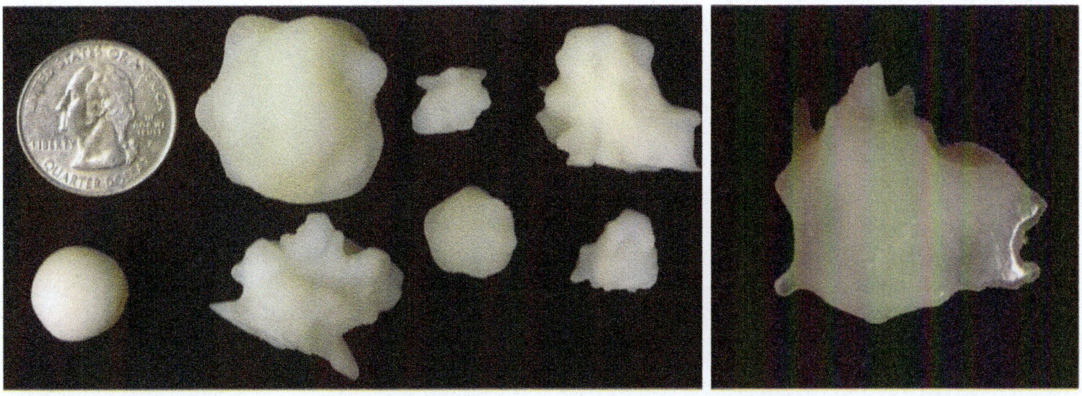

Fig. 15.3 (Left) Examples of 3D printed textured lesion models of different sizes with anatomically informed texture and morphology. The lesion models are shown next to a quarter for size comparison. (Right) A cross section of a textured lesion model which was cut to show the internal heterogeneity of the two materials

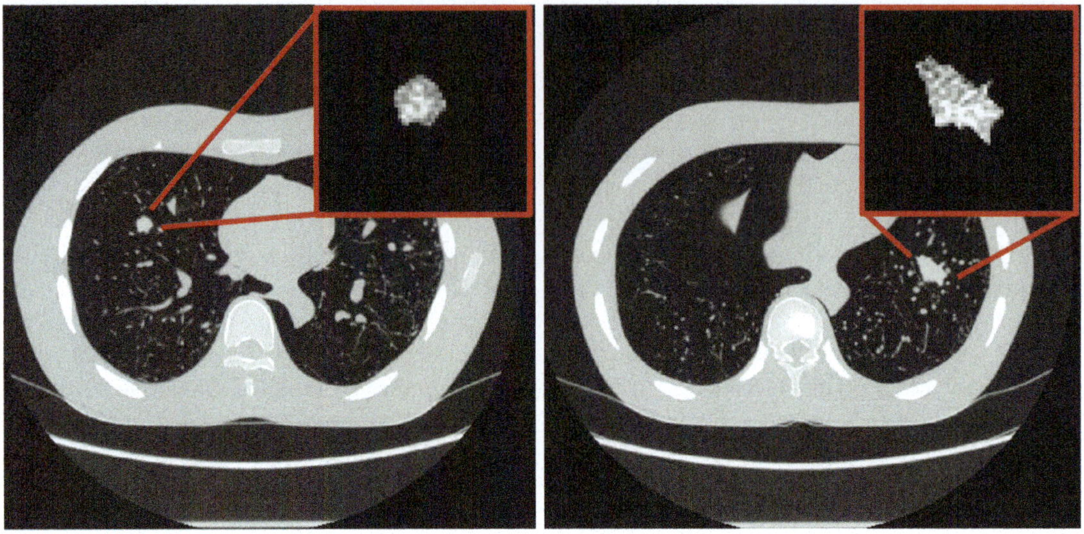

Fig. 15.4 Example cross-sectional CT images (scanned with GE Revolution, FBP Standard Reconstruction) of heterogenous and morphologically realistic 3D printed nodules imbedded within the anthropomorphic chest phantom

truth object. In cases of 3D printing, theoretically the ground truth object is a known quantity because it is 3D printed, and therefore the size, shape, materials, etc. should be exactly known. These objects which are exactly known can be inserted into anthropomorphic phantoms and scanned with commercial CT scanners (Fig. 15.4). While 3D printing is incredibly powerful, the 3D printing process itself is not always exact. The 3D prints themselves need to be validated and verified for their accuracy, both geometrically [22] and in terms of material density; the current 3D printed materials have a limited range of radiodensity for soft tissue representation, making it difficult to represent realistic anatomical heterogeneity. Using computational models and simulation through so-called virtual clinical trials offer advantages that remedy these limitations.

In summary, quantification should be objective to give information about the ground truth anatomy of the patient. Any quantification should be reflective of the true state of the patient rather than the imaging technology used to obtain images. Objectivity can be assessed by quantifying the bias between the ground truth and the CT representation of the ground truth. In creating a ground truth reference object, ether physical or computational, it is important to ensure that it is designed with materials and morphology which is representative of patients. It is also important to verify that the objects created are exactly known and are not altered over time or during the creation process.

Robustness

Once we have identified a relevant attribute of a patient to which we want to assign an objective quantification, what is the best way to quantify the attribute? For example, we know that lesion size is a relevant attribute of a lesion indicative of patient outcome, but how do we quantify it? Volume, area, and in-plane diameter are all different ways to assign a number to lesion size, but which is the best quantification that can be made most objective and most precise? There may even be a better metric that quantifies size. With all the different options for quantifying an attribute, it is challenging to determine which quantification will be the best one which will ensure objectivity but will also be able to be measured robustly.

Quantifications are considered robust when they can be done precisely with low amount of variability. Ensuring robustness is all about ascertaining the imprecision in any measurement and identifying, and possibly mitigating, the sources of variability. Variability can be measured between different scanners, within the same scanner across different patients or even within the same scanner and same patient over time or on the same day, after a so-called coffee break. There are many sources of variability in the quantification process including the quantification metric itself, the inherent noise properties of the scanner, the variability between different imaging conditions, the variability in the ground truth of the patient day-to-day, the operator or segmentation algorithm used to identify the object or region of interest in the image, the amount and type of contrast given, the background anatomy interfering with isolating the object, and the extent of motion in the patient. Figure 15.5 gives an example of how the same lesion may look different on a CT scan based on different resolution and noise properties alone.

The first variability which must be understood is that caused by image noise which is always present in CT imaging. Noise in CT images never presents in the same way from scan to scan and can significantly impact the robustness of certain quantifications. The variability due to image noise can be assessed by re-scanning the exact same object or patient under the exact same conditions consecutively in what is known as a test-retest or a "coffee break" study design. The consecutive images can be analyzed by extracting the same quantitative feature, such as volume, texture, or contrast. The two extracted measurements from the two consecutive images will never be the same due to the inherent noise in the image. If the same object were scanned 100 s of times in a row and the feature was measured every time, it would be possible to measure a standard deviation for the quantification which is due strictly

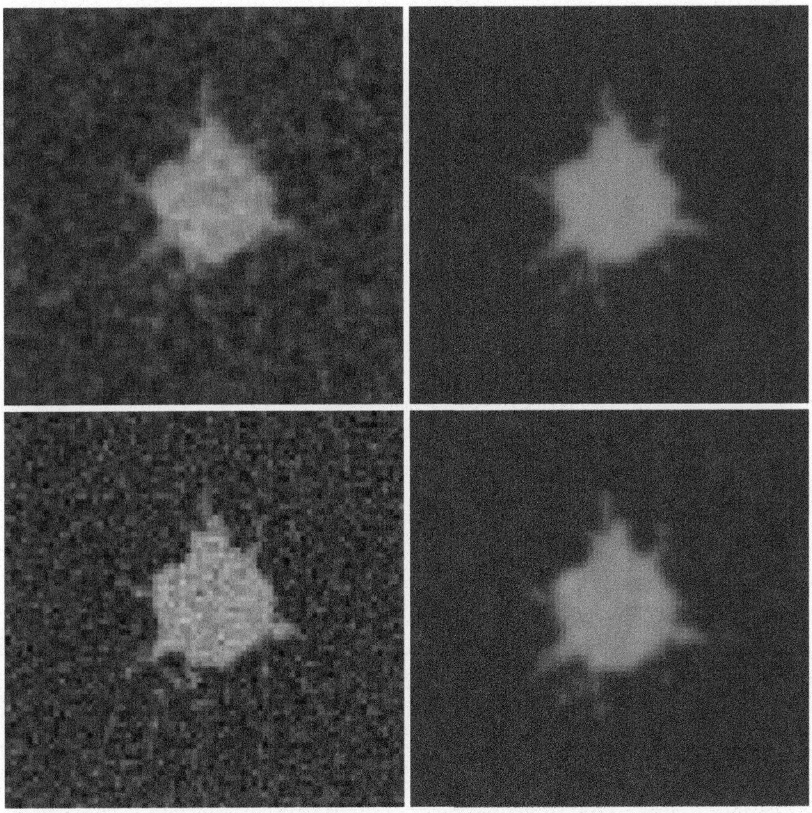

Fig. 15.5 The same lesion model presented with different noise and resolution properties of commercial CT scanners

to the noise alone. This is the fundamental first level of variability which underlies the process of image quantification and is specific to each acquisition setting and noise level in the image.

The next level of variability is caused by the different settings which could be used to acquire CT scans. The variability due to different scanning conditions can be assessed by scanning the same object multiple times using multiple different scanning settings. The quantitative measurement can then be extracted from the images. A standard deviation of the quantitative features can be calculated to describe the variability due to scanning conditions. This variability can potentially be considered a systematic effect that can be mitigated by calibrations or corrections, but when many clinical applications use imaging generically without respect to this effect, it is important to understand it as a source of random variability in the quantitative feature measurement. If this variability is large, then it may be necessary to define specific scanning protocols, such as specific slice thickness, image noise, and reconstruction method, which limit the variability in the final quantification measurement. For example, texture measurements of lesions may be significantly affected by the image noise, slice thickness, and reconstruction settings [23]. To limit the variability in this space, it may be necessary to define specific protocols which render extracted features with a controlled level of variability.

Another level of variability which is important clinically is the variability in a feature due to different readers and segmentation algorithms [24, 25]. To illustrate the importance of this variability, consider a patient with a lung lesion being treated and monitored over time to assess the effectiveness of the therapy. If the patient is scanned and the volume of a lesion is measured by one radiologist, and 6 months later, the patient returns to the clinic and is scanned again and the lesion volume is measured by a different radiologist, we want to be sure that the variability between different radiologists is low so that we can trust that the measurements are precise descriptions of the patient disease status. This interobserver variability can be assessed by giving different observers the same sets of images for analysis [25]. Each observer is asked to process the relevant anatomy and measure the quantitative feature. A standard deviation can then be calculated to quantify the variability due to different observers. The same methods can also be applied to different segmentation algorithms which can be manual, automatic, or semiautomatic. It is likely that some segmentation algorithms will be less variable than others, and therefore, the segmentation algorithms which are less variable should be used for quantitative purposes to ensure precision in quantification. However, it is always important to note that segmentation algorithms which are more precise might also be biased – and if so, the bias should be mitigated.

While sources of variability are naturally present in the process of quantification in CT, there are ways to determine the quantification of an attribute which is most robust across different sources of variability. For example, the feature compactness is a metric that takes the ratio of volume to surface area to describe how similar or different an object is from a sphere. There are several equations used to measure compactness, and some measures are less variable than others when applied to CT images which contain voxelized depictions of objects. Voxelized objects have inherent variability at the edges due to partial volume averaging which leads to a variable determination at the edges of an object, i.e., whether a pixel should be included or excluded from the segmentation mask. The variability at the edges might be different if the object were scanned differently or if the boundary of the object was assessed by different people. This variability can either be magnified or suppressed depending on how compactness is calculated.

One method, which magnifies the variability in compactness, uses calculations of volume and surface area which are made directly from the voxelized segmentation mask. The voxelized surface area is very misleading, because the surface area of a voxelized object is the sum of all the external faces of the cubes that make up the object. Since anatomy is not made up of cubic faces, the cubic calculation of surface area tends to lead to an overestimation of the surface area and also to a more variable measure of surface area depending on which specific boundary voxels do or do not get included in the segmentation mask. Another method of calculating compactness uses the volume and surface area of meshes which are fit to the voxelized object. This method is less variable than the previous method because the mesh fit takes out the systematic overestimation of surface area and reduces some of the variability of included and excluded voxels at the edges of the object. Yet, another way to measure compactness is using the equation for discrete compactness [26] which calculates compactness on a voxelized object using a formula based on the number of voxels included in the segmentation mask. This discrete compactness method was shown to be less variable than other metrics in the case of voxelized objects [26]. This example illustrates that the method of quantification of an attribute can affect the robustness of the measurement and that quantification methods should be chosen carefully to minimize sources of variability.

Variability in quantification can also be due to variations in the biology of a patient. For example, in the quantification of coronary stenosis, patient heart rate can affect the stenosis quantification such that patients with higher heart rates have less precise quantification of stenosis than patients with lower heart rates [15]. Another example of biologic variability is the variability in lesion measures due to confluence of the features of the lesion and the segmentation process. For instance, if the lung lesions have well-defined margins, they may be able to be segmented with less variability than lesions which are more spiculated and have unclear boundaries between cancerous tissue and healthy tissue. In this case, spiculated lesions may result in volume measurements which are less robust and less precise than well circumscribed lesions. A third example of biologic variability is the degree of motion-induced blurring affecting the quantification of radiomics features [27]. A final example of biologic variability is the case of metal in the patient. Patients with metal implants which are located near relevant anatomy may have more variable quantification of features because of variations in how the metal artifact presents itself in the image. The metal artifact induced variability also may be impacted by any metal artifact reduction algorithms used.

Study designs for ascertaining measurement robustness can be performed in patients, physical phantoms, computational, and hybrid datasets, each with their relative strengths and weaknesses. Test-retest studies in patients [28, 29] are useful for providing realistic anatomic geometry and material properties; however, these studies lack ground truth, are expensive, and subject patients to ionizing radiation. Studies of robustness in phantoms [30, 31] are useful for knowing the ground truth and overcoming radiation exposure limitations; however, they have the added challenge of utilizing phantom geometry and materials which may not be realistic and complex compared with patients. In addition, physical phantom studies only allow for a finite number of different objects and scan repeats [32] due to resource constraints in creating different combinations of physical phantom characteristics and scans. Hybrid datasets [33], which are created by inserting computational models of lesions into patient data, can be created to ascertain robustness. Hybrid datasets have been shown to yield similar conclusions to real CT datasets [34], with added benefit of knowing the ground truth of the inserted lesion. The downside of hybrid datasets, however, is that they are often limited to study imaging acquisition protocols which have been previously used to image patients. Finally, simulation studies of CT imaging systems through virtual clinical trials [11, 12, 32] can be useful for quantifying variability across a larger range of possible scenarios with known ground truth. While simulation studies are fast and cost-effective, they have the caveat that they need to be validated to ensure realism. Each study design has its relative strengths and weaknesses, ranging on a spectrum from controlled experimentation to clinical realism (Fig. 15.6). In the process of ascertaining the robustness of a quantitative feature, it may be necessary to use a combination of patient, phantom, hybrid, or

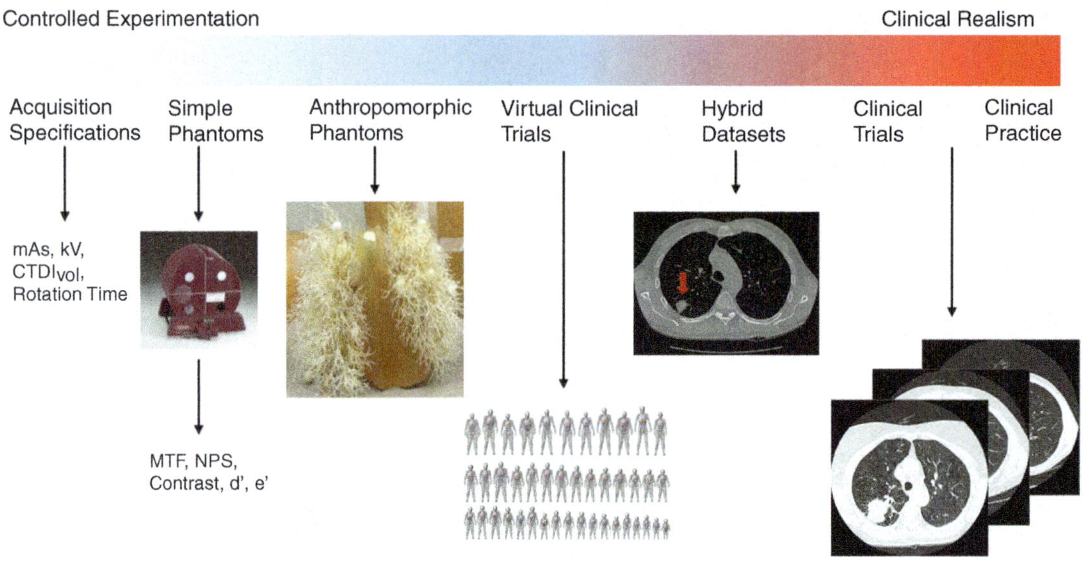

Fig. 15.6 The range of possible studies to ascertain variability ranges from controlled experimentation to clinical realism. Each type of study has its relative merits and drawbacks

simulation studies to fully understand and validate the expected degree of variability.

It is important to understand the degree of variability of a feature because it is important to be able to differentiate between real biological change in a quantitative feature over time and an artifactual change due to the quantification process itself. For example, consider a case where a patient with a liver lesion is being monitored over time. At each time point, the liver lesion volume is measured. It is important to know the expected variability in liver lesion volume due to different acquisition settings, image noise, segmentations, etc. so that we can say with confidence either that the patient's liver lesion is truly getting larger or that the change is likely due to inherent variability in the imaging and quantification process. By knowing the variability, a minimum detectable change in liver lesion volume can be calculated with, for example, 95% confidence. The concept of minimum detectable difference, which has been previously applied to iodine concentration [35] and lung nodule volume estimation [36], can be a powerful tool to aid decision-making about when the differences in a quantification are real and when they are due to other imaging factors.

In summary, ideal CT-based quantification should be robust across different sources of variability present in CT. The fundamental underlying variability in CT imaging is due to different instances of image noise. Other sources of variability come from differences in CT acquisition protocols and scanners, in observes and segmentation algorithms, in methods of quantifying a given biological phenomena, and in the patient anatomy and biology. Variability can be assessed by imaging the same object across the different sources of variability. After variability has been assessed, it is necessary to ensure that the quantification process is done in the most robust way to limit the impact of variability. This may involve choosing specific CT imaging protocols and segmentation algorithms which minimize variability of a specific quantitative feature. It may also involve choosing the quantification method which is most precise and robust in the context of voxelized images of human anatomy. It will never be possible to eliminate variability entirely; however, if variability is known, then it can be used to give a lower limit on the ability to detect a change in quantitative features, i.e., a lower minimum detectable change.

Implementation

While it is essential that the extraction of quantitative measures from CT images be relevant to biology, objective, and robust, it is also essential that the process be implementable in a clinical workflow. Quantification will not ultimately improve patient care if it is too difficult to implement or if the process of calculating quantitative features takes too long compared with the clinical demands. For example, if the time needed to compute a quantitative metric is too long, it may be impractical. If the quantification requires an in-depth interaction between a clinician and a quantification user interface, this may also be impractical. It is therefore necessary to integrate quantification into the clinical software and to make the process of quantification as automated and as intuitive as possible.

Integration and automation of quantification into clinical software has several potential benefits for patient care. One benefit of automation is that it makes the process less dependent on specific members of the clinical care team to take time out of their schedules to initiate a quantification workflow. Automation also has the benefit of being less prone to inter- and intra-observer differences and would therefore be more likely to be robust. For example, if the clinical implementation of a volume measurement requires a radiologist to manually segment multiple slices of a lesion, this may become too time-consuming for the clinical workflow and may also lead to a high degree of variability between different radiologists. However, if the process of segmentation can be semiautomatic so that the radiologist just needs to do minimal manual segmentation in a single slice, this will save time.

There will of course be more time-saving by implementing automatic algorithms which segment the desired anatomy independent of human input. Automatic segmentation can further send the results to the electronic record; this would allow the radiologist to see quantitative results while reading the images. The challenge with automatic segmentation, however, is that it will be necessary to ensure that the segmentation worked in all cases the way it was intended. Some patients have conditions which make the automatic detection of their anatomy challenging. Examples include lung and spine segmentation in patients with collapsed lungs and severe scoliosis. In these cases, when the anatomy is significantly different from what is expected, the algorithm may fail to work as intended. Therefore, it may be necessary to have a user interface which can display the segmentation to a clinician to ensure proper quantification. It will also be ideal to design the interface such that it gives the clinicians the variability surrounding the extracted quantification so that they know the imprecision of any quantity that they may use to make clinical decisions. The advances in machine-learning and AI methods in image segmentation and quantification can address some of the current limitations, but that will take time.

Some other key considerations for implementation include designing a quantification tool which is efficient without compromising patient care and designed to allow for the most efficient and intuitive interactions between caregivers and the technology. For example, if the quantification tool calculates quantitative features but displays them in a confusing way or makes the clinicians work to find the desired results, then the technology is likely to be under-utilized clinically. A well-designed user interface would be intuitive for clinicians to use, making it easy for them to find and interpret the quantitative results they need to make clinical decisions.

In summary, CT-based quantification should be implementable clinically. Clinically implementable quantification tools should operate with high speed and be integrated into the clinical workflow. Automation of segmentation in clinical software will make quantification less prone to inter- and intra-observer differences and will save time that would have been spent by clinicians in segmenting and calculating features. One challenge with automation of segmentation and feature calculation is the need to validate the segmentation and calculation. If quantitative features are presented to radiologists while they are reading, the interface which displays the quantitative results should be intuitive to understand and to use. The machine-learning and AI methods can provide significant advantages in improving the robustness and implementability of quantitative CT.

Interactions

While we present the relevance, objectivity, robustness, and implementation as four distinct aspects of quantification, these aspects are closely related and inform one another. For instance, it is uncertain if a metric is relevant until it is robust enough for this to be ascertained. As such, it is difficult to discern if it is better to start by identifying relevant metrics and then later test their objectivity and robustness or if it is better to identify robust and objective metrics and then later determine if they are relevant. For example, if we consider quantification of texture features, it may be possible that texture features derived from gray level co-occurrence and gray level run length matrices are relevant metrics which correlate with patient outcomes. However, until researchers and clinicians can identify a quantification protocol which reduces the variability and bias, it may appear that the metrics are not correlated with patient outcomes. It may be the case that metrics which are not robust and objective are also less likely to be clinically relevant, and as a result, the attributes feed into and inform each other (Fig. 15.7).

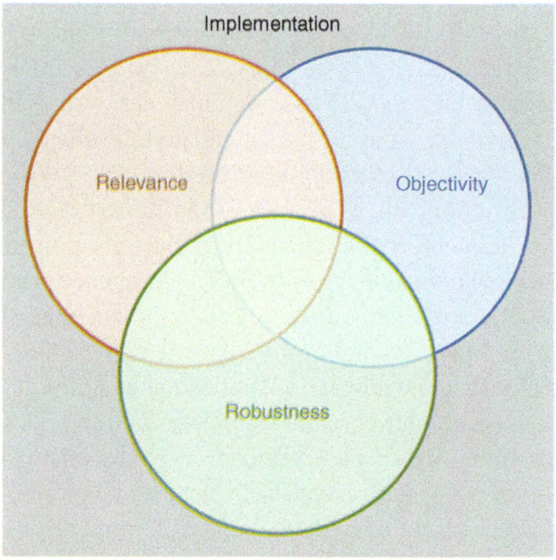

Fig. 15.7 The aspects of relevance, objectivity, and robustness are at times interrelated and feed into each other. Implementation is shown on the outside because it can only be achieved effectively once the other three aspects have been established

Conclusions

While CT-based quantification has not been the historical norm in radiology, its continued and expanded use allows for patient care to be more consistent and evidence-based. For CT-based quantification to be effective, it will be necessary to ensure that quantification is clinically and biologically relevant, objective, robust, and finally implementable clinically. Biological and clinical relevance is the overall end goal of quantification in CT because the metrics measured from CT scans must be useful clinically. Once metrics have been identified which are biologically and clinically relevant, then it is necessary to make sure that those measurements capture the physical quantity they are intended to measure and that they do so in a way that is objective and robust. Ideal quantifications are done with low variability and with a high degree of accuracy. To verify the accuracy and variability, it is necessary to have biologically relevant reference ground truth. Finally, quantification must be implementable in a clinical workflow and therefore must have sufficiently fast computation time and must be presented in a way which is intuitive for clinicians to understand and to use.

Not addressed in this chapter is the provision of approaching quantitative CT without the medium of radiomics biomarkers – taking advantages of machine-learning and AI methods operating on large datasets to ascertain the disease condition directly from the data. This is an exciting prospect with much potential. However, this development requires large amount of "clean" data, with established ground truth, so the training process can be trusted. Further the results should ultimately be understood and related to the biological reality of the disease, provisioned through radiomics. And finally, many sources of variabilities noted above can limit the reach of radiomics-less methodologies as well. As such, we expect that in the decades to come, quantitative CT will be advanced along both the principle-driven/radiomics and data-driven approaches. Ultimately, as in all medical developments, the goal is never the tool, but the good that it is expected to provide to advance human health.

References

1. Radiologic Society of North America. Quantitative imaging biomarkers alliance. 2017. Available: https://www.rsna.org/QIBA/.
2. Gillies RJ, Kinahan PE, Hricak H. Radiomics: images are more than pictures, they are data. Radiology. 2015;278:563–77.
3. Aerts HJ, Velazquez ER, Leijenaar RT, Parmar C, Grossmann P, Cavalho S, et al. Decoding tumour phenotype by noninvasive imaging using a quantitative radiomics approach. Nat Commun. 2014;5:4006.
4. Kumar V, Gu Y, Basu S, Berglund A, Eschrich SA, Schabath MB, et al. Radiomics: the process and the challenges. Magn Reson Imaging. 2012;30:1234–48.
5. Motta G, Carbone E, Spinelli E, Nahum M, Testa T, Flocchini G. Considerations about tumor size as a factor of prognosis in NSCLC. Ann Ital Chir. 1999;70:893–7.
6. Eisenhauer EA, Therasse P, Bogaerts J, Schwartz LH, Sargent D, Ford R, et al. New response evaluation criteria in solid tumours: revised RECIST guideline (version 1.1). Eur J Cancer. 2009;45:228–47.
7. Zwirewich CV, Vedal S, Miller RR, Müller NL. Solitary pulmonary nodule: high-resolution CT and radiologic-pathologic correlation. Radiology. 1991;179:469–76.
8. Huang Y-H, Chang Y-C, Huang C-S, Wu T-J, Chen J-H, Chang R-F. Computer-aided diagnosis of mass-like lesion in breast MRI: differential analysis of the 3-D morphology between benign and malignant tumors. Comput Methods Prog Biomed. 2013;112:508–17.
9. Gilhuijs KG, Giger ML, Bick U. Computerized analysis of breast lesions in three dimensions using dynamic magnetic-resonance imaging. Med Phys. 1998;25:1647–54.
10. Chalkidou A, O'Doherty MJ, Marsden PK. False discovery rates in PET and CT studies with texture features: a systematic review. PLoS One. 2015;10:e0124165.
11. Abadi E, Harrawood B, Sharma S, Kapadia A, Segars WP, Samei E, DukeSim: a realistic, rapid, and scanner-specific simulation framework in computed tomography. IEEE Trans Med Imaging. 2018.
12. Hoye J, Solomon J, Sauer TJ, Robins M, Samei E. Systematic analysis of bias and variability of morphologic features for lung lesions in computed tomography. J Med Imaging. 2019;6:013504.
13. Zheng Y, Solomon J, Choudhury K, Marin D, Samei E. Accuracy and variability of texture-based radiomics features of lung lesions across CT imaging conditions. In SPIE Medical Imaging. Bellingham, Washington; 2017. p 101325F-101325F-7.
14. Mackin D, Fave X, Zhang L, Fried D, Yang J, Taylor B, et al. Measuring CT scanner variability of radiomics features. Investig Radiol. 2015;50:757.
15. Richards T, Sturgeon GM, Ramirez-Giraldo JC, Rubin GD, Koweek LH, Segars WP, et al. Quantification of uncertainty in the assessment of coronary plaque in CCTA through a dynamic cardiac phantom and 3D-printed plaque model. J Med Imaging. 2018;5:013501.
16. Huang JY, Kerns JR, Nute JL, Liu X, Balter PA, Stingo FC, et al. An evaluation of three commercially available metal artifact reduction methods for CT imaging. Phys Med Biol. 2015;60:1047.
17. Solomon J, Ba A, Bochud F, Samei E. Comparison of low-contrast detectability between two CT reconstruction algorithms using voxel-based 3D printed textured phantoms. Med Phys. 2016;43:6497–506.
18. Castella C, Kinkel K, Descombes F, Eckstein MP, Sottas P-E, Verdun FR, et al. Mammographic texture synthesis: second-generation clustered lumpy backgrounds using a genetic algorithm. Opt Express. 2008;16:7595–607.
19. Abadi E, Segars WP, Sturgeon GM, Roos JE, Ravin CE, Samei E. Modeling lung architecture in the XCAT series of phantoms: physiologically based airways, arteries and veins. IEEE Trans Med Imaging. 2018;37:693–702.
20. Graff CG. A new, open-source, multi-modality digital breast phantom. In: Medical imaging 2016: physics of medical imaging. Bellingham, Washington; 2016. p. 978309.
21. Solomon J, Samei E. A generic framework to simulate realistic lung, liver and renal pathologies in CT imaging. Phys Med Biol. 2014;59:6637.
22. Bortolotto C, Eshja E, Peroni C, Orlandi MA, Bizzotto N, Poggi P. 3D printing of CT dataset: validation of an open source and consumer-available workflow. J Digit Imaging. 2016;29:14–21.
23. Ger RB, Zhou S, Chi P-CM, Lee HJ, Layman RR, Jones AK, et al. Comprehensive investigation on controlling for CT imaging variabilities in radiomics studies. Sci Rep. 8:13047.. 2018/08/29 2018
24. Buckler AJ, Danagoulian J, Johnson K, Peskin A, Gavrielides MA, Petrick N, et al. Inter-method performance study of tumor volumetry assessment on computed tomography test-retest data. Acad Radiol. 2015;22:1393–408.
25. Robins M, Solomon J, Hoye J, Smith T, Zheng Y, Ebner L, et al. Interchangeability between real and three-dimensional simulated lung tumors in computed tomography: an interalgorithm volumetry study. J Med Imaging. 2018;5:035504.

26. Bribiesca E. A measure of compactness for 3D shapes. Comput Math Appl. 2000;40:1275–84.
27. Lafata K, Cai J, Wang C, Hong J, Kelsey CR, Yin F-F. Spatial-temporal variability of radiomic features and its effect on the classification of lung cancer histology. Phys Med Biol. 2018;63:225003.
28. Balagurunathan Y, Kumar V, Gu Y, Kim J, Wang H, Liu Y, et al. Test–retest reproducibility analysis of lung CT image features. J Digit Imaging. 2014;27:805–23.
29. Wormanns D, Kohl G, Klotz E, Marheine A, Beyer F, Heindel W, et al. Volumetric measurements of pulmonary nodules at multi-row detector CT: in vivo reproducibility. Eur Radiol. 2004;14:86–92.
30. Chen B, Barnhart H, Richard S, Colsher J, Amurao M, Samei E. Quantitative CT: technique dependence of volume estimation on pulmonary nodules. Phys Med Biol. 2012;57:1335.
31. Gavrielides MA, Kinnard LM, Myers KJ, Petrick N. Noncalcified lung nodules: volumetric assessment with thoracic CT. Radiology. 2009;251:26–37.
32. Li Q, Gavrielides MA, Zeng R, Myers KJ, Sahiner B, Petrick N. Volume estimation of low-contrast lesions with CT: a comparison of performances from a phantom study, simulations and theoretical analysis. Phys Med Biol. 2015;60:671.
33. Robins M, Solomon J, Sahbaee P, Sedlmair M, Choudhury KR, Pezeshk A, et al. Techniques for virtual lung nodule insertion: volumetric and morphometric comparison of projection-based and image-based methods for quantitative CT. Phys Med Biol. 2017;62:7280.
34. Robins M, Kalpathy-Cramer J, Obuchowski NA, Buckler A, Athelogou M, Jarecha R et al. Evaluation of Simulated Lesions as Surrogates to Clinical Lesions for Thoracic CT Volumetry: The Results of an International Challenge. Academic radiology. 2019; 26(7):e161–e173.
35. Euler A, Solomon J, Mazurowski MA, Samei E, Nelson RC. How accurate and precise are CT based measurements of iodine concentration? A comparison of the minimum detectable concentration difference among single source and dual source dual energy CT in a phantom study. European radiology. 2019;29(4):2069–78.
36. Gavrielides MA, Li Q, Zeng R, Myers KJ, Sahiner B, Petrick N. Minimum detectable change in lung nodule volume in a phantom CT study. Acad Radiol. 2013;20:1364–70.

CT Material Identification

16

Federica Vernuccio and Daniele Marin

Introduction

Material identification with conventional computed tomography (CT) is based on x-ray attenuation as quantified in Hounsfield Units and displayed in shades of gray at different window levels. However, material identification with conventional CT is limited by the dependence of the linear attenuation coefficient μ – and subsequently the CT number – on mass density, material type (effective atomic number, Z), beam energy, and CT scanner. Above all, CT number only provides an estimated average of the x-ray attenuation of different materials at a given kVp within a selected voxel, and different materials with similar attenuation coefficients (e.g., calcium and iodine) have similar CT numbers, even if they differ in mass attenuation coefficients and elemental compositions [1].

In contrast to a single-energy acquisition, dual-energy CT (DECT) allows for the selective identification of materials in tissues. This has important clinical implications as precise material identification with DECT is nowadays a mainstay for detection and characterization of different diseases, from head (e.g., differentiation of intracranial hemorrhage from iodinated contrast material staining) to toe (e.g., characterization of monosodium urate deposits in tophaceous gout) [2]. A more recent approach for material identification is represented by photon-counting computed tomography (PCCT), which is currently under research and technological development, and is being translated into clinical studies.

Material Identification: General Principles

The attenuation coefficient μ of any material can be described as the linear combination of two independent functions – the photoelectric effect and the Compton (incoherent) scattering. Compton scattering is relatively similar across most materials; conversely, the likelihood of photoelectric absorption varies considerably, depending mainly on the material and on the x-ray energy. When an atom undergoes the photoelectric effect, the innermost shell (the k-shell) electron is ejected via the incident photon. Photoelectric absorption depends strongly on the unique binding energy of any k-shell electron for a particular material. The k-edge is the minimum energy required for the photoelectric event to occur with a k-shell

F. Vernuccio (✉)
Department of Radiology, Duke University Medical Center, Durham, NC, USA

Department of Health Promotion, Mother and Child Care, Internal Medicine and Medical Specialties, University of Palermo, Palermo, Italy

D. Marin
Department of Radiology, Duke University Medical Center, Durham, NC, USA
e-mail: daniele.marin@duke.edu

© Springer Nature Switzerland AG 2020
E. Samei, N. J. Pelc (eds.), *Computed Tomography*, https://doi.org/10.1007/978-3-030-26957-9_16

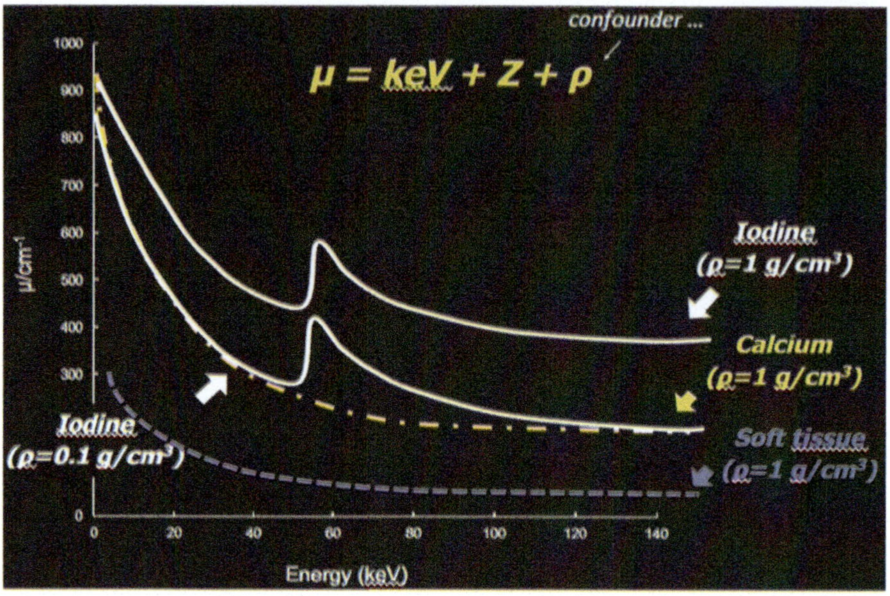

Fig. 16.1 Graph of linear attenuation coefficients for iodine at two different densities (assuming ρ = 1 g/cm^3) (white), calcium (assuming ρ = 1 g/cm^3) (yellow), and soft tissue (assuming ρ = 0.1 g/cm^3) (violet) as a function of energy (in kiloelectron volts). (Adapted from McCollough et al. [2])

electron. The k-edge varies for each material and is higher with increasing atomic numbers (Z). The closer the x-ray energy level is to the k-edge of a material, the more the material attenuates. By analyzing photoelectric absorption properties of different materials at different x-ray energies, it is possible to identify materials with sufficiently different atomic numbers *Z irrespective of their material density* (Fig. 16.1) [3]. This basic principle, known as material decomposition, can be exploited for material identification using either DECT or PCCT.

Dual-Energy CT: Material Identification with Single- and Dual-Source Systems

DECT operates with low-energy (between 70 kVp and 100 kVp depending on the dual energy platform) and high-energy (between 140 kVp and 150 kVp depending on the dual energy platform) x-ray spectra, obtaining the relative attenuation of voxels in the imaged volume at these two energies [2]. DECT technology includes simultaneous (i.e., dual-layer detector DECT) and near-simultaneous (i.e., single-source rapid KV-switching DECT [rsDECT] and dual-source DECT [dsDECT]) low- and high-energy acquisition. The relative difference in attenuation at the two energies forms the basis for material decomposition with DECT. The ability of DECT to discriminate between two materials depends strongly on the difference between the characteristic CT number ratio (or index) for each material defined as the low- to high-kVp CT number ratio of a given material (Fig. 16.2) [4].

Single-source DECT systems create material-specific images using a two-material decomposition algorithm. Though any two materials can be selected for two-material decomposition, if the basis pair includes two materials with similar spectral properties the resulting information will be limited as the mass density images would be nearly identical. In clinical practice, the typical basis pair for two-material decomposition comprises water and iodine because of the large difference in the attenuation-energy curves between these two materials.

Dual-source DECT systems typically create material-specific images using a three-material decomposition algorithm. Owing to the assumption of volume and mass conservation, the three-material decomposition algorithm

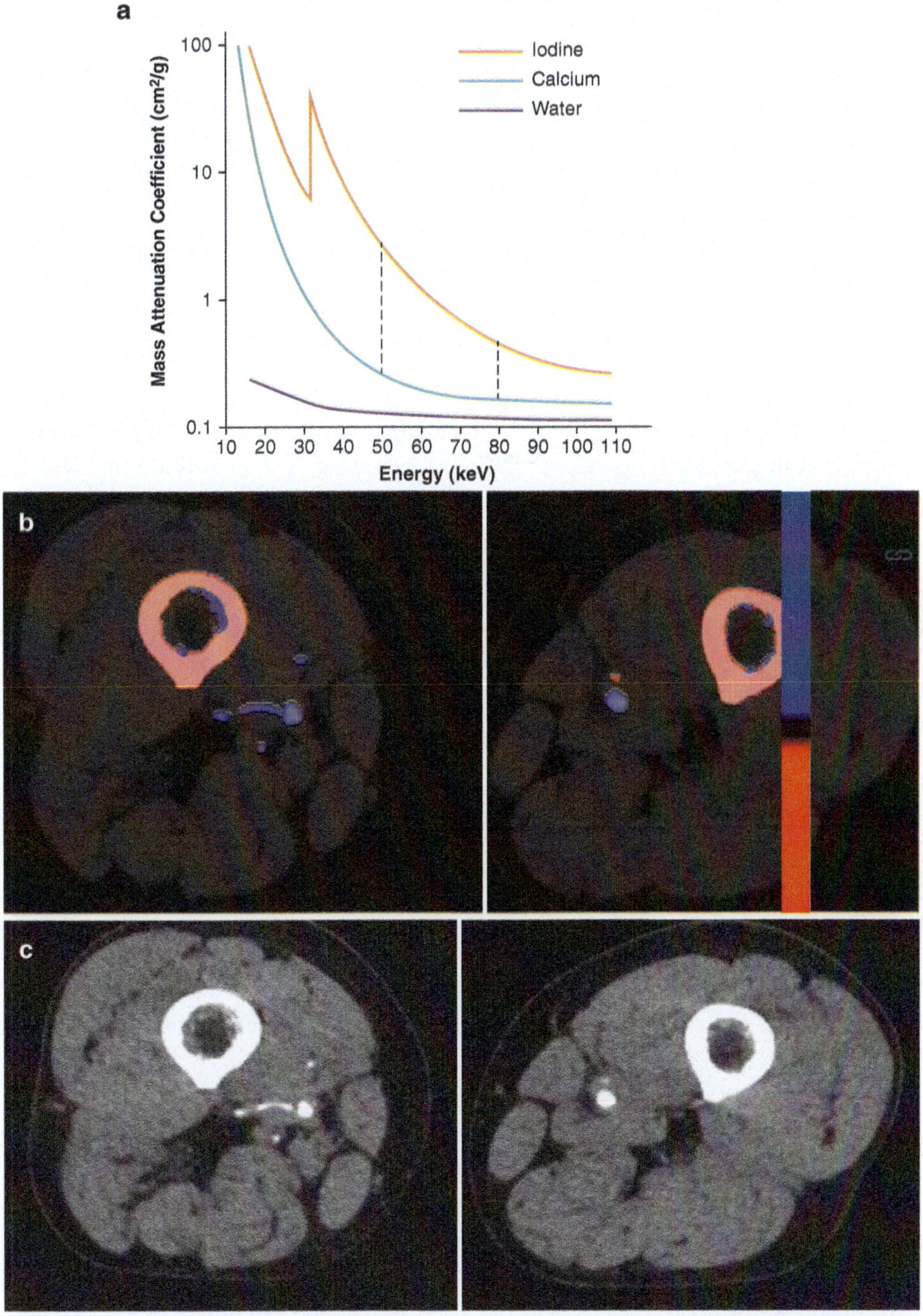

Fig. 16.2 (**a**) CT Number of iodine (yellow), calcium (green), and water (violet) at different x-ray energies (**a**). Each material has its own characteristic changing pattern at low and high kilovoltage: at a low kilovoltage, materials with a high molecular weight (mainly iodine) show greater x-ray absorption due to a greater likelihood of the photoelectric effect occurring. The change in measurement of CT attenuation between low and high kilovoltage will enable differentiating iodine and calcium as demonstrated in (**b**) and (**c**). Color-coded dual-energy post-processed axial CT scan (**b**) demonstrates the bone in red owing to the presence of calcium and the vessels in blue owing to the presence of iodine. In the left femoral artery, the color-coded images allow to easily recognize the presence of calcified parietal atherosclerosis in red. The presence of calcified parietal atherosclerosis shows a similar hyperattenuation as compared to the lumen of the vessel in the axial CT scan in the arterial phase (**c**), thus preventing from easy differentiation between calcium and iodine on conventional CT

allows to estimate the concentration of three materials with known elemental compositions in a voxel. In the post-processing, the three-material decomposition algorithm allows the suppression or the enhancement of one of the materials, depending on the desired clinical application. In particular, by erasing iodine contrast material, it is possible to produce a virtual non-contrast (VNC) image; conversely, the enhancement of iodine contrast material will result in a color-coded iodine series. More recently, a multimaterial decomposition algorithm has been developed for fast kilovolt-peak-switching DECT and seems to be promising for fat quantification [5].

One of the main questions regarding VNC has been its clinical acceptability as a replacement of true non-contrast images. It is important to realize that the necessary assumption for accepting VNC in clinical practice is demonstration of an equivalence of these two image reconstructions. Previous studies have shown that VNC can provide reliable quantitative information regarding baseline tissue attenuations in HU, suggesting that these images may obviate the need of a separate nonenhanced acquisition during multiphasic CT protocols with substantial radiation dose savings (Fig. 16.3) [6, 7]. However, DE-based iodine subtraction is not always perfect. In the assessment of renal enhancement, lower attenuation values may be encountered in the dorsal portion of the kidneys next to the spine, owing to

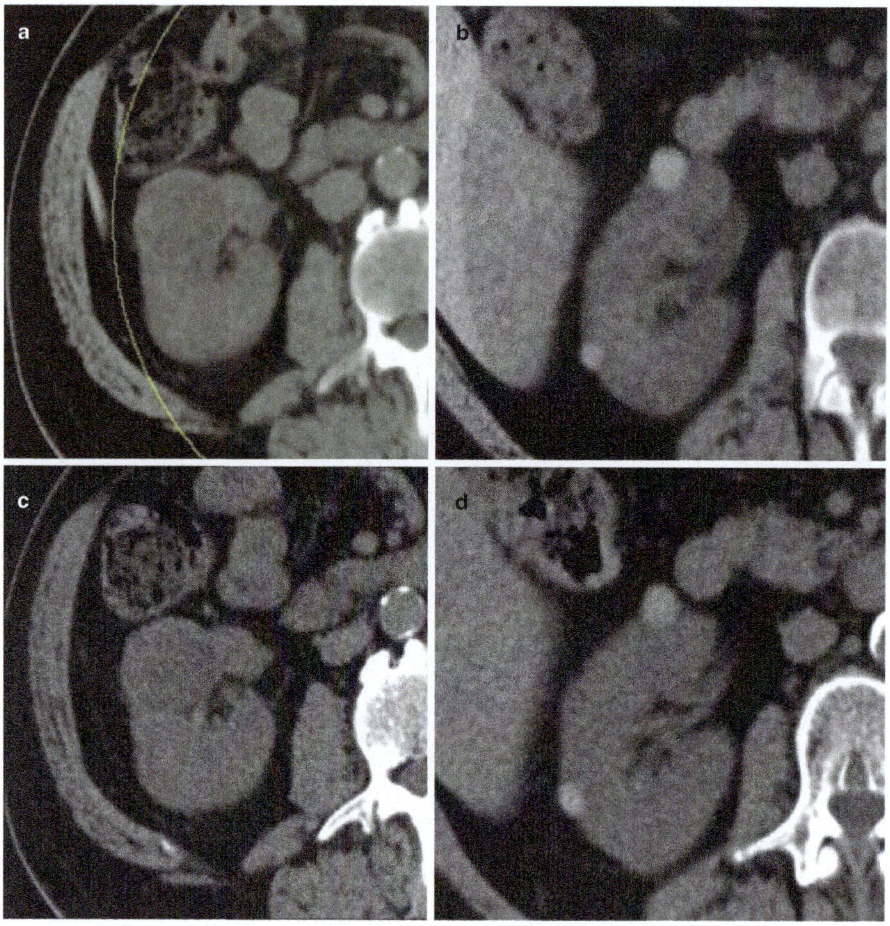

Fig. 16.3 Post-processed virtual non-contrast axial CT images of a simple renal cyst (**a**) and of an hemorrhagic renal cyst (**b**) show almost the same density as compared to the respective true non-contrast images (**c** and **d**, respectively), thus allowing a confident diagnosis

beam hardening affecting the low-kilovoltage images. Additional potential drawbacks of the VNC include erroneous subtraction of calcium (e.g., small renal calculi), as well as higher image noise.

Color-coded iodine images have several potential benefits. First, because these images are reconstructed from the same contrast-enhanced dual-energy dataset, they are not prone to motion and/or breathing artifacts and eliminate any potential variability that can occur during two separate acquisitions with a single-energy conventional multiphasic CT protocol. As such, quantitative information regarding the iodine uptake can be conveniently obtained from a single region of interest manually placed on the color-coded iodine map.

In addition, DECT allows for reconstruction of simulated monoenergetic images, which can be viewed through a broad range of energies, yielding increased consistency and precision of calculated CT numbers. Simulated monoenergetic images are generated through basis material decomposition, but the approach depends on the DECT platform – including an image-based method for the dsDECT and a projection-based method for rsDECT platform [8]. The different DECT hardware implementations may lead to potential significant differences in virtual monochromatic CT numbers from the same lesion examined with these two different methods [8]. In clinical practice, 70–75 KeV has been validated for routine adoption in many clinical contexts [9]. The adjustment of window and level values of simulated monoenergetic images may improve perceived conspicuity of lesions and the perception of image quality [10].

Unfortunately, one of the main limitations of DECT for material identification is represented by a high degree of overlap between the x-ray energy spectra generated at low (from 70 to 100 kVp) and high (140 or 150 kVp) peak tube potentials [11]. In addition, accuracy of material quantification may be significantly impacted by patient size and DECT parameters [12].

Photon-Counting CT: An Emerging Approach for Material Identification

PCCT is an emerging technology based on the adoption of photon-counting detectors (PCDs) to directly count individual photon interactions [13]. While in energy-integrating detectors (EIDs) – currently used in clinical CT scanners – each detector element measures the total x-ray energy deposited in the detector during each measurement interval, PCDs directly convert individual x-ray photons into an electric pulse in the detector readout electronics, with the height of each pulse proportional to the individual photon energy. This improved PCCT technology potentially yields improved contrast-to-noise ratio, dose reductions of x-ray radiation and contrast agents, improved spatial resolution, reduction of beam hardening artifacts, and, above all, an improved material identification owing to a more accurate K-edge imaging compared to DECT [14]. However, the clinical adoption of PCCT is limited by technical challenges (i.e., cross talk, pulse pileup, charge charging, K-escape x-rays, and charge trapping) resulting in a performance degradation of PCDs [13, 14].

Clinical Applications of Material Identification with DECT

Post-processed images from DECT – including virtual monochromatic images, color-coded iodine overlay, and iodine-only images – may improve the detection and characterization of diffuse and focal diseases and contrast enhancement with a wide spectrum of potential benefits in different clinical settings.

Material Identification with DECT: Hepatic Applications

DECT has proved its role in the identification and characterization of focal and diffuse liver diseases. The exact knowledge of the number of hepatic lesions may modify the therapeutical approach at diagnosis and at follow-up for both primary and secondary tumors. Low-energy simulated monoenergetic and material density iodine DECT images outperform conventional single-energy CT yielding increased conspicuity and detection rates for both hypervascular and hypovascular hepatic lesions, including metastases and hepatocellular carcinoma [15–17].

The use of DECT iodine maps allows for improved diagnostic accuracy in the diagnosis of neoplastic portal vein thrombosis. According to one study, an iodine concentration of 0.9 mg/ml during the late hepatic arterial phase results results in a sensitivity of 100% and specificity of 95.2% in the diagnosis of neoplastic thrombosis in patients with hepatocellular carcinoma [18]. Owing to the possibility of quantifying iodine content in the iodine maps, DECT may be also used for the characterization of small incidental hypoattenuating hepatic lesions deemed indeterminate with conventional CT images [19]. In our experience, an iodine concentration of 1.2 mg I/mL may differentiate benign from malignant indeterminate hypoattenuating hepatic lesions between 5 and 20 mm with a sensitivity of 94% and a specificity of 93% (Fig. 16.4) [19]. Finally, iodine maps may help in the assessment of intratumoral vital tumor burden after different therapies for primary or secondary liver tumors (Fig. 16.5) [20, 21].

In addition to the detection and characterization of focal hepatic lesions, DECT material

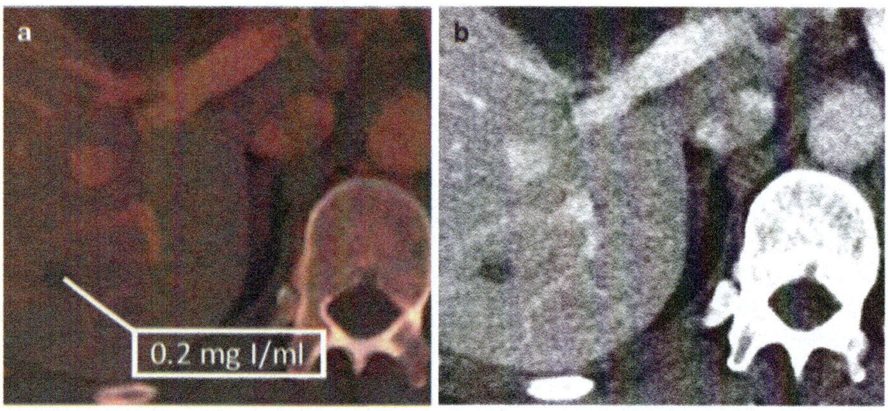

Fig. 16.4 Iodine material attenuation map (**a**) shows absence of significant iodine uptake of a 0.9 cm hypoattenuating lesion on contrast-enhanced CT on portal venous phase (**b**) deemed indeterminate 68-year-old male with history of previous malignancy. Based on the optimized thresholds of 1.2 mg I/mL, the lesion is correctly diagnosed as benign

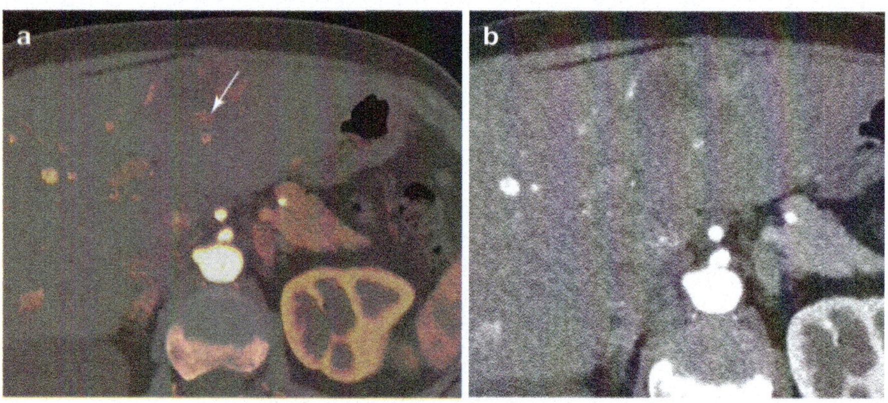

Fig. 16.5 Post-processed contrast map (**a**) shows peripheral viable tissue (arrow) in a hypodense lesion in the left liver lobe, improving the detection of the peripheral enhancement compared to contrast-enhanced CT in the arterial phase (**b**)

decomposition analysis may have a clinical role in the assessment of diffuse liver diseases such as steatosis, liver fibrosis, and hemochromatosis. Quantification of hepatic fat is becoming increasingly important as it represents the reversible stage in nonalcoholic fatty liver disease before progression to fibrosis and cirrhosis. Owing to the decreased attenuation at lower energy levels in presence of fat content, the spectral curve for hepatic steatosis shows an increase in the attenuation of fat with an increase in tube potential. An attenuation change greater than 10 HU between 80 and 140 kVp may be suggestive of at least 25% fatty infiltration. To date, unenhanced single-energy CT remains more accurate than unenhanced DECT for hepatic fat quantification, probably because of the small difference in the attenuation-energy curves between water and fat [22]. Nowadays, it is possible to generate the fat volume fraction (i.e., fat content in units of percentage volume) from the contrast-enhanced scan potentially eliminating the need for a separated non-contrast CT scan. The technical solutions for the fat volume fraction quantification include a three-material decomposition algorithm which assumes fat, soft tissue, and iodine as the main components [4] or a multimaterial decomposition algorithm using fast-kilovolt-peak switching DECT which allows to quantify fat with a convex constrained least-squares problem [5].

In addition to fat quantification, other biopsy-related indicators – including lobular inflammation, hepatocyte ballooning, and fibrosis – are often necessary for proper diagnosis and management in patients with chronic liver disease. The increase in collagen deposition – which is typical in patients with chronic liver disease with progressing fibrosis – results in the expansion of the extravascular extracellular space with a larger volume distribution for the contrast agent within the liver parenchyma. Using iodine maps, DECT may be used to estimate the increased distribution of the contrast agent in the extracellular space. During the equilibrium phase, the concentration of contrast agent within the intravascular space approximately equals that within the extravascular extracellular space. Iodine concentrations on the equilibrium phase images correlates with higher stages of fibrosis, and the iodine concentration (liver/aorta) ratio may be used for differentiating quantitatively healthy liver from cirrhotic liver and to estimate the severity of the disease [23, 24]. Estimated cutoff values that yield good accuracy for discriminating METAVIR fibrosis stages in chronic liver disease are 0.260 for F1 stage (sensitivity 71%, specificity 100%), 0.274 for F2 (sensitivity 79%, specificity 77%), 0.286 for F3 (sensitivity 76%, specificity 82%), and 0.299 for F4 (sensitivity 90%, specificity 73%) [24].

The detection and quantification of hepatic iron overload in primary or secondary hemochromatosis are clinically relevant because iron accumulation may cause oxidative hepatocellular injury, progressive fibrosis, and, ultimately, hepatocellular carcinoma. MR imaging based on the transverse relaxation rates ($R2* = 1/T2*$) is routinely used to quantify liver and heart iron concentrations. Owing to the possibility of three-material decomposition algorithm, DECT may identify hepatic iron overload over 3.2 mg of iron per gram or higher with a diagnostic performance comparable to $R2*$, yielding 100% specificity at thresholds of 7.0 mg of iron per gram of dry tissue or higher [25].

Material Identification with DECT: Pancreatic Applications

Pancreatic cancer is the fourth leading cause of cancer death, with better survival in patients diagnosed at an early stage. Conventional CT has been considered for years the most accurate imaging modality for diagnosis and staging of pancreatic cancer, with a sensitivity for small tumors ranging from 63% to 85%. The adoption of a low-tube-voltage (80 kVp) DECT technique and iodine-specific images may increase the detection rate by improving tumor conspicuity and tumor-to-parenchyma contrast and reducing streak artifacts caused by metal implants (Fig. 16.6) [26, 27]. Nonetheless, these improvements come at the cost of decreased perceived image quality owing to increased image noise [26]. DECT may also prove to be useful in differentiating an enhanc-

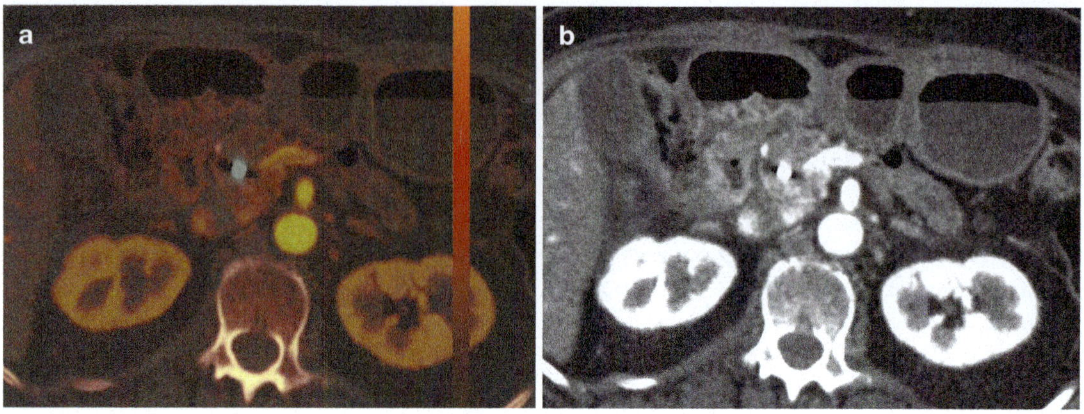

Fig. 16.6 Iodine material attenuation map (**a**) post-processed axial CT scan demonstrates a pancreatic head carcinoma (**a**) which corresponds to the hypoattenuating lesion in the contrast-enhanced axial CT scan in the portal venous phase (**b**)

ing pancreatic mass from a cystic lesion and in avoiding false-positive diagnosis of pancreatic mass in cases of pseudolesions, such as focal fatty change [28]. Finally, VNC images obtained from contrast-enhanced images can be used to identify calcifications and necrosis without additional unenhanced scans, thus reducing dose exposure in patients undergoing repetitive examinations.

Material Identification with DECT: Genitourinary Applications

Material decomposition analysis for genitourinary diseases represents a major area of opportunity of DECT. VNC images allow the detection of urinary calculi with a sensitivity of 53–87%, without the need for a true unenhanced phase [4, 29]. However, the main benefit of DECT in the assessment of urinary calculi is the possibility of ascertain their mineral composition using the CT number ratio:

- A CT number ratio <1.13 guides for uric acid stones.
- A CT number ratio between 1.13 and 1.24 guides for cystine stones.
- A CT number ratio >1.24 guides for calcium oxalates/phosphate stones.

Nonetheless the detection and characterization of urinary calculi is limited by the size and attenuation of the calculi, with decreased accuracy for smaller (<3 mm) stones, and by noise and artifacts occurring in large patients [29].

DECT proves to be particularly useful in the characterization of indeterminate renal masses [30]. VNC images can be confidently used to appreciate baseline characteristics of the mass, and virtual monochromatic images at an optimal energy level can overcome renal cyst pseudoenhancement [31]. Color-coded iodine overlay images allow for qualitative and quantitative assessment of contrast enhancement. An iodine concentration >2 mg/mL for rsDECT and >0.5 mg/mL for dsDECT is defined as contrast enhancement. Color-coded iodine overlay images and iodine maps can be used not only for the differentiation of benign and malignant renal lesions (Fig. 16.7) but also for the differentiation between clear cell and papillary renal cell carcinoma as well as for the assessment of response to treatment for metastatic renal cell carcinoma [29, 32, 33]. However, optimal cutoffs to discriminate clear cell and papillary renal cell carcinoma differ among different DECT systems, thus rendering difficult their routine adoption.

Material Identification with DECT: Other Abdominal Applications

Incidental adrenal nodules are detected in approximately 4–5% of patients undergoing CT, with most of these nodules being benign adenomas. However, if the nodule has a density over 10 UH

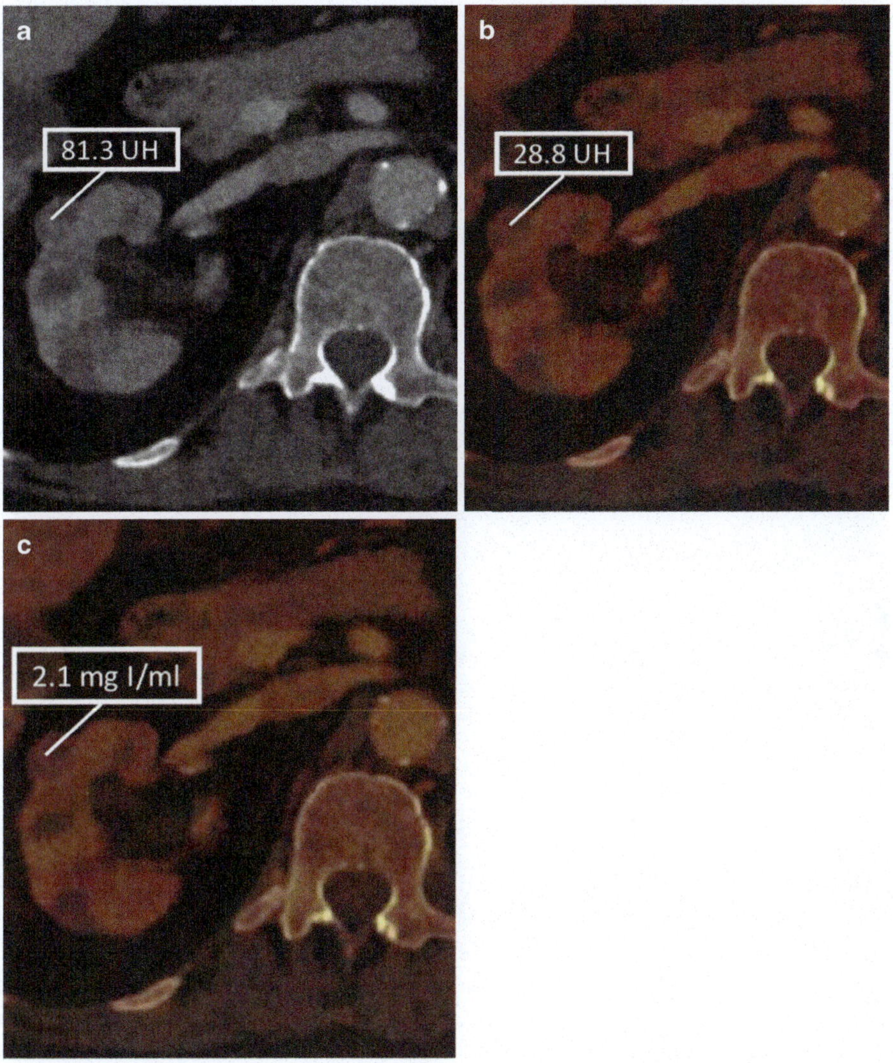

Fig. 16.7 Blended 120-kVp (**a**), contrast map (**b**), and iodine material attenuation (**c**) CT images show a hypervascular lesion in the right kidney, with an iodine uptake of 1.4 mg I/ml, accurately classified as renal cell carcinoma

on unenhanced scan or a relative or absolute washout less than 40% and 60%, respectively, then the lesion is indeterminate, and further work-up – including biopsy or MR – is needed. DECT may overcome the need for an true unenhanced scan for adrenal lesions and offers the great advantage of differentiating both lipid-rich and lipid-poor adenomas from nonadenomas using material density analysis with a 96% sensitivity and 100% specificity (Fig. 16.8) [34, 35].

DECT may be used as a further aid to evaluate various bowel disorders [36]. The increased conspicuity of subtle enhancement differences on iodine maps, overlay images, or low-kiloelectron volt imaging may allow for identification in patients with inflammatory, ischemic, or neoplastic bowel diseases – allowing accurate differentiation of tumor from stool – as well as depiction of active gastrointestinal bleeding as intraluminal hyperattenuation that persists on the iodine map but disappears on VNC [37]. Owing to the increased detectability of parenchymal lesions, it is expected that DECT may also have a great potential to assist the interpreting radiologist in the detection of solid organ injuries [37]. Though there is scant literature on DECT detectability of

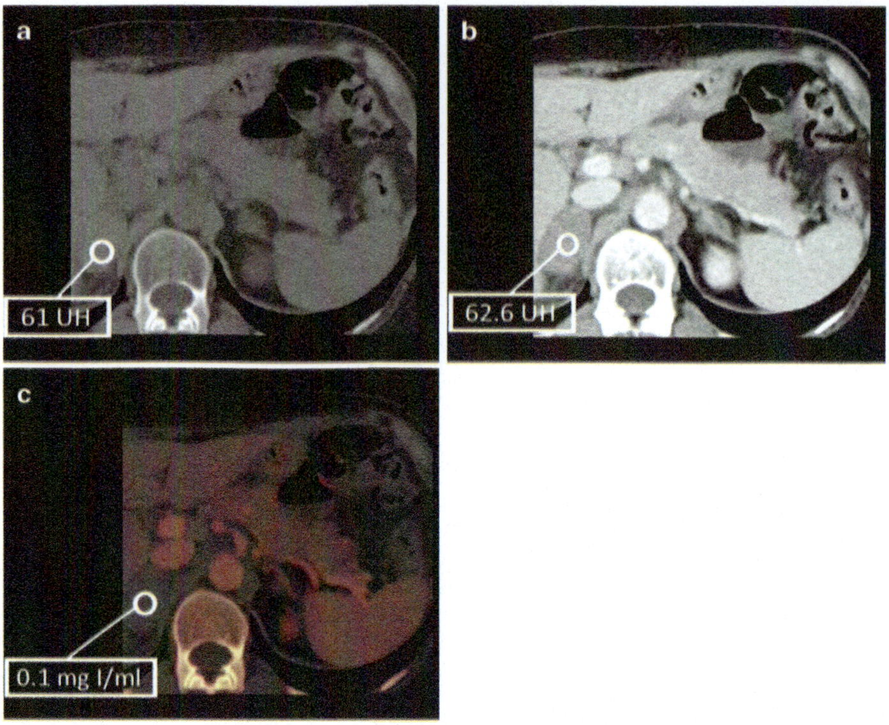

Fig. 16.8 Virtual non-contrast (**a**), contrast-enhanced CT in the venous phase (**b**), and post-processed iodine map (**c**) show a spontaneously hyperattenuating right adrenal lesion without significant contrast enhancement or iodine uptake (0.1 mg I/mL), accurately diagnosed as adrenal hematoma

traumatic abdominopelvic lesions, post-processed DECT images have also the potential to detect areas of altered bowel wall enhancement, as well as vascular injuries and active extravasation [37]. Iodine-selective, simulated monoenergetic, and VNC images may potentially improve the detection of the so-called posttraumatic "shock bowel" by differentiating intramural hemorrhage, mucosal hyperenhancement, and hyperattenuating ingested content in the bowel lumen [37]. By analyzing VNC and iodine overlay images, active extravasation and its origin may also be confidently detected. However, further studies on applicability of DECT in bowel disorders and abdominopelvic injuries are still needed.

Material Identification with DECT: Chest Applications

The main application of DECT in chest pathologies is pulmonary embolism. Though widely used for detection of pulmonary embolism, conventional CT pulmonary angiography has a limited sensitivity (83%) for pulmonary emboli [38], with major challenges for small segmental and subsegmental emboli. Compared to CT pulmonary angiography, DECT iodine maps show a small incremental benefit in sensitivity for the detection of occlusive small (i.e., segmental and subsegmental) pulmonary emboli [39]. The simultaneous detection of a clot in a pulmonary artery on pulmonary conventional CT pulmonary angiography and of a corresponding wedge-shaped perfusion defect on DECT-based blood pool imaging indicates occlusive pulmonary embolism. However, other potential causes of perfusion defects on iodine maps – including aberrant vascular supply, beam-hardening artifacts or motion artifacts, or parenchymal diseases – must be kept in mind to avoid false-positive diagnosis of pulmonary embolism [40]. Iodine-selective and simulated monoenergetic images at low keV may also improve the detection of aortic dissection, aortic endoleaks, arteriovenous malformations, and contrast uptakes in lung malignancies [39–41]. DECT has also huge potential for evaluating the hemodynamic significance of coronary disease (i.e., myocardial perfusion) using myocardial iodine map as an addition to coronary artery assessment with plaque characterization as lipid-rich, fibrous-rich, calcified, or noncalcified plaque.

Material Identification with DECT: Musculoskeletal Applications

Though a comprehensive evaluation of CT in musculoskeletal applications goes beyond the purpose of this chapter, the application of the material decomposition algorithms for material identification is increasingly used for detection and characterization of musculoskeletal diseases. Applications of DECT in musculoskeletal imaging include gout, bone marrow edema, tendons, and ligaments and the use of monoenergetic techniques to minimize metal prosthesis beam-attenuating artifacts. DECT provides good diagnostic accuracy for detection of monosodium urate deposits in patients with gout, with a sensitivity of 90% [42]. False-negative diagnosis may occur in patients with recent-onset disease or on allopurinol with serum uric acid <6 mg/dl) [42]. To date, DECT may be indicated as second-line diagnostic technique in patients with possible gouty arthritis in whom polarizing microscopy of synovial fluid has failed to confirm a diagnosis.

More recently, DECT proved its clinical importance in traumatic patients. The detection of bone marrow edema (i.e., "bone bruise") in traumatic patients is of utmost importance. Single-energy CT is limited by overlying trabecular bone, and MR imaging is considered the reference standard for the detection of bone marrow edema. However, thanks to the possibility of removing the confounding effect of trabecular bone, DECT provides a visual representation of the bone marrow composition with a sensitivity of 82% for bone marrow edema [28]. This has been shown to be particularly beneficial for nondisplaced fractures, such as the knee and hip or spine [43, 44]. In order to preserve the anatomical information of the CT scan, the VNC image may also be presented as a color-coded map superimposed on the conventional CT image. Some limitations pertain to the DECT analysis of bone marrow edema including the difficulties in demonstrating bone marrow lesions adjacent to cortical bone owing to "masking" of the nearby cortex or in significantly sclerotic vertebral bodies [44].

The huge possibility offered by DECT to reduce streak artifacts caused by metal implants is of fundamental importance in the study of bone and soft tissue diseases in patients with metallic implants – i.e., in patients with knee or femoral prosthesis – yielding improved detection of lesions obscured by the metal artifacts [44].

Soft tissue characterization of collagenous structures – including ligaments, tendons, and intervertebral disks – has generally been limited with conventional CT due to lack of attenuation contrast and in some cases increased beam hardening artifacts obscuring fine details. Due to the presence of dense hydroxylysine and hydroxyproline side chains within the collagen molecules, DECT can be potentially used to differentiate soft tissue collagenous structures (ligaments and tendons) due to their relatively high density. Once identified, they can be color-coded and combined with gray-scale CT images to help with anatomic localization and detection of pathologic conditions [44].

Material Identification with DECT: Head and Neck Applications

Though the literature on DECT for neck imaging is still scanty, DECT seems to be promising also in the detection of cartilage invasion by laryngeal and hypopharyngeal squamous cell carcinoma, a fundamental information for determining the appropriate treatment strategies for laryngeal and hypopharyngeal cancer [45].

Promising applications of DECT in brain diseases include bone removal in CT angiography of intracranial vessels and evaluation of vascular malformations, an accurate differentiation of high attenuation areas after mechanical revascularization in acute ischemic stroke, which may be related to contrast staining or brain hemorrhage. High keV monoenergetic images are also advantageous during the evaluation of brain aneurysms remnants after surgical clipping owing to the possibility of reducing metal artifacts.

Clinical Applications of Material Identification with PCCT

PCCT scanners are not yet commercially available, because their clinical use is still limited by many intrinsic technical challenges above described. However, the gaining obtained with PCCT will likely allow for improved spatial resolution with already proven added value for breast CT and potential value for cardiac, lung, orthopedic, and vascular applications, reduced iodine concentrations – which could be particularly important in patients with impaired renal function – and use of contrast agents other than iodine or barium, including gadolinium, gold, and platinum, which could be beneficial for patients with iodine allergies. Compared to conventional CT, PCCT offers lower noise with better contrast-to-noise resolution, reduction of beam-hardening and blooming artifacts allowing for more accurate estimation of HU value and improved luminal vessel evaluation, and decrease of radiation doses by at least 30–40%. The potential possibility of simultaneous multi-contrast agent imaging with PCCT could further reduce radiation doses and provide the possibility to match perfectly images from different phases enabling the detection and characterization of small lesions.

Discussion and Conclusion

Material density analysis through DECT overcomes ambiguity of HU measurements using single-energy CT. Material-specific images obtained with DECT provide qualitative and quantitative information about tissue composition and contrast agent distribution. The main contribution of DECT-based material characterization comes from iodine-specific images, which yield increased tissue contrast facilitating discrimination between normal and abnormal tissues. This will ultimately result in increased sensitivity for lesion detection and better characterization of tissue composition compared to single-energy CT. Several other materials, including calcium, fat, and uric acid, can be characterized using material decomposition techniques, which expands the clinical utility of DECT. The ability of DECT to discriminate different tissues is largely dependent of the energy spectral separation of the two energies, as well as the patient body size. These limitations will likely be mitigated with the potential introduction into clinical practice of PCCT systems.

References

1. Patino M, Prochowski A, Agrawal MD, et al. Material separation using dual-energy CT: current and emerging applications. Radiographics. 2016;36:1087–105.
2. McCollough CH, Leng S, Yu L, Fletcher JG. Dual- and multi-energy CT: principles, technical approaches, and clinical applications. Radiology. 2015;276:637–53.
3. Alvarez RE, Macovski A. Energy-selective reconstructions in x-ray computerized tomography. Phys Med Biol. 1976;21:733–44.
4. Marin D, Boll DT, Mileto A, Nelson RC. State of the art: dual-energy CT of the abdomen. Radiology. 2014;271:327–42.
5. Hyodo T, Yada N, Hori M, et al. Multimaterial decomposition algorithm for the quantification of liver fat content by using fast-kilovolt-peak switching dual-energy CT: clinical evaluation. Radiology. 2017;283:108–18.
6. Sauter AP, Muenzel D, Dangelmaier J, et al. Dual-layer spectral computed tomography: virtual non-contrast in comparison to true non-contrast images. Eur J Radiol. 2018;104:108–14.
7. Ho LM, Yoshizumi TT, Hurwitz LM, et al. Dual energy versus single energy MDCT: measurement of radiation dose using adult abdominal imaging protocols. Acad Radiol. 2009;16:1400–7.
8. Mileto A, Barina A, Marin D, et al. Virtual monochromatic images from dual-energy multidetector CT: variance in CT numbers from the same lesion between single-source projection-based and dual-source image-based implementations. Radiology. 2016;279:269–77.
9. Schabel C, Patel B, Harring S, et al. Renal lesion characterization with spectral CT: determining the

optimal energy for virtual monoenergetic reconstruction. Radiology. 2018;287:874–83.
10. Fu W, Marin D, Ramirez-Giraldo JC, et al. Optimizing window settings for improved presentation of virtual monoenergetic images in dual-energy computed tomography. Med Phys. 2017;44:5686–96.
11. Patel BN, Marin D. Strategies to improve image quality on dual-energy computed tomography. Radiol Clin N Am. 2018;56:641–7.
12. Marin D, Pratts-Emanuelli JJ, Mileto A, et al. Interdependencies of acquisition, detection, and reconstruction techniques on the accuracy of iodine quantification in varying patient sizes employing dual-energy CT. Eur Radiol. 2015;25:679–86.
13. Willemink MJ, Persson M, Pourmorteza A, Pelc NJ, Fleischmann D. Photon-counting CT: technical principles and clinical prospects. Radiology. 2018;289:293–312.
14. Taguchi K, Iwanczyk JS. Vision 20/20: single photon counting x-ray detectors in medical imaging. Med Phys. 2013;40:100901. https://doi.org/10.1118/1.4820371.
15. Muenzel D, Lo GC, Yu HS, et al. Material density iodine images in dual-energy CT: detection and characterization of hypervascular liver lesions compared to magnetic resonance imaging. Eur J Radiol. 2017;95:300–6.
16. Shuman WP, Green DE, Busey JM, et al. Dual-energy liver CT: effect of monochromatic imaging on lesion detection, conspicuity, and contrast-to-noise ratio of hypervascular lesions on late arterial phase. Am J Roentgenol. 2014;203:601–6.
17. Marin D, Nelson RC, Samei E, et al. Hypervascular liver tumors: low tube voltage, high tube current multidetector CT during late hepatic arterial phase for detection–initial clinical experience. Radiology. 2009;251:771–9.
18. Ascenti G, Sofia C, Mazziotti S, et al. Dual-energy CT with iodine quantification in distinguishing between bland and neoplastic portal vein thrombosis in patients with hepatocellular carcinoma. Clin Radiol. 2016;71:938.e1–9.
19. Patel BN, Rosenberg M, Vernuccio F, et al. Characterization of small incidental indeterminate hypoattenuating hepatic lesions: added value of single-phase contrast-enhanced dual-energy CT material attenuation analysis. Am J Roentgenol. 2018;211:571–9.
20. Dai X, Schlemmer HP, Schmidt B, et al. Quantitative therapy response assessment by volumetric iodine-uptake measurement: initial experience in patients with advanced hepatocellular carcinoma treated with sorafenib. Eur J Radiol. 2013;82:327–34.
21. Vandenbroucke F, Van Hedent S, Van Gompel G, et al. Dual-energy CT after radiofrequency ablation of liver, kidney, and lung lesions: a review of features. Insights Imaging. 2015;6:363–79.
22. Raptopoulos V, Karellas A, Bernstein J, Reale FR, Constantinou C, Zawacki JK. Value of dual-energy CT in differentiating focal fatty infiltration of the liver from low-density masses. Am J Roentgenol. 1991;157:721–5.
23. Horowitz JM, Venkatesh SK, Ehman RL, et al. Evaluation of hepatic fibrosis: a review from the society of abdominal radiology disease focus panel. Abdom Radiol. 2017;42:2037–53.
24. Sofue K, Tsurusaki M, Mileto A, et al. Dual-energy computed tomography for non-invasive staging of liver fibrosis: accuracy of iodine density measurements from contrast-enhanced data. Hepatol Res. 2018; https://doi.org/10.1111/hepr.13205. [Epub ahead of print].
25. Luo XF, Xie XQ, Cheng S, et al. Dual-energy CT for patients suspected of having liver iron overload: can virtual iron content imaging accurately quantify liver iron content? Radiology. 2015;277:95–103.
26. Marin D, Nelson RC, Barnhart H, et al. Detection of pancreatic tumors, image quality, and radiation dose during the pancreatic parenchymal phase: effect of a low-tube-voltage, high-tube-current CT technique – preliminary results. Radiology. 2010;256:450–9. https://doi.org/10.1148/radiol.10091819.
27. Macari M, Spieler B, Kim D, et al. Dual-source dual-energy MDCT of pancreatic adenocarcinoma: initial observations with data generated at 80 kVp and at simulated weighted-average 120 kVp. Am J Roentgenol. 2010;194:W27–32.
28. Agrawal MD, Pinho DF, Kulkarni NM, Hahn PF, Guimaraes AR, Sahani DV. Oncologic applications of dual-energy CT in the abdomen. Radiographics. 2014;34:589–612. https://doi.org/10.1148/rg.343135041.
29. Vernuccio F, Meyer M, Mileto A, Marin D. Use of dual-energy computed tomography for evaluation of genitourinary diseases. Urol Clin North Am. 2018;45:297–310.
30. Patel BN, Bibbey A, Choudhury KR, Leder RA, Nelson RC, Marin D. Characterization of small (< 4 cm) focal renal lesions: diagnostic accuracy of spectral analysis using single-phase contrast-enhanced dual-energy CT. Am J Roentgenol. 2017;209:815–25.
31. Mileto A, Nelson RC, Samei E, et al. Impact of dual-energy multi-detector row CT with virtual monochromatic imaging on renal cyst pseudoenhancement: in vitro and in vivo study. Radiology. 2014;272:767–76.
32. Mileto A, Marin D, Alfaro-Cordoba M, et al. Iodine quantification to distinguish clear cell from papillary renal cell carcinoma at dual-energy multidetector CT: a multireader diagnostic performance study. Radiology. 2014;273:813–20.
33. Marin D, Davis D, Roy Choudhury K, et al. Characterization of small focal renal lesions: diagnostic accuracy with single-phase contrast-enhanced dual-energy CT with material attenuation analysis compared with conventional attenuation measurements. Radiology. 2017;284:737–47.
34. Mileto A, Nelson RC, Marin D, Roy Choudhury K, Ho LM. Dual-energy multidetector CT for the characterization of incidental adrenal nodules: diagnostic performance of contrast-enhanced material density analysis. Radiology. 2015;274:445–54.

35. Ho LM, Marin D, Neville AM, et al. Characterization of adrenal nodules with dual-energy CT: can virtual unenhanced attenuation values replace true unenhanced attenuation values? Am J Roentgenol. 2012;198:840–5.
36. Fulwadhva UP, Wortman JR, Sodickson AD. Use of dual-energy CT and iodine maps in evaluation of bowel disease. Radiographics. 2016;36:393–406.
37. Wortman JR, Uyeda JW, Fulwadhva UP, Sodickson AD. Dual-energy CT for abdominal and pelvic trauma. Radiographics. 2018;38:586–602.
38. Stein PD, Fowler SE, Goodman LR, et al. Multidetector computed tomography for acute pulmonary embolism. N Engl J Med. 2006;354:2317–27.
39. Weidman EK, Plodkowski AJ, Halpenny DF, et al. Dual-energy CT angiography for detection of pulmonary emboli: incremental benefit of iodine maps. Radiology. 2018;11:180594. https://doi.org/10.1148/radiol.2018180594.
40. Kang MJ, Park CM, Lee CH, Goo JM, Lee HJ. Dual-energy CT: clinical applications in various pulmonary diseases. Radiographics. 2010;30:685–98.
41. Otrakji A, Digumarthy SR, Lo Gullo R, Flores EJ, Shepard JA, Kalra MK. Dual-energy CT: spectrum of thoracic abnormalities. Radiographics. 2016;36:38–52.
42. Bongartz T, Glazebrook KN, Kavros SJ, et al. Dual-energy CT for the diagnosis of gout: an accuracy and diagnostic yield study. Ann Rheum Dis. 2015;74:1072–7.
43. Yang P, Wu G, Chang X. Diagnostic accuracy of dual-energy computed tomography in bone marrow edema with vertebral compression fractures: a meta-analysis. Eur J Radiol. 2018;99:124–9.
44. Mallinson PI, Coupal TM, McLaughlin PD, Nicolaou S, Munk PL, Ouellette HA. Dual-energy CT for the musculoskeletal system. Radiology. 2016;281:690–707.
45. Kuno H, Onaya H, Iwata R, et al. Evaluation of cartilage invasion by laryngeal and hypopharyngeal squamous cell carcinoma with dual-energy CT. Radiology. 2012;265:488–96.

CT Texture Characterization

17

Samuel G. Armato III, Maryellen L. Giger, and Joseph J. Foy

Introduction

The phrase "A picture is worth a thousand words" is not quite true for images from a computed tomography (CT) scan. Consider that a single image (or "slice" or "section") acquired during a CT scan is a 512×512 matrix of pixels, each of which is allocated 2 bytes of computer memory to store the numeric value generated at that spatial location by the CT scanner. A single CT section, therefore, requires $512 \times 512 \times 2 = 524{,}288$ bytes of storage on the computer. If the average English word is 4.5 letters long (and each letter requires one byte of computer storage), then a single CT image is, in fact, equivalent to 120,953 words—and a complete CT scan typically comprises hundreds of sections.

The purpose of this mathematical exercise is to illustrate that an image (specifically a CT scan) is nothing more than a two-dimensional array of numeric values (Fig. 17.1)—it is inherently a quantitative construct. How those specific values came to exist at any specific element of the array is a complex interplay of the biology of the patient being imaged, the physics and engineering of the scanner, and the mathematics of the employed image reconstruction algorithms. But given that an image (the specific array of numbers) has been generated within a CT scanner, the image itself now presents an opportunity for mathematical manipulation of its constituent numeric values—the data contained within the image.

Post-acquisition mathematical analysis of medical images can range from simple image processing to complex computer-aided diagnosis. The intent of such manipulation can range from the enhancement of aspects of the image for improved human visualization (e.g., "sharpening" of edges within the image or reduction of image noise) to artificial intelligence (e.g., disease detection or assessment of cancer risk). The tools available for image analysis span the fields of mathematics, statistics, and computer science. This chapter explores the concepts and practical implementation of one specific form of mathematical manipulation of CT images: texture analysis. The quantification of image textures attempts to capture underlying (and often not visually discernible) relationships among the values and spatial distributions of pixels (the elements of the two-dimensional matrix of values that represents an image). Texture analysis has proven to be a powerful tool over a broad array of CT applications, several of which will be reviewed.

S. G. Armato III (✉) · M. L. Giger · J. J. Foy
Department of Radiology, The University of Chicago, Chicago, IL, USA
e-mail: s-armato@uchicago.edu; m-giger@uchicago.edu; joefoy@uchicago.edu

© Springer Nature Switzerland AG 2020

E. Samei, N. J. Pelc (eds.), *Computed Tomography*, https://doi.org/10.1007/978-3-030-26957-9_17

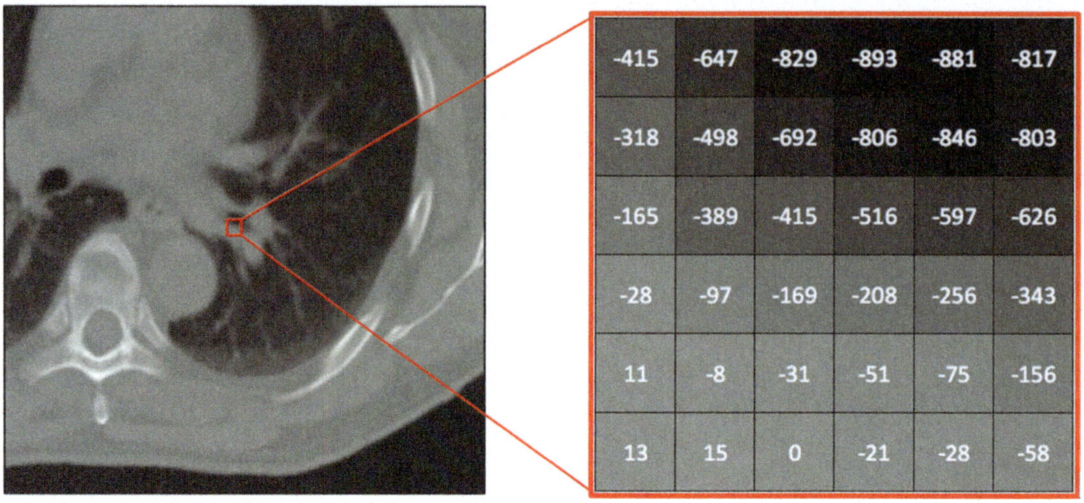

Fig. 17.1 A medical image is a matrix of numeric values, with each pixel represented by a single value. The magnitude of this value is translated to the brightness of that pixel, and the spatial variations in these values give the image texture

Image Texture

Texture refers to the local spatial variations in the pixel values ("brightness") within an image. The values in the two-dimensional array that underlies an image may be depicted as elevation in a three-dimensional surface representation of that data. Texture, then, may be interpreted as the "roughness" of that surface.

In many cases roughness may be qualitatively described by a human observer from its perceived visual impression. Image texture may be described as "fine," "coarse," "grained," or "smooth," for example. An image region with "fine" texture would contain small texture elements with high spatial frequency, while an image region with "coarse" texture would contain large texture elements with low spatial frequency. Terms that may be found in the radiology reports of chest CT scans, such as "ground glass opacity," "honeycombing," and "mosaic attenuation pattern," convey subjective assessments of textures within the lung regions of the scan; these qualitative assessments of texture, when combined with other imaging and nonimaging information through the lens of a radiologist's vast knowledge and experience, aid in the medical decision-making process. A more objective, quantitative approach to the characterization of texture can be achieved through mathematical texture analysis.

Texture as a mathematical entity possesses magnitude, spatial frequency content, and direction. The magnitude is the value of the specific texture quantity, while the spatial frequency content and directionality capture the spatial distribution and orientation dependence associated with some texture quantities. Importantly, although texture is a single concept, texture is not characterized by a single mathematical construct. Instead, different families of equations exist to capture different elements of image texture. Some more commonly used classes of texture analysis are histogram analysis, co-occurrence matrices, Fourier analysis, Laws' textures analysis, and fractal analysis, each of which deserves a brief summary of the concepts on which they are based and the calculations required to extract quantitative information from images to which they are applied.

Histogram Analysis

Histogram analysis (sometimes referred to as first-order texture analysis) is the most basic form of texture analysis. The basis for histogram analysis is construction of a pixel-value histogram (i.e., a frequency distribution of the numbers of pixels in the image with different values). The texture features computed from histogram analysis, then, are quantitative characteristics of that histogram: maximum and minimum pixel values, mean and standard deviation of the pixel values, percent threshold (the pixel value at which a specified percentage of the area under the histogram lies below that pixel value), balance, skewness, kurtosis, and other histogram moments. Each of these quantitative descriptors can be used to describe the distribution of pixel values within an image.

In a strict sense, histogram analysis does not actually capture "texture," which was described previously as local spatial variations in the pixel values of an image, since the constructed histogram ignores any information about spatial location. Only the values of the pixels are used to generate a pixel-value histogram, as demonstrated in Fig. 17.2, in which two images with the

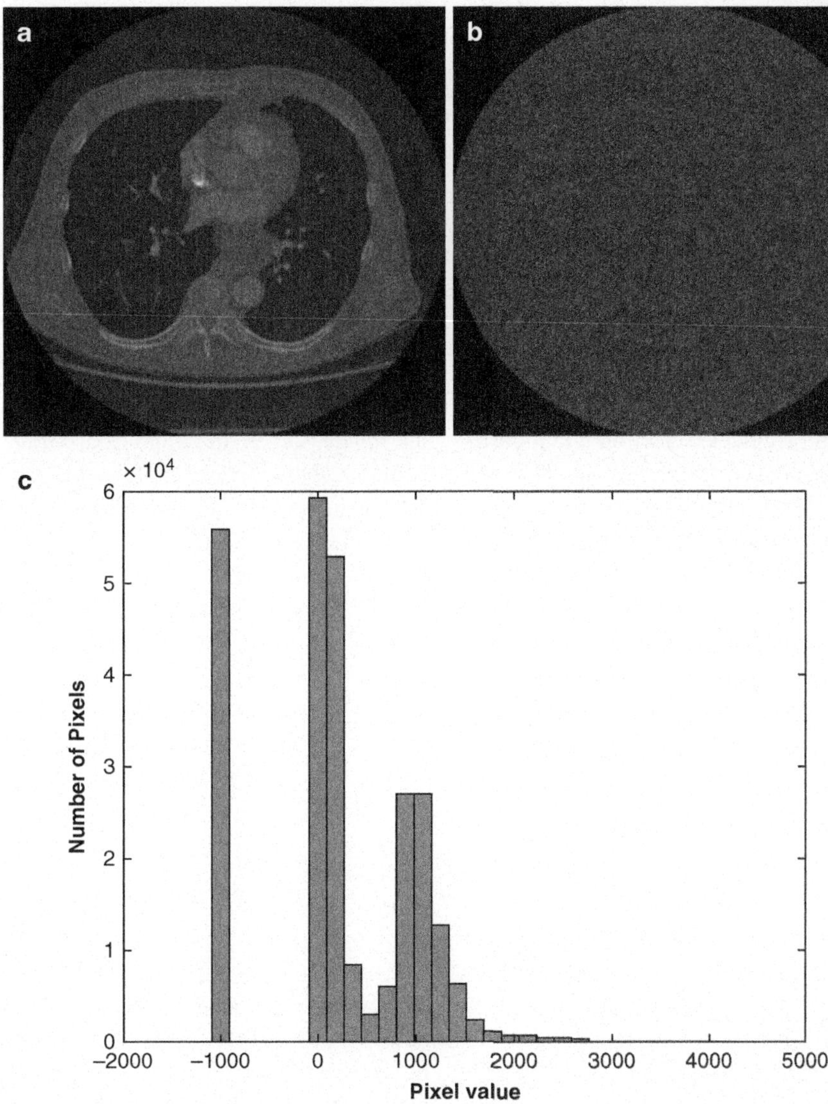

Fig. 17.2 (**a**) A single section of a thoracic CT scan along with (**b**) the same image with the pixels within the reconstructed field of view randomly placed. Since histogram analysis does not capture information regarding the spatial relationship among pixels, both images result in the same pixel-value histogram (**c**)

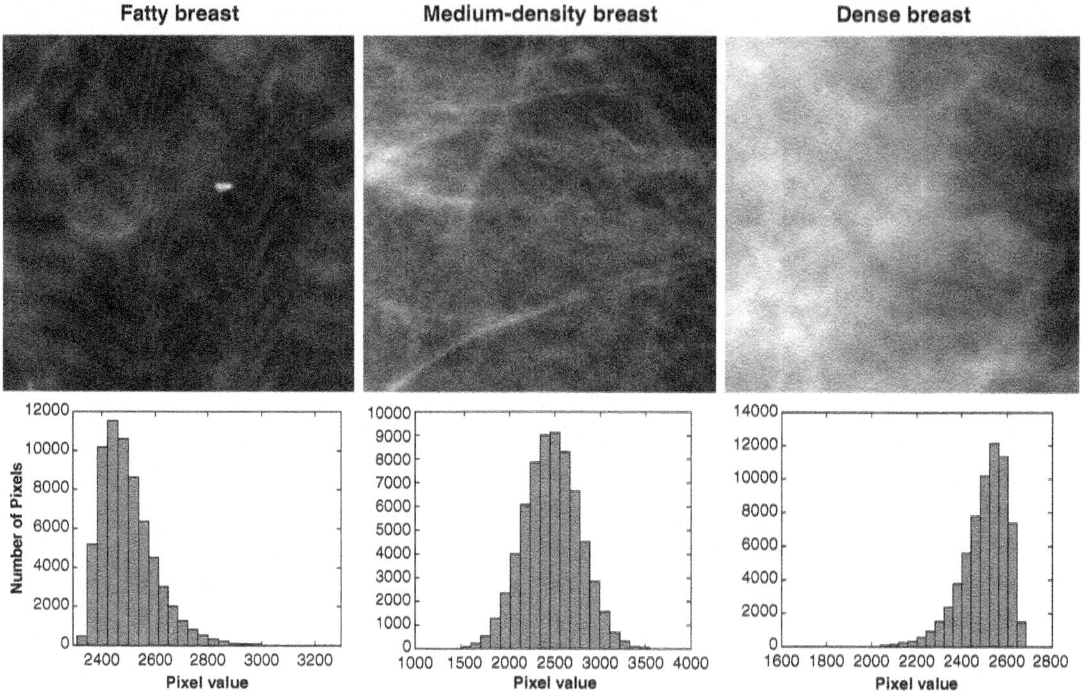

Fig. 17.3 First-order histogram features can be used to differentiate various kinds of tissues such as fatty and dense breast tissue based on the pixel-value distribution

same pixels (an original CT section and a corresponding image created from the original pixels placed in random spatial positions) are shown to yield the same histogram and hence identical histogram-based features. Nevertheless, histogram analysis has potential value for radiologic tasks such as distinguishing among mammographically dense, mixed, and fatty regions [1, 2], which tend to exhibit left-skewed, symmetric, and right-skewed histograms, respectively (Fig. 17.3).

Gray-Level Co-occurrence Matrix

One of the most commonly used tools of texture analysis is the gray-level co-occurrence matrix (GLCM). This matrix is constructed based on the spatial relationships among pixels with different relative values. Essentially the GLCM is based on the repeated occurrence of certain gray-value configurations within the texture of the image. Given an image of arbitrary size that contains G distinct gray levels, the GLCM specified by distance d and orientation ϕ will be a $G{\times}G$ matrix such that the value at matrix location (row=i, column=j) is the number of times in the image that a pixel with gray level j exists d pixels away from a pixel with gray level i in direction ϕ.

An image does not yield a single GLCM, but rather a family of GLCMs may be generated from a single image by varying the distance (d) and orientation (ϕ) parameters. The choice of parameters will be task dependent. The GLCM is calculated from the pixels in an image, but the quantitative texture features used for texture analysis are derived from mathematical manipulation of the GLCM itself. Texture features that may be obtained from the GLCM include energy, entropy, correlation, contrast, maximum probability, and inverse different moment [3], many of which describe the heterogeneity of the distribution of image pixel values.

Fourier Analysis

The Fourier transform decomposes a function into the sum of superimposed sine and cosine waves of varying amplitude, frequency, and phase. The Fourier transform of a two-dimensional function (e.g., an image) may be expressed as

$$F(u,v) = \iint f(x,y)e^{-2\pi i(ux+vy)}\,\mathrm{d}x\,\mathrm{d}y,$$

where u and v are the spatial frequency dimensions that correspond to the x and y spatial dimensions (the columns and rows of the image), respectively. This equation effectively "transforms" an image from the conventional spatial representation of data into a spatial frequency-based representation of that data. Images that contain fine structural details of objects will have a greater amount of high spatial frequency content. Information regarding spatial frequency, which contains both a magnitude and a direction, may be exploited through, for example, texture features based on the power spectrum of an image ($|F(u,v)|^2$) such as the root mean square (RMS)

$$\mathrm{RMS} = \sqrt{\iint |F(u,v)|^2\,\mathrm{d}u\,\mathrm{d}v}$$

and the first moment of the power spectrum (FMP)

$$\mathrm{FMP} = \frac{\iint \sqrt{u^2+v^2}\,|F(u,v)|^2\,\mathrm{d}u\,\mathrm{d}v}{\iint |F(u,v)|^2\,\mathrm{d}u\,\mathrm{d}v}.$$

1.4 Laws' Textures Analysis

Laws' filter features are designed to emphasize local region microstructure within an image such as regions exhibiting spot, wave, ripple, edge, or level surface patterns (Fig. 17.4). Mathematically,

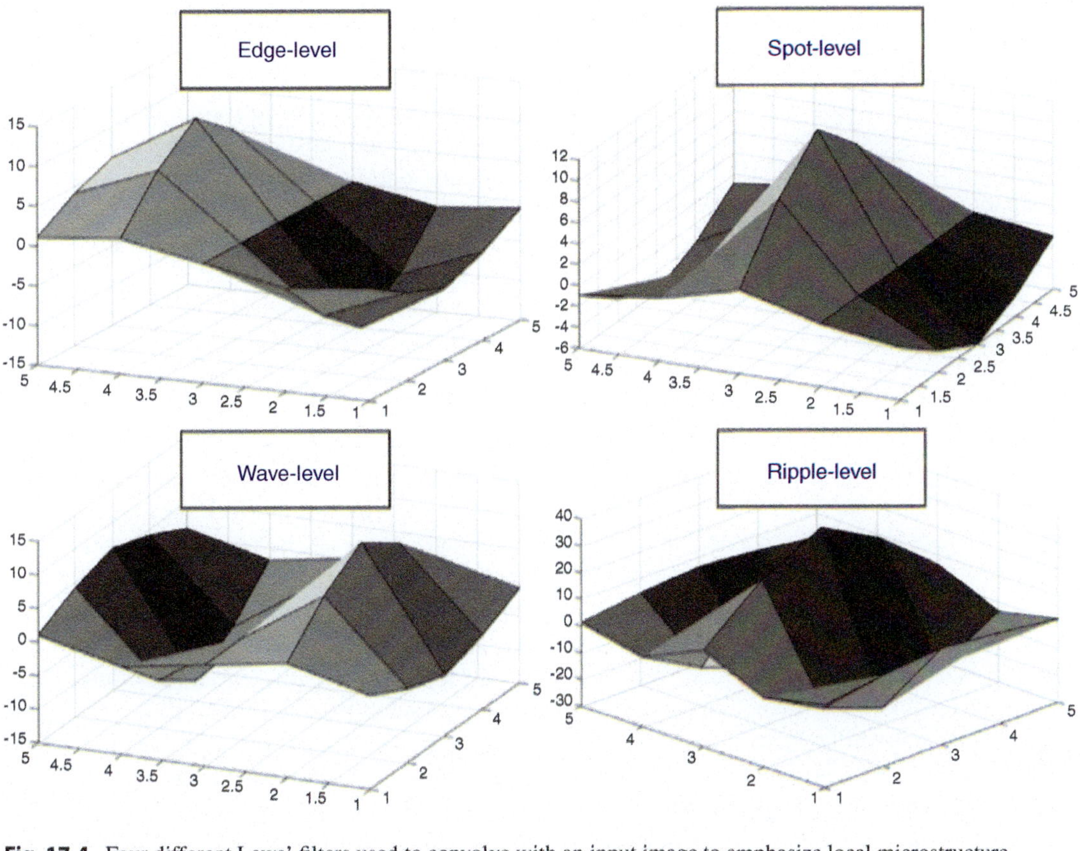

Fig. 17.4 Four different Laws' filters used to convolve with an input image to emphasize local microstructure

these patterns are represented as vectors, where the length of the vector is dependent on the pattern sought, and the outer product of these vectors is calculated to generate a two-dimensional filter for each pairwise combination of these vectors. Each filter is convolved with an input image to emphasize the patterns associated with the filter. Using the resulting filtered image, various first-order features can then be calculated to quantify these textural variations [4].

Fractal Analysis

Fractal features describe the self-similarity of a region at different scales and relate to the complexity of these regions. This self-similarity can typically be quantified using a single value called the fractal dimension, but the fractal dimension can be calculated in a number of ways including the box-counting method, the Brownian motion method, and the blanket method. Each of these methods aims to measure the same concept: if one were to break a figure into equal parts, at what scale would the parts have to be magnified to obtain the original figure, thus quantifying the self-similarity of the figure [5]? For example, a square may be broken into N^2 self-similar pieces with each piece requiring a magnification factor of N. The fractal dimension is then quantified using the equation

$$F = \frac{\log(\text{Number of Self-Similar Pieces})}{\log(\text{Magnification Factor})}.$$

Substituting N^2 and N for the corresponding terms in the above equation, the fractal dimension of a square is 2. Expanding on this logic, the fractal dimension of a cube is 3. For more complicated figures, such as medical images characterized by large variations in pixel values, more sophisticated methods (e.g., the Brownian method or box-counting method) can be used to quantify this self-similarity [5, 6], as can methods that incorporate morphological opening and closing operations (e.g., for descriptions of the parenchyma within mammograms or other radiographic images [7, 8]).

Practical Considerations

Regions of Interest

A single image often is comprised of multiple textures, so that image texture is most useful when computed from within localized regions of interest (ROIs), which may be a square neighborhood of pixels or a region defined to capture a specific structure (e.g., organ or abnormality) within the image. Quantitative differences among the local textures computed across the spatial extent of an image then can become a powerful signature of an abnormality.

Image Acquisition

The data contained within an image is a representation of the physical object that underwent the imaging examination. The same anatomy imaged through a different imaging modality will appear different in the resulting image, and that image, furthermore, will contain different textures both qualitatively and quantitatively. The same is true of anatomy imaged through the same imaging modality but with different image acquisition parameters used to generate the image. CT has a number of parameters that may be modified to optimize the visualization of the anatomy or suspected disease under consideration. These parameters include slice thickness, pixel size, mA, kV, and reconstruction algorithm. Moreover, engineering differences among the scanners of different CT manufacturers (e.g., detector dimension and composition, x-ray beam filtration, and electronic noise signature) further impact the appearance and quality of the resulting images. These factors may all contribute to differences in image texture and must be carefully understood to ensure the accurate interpretation of the computed textures and differences in texture across serial CT scans [9–17].

Any practical application of texture analysis algorithms, like statistical software, requires a user's domain knowledge of the input data sets (i.e., images) in order to correctly understand the output of the software. Consequently, texture analysis methods designed for images acquired from one modality, for one anatomic region, or for one disease state should not be assumed to transfer to any other modality, region, or disease without substantial modification and validation to accommodate the expected differences in texture. CT presents a further challenge in this regard, since a single CT scan typically contains multiple series with different image reconstruction implementations; therefore, texture is not computed on the "CT scan" but rather on a specific series within the scan, and this series must be specified for future reference and for consistent comparisons across scans.

Image Manipulation

Post-acquisition manipulation of images will almost certainly alter the textural composition of the images, with implications for computed texture features. Image rescaling to match a desired image pixel size, image interpolation along the axial (z) axis of a CT scan volume to generate images with a desired section spacing, and nonlinear image registration to compare anatomically matched regions across temporally sequential CT scans will all impact image texture. Cunliffe et al. [18] investigated texture features that were robust to image registration across normal CT scans acquired at two time points and quantified the extent of textural change introduced into images transformed by four different registration methods. Examples of the texture change introduced by two deformable registration methods are shown in Fig. 17.5. Further findings suggested that anatomically matched regions across serial CT scans that will be subjected to texture analysis should be identified based on the vector deformation field generated by the image registration software rather than nonlinearly warping the images to achieve the same spatial coordinate system [19].

Texture Software Packages

Aside from the impact of image acquisition on computed texture features, the actual algorithms used to compute texture features can vary across software packages so that the same input image could yield a range of output texture feature values from different packages. Common reasons for such variability include differences in the way images are preprocessed by the software prior to the mathematical computations, differences in the default settings of parameters for features that require defined parameters (and some packages may not even allow for user adjustment of these default settings), varying approaches to computational implementation within the coded algorithms, and different package-specific mathematical definitions for the same texture feature. Furthermore, some pack-

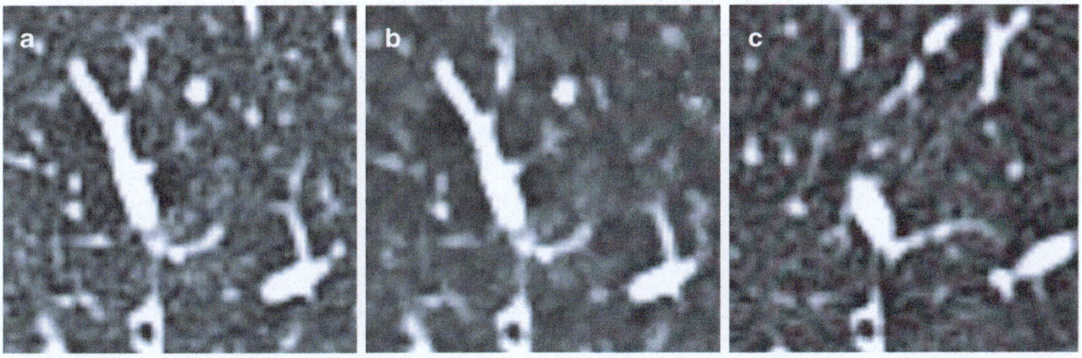

Fig. 17.5 Texture change of normal lung parenchyma in anatomically matched ROIs acquired at two time points. The baseline scan (**a**) was well matched with the follow-up scan when registered using demons deformable registration (**b**), but the texture was smoothed. When registered with B-splines deformable registration (**c**), texture was preserved, but the anatomy was not well matched. (Reprinted with permission from [18])

ages accommodate the three-dimensional extraction of certain texture features, while other packages compute features only in two dimensions.

The fundamental reason for software differences is the basic notion that most texture packages were developed for a specific application (e.g., CT scans of the chest or natural scene images) and thus lack generalizability to images from other domains (or even from other modalities within the medical imaging domain). A study by Foy et al. [10] investigated 4 texture analysis software packages (2 in-house packages and 2 open-source packages) applied to 40 ROIs from distinct mammograms and 39 manually delineated regions of interest from distinct head and neck CT scans. All first-order features computed from the mammography and CT regions (with the exception of one feature) were significantly different across all four packages due to package-specific systematic biases; all second-order features were significantly different across all four packages due predominantly to differences in package-specific default GLCM parameters—differences that likely would have remained undiscovered if not the specific target of the study being conducted. Other observed differences in texture feature values were caused by varying approaches to image preprocessing, algorithm implementation, and feature naming conventions. The authors concluded that such large variations in computed feature values across software packages support the efforts of groups such as the Image Biomarker Standardisation Initiative (IBSI) seeking to standardize radiomics processes.

Applications of Image Texture in CT Scans

The computation of image texture from structures (anatomic or pathologic) in CT scans is not interesting in itself. The power of image texture quantification lies in the potential for texture to differentiate between normal anatomy and disease, to capture a phenotypical distinction among tumors with different genetic variations, to serve as a prognostic marker, to provide early assessment of response, or to generate a correlate with patient outcomes. Applications of CT texture analysis have been increasing in the literature and span topics such as segmentation, tumor heterogeneity, lesion classification, tumor response prediction and prognosis, assessment of nonfocal lesions, content-based image retrieval, and image quality assessment [9, 20–28].

Bladder Lesion Response

Texture-based analyses of lesions on CT commonly begin with some form of automated or semiautomated lesion segmentation. Pixels within the segmented tumor (and sometimes pixels in the peritumoral region) then become the basis for computations of image texture. Cha et al. [29] computed the texture of bladder cancers to differentiate between those with and without complete response to chemotherapy. The lesions were segmented from paired CT scans (pre- and post-therapy), and a random forest classifier was trained to distinguish between lesions that fully responded and those that did not based on shape, size, and texture features. The method achieved an area under the receiver operating characteristic (ROC) curve of 0.77 in this response-assessment task. This study is representative of many studies that combine texture analysis with the larger concept of radiomics, merging an array of image-based characteristics (beyond texture alone) through an automated classifier (or, more recently, through a deep learning-based convolutional neural network) to perform a defined radiologic task.

Lung Lesion Classification

The use of image texture to classify lung nodules on chest imaging examinations has been reported in the literature for over 20 years [25, 30, 31]. Choi et al. [32] developed a prediction model to improve the classification of lung nodules in low-dose CT scans. This study merged texture features with other radiomics features to create a prediction model by using a support vector machine classifier (SVM) coupled with a least

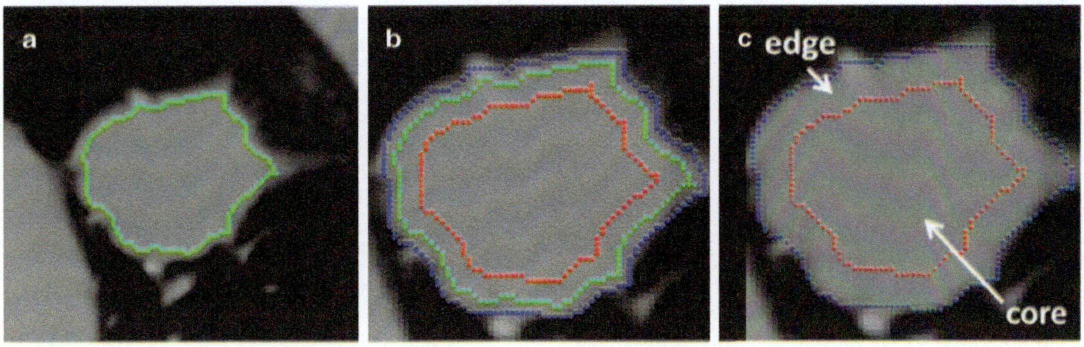

Fig. 17.6 A segmented lung nodule (**a**) was eroded and dilated (**b**) to obtain the edge and core regions (**c**). Texture features were calculated in both regions, and differences in certain features corresponded to malignancy status. (Reprinted with permission from [33])

absolute shrinkage and selection operator (LASSO). The model achieved an accuracy of 84.6%, which was 12.4% higher than the corresponding accuracy of the American College of Radiology's Lung CT Screening Reporting and Data System (Lung-RADS).

Texture analysis may be applied on an even more local basis. For example, Suo et al. [33] evaluated the image texture differences between the periphery and the core of lung lesions on CT for differentiation of malignant from inflammatory lung nodules and masses (Fig. 17.6). When combined with lesion volume, the computed texture features achieved an area under the ROC curve of 0.86 in this task.

Lesion classification is not limited to decisions regarding malignancy status. Other classification decisions include predicting whether a specific patient will respond to a given therapy. Hunter et al. [34] developed a quantitative image feature model to predict the volume shrinkage of malignant lung nodules from the patient's preradiotherapy CT scan. Principal component regression was used to create prediction models, the most optimal of which yielded strong correlation between the observed and predicted tumor shrinkage ($r = 0.81$, mean squared error = 0.0086). The authors concluded that "quantitative image features extracted from existing pre-treatment CT images can successfully predict tumor shrinkage and provide additional information for clinical decisions regarding patient risk stratification, treatment, and prognosis."

Normal Tissue Complications

Quantitative assessment of disease on CT through texture analysis can provide powerful objective information regarding treatment response. Equally important, however, is the impact of a treatment regimen on surrounding normal tissue (the concept of "normal tissue complications"). Cunliffe et al. [35] demonstrated correlation between radiologist-defined severity of normal tissue damage following radiation therapy for lung cancer and a set of CT texture features (along with change in the values of these texture features between pre- and post-therapy scans), thus establishing a relationship between the qualitative interpretation of a human observer and the quantitative computation of mathematical features in this context.

This group later used these features to assess the relationship between radiation dose and texture feature change to determine the ability of texture analysis to identify patients who develop radiation pneumonitis as a side effect of radiation therapy. For all 20 features considered, a significant change in value was observed within CT regions that received increasing radiation dose. Twelve of these features changed significantly for patients who had radiation pneumonitis. Combining various features through a classifier achieved areas under the ROC curve that ranged from 0.59 to 0.84 in the task of distinguishing patients with and without pneumonitis. The authors concluded that their study "demonstrated the ability of radiomics to provide a quantitative, individualized measurement of patient lung tissue reaction to radiation therapy and assess radiation pneumonitis development" based on CT scan texture [26].

Conclusions

Texture refers to the magnitude, spatial orientation, and spatial frequency content of gray-level fluctuations within an image. Texture analysis mathematically captures various aspects of these fluctuations and provides a way to objectively extract quantitative information from CT scans. The power of CT image texture quantification lies in the potential for texture to differentiate between normal anatomy and disease, to capture a phenotypical distinction among tumors with different genetic variations, to serve as a prognostic marker, to provide early assessment of response, or to generate a correlate with patient outcomes. Applications of CT texture analysis have been increasing in the literature and hold promise for a wide range of radiologic tasks in CT. An important caveat for the eventual clinical use of CT texture analysis is its dependence on CT image acquisition parameters, transformations to which an image might be subjected post-acquisition, and algorithmic details of the texture software package employed. The expectation is that quantitative image texture features will augment the qualitative interpretation of CT scans provided by radiologists to enhance patient care and further extend the role of imaging in the medical decision-making process.

References

1. Huo Z, Giger ML, Wolverton DE, Zhong W. Computerized analysis of mammographic parenchymal patterns for breast cancer risk assessment: feature selection. Med Phys. 1998;27:4–12.
2. Li H, Giger ML, Olopade O, Margolis A, Lan L, Chinander MR. Computerized texture analysis of mammographic parenchymal patterns of digitized mammograms. Acad Radiol. 2005;12:863–73.
3. Haralick RM, Shanmugam S, Sinstein I. Texture features for image classification. IEEE Trans Syst Man Cybern. 1973;SMC-3:610–21.
4. Laws KI: Textured image segmentation. USCIPI Technical Report No. 940, University of Southern California, 1980.
5. Mandelbrot BB, Van Ness JW. Fractal Brownian motions, fractal noise and applications. SIAM Rev. 1968;10:422–37.
6. Creutzburg R, Ivanov E. Fast algorithm for computing fractal dimensions of image segments. In: Cantoni V, Creutzburg R, Levialdi S, Wolf G, editors. Recent issues in pattern analysis and recognition. Lecture notes in computer science, vol. 399. Berlin, Heidelberg: Springer; 1989. p. 42–51..
7. Li H, Giger ML, Lan L, Brown JB, MacMahon A, Mussman M, Olopade OI, Sennett C. Computerized analysis of mammographic parenchymal patterns on a large clinical dataset of full-field digital mammograms: robustness study with two high-risk datasets. J Digit Imaging. 2012;25:591–8.
8. Jiang C, Giger ML, Chinander MR, Martell JM, Kwak S, Favus MJ. Characterization of bone quality using computer-extracted radiographic features. Med Phys. 1999;26:872–9.
9. Gillies RJ, Kinahan PE, Hricak H. Radiomics: images are more than pictures, they are data. Radiology. 2016;278:563–77.
10. Foy JJ, Robinson KR, Li H, Giger ML, Al-Hallaq H, Armato SG. Variation in algorithm implementation across radiomics software. J Med Imaging. 2018;5:044505.
11. Oliver JA, Budzevich M, Zhang GG, Dilling TJ, Latifi K, Moros EG. Variability of image features computed from conventional and respiratory-gated PET/CT images of lung cancer. Transl Oncol. 2015;8:524–34.
12. Galavis PE, Hollensen C, Jallow N, Paliwal B, Jeraj R. Variability of textural features in FDG PET images due to different acquisition modes and reconstruction parameters. Acta Oncol. 2010;49:1012–6.
13. Cheng NM, Fang YH, Yen TC. The promise and limits of PET texture analysis. Ann Nucl Med. 2013;27:867–9.
14. Leijenaar RT, Nalbantov G, Carvalho S, van Elmpt WJ, Troost EG, Boellaard R, Aerts HJ, Gillies RJ, Lambin P. The effect of SUV discretization in quantitative FDG-PET Radiomics: the need for standardized methodology in tumor texture analysis. Sci Rep. 2015;5:11075.
15. Shafiq-Ul-Hassan M, Zhang GG, Latifi K, Ullah G, Hunt DC, Balaguranathan Y, Abdalah MA, Goldorf DG, Mackin D, Court LE, Gillies RJ, Moros EG. Intrinsic dependencies of CT radiomic features on voxel size and number of gray levels. Med Phys. 2017;44:1050–62.
16. Mackin D, Fave X, Zhang L, Fried D, Taylor B, Rodriguez-Rivera E, Dodge C, Jones AK, Court L. Measuring computed tomography scanner variability of radiomics features. Investig Radiol. 2015;50:757–65.

17. Mendel KR, Li H, Lan L, Cahill CM, Rael V, Abe H, Giger ML. Quantitative texture analysis: robustness of radiomics across two digital mammography manufacturers' systems. J Med Imaging. 2017;5:011002.
18. Cunliffe AR, Al-Hallaq HA, Labby ZE, Pelizzari CA, Straus C, Sensakovic WF, Ludwig M, Armato SG III. Lung texture in serial thoracic CT scans: assessment of change introduced by image registration. Med Phys. 2012;39:4679–90.
19. Cunliffe AR, Armato SG III, Fei XM, Tuohy RE, Al-Hallaq HA. Lung texture in serial thoracic CT scans: registration-based methods to compare anatomically matched regions. Med Phys. 2013;40:061906. (9 pages).
20. Rizzo S, Botta F, Raimondi S, Origgi D, Danciullo C, Morganti AG, Bellomi M. Radiomics: the facts and challenges of image analysis. Eur Radiol Exp. 2018;2:36. (8 pages).
21. Owens CA, Peterson CB, Tang C, Koay EJ, Yu W, Mackin DS, Li J, Salehpour MR, Fuentes DT, Court LE, Yang J. Lung tumor segmentation methods: impact on the uncertainty of radiomics features for non-small cell lung cancer. PLoS One. 2018;13:e0205003. (22 pages).
22. Nougaret S, Tardieu M, Vargas HA, Reinhold C, Vande Perre S, Bonanno N, Sala E, Thomassin-Naggara I. Ovarian cancer: an update on imaging in the era of radiomics. Diagnostic Interventional Imaging, DII-1134 (9 pages). 2018.
23. Shi L, He Y, Yuan Z, Benedict S, Valicenti R, Qiu J, Rong Y. Radiomics for response and outcome assessment for non-small cell lung cancer. Technol Cancer Res Treat. 2018;17:1–14.
24. Liu Z, Wang S, Dong D, Wei J, Fang C, Zhou X, Sun K, Li L, Li B, Wang M, Tian J. The applications of radiomics in precision diagnosis and treatment oncology: opportunities and challenges. Theranostics. 2019;9:1303–22.
25. Giger ML, Chan HP, Boone J. Anniversary paper: history and status of CAD and quantitative image analysis: the role of medical physics and AAPM. Med Phys. 2008;35:5799–820.
26. Cunliffe AR, Armato SG III, Castillo R, Pham N, Guerrero T, Al-Hallaq HA. Lung texture in serial thoracic computed tomography scans: correlation of radiomics-based features with radiation therapy dose and radiation pneumonitis development. Int J Radiat Oncol Biol Phys. 2015;91:1048–56.
27. Aerts HJ, Velazquez ER, Leijenaar RT, Parmar C, Grossmann P, Cavalho S, Bussink J, Monshouwer R, Haibe-Kains B, Rietveld D, Hoebers F, Rietbergen MM, Leemans CR, Dekker A, Quackenbush J, Gillies RJ, Lambin P. Decoding tumour phenotype by noninvasive imaging using a quantitative radiomics approach. Nat Commun. 2014;5:1–8.
28. Kumar V, Gu Y, Basu S, Berglund A, Eschrich SA, Schabath MB, Forster K, Aerts HJ, Dekker A, Fenstermacher D, Goldgof DB, Hall LO, Lambin P, Balagurunathan Y, Gatenby RA, Gillies RJ. Radiomics: the process and the challenges. Magn Reson Imaging. 2012;30:1234–48.
29. Cha KH, Hadjiiski L, Chan HP, Weizer AZ, Alva A, Cohan RH, Caoili EM, Paramagul C, Samala RK. Bladder cancer treatment response assessment in CT using radiomics with deep-learning. Sci Rep. 2017;7:8738.
30. Vittitoe NF, Baker JA, Floyd CE Jr. Fractal texture analysis in computer-aided diagnosis of solitary pulmonary nodules. Acad Radiol. 1997;4:96–101.
31. McNitt-Gray MF, Hart EM, Wyckoff N, Sayre JW, Goldin JG, Aberle DR. A pattern classification approach to characterizing solitary pulmonary nodules imaged on high resolution CT: preliminary results. Med Phys. 1999;26:880–8.
32. Choi W, Oh JH, Riyahi S, Liu CJ, Jiang F, Chen W, White C, Rimner A, Mechalakos JG, Deasy JO, Lu W. Radiomics analysis of pulmonary nodules in low-dose CT for early detection of lung cancer. Med Phys. 2018;45:1537–49.
33. Suo S, Cheng J, Cao M, Lu Q1, Yin Y1, Xu J2, Wu H. Assessment of heterogeneity difference between edge and core by using texture analysis: differentiation of malignant from inflammatory pulmonary nodules and masses. Acad Radiol. 2016;23:1115–22.
34. Hunter LA, Chen YP, Zhang L, Matney JE, Choi H, Kry SF, Martel MK, Stingo F, Liao Z, Gomez D, Yang J, Court LE. NSCLC tumor shrinkage prediction using quantitative image features. Comput Med Imaging Graph. 2016;49:29–36.
35. Cunliffe AR, Armato SG III, Straus C, Malik R, Al-Hallaq HA. Lung texture in serial thoracic CT scans: correlation with radiologist-defined severity of acute changes following radiation therapy. Phys Med Biol. 2014;59:5387–98.

Part VI

Functional CT

CT as a Functional Imaging Technique

18

Jonathan W. Revels and Achille Mileto

Introduction

Development and clinical inception of CT have profoundly changed the contemporary practice of medicine. Since the first CT system fabricated in the 1970s by Sir Godfrey Hounsfield and branded by the Electric and Musical Industries (EMI CT scanner), CT equipment have dramatically changed and evolved into the multi-detector row CT technology capable of providing high spatial and temporal resolution, wide coverage, and isotropic voxels with three-dimensional anatomic visualization abilities. These characteristics have enabled a better understanding and depiction of human diseases, including measurements of tumor morphology and staging or recognition of pathognomonic patterns of diseases in certain organs.

The profound paradigm shift in medical practice toward the need for individualized, precision medicine has spurred diagnostic imaging to pursue new avenues for improved disease detection and characterization, with earlier diagnosis of pathologic processes and more precise phenotypical profiling of them. This change is particularly affecting CT that has long been the work-horse modality in diagnostic imaging, relying upon visualization of merely morphological-structural or dimensional changes. Tremendous advances in multi-detector CT systems afforded by sophisticated hardware and software infrastructures enabled engineering of novel CT techniques such as PET/CT, texture analysis, perfusion CT, dual-energy CT and spectral imaging techniques, and CT volumetry. These techniques are marking the change in the way CT imaging is performed, transitioning from pristinely morphologic/anatomical technique to a semi-functional technique. In this chapter, we provide the readership with an overview on main techniques best representing this paradigm shift in CT imaging toward a functional quantitative imaging technique.

PET/CT

One of the more commonly known functional imaging modalities among medical specialties is positron emission tomography/computed tomography (PET/CT). Until recently, the breadth of PET/CT in clinical use was based on glucose uptake, 18-fludeoxyglucose (18-FDG), which allowed a measurable metabolic activity of pathologic tissues. Patient motion and tissue of interest size are more common limitations of

J. W. Revels (✉)
Department of Radiology, Division of Body and Thoracic Imaging, University of New Mexico, Albuquerque, NM, USA

A. Mileto
Department of Radiology, Division of Body Imaging, University of Washington, Seattle, WA, USA
e-mail: amileto@uw.edu

© Springer Nature Switzerland AG 2020

E. Samei, N. J. Pelc (eds.), *Computed Tomography*, https://doi.org/10.1007/978-3-030-26957-9_18

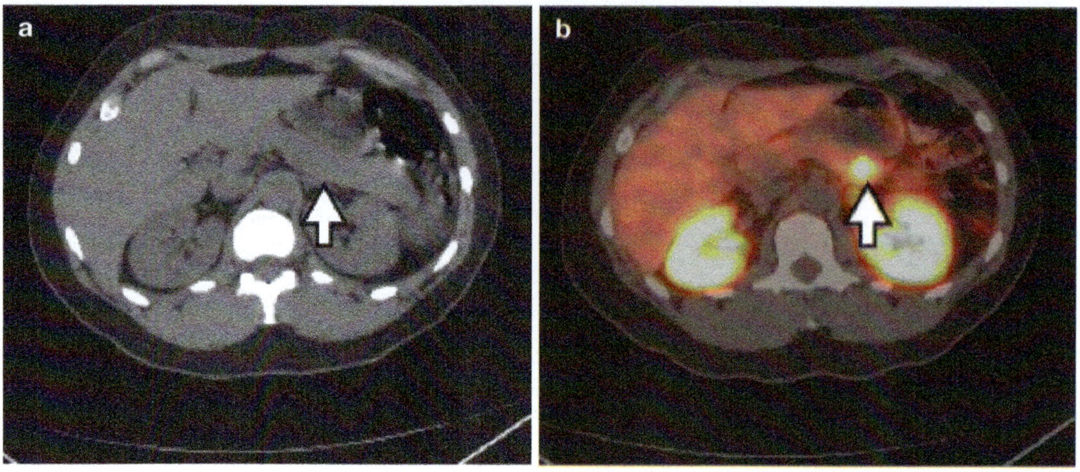

Fig. 18.1 PET/CT. DOTATATE PET/CT of a patient with suspected neuroendocrine tumor due to multiple endocrine neoplasia (MEN) type 1. Non-contrast CT at the level of the pancreas (arrow), without an obvious abnormality (**a**). Fused PET and CT image at the same level demonstrating radiotracer localization at the pancreatic tail (arrow head) that is indicative of a focal neuroendocrine tumor that contains somatostatin receptors (**b**)

PET/CT and should always be considered during the protocol process.

The concept of PET/CT was first envisioned in the 1990s by Townsend, Nutt, and colleagues as a means to provide anatomic information more familiar to surgeons and clinicians. The University of Pittsburgh Medical Center was the location of the first prototype PET/CT, becoming operational in 1998. The result of the combined anatomic and functional information improved imaging interpretation accuracy and confidence among interpreting radiologic and nuclear medicine physicians and made way for the design of commercially available PET/CT scanners [1].

Until recent years, the use of PET/CT radiopharmaceuticals had been limited to 18-FDG. Tumor cells tend to require a disproportionately increased amount of glucose to sustain growth, by comparison to normal tissues. This physiology is exploited through the use of 18-FDG, which is analogous to glucose, and once 18-FDG is phosphorylated, it does not undergo further metabolism and remains trapped intracellularly allowing for localized positron emission and imaging detection [2]. The uptake of 18-FDG by tumors can then be measured and semiquantitated in terms of standardized uptake value (SUV). The SUV can be reflected as a minimum, mean, or maximum value. These SUV measurements can be compared to normal soft tissue, trended to determine tumor treatment response to systemic therapy or aid in the detection of viable tumor postoperatively [2].

A complete discussion of the newer PET agents and their mechanisms is beyond the scope of this text. Each of these newer radiopharmaceuticals targets unique cellular types and/or pathways that improve radiologic diagnosis and provide similar trending abilities for posttreatment exams as 18-FDG. For example, choline radiopharmaceuticals can be radiolabeled with one of two positron-emitting isotopes (11C or 18F) and become integrated into cellular membranes. As cancer cells possess increased cellular membrane synthesis, there is a preferential localization for radiolabeled choline [3]. Somatostatin receptors may be present in neuroendocrine tumors, which can be assessed with a somatostatin analog, tyrosine type compound, such as DOTA-octreotide (DOTATATE) (Fig. 18.1).

CT Texture Analysis

CT at baseline provides clinically relevant and validated objective information based on anatomic findings such as size, as well as attenuation and enhancement. CT texture analysis (CTTA) is a post-processing analytical technique that assesses tissue heterogeneity through assessment of image voxel and pixel values/gray levels. The gray values can be graphed and measured in a statistics manner, as well as displaced visually to provide additional understanding of tissue homo- or heterogeneity. Though still under investigation, publications regarding CTTA show promise with regard to helping improve tumor assessment with regard to histopathologic diagnosis and treatment response [4].

CTTA is a post-processing technique, which requires specific software to perform. The advantage of post-processing is that (1) processing is done retrospectively using the display images, which means it can be done on studies that may have not been performed in your institution, and (2) many software programs are vendor neutral. Processing can be performed either 2D or 3D, though there is no consensus as to which method is best and the published literature is quite heterogenous [4, 5].

Once a region of interest is identified and marked, CTTA processes the levels of gray using various statistics methods that can provide information on a first order, second order, or higher order. First-order CTTA provides a graphed display of the overall region of interest, such as mean gray level intensity, threshold, standard deviation, skewness, and kurtosis; however, first-order models do not provide spatial information with regard to where the pixels of higher intensity reside on the image. Second-order statistics begin to provide some spatial information, as well as expand upon features of first-order models. Higher-order statistics considers a voxel's location and its relationship to adjacent voxels [4]. Through the use of filtration, image noise can be removed, and the pixel signal can be altered so as to emphasize the relevant data, such as enhancement.

CT Perfusion in the Oncologic Setting

A universally understood requirement for cellular growth and organ sustainability is blood perfusion. In cellular growth and development, this is accomplished through angiogenesis, which is a complex pathway stimulated in part by vascular endothelial growth factor (VEGF). By targeting the vascular proliferation pathways, certain chemotherapies aim to disrupt, and/or prevent, tumoral growth [6, 7]. Computed tomography perfusion imaging allows for qualitative and quantitative evaluation of regional blood flow that can be measured prior to and following treatment initiation. Additionally, CT perfusion imaging aids in assessment of organ hypoperfusion, such as myocardial infarction and cerebral vascular accidents, discussed later. In either case, the clinical applications of CT perfusion can significantly aid in patient care by providing an objective means to assess tissue before and after treatment and yield information that goes beyond size measurement. As the oncologic applications are more broadly applicable, this is where the focus of this topic will begin.

With CT being a widely available modality already well engrained in the assessment of tumoral changes, implementation of CT perfusion into the oncologic radiologist's armamentarium can greatly aid in patient care. The basic principle underscoring CT perfusion is the ability to temporally assess changes in tissue attenuation following in intravenous contrast administration beyond the traditional arterial, portal venous, and delayed time intervals. With dynamic acquisition, an understanding of how much and how quickly contrast flows to and through a region of interest can be calculated, as can the peak concentration of contrast. The calculated values reflect blood flow, blood volume, and tumoral vessel permeability. The features can be correlated to understanding a tumor's underlying structure (vascular organization, or order), as well as a tumor functionality (high permeability, or vascular shunting) [6].

Perfusion imaging begins with a baseline, non-contrast-enhanced image, followed by dynamic imaging at preestablished time intervals. This allows for subtraction of baseline tissue attenuation from a more precise determination of contrast enhancement, which is then graphically represented on a time-density curve. The protocols employed in CT perfusion are dependent on the organ of interest, the kinetic model used, and the CT scanner's configuration. High temporal resolution is a requirement of all perfusion imaging (CT, MR, fluoroscopy, ultrasound, etc.). The initial phase, or first pass, of contrast is less than a minute in duration and reflects the amount of contrast within the intravascular space, and acquisitions are typically obtained at less than 2 s intervals. This is followed by interstitial phase, which reflects the amount of contrast within the interstitium, and is related to vascular permeability. The second phase does not necessarily require as high an acquisition time, and the duration for this phase is based on the utilized kinetic model [6].

Two broadly categorized kinetic models include compartmental or deconvolution models. Each model can yield different functions and has its own set of advantages and disadvantages based on conceptual assumptions. A complete review of these models is beyond the scope of this text and will be discussed in broad senses. Compartmental analysis can be approached by two means: single or double compartment methods. The single compartmental method assumes both the intravascular and extravascular compartments exist as one entity, which is ideal to determine blood flow, and yields a maximum value of attenuation that is directly related to the quantity of contrast present. However, the disadvantage comes by assuming that no venous outflow is occurring during the exam, which is a non-physiologic assumption, and in instance of high venous outflow may underestimate the true peak. The two-compartment method assumes that the vascular and extravascular compartments exist separately, and contrast passes between the two compartments at rate constants. The two-compartment method therefore allows calculation of how much blood volume (BV) is present in a tissue of interest as well as the rate of contrast extraction (Fig. 18.2). Deconvolution analysis takes advantage of multiple data points acquired during the exam: arterial perfusion and contrast concentration. A disadvantage of deconvolution is the assumption that there is no contrast diffusing into the extracellular space, i.e., the contrast is merely traveling from arteries, to capillaries, and then into veins [6].

Regardless of the kinetic model utilized, it is important to have a general understanding of the result parameters and their potential pathologic correlation. Microvascular density tends to increase within tumors as a result of angiogenesis, as discussed previously. Therefore, any changes in microvascular density will be reflected in blood volume and blood flow (Fig. 18.2), though blood volume tends to be better correlated as blood flow can be altered as a result of cardiac dysfunction. A decrease in mean transit time can reflect changes related to abnormal arterial venous shunting, which tumors tend to possess. The two-compartment models allow for characterization of the extracellular space, and as tumor vessels tend to be malformed and "leaky," an increased vascular permeability and contrast extraction rate can be calculated. Research validating the implications of perfusion changes and tumor viability remains ongoing but remains of high interest in the medical field.

CT perfusion becomes more complicated in the case of the liver. With a unique dual blood supply, arterial and portal venous, the analytic models used to assess the liver possess their own unique limitations and drawbacks, and various pathologies can alter which vessel functions as the dominant means of perfusion [7]. In cases of neoplasia, not all tumors within the liver utilize the same means of perfusion. For instance, in cases of hepatocellular carcinoma, the tumor generates arteries that are not associated with the hepatic sinusoids and communicate directly to the hepatic artery, and lack portal venous communication to allow for portal venous perfusion. Whereas some hepatic metastases stimulate native hepatic arteries and portal veins to proliferate, thereby still possess an association with the portal triad. These neovascular changes become even more complicated to interpret by perfusion imaging in the presence of cirrhosis, which results in an increased arterial perfusion of the liver and decreased portal venous perfusion.

While CT perfusion in the oncologic setting provides benefits of improved tumor detection and objective physiologic changes/tumor

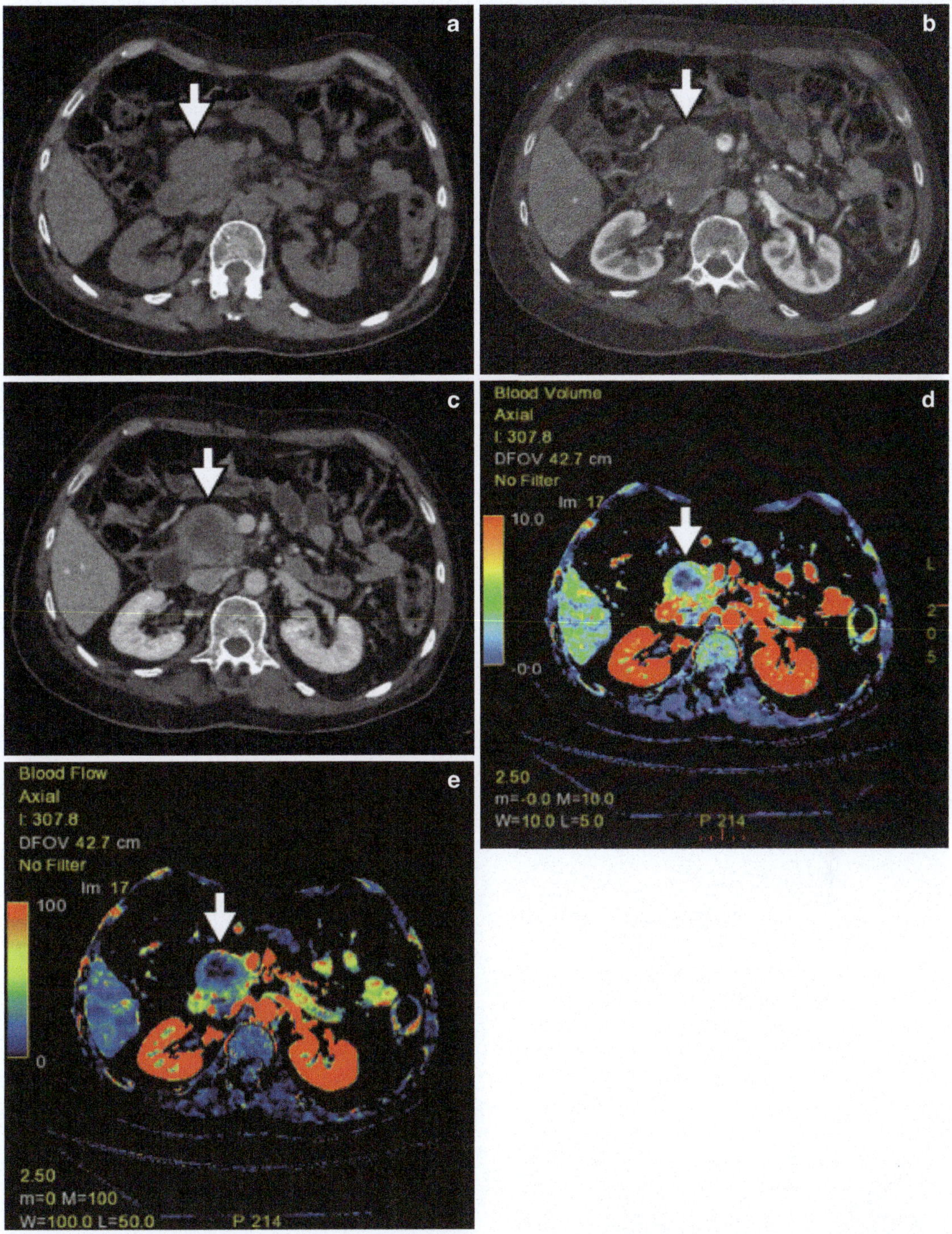

Fig. 18.2 CT perfusion. Seventy-year-old patient with pancreatic head adenocarcinoma. The non-perfusion images demonstrate a 5 cm soft tissue mass (arrows) that minimally enhances when comparing non-contrast images (**a**) to the arterial (**b**) and portal venous (**c**) phases. Post-processing was performed to assess perfusion features, which confirm hypoperfusion on both blood volume (**d**) and blood flow (**e**) images (Case contributed by Dr. Ryan O'Malley, University of Washington, Department of Radiology, Seattle, Washington)

response, it has drawbacks and limitation. First, CT perfusion has higher radiation exposure to the patient; some publications report doses for a single exam as high as 30 mSv, and in clinical trial situations, the patient may require multiple perfusion exam. Alterations to the CT acquisition technique can be applied to decrease radiation exposure (decreased kV and mA), but these come at the expense of increased image noise. Use of iterative reconstruction can assist in noise reduction and pixel variation without compromising spatial resolution. The practice of CT perfusion lacks a universal adopted standardization for performance and reporting, which limits reproducibility across the medical community.

CT Functional Assessment in Cardiac Imaging

Heart disease is a multifactorial disease and is one of the leading causes of death in the USA [8]. With continuous data demonstrating the health benefits of medical intervention in patients with heart disease, imaging is becoming increasingly in demand to provide a noninvasive means of screening those patients at risk for heart disease, as well as evaluating symptomatic patients in both the acute and outpatient setting. Improvements in CT technology have allowed the radiologist to provide a service of noninvasive coronary artery evaluation in recent years. CT angiography of the coronary arteries is now a recommended modality in evaluation of acute chest pain in patients with low to intermediate risk for acute coronary syndrome by multiple organizations [8]. Further improvements in CT now allow for an even greater breath of myocardial information to be gained that previously required multimodality assessment. With improvements in temporal resolution and electrocardiogram gating, CT is capable of assessing for regional wall motion abnormalities, as well as myocardial perfusion differences (Fig. 18.3), all in a single exam [9]. The limitations of the noninvasive, non-CT modalities are their inability to provide a simultaneous coronary artery anatomic assessment [10]. The following discussion is primarily directed toward the use of CT in the functional evaluation of coronary artery disease. The functional assessment of myocardium is clinically important as it provides clinical insight into the bur-

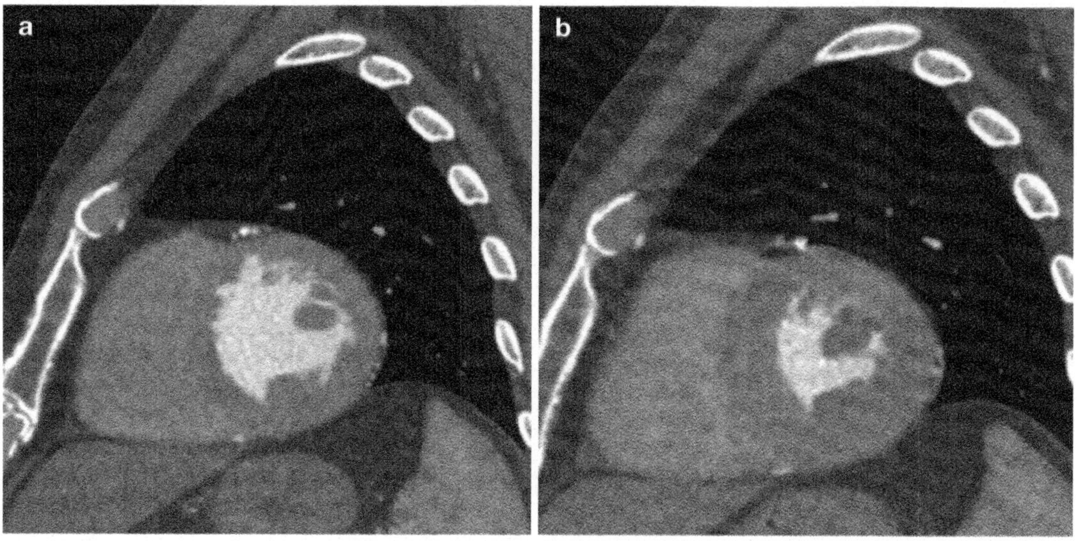

Fig. 18.3 Cardiac CT. Gated cardiac CT obtained for an 86-year-old male patient with chest pain that also has a history of aortic stenosis. The images are centered at the left ventricle mid-myocardial level in phases of diastole (**a**) and systole (**b**). Note the normal, uniform, circumferential contraction between diastole and systole

den of myocardium affected by coronary artery disease and correlates with clinical outcomes.

Previously the evaluation of myocardial perfusion was dominated by nuclear scintigraphy, which has well-established degrees of sensitivity and specificity, and risk stratification models of clinical outcomes. However, through the measurement of myocardial iodine concentration, one can similarly assess coronary artery perfusion using CT methods. Myocardial iodine concentration can be evaluated both qualitatively and quantitatively, the latter through use of post-processing software. There are two primary means of acquiring CT data for myocardial perfusion assessment: static and dynamic. Static acquisition is performed during the contrast bolus first pass, which directly reflects the coronary arterial supply to the myocardium, and regions of hypoperfusion will be less enhancing, and can be performed using single energy or dual energy. Both static acquisition technique suffers from being mere "snapshots" of myocardial iodine distribution at a single time point that must assume uniformity in the image, i.e., all of the myocardium must be in the exact same phase of the cardiac cycle at the moment the data was acquired, as well as the assumption that imaging was performed at peak contrast enhancement. Static assessment allows for quantitative calculation of iodine concentration and has the benefit of simultaneous acquisition during routine coronary artery CT angiography. Dynamic acquisition during the first pass allows for a truer assessment of myocardial perfusion because information is acquired through the cardiac cycle, as opposed to merely a single time point. As a result of the increased information obtained from dynamic perfusion imaging, blood flow can be calculated, in addition to quantitative assessment of myocardial iodine concentration. The high degree of temporal resolution that is required for dynamic myocardial CT perfusion assessment requires very specific CT scanner technology, which limits its widespread implementation. High-dose radiation exposure is another limitation to dynamic myocardial CT perfusion and is the result of the required increased imaging time intervals to obtain perfusion information and the additional scanning required for dedicated assessment of the coronary arteries [11].

Coronary artery disease does not always involve a single site and can occur in tandem within the same vessel (single artery with multiple sites of disease). Additionally, not all sites of disease result in a hemodynamic significant stenosis that would warrant coronary intervention, such as angioplasty and/or stenting. Similarly, a site of stenosis that may be considered minimal or mildly stenotic on CT (<50%) may actually have hemodynamic significance [12]. To determine which stenosis requires treatment, cardiologists measure the fractional flow reserve. Fractional flow reserve measures the pressure gradient across a coronary lesion that may be "flow-limiting" based on differences in arterial pressures pre- and post-stenosis, obtained during maximum perfusion, and reflects maximum blood flow in a vessel as a ratio of measure compared to expected. Fractional flow reserve values equal to or less than <0.80, less than 80% expected flow, are considered myocardial ischemic-inducing lesions, whereas those measuring >0.80 are unlikely to be ischemia inducing. Fractional flow reserve cutoff values may differ by institution [13]. The modern features of CT and post-processing now allow for fractional flow reserve calculation to be obtained noninvasively during routine coronary artery CT angiography, even in cases not performed with pharmacologic stress agents. The mathematics and physics that underscore this significant advancement are far beyond the scope of this writing and range from fluid dynamics to computer image-based modeling. Suffice it to say, when fractional flow reserve is coupled with CT coronary angiography there is a high diagnostic accuracy in determining clinically significant coronary artery disease [14].

Volumetric CT Measurements

Accurate measurement of in vivo soft tissue, whether an organ or a tumor, is paramount for noninvasive clinical assessments ranging from deciding who qualifies for organ donation to determining if an oncologic treatment is effective. Understanding how tissue volume is calculated is a basic concept that radiologists should possess in order to best serve the referral population and ensure accurate reporting.

Early CT scanner technology was hindered in its ability to provide accurate volume measurements due to poor z-axis resolution related to motion, as well as limitations in detector size. However, continued improvements gave birth to helical CT, fast pitch technologies, and detectors capable of submillimeter resolution. From these advances came post-processing software and, moreover, research supporting the accuracy of radiologic assessment of tissue sizes.

With regard to oncology, tumors are usually measured in their greatest dimension, with or without an additional perpendicular measurement obtained on the same image. This approach assumes that tumors change merely in two dimensions and has intrinsic limitations in demonstrating change. The ability to provide a three-dimensional representation of a tumor can convey substantial differences in size across examinations, as has been demonstrated in the evaluation of lung nodules. The Response Evaluation Criteria in Solid Tumors (RECIST) allows interval size differences of 20–30% or less to be termed stable; however, in cases of small lung nodules, a size difference of 1 mm can result in a marked increase in tumor volume, i.e., a volume change of greater than 100%. In some studies, a volumetric measurement may more accurately detect tumor response to treatment than two-dimensional measurements [15]. Tissue measurements can be performed manually or using automated/semiautomated methods. Regardless of how the region of interest is measured, ensuring accuracy of a lesion's borders is key for measurements. Voxels may be subject to partial volume effect related to the limitations of a CT scanner's resolution, which can lead to over- or underestimation [16]. Factors that can contribute toward partial volume effect include slice thickness and the reconstruction kernel. While thicker image slices reduce the overall number of images to review and improve workflow, it can lead to overestimating nodule volume [17]. Adjacent structures (vessel or airspace disease) can also affect accurate pulmonary nodule measurements due to obscuration of the nodule's borders. Inter- and intra-variability studies have previously demonstrated the differences that exist among pulmonary nodule volume measurements, and it has been reported that a volume change of more than 55% would be needed to have a minimum 95% confidence that a measured change were true and not the result of error [16]. Though variability remains in reporting of tumor volume measurements, ongoing research continues to demonstrate improvement in the fidelity of measurements across multiple CT scanner and post-processing platforms [18].

The application of volumetric measurements extends beyond oncologic applications and has also been applied in screening evaluation of organ transplants, examining correlation of organ volume changes and medical conditions (Fig. 18.4), as well as providing a means for research in less often considered medical ailments. For instance, there is ongoing research in the use of CT for predication of diabetes mellitus, where lower pancreatic volumes have been reported in patients with diabetes compared to those without diabetes [19]. This decrease in volume loss may even occur prior to the clinical manifestations of diabetes. Volumetric CT has also been utilized in monitoring urinary stones; both in predicting stones that may become symptomatic and providing a means to monitor changes in size during noninvasive medical treatment [20, 21].

Material Decomposition

Not all tissue within an organ is necessarily composed of the same materials, for example, a tumor compared to adjacent normal tissue. This difference, however, may prove difficult to visualize on single-energy CT if the two tissues have similar linear attenuation coefficients. One means of assessing tissue differences is through the use of intravenous contrast material and determines how a tissue of interest enhances when compared to normal tissue, which is the more traditional

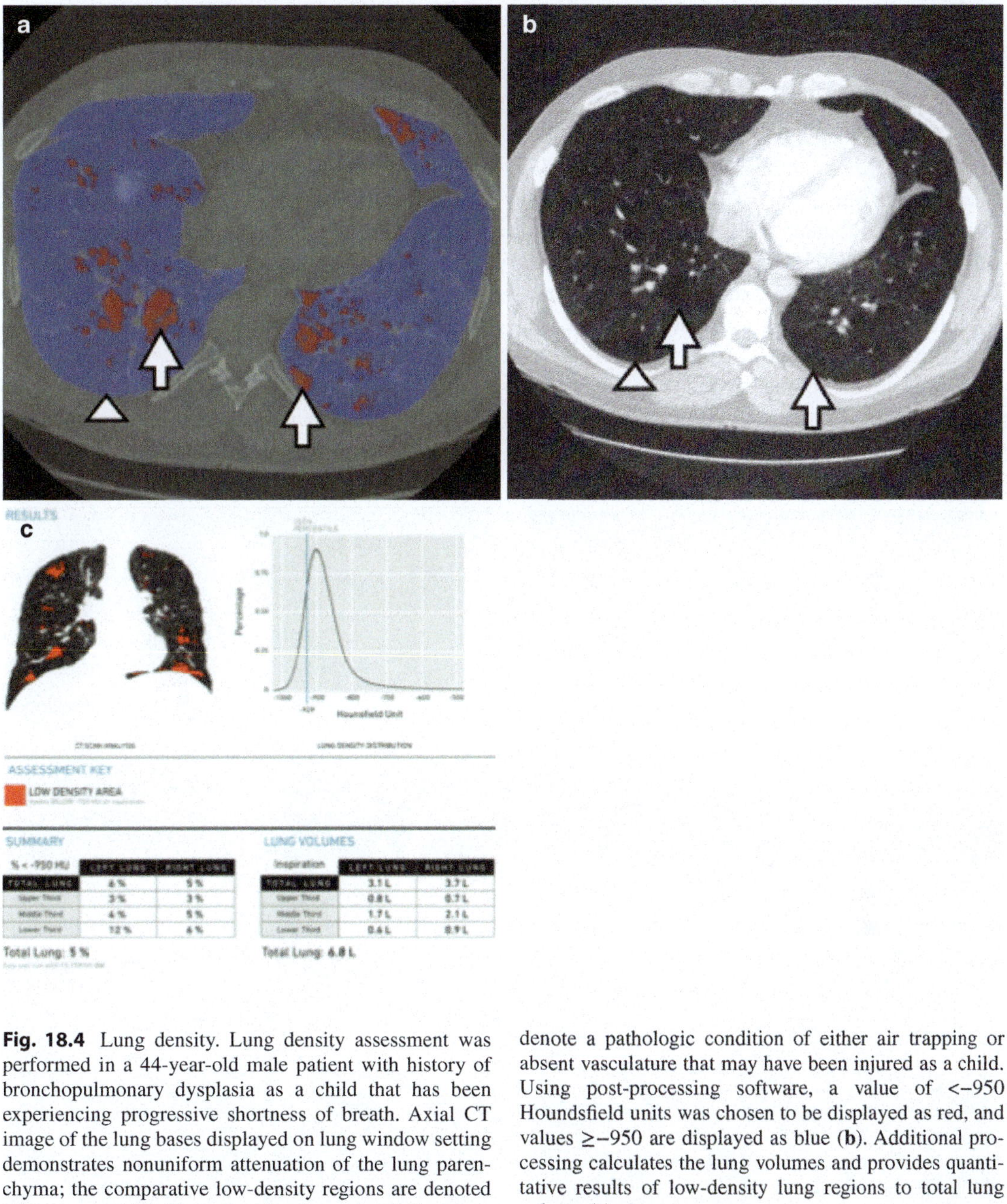

Fig. 18.4 Lung density. Lung density assessment was performed in a 44-year-old male patient with history of bronchopulmonary dysplasia as a child that has been experiencing progressive shortness of breath. Axial CT image of the lung bases displayed on lung window setting demonstrates nonuniform attenuation of the lung parenchyma; the comparative low-density regions are denoted with an arrow (**a**). These low-density regions of concern denote a pathologic condition of either air trapping or absent vasculature that may have been injured as a child. Using post-processing software, a value of <–950 Houndsfield units was chosen to be displayed as red, and values ≥–950 are displayed as blue (**b**). Additional processing calculates the lung volumes and provides quantitative results of low-density lung regions to total lung volume (**c**)

approach to contrast-enhanced CT. However, the information gained in this more common practice is a mere fraction of what the current technology of CT can provide. Born from dual-energy CT, material decomposition is based in evaluation of material interaction with varying x-ray energies and exploiting differences in atoms as a result of the photoelectric effect which is dependent on a material's k-edge [22, 23]. The more commonly used applications in clinical practice include improvement in visualization of iodine on contrast-enhanced images, characterization of renal stones, or uric acid assessment; however, with the continued research and development in targeted contrast agents, such as tissue-specific gold nanoparticles, CT material decomposition has the potential to improve clinical assessment of multiple tissues simultaneously with a previously dreamed specificity. Herein, the more common applications of dual-energy CT imaging techniques in functional imaging are material differentiation and quantification.

The complete theoretical concept of material decomposition is beyond the scope of this chapter. Rather, the focus of this section is on the current applications and translational research underway to bring material decomposition to clinical practice and its use in providing functional information. Briefly, to differentiate two materials using dual-energy CT, ideally the materials should be composed of atoms of largely different atomic numbers, such as iodine and calcium, so as to have greater differences in attenuation when the materials are exposed to x-rays of different keV [23, 24]. Measuring the change in attenuation then allows for mathematical calculation (decomposition) of a voxel into its elemental makeup (fat, iodine, soft tissue, etc.), and by applying the laws of conservation, the estimated sum of each material within the voxel can be determined (Fig. 18.5) [24].

The goal of any imaging contrast agent is to improve radiologic conspicuity of the target when compared to the background tissue. In the onco-

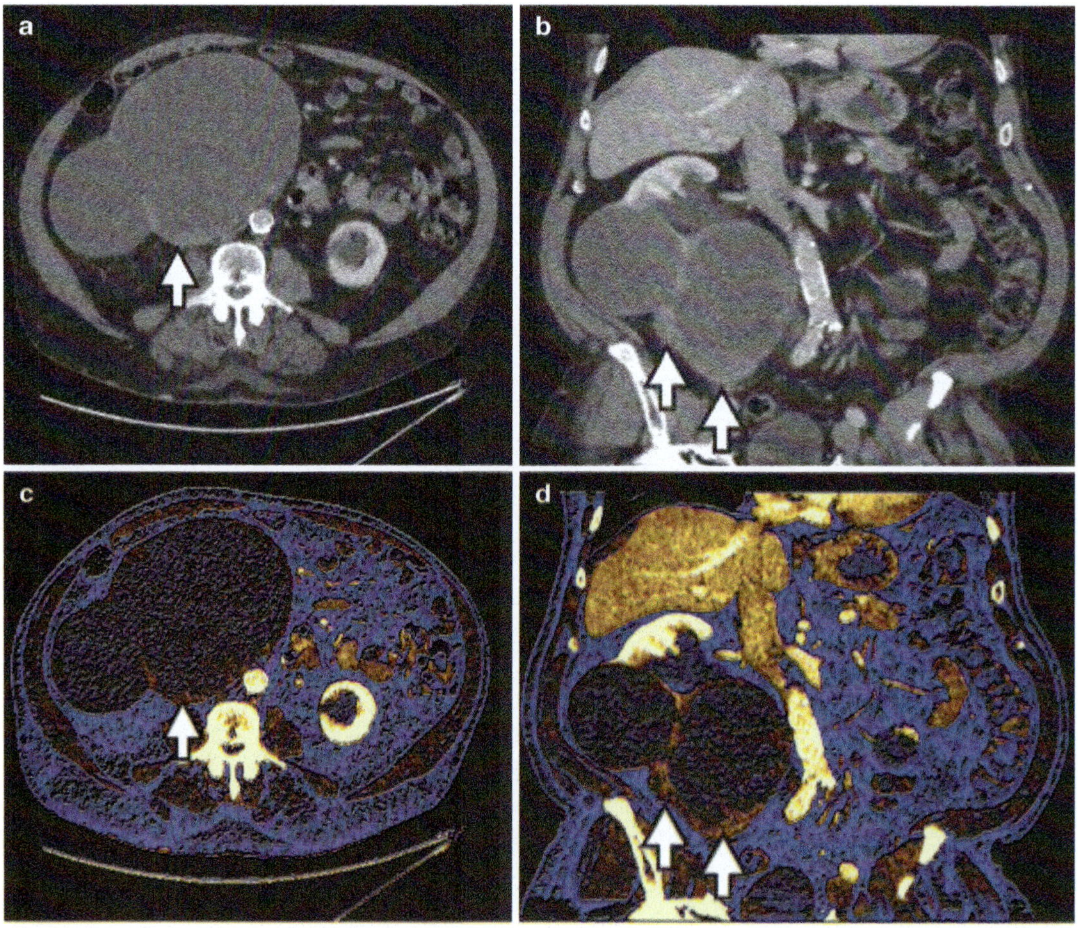

Fig. 18.5 Renal cyst iodine. Contrast-enhanced CT was performed in a 64-year-old man with large complex cystic right renal mass. 70 keV axial (**a**) and coronal reformat (**b**) show high density components within the renal lesion (arrows). Note that axial (**c**) and coronal (**d**) iodine maps allow for identifying solid enhancing components visualized as foci of color-coded iodine uptake (arrows) within the mass, consistent with a Bosniak category 4

logic field, the target would be a tumoral tissue, though the application is limitless. Computed tomography contrast agents can be broadly placed into one of two categories: general use and targeted contrast agents. It is important to remember that no "targeted" contrast agents have been approved for CT imaging by the FDA [23]. In either category a consideration, and somewhat limitation, of CT is the elemental concentration requirement needed to function as a contrast agent, typically 2 mg/mL in single-energy CT, but can be decreased to near 1 mg/mL in dual-energy CT, or in terms of molarity, CT detection limits approach 10^{-3} M compared to MRI 10^{-5} M and nuclear medicine 10^{-10} M [23, 25]. An example of general use contrast would be the currently available iodinated contrast agents. Increasing the elemental concentration within the chemical contrast agent can be achieved through modification of the polymeric backbone molecule to allow for greater elemental binding or by packing larger quantities of elemental particles such as iodine within liposome and nanoparticle agents [26, 27]. Chemical modifications not only allow for increased elemental concentration, but moiety modifications can also be made to improve tissue targeting specificity [28]. As mentioned previously, the FDA has yet to approve any targeted CT contrast agents; however, some are currently in clinical trial that could prove more sensitive in identifying tumors and monitoring response to therapy through increased microvascular permeability [26]. If the element used in the targeted contrast agent is not iodine, targeted agent exclusive radiologic images can be generated to increase target tissue conspicuity, which could improve volumetric assessment, as well as the potential to improve/expand upon other functional imaging techniques.

With growing interest in cellular-based therapies, such as stem cell therapies, comes the need for a means of determining whether the treatment cells (1) correctly implant at the organ of interest and (2) exert their intended effect (cancer treatment or tissue regeneration). Cell tracking provides a noninvasive imaging approach of evaluating tissue changes after initiating cellular therapy. Cells can be labeled with CT contrast agents directly (incubate with contrast in vitro) or indirectly (such as genetic modification which allows for transfer of genetic material to future cell lines during in vivo replication) [25, 29, 30]. Nanoparticles can also function as a cage to house transplanted cells, and the contrast agent (iodine, gold, barium, etc.) can reside either with the cells or an outer core ("capsule-in-capsule) can be created to sequester the two from one another preventing any potential reaction the cells may have to the contrast [31]. Similar structures can be synthesized to attach to tumor cells allowing for earlier detection than what current CT imaging provides, as well as delivery of therapeutic medications [25, 32].

While the potential of these future contrast agents and their role in functional CT imaging is alluring, they remain experimental. Given that current iodinated intravenous contrast agents have decades of clinical use, any new agents must demonstrate similar safety profiles. With regard to nanoparticle agents and cellular tracking, current research has yet to correlate changes of in vivo CT attenuation with cellular viability and/or function changes [25]. As mentioned previously, the use of dual-energy CT and material decomposition would allow simultaneous use of traditional and experimental contrast agents, which may prove helpful in overcoming some of the aforementioned limitations.

Conclusion

State-of-the-art CT imaging hardware and software solutions have enabled a paradigm transition in clinical imaging. Improved and more timely detection of diseases, assessment of tumor perfusion, and viability can render a better substrate for clinicians' decision-making algorithms (e.g., early identification of responders versus nonresponders). Coupling with metabolic techniques, in vivo quantification of highly effective atomic number materials (e.g., iodine), texture analysis techniques, and utilization of novel contrast media can open up a new season for diagnostic CT imaging where disease can be precisely tagged and tracked. In the near future CT will likely be able to provide a wealth of quantitative, minable data and features for routine and more robust application of machine learning/artificial intelligence techniques.

Acknowledgments Thank you to Dr. Ryan O'Malley for contributing a CT case of pancreatic tumor perfusion.

References

1. Townsend DW. Combined PET/CT: the historical perspective. Semin Ultrasound CT MR. 2008;29(4):232–5. https://doi.org/10.1053/j.sult.2008.05.006.
2. Kapoor V, McCook BM, Torok FS. An introduction to PET-CT imaging. Radiographics. 2004;24(2):523–43. https://doi.org/10.1148/rg.242025724.
3. Welle CL, Cullen EL, Peller PJ, Lowe VJ, Murphy RC, Johnson GB, et al. 11C-choline PET/CT in recurrent prostate cancer and nonprostatic neoplastic processes. Radiographics. 2016;36(1):279–92. https://doi.org/10.1148/rg.2016150135.
4. Lubner MG, Smith AD, Sandrasegaran K, Sahani DV, Pickhardt PJ. CT texture analysis: definitions, applications, biologic correlates, and challenges. Radiographics. 2017;37(5):1483–503. https://doi.org/10.1148/rg.2017170056.
5. Shen C, Liu Z, Guan M, Song J, Lian Y, Wang S, et al. 2D and 3D CT radiomics features prognostic performance comparison in non-small cell lung cancer. Transl Oncol. 2017;10(6):886–94. https://doi.org/10.1016/j.tranon.2017.08.007.
6. Garcia-Figueiras R, Goh VJ, Padhani AR, Baleato-Gonzalez S, Garrido M, Leon L, et al. CT perfusion in oncologic imaging: a useful tool? AJR Am J Roentgenol. 2013;200(1):8–19. https://doi.org/10.2214/ajr.11.8476.
7. Kim SH, Kamaya A, Willmann JK. CT perfusion of the liver: principles and applications in oncology. Radiology. 2014;272(2):322–44. https://doi.org/10.1148/radiol.14130091.
8. Taylor AJ, Cerqueira M, Hodgson JM, Mark D, Min J, O'Gara P, et al. ACCF/SCCT/ACR/AHA/ASE/ASNC/NASCI/SCAI/SCMR 2010 appropriate use criteria for cardiac computed tomography. A report of the American College of Cardiology Foundation appropriate use criteria task force, the Society of Cardiovascular Computed Tomography, the American College of Radiology, the American Heart Association, the American Society of Echocardiography, the American Society of Nuclear Cardiology, the North American Society for Cardiovascular Imaging, the Society for Cardiovascular Angiography and Interventions, and the Society for Cardiovascular Magnetic Resonance. Circulation. 2010;122(21):e525–55. https://doi.org/10.1161/CIR.0b013e3181fcae66.
9. Han R, Sun K, Lu B, Zhao R, Li K, Yang X. Diagnostic accuracy of coronary CT angiography combined with dual-energy myocardial perfusion imaging for detection of myocardial infarction. Exp Ther Med. 2017;14(1):207–13. https://doi.org/10.3892/etm.2017.4485.
10. Yang DH, Kim YH. CT myocardial perfusion imaging: current status and future perspectives. Int J Cardiovasc Imaging. 2017;33(7):1009–20. https://doi.org/10.1007/s10554-017-1102-6.
11. Rossi A, Merkus D, Klotz E, Mollet N, de Feyter PJ, Krestin GP. Stress myocardial perfusion: imaging with multidetector CT. Radiology. 2014;270(1):25–46. https://doi.org/10.1148/radiol.13112739.
12. Duran Karaduman B, Akcay M, Ayhan H, Kasapkara HA, Guney MC, Durmaz T, et al. Comparison between fractional flow reserve and visual assessment for moderate coronary artery stenosis. Kardiol Pol. 2017;75(6):545–53. https://doi.org/10.5603/KP.a2017.0037.
13. Lotfi A, Jeremias A, Fearon WF, Feldman MD, Mehran R, Messenger JC, et al. Expert consensus statement on the use of fractional flow reserve, intravascular ultrasound, and optical coherence tomography: a consensus statement of the Society of Cardiovascular Angiography and Interventions. Cathet Cardiovasc Interv: Off J Soc Card Angiography Interv. 2014;83(4):509–18. https://doi.org/10.1002/ccd.25222.
14. Tesche C, Cecco CND, Albrecht MH, Duguay TM, II RRB, Litwin SE, et al. Coronary CT angiography–derived fractional flow reserve. Radiology. 2017;285(1):17–33. https://doi.org/10.1148/radiol.2017162641.
15. Hayes SA, Pietanza MC, O'Driscoll D, Zheng J, Moskowitz CS, Kris MG, et al. Comparison of CT volumetric measurement with RECIST response in patients with lung cancer. Eur J Radiol. 2016;85(3):524–33. https://doi.org/10.1016/j.ejrad.2015.12.019.
16. Gavrielides MA, Kinnard LM, Myers KJ, Petrick N. Noncalcified lung nodules: volumetric assessment with thoracic CT. Radiology. 2009;251(1):26–37. https://doi.org/10.1148/radiol.2511071897.
17. Winer-Muram HT, Jennings SG, Meyer CA, Liang Y, Aisen AM, Tarver RD, et al. Effect of varying CT section width on volumetric measurement of lung tumors and application of compensatory equations. Radiology. 2003;229(1):184–94. https://doi.org/10.1148/radiol.2291020859.
18. Samei E, Robins M, Chen B, Agasthya G. Estimability index for volume quantification of homogeneous spherical lesions in computed tomography. J Med Imaging (Bellingham, Wash). 2018;5(3):031404. https://doi.org/10.1117/1.Jmi.5.3.031404.
19. Almeida RR, Lo GC, Patino M, Bizzo B, Canellas R, Sahani DV. Advances in pancreatic CT imaging. Am J Roentgenol. 2018;211(1):52–66. https://doi.org/10.2214/AJR.17.18665.
20. Planz VB, Posielski NM, Lubner MG, Li K, Chen G-H, Nakada SY, et al. Ultra-low-dose limited renal CT for volumetric stone surveillance: advantages over standard unenhanced CT. Abdom Radiol. 2018; https://doi.org/10.1007/s00261-018-1719-5.

21. Selby MG, Vrtiska TJ, Krambeck AE, McCollough CH, Elsherbiny HE, Bergstralh EJ, et al. Quantification of asymptomatic kidney stone burden by computed tomography for predicting future symptomatic stone events. Urology. 2015;85(1):45–50. https://doi.org/10.1016/j.urology.2014.08.031.
22. Patino M, Prochowski A, Agrawal MD, Simeone FJ, Gupta R, Hahn PF, et al. Material separation using dual-energy CT: current and emerging applications. Radiographics. 2016;36(4):1087–105. https://doi.org/10.1148/rg.2016150220.
23. Yeh BM, FitzGerald PF, Edic PM, Lambert JW, Colborn RE, Marino ME, et al. Opportunities for new CT contrast agents to maximize the diagnostic potential of emerging spectral CT technologies. Adv Drug Deliv Rev. 2017;113:201–22. https://doi.org/10.1016/j.addr.2016.09.001.
24. Fornaro J, Leschka S, Hibbeln D, Butler A, Anderson N, Pache G, et al. Dual- and multi-energy CT: approach to functional imaging. Insights Imaging. 2011;2(2):149–59. https://doi.org/10.1007/s13244-010-0057-0.
25. Kim J, Chhour P, Hsu J, Litt HI, Ferrari VA, Popovtzer R, et al. Use of nanoparticle contrast agents for cell tracking with computed tomography. Bioconjug Chem. 2017;28(6):1581–97. https://doi.org/10.1021/acs.bioconjchem.7b00194.
26. Raatschen HJ, Fu Y, Brasch RC, Pietsch H, Shames DM, Yeh BM. In vivo monitoring of angiogenesis inhibitory treatment effects by dynamic contrast-enhanced computed tomography in a xenograft tumor model. Investig Radiol. 2009;44(5):265–70. https://doi.org/10.1097/RLI.0b013e31819f1b60.
27. Bhavane R, Badea C, Ghaghada KB, Clark D, Vela D, Moturu A, et al. Dual-energy computed tomography imaging of atherosclerotic plaques in a mouse model using a liposomal-iodine nanoparticle contrast agent. Circ Cardiovasc Imaging. 2013;6(2):285–94. https://doi.org/10.1161/circimaging.112.000119.
28. Ashton JR, West JL, Badea CT. In vivo small animal micro-CT using nanoparticle contrast agents. Front Pharmacol. 2015;6:256. https://doi.org/10.3389/fphar.2015.00256.
29. Kircher MF, Gambhir SS, Grimm J. Noninvasive cell-tracking methods. Nat Rev Clin Oncol. 2011;8(11):677–88. https://doi.org/10.1038/nrclinonc.2011.141.
30. Srivastava AK, Bulte JW. Seeing stem cells at work in vivo. Stem Cell Rev. 2014;10(1):127–44. https://doi.org/10.1007/s12015-013-9468-x.
31. Kim J, Arifin DR, Muja N, Kim T, Gilad AA, Kim H, et al. Multifunctional capsule-in-capsules for immunoprotection and trimodal imaging. Angew Chem Int Ed Engl. 2011;50(10):2317–21. https://doi.org/10.1002/anie.201007494.
32. Menk RH, Schultke E, Hall C, Arfelli F, Astolfo A, Rigon L, et al. Gold nanoparticle labeling of cells is a sensitive method to investigate cell distribution and migration in animal models of human disease. Nanomed: Nanotechnol Biol Med. 2011;7(5):647–54. https://doi.org/10.1016/j.nano.2011.01.010.

19 CT Perfusion Techniques and Applications in Stroke and Cancer

Ting-Yim Lee, Dae Myoung Yang, Fiona Li, and Raanan Marants

Introduction

Stroke is the second leading cause of death and third leading cause of disability worldwide according to the World Health Organization [1]. Overall, stroke mortality rates have declined over the last 30 years in the United States [2] and Canada [3], due to a decrease in the number of fatal strokes [4], rather than a decrease in stroke incidence, which is projected to more than double over the next 30 years, with most of the increase coming from people aged 75 years or older [5]. Approximately half the survivors of stroke are institutionalized or disabled within 5 years [6], and due to the aging population, the number of individuals living with disability resulting from stroke is projected to almost double in the next two decades [7]. Long-term care for these patients will further increase the socioeconomic burden of cerebrovascular disease [8]. CT perfusion (CTP) is a minimally invasive imaging technique that produces quantitative maps of hemodynamic parameters which are useful for assessing tissue viability [9, 10]. CTP could improve stroke outcome by helping to select the optimal treatment for individual patients. For example, among the five (ESCAPE, EXTEND-IA, MR CLEAN, REVASCAT, and SWIFT-PRIME [11–15]) successful trials of treating large vessel occlusion within 6–8 h of symptom onset with mechanical thrombectomy (MT), EXTEND-IA and SWIFT-PRIME, which used thresholds applied to parameter maps from CTP to exclude patients with large infarct volumes and/or small penumbra volumes [11, 13], had higher rates of good functional outcome in the MT group (53% to 71%) than MR CLEAN and REVASCAT, which did not use CTP (33% to 44%) [14, 15]. The utility of CTP to select patients for MT was further confirmed by DEFUSE 3 [16] which extended the treatment time window to 16 h. DEFUSE 3 used threshold applied to CTP-derived CBF and T_{max} map to estimate infarct core and penumbral volume. Patients were eligible for treatment if penumbra volume was 1.8 times larger than the infarct, infarct volume was <70 mL, and penumbra volume was >15 mL [16].

Application of CTP in cancer is to image tumor-associated angiogenesis [17] which has significant implications in the diagnosis and treatment of various solid tumors [18] including lesion characterization and staging; response prediction

T.-Y. Lee (✉)
Imaging Program, Lawson Health Research Institute & Robarts Research Institute, Medical Biophysics, Medical Imaging and Oncology, The University of Western Ontario, London, ON, Canada
e-mail: tlee@robarts.ca

D. M. Yang · F. Li · R. Marants
Medical Biophysics, The University of Western Ontario, London, ON, Canada
e-mail: dyang27@uwo.ca; fli222@uwo.ca; rmarant@uwo.ca

© Springer Nature Switzerland AG 2020

E. Samei, N. J. Pelc (eds.), *Computed Tomography*, https://doi.org/10.1007/978-3-030-26957-9_19

to chemotherapy, radiotherapy, antiangiogenic therapy, and other newer targeted therapies (e.g., immunotherapy); evaluation of relapse; and resistance to treatment. For example, a recent multicenter Phase 3 trial [19] demonstrated that for advanced ovarian cancer patients who were treated with carboplatin/paclitaxel plus optional bevacizumab, blood flow increase was associated with shorter progression-free survival (HR 2.9, 95% CI, 1.3–6.4, $P = 0.008$) and remained significant after adjusting for age, change in tumor volume, and surgery status.

In this chapter we discuss the basic principles of CTP and application examples in stroke and cancer.

Theory of Contrast Transport

There are two approaches in describing contrast transport in tissue. The model-independent approach relies on the conservation of mass (Fick principle) and the principle of superimposition, while the modeling approach explicitly models how contrast is transported in blood vessels and permeates the endothelial barrier between blood and tissue.

Model-Independent Approach

If $C_a(t)$ and $C_v(t)$ are the arterial and venous contrast concentration, respectively, and $Q(t)$ is the tissue contrast concentration, then by the conservation of mass or Fick principle:

$$Q(t) = F\int_0^t \left[C_a(u) - C_v(u)\right]\mathrm{du} \qquad (19.1)$$

where F is the blood flow carrying contrast into and out of the tissue. If contrast transport is stationary (i.e., time invariant), then by the principle of superimposition,

$$C_v(t) = C_a(t) \otimes h(t) \qquad (19.2)$$

where $\otimes$ is the convolution operator, and $h(t)$ is probability density function of contrast transit time through the tissue or transit time spectrum. Substituting Eq. (19.2) into Eq. (19.1) and simplifying leads to:

$$Q(t) = C_a(t) \otimes \mathrm{FR}(t) = C_a(t) \otimes R_F(t) \qquad (19.3)$$

where

$$R(t) = 1 - \int_0^t h(u)\,du \qquad (19.4)$$

$R(t)$ is the impulse residue function (IRF) of the tissue. IRF is the idealized tissue time-density (concentration) curve (TDC) measured by the scanner if a unit amount of contrast is injected as a sharp bolus into the arterial inlet of the tissue. In a CTP study, both $Q(t)$ and $C_a(t)$ are measured, and then Eq. (19.3) suggests that FR(t) or the flow-scaled IRF, $R_F(t)$, can be calculated by deconvolving $C_a(t)$ from $Q(t)$. The tissue blood flow, F, and volume, V, are estimated as the maximum and area under the curve (AUC) of $R_F(t)$, respectively [20]. Then by the central volume principle [20], the mean transit time, MTT, is the ratio of V to F (or area over height of $R_F(t)$). Contrast remains intravascular in the brain where the blood-brain barrier (BBB) is intact; however, in other organs as well as when the BBB is disrupted as in intracerebral hemorrhage and brain tumor, contrast does leak into the extravascular interstitial space. Equations (19.1, 19.2, 19.3, and 19.4) apply, and tissue blood flow (F) is always equal to the peak height of tissue blood flow (F) regardless of whether the contrast remains intravascular or leaks out into the extravascular interstitial space. When contrast is intravascular, the AUC of $R_F(t)$ is the vascular blood volume, V_b, and the ratio of AUC to maximum height of $R_F(t)$ is the vascular mean transit time (MTT_v). When contrast leaks from blood vessels into tissue, the AUC of $R_F(t)$ is the total contrast distribution volume, V_D, which includes V_b, while the area over height is the tissue mean transit time, MTT_t [21]. When contrast is intravascular and if only tissue blood flow and volume and vascular mean transit time are required, then the model-independent approach is preferred because of its conceptual simplicity.

For the time period before contrast exits from the tissue via the venous outlets, Eq. (19.1) simplifies to:

$$Q(t) = F\int_0^t C_a(u)\,\mathrm{du}$$

differentiating to obtain:

$$\frac{\mathrm{dQ}(t)}{\mathrm{dt}} = \mathrm{FC}_a(t)$$

In particular, the maximum front slope of the tissue time-density curve, $Q(t)$, is:

$$\left[\frac{\mathrm{dQ}(t)}{\mathrm{dt}}\right]_{\max} = F\left[C_a(t)\right]_{\max}$$

and the tissue blood flow is equal to:

$$F = \left[\frac{\mathrm{dQ}(t)}{\mathrm{dt}}\right]_{\max} \Big/ \left[C_a(t)\right]_{\max} \qquad (19.5)$$

Equation (19.5) is the basis for the maximum front slope method for the measurement of tissue blood flow [22]. While simplicity is the appeal of this method, its validity is dependent on the no venous outflow of contrast assumption which may not hold in general, particularly for the brain where MTT_v is typically less than 4–6 s; when the assumption is violated, this method will underestimate blood flow because of the washout of contrast from the tissue.

Modeling Approaches

X-ray contrast is inert and extracellular meaning after permeating the endothelial barrier at the blood-tissue interface, it neither binds to any target nor enters cells and distributes only in the interstitial space. As such, in all modeling approaches, the interstitial space is represented as a compartment, namely, contrast is uniformly distributed in the space, and its concentration is only dependent on time. The main distinguishing feature among the modeling approaches is whether the blood vessels are treated as a compartment or not as discussed below.

Blood Vessels as a Compartment: Two-Compartment Model

This approach is exemplified by the two-compartment model shown in Fig. 19.1. In this model, how contrast is delivered to the blood vessels in the tissue voxel is not modeled. Contrast concentration in blood vessels is assumed to be a time function only, $C_a(t)$, as measured in an artery. No contrast concentration gradient along blood vessels, as would be expected when contrast is leaking from the vessels, is modeled; instead the permeation of the blood vessels is lumped together as two model parameters: K_1 (K_{trans}) and k_2 – the influx and efflux rate constant from bidirectional passive diffusion of inert contrast through the endothelial barrier. The governing equations of the two-compartment model in Fig. 19.1 are:

$$\frac{\mathrm{dQ}(t)}{\mathrm{dt}} = K_1 C_a(t) - k_2 C_e(t)$$

$$Q(t) = V_b C_a(t) + C_e(t)$$

Solving the above two equations together with the initial condition $[C_e(t)]_{t=0} = 0$:

$$\begin{aligned} Q(t) &= V_b C_a(t) + K_1 C_a(t) \otimes e^{-k_2 t} \\ &= C_a(t) \otimes \left[V_b \delta(t) + K_1 e^{-k_2 t}\right] \end{aligned} \qquad (19.6)$$

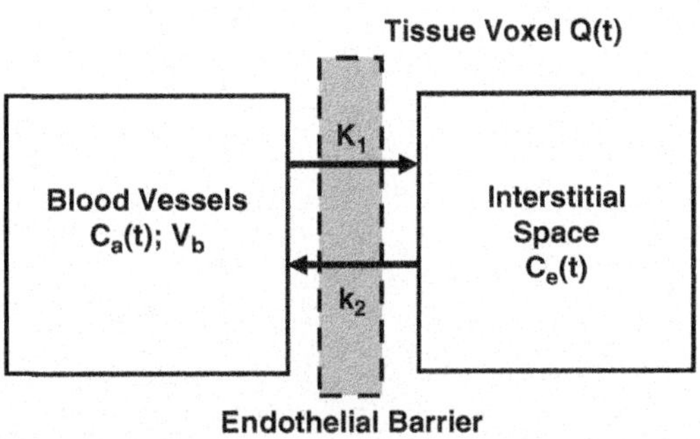

Fig. 19.1 Model of contrast distribution in tissue with both blood vessel and interstitial space treated as compartments. $C_a(t)$, $C_e(t)$, and $Q(t)$ are the contrast concentration in blood vessels, interstitial space, and tissue voxel, respectively. V_b is the blood volume

where $\delta(t)$ is the delta function. Comparing Eqs. (19.3) and (19.6), we can identify the flow-scaled IRF of the two-compartment model as:

$$R_F^{2C}(t) = V_b \delta(t) + K_1 e^{-k_2 t} \quad (19.7)$$

In CT perfusion studies, $C_a(t)$ is usually measured in a large blood vessel (to avoid partial volume averaging leading to underestimation of the true arterial concentration) upstream from the tissue; therefore there is a delay, T_o, in the arrival of contrast at the tissue relative to the artery. Equations (19.6) and (19.7) can be modified to account for this delay as follows:

$$Q(t) = C_a(t) \otimes \left[V_b \delta(t - T_o) + K_1 e^{-k_2 (t - T_o)} \right] \quad (19.6a)$$

$$R_F^{2C}(t) = V_b \delta(t - T_o) + K_1 e^{-k_2 (t - T_o)} \quad (19.7a)$$

Equation (19.6) suggests that deconvolving $C_a(t)$ from $Q(t)$ according to the two-compartment model in Fig. 19.1 would allow determination of the model parameters: V_b, K_1, k_2, and T_o. As expected, because blood flow delivery of contrast to the tissue is not modeled in the two-compartment model, perfusion is not explicitly estimated in the deconvolution. However, as shown in the next section, K_1 is related to blood flow.

Plug (Non-dispersive) Flow in Blood Vessels: Johnson-Wilson-Lee Model

The simplest model to describe the blood flow delivery of contrast to the blood vessels and leakage into the interstitial space (treated as a compartment) is the Johnson-Wilson-Lee model as shown in Fig. 19.2. In this model, all blood vessels in the tissue region (voxel) are "collapsed" into a single tube of volume V_b, the blood volume. Blood carrying contrast flows as a "plug" into and out of the vessels without dispersion (that is *not* laminar flow with parabolic flow profile) with transit time equal to W. During the initial transit of contrast through the vessels, contrast leaks into the interstitial space from vessels, so there is a contrast gradient from the venous exit to the arterial inlet (or the vessels are no longer treated as a compartment). After the passage of contrast, then the extravasated contrast in the interstitial space leaks back into the vessels. We introduced the adiabatic approximation [23] to derive a closed form solution for the flow-scaled impulse residue function of the JWL model, $R_F^{JWL}(t)$, as follows:

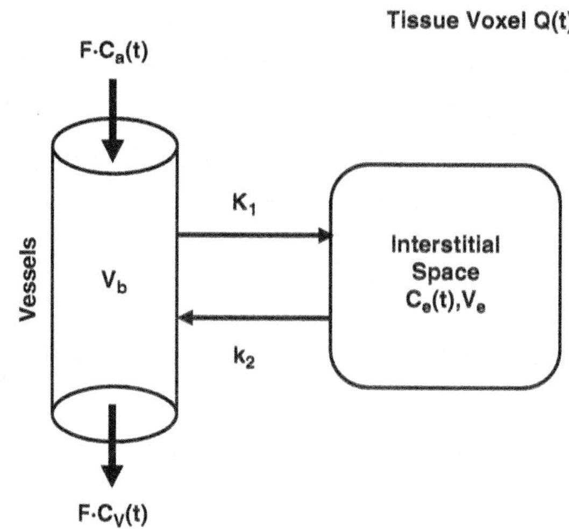

Fig. 19.2 The Johnson-Wilson-Lee (JWL) model for the distribution of contrast in a tissue region (voxel). $C_a(t)$ and $C_v(t)$ are the contrast concentration in arterial and venous blood entering and exiting the voxel via the vessels. K_1 is the influx and efflux rate constant of contrast as in the two-compartment model (Fig. 19.1). $C_e(t)$ and $Q(t)$ is the contrast concentration in the interstitial space and the voxel. V_e is the contrast distribution volume in the interstitial space

$$R_F^{\text{JWL}}(t)=\begin{cases}0.0 & 0<t<T_o\\ F & T_o\le t<T_o+W\\ K_1e^{-k_2(t-T_o-W)} & t\ge T_o+W\end{cases} \quad (19.8)$$

In addition, we showed that [23]:

$$K_1=\text{FE}; E=1-e^{-\frac{\text{PS}}{F}}; k_2=\frac{K_1}{V_e} \quad (19.9)$$

where E is the extraction efficiency of contrast by the tissue [24] and PS is permeability surface area product of perfused vessels [17, 25]. Using Eqs. (19.3) and (19.8), the JWL model tissue (voxel) time-density curve is evaluated as:

$$Q(t)=\begin{cases}0.0 & 0\le t<T_o\\ \text{FD}(t-T_0) & T_o\le t<T_o+W\\ \text{FD}(t-T_0)-\text{FD}(t-T_0-W)+\text{FEC}_a(t-T_o-W)*e^{-k_2(t-T_o-W)} & t\ge T_o+W\end{cases}$$

where $D(t)=\int_0^t C_a(u)\text{du}$ and can be further simplified to (noting $V_b=\text{FW}$):

$$Q(t)=\begin{cases}0.0 & 0<t<T_o\\ \text{FD}(t-T_{o)} & T_o\le t<T_o+W\\ V_bC_a(t-T_o-\theta W)+K_1C_a(t-T_o-W)*e^{-k_2(t-T_o-W)} & t\ge T_o+W\end{cases} \quad (19.10)$$

where $0<\theta<1$. Comparing Eq. (19.10) for the case of $t\ge T_o+W$ with Eq. (6a) allows the identification that K_1 and k_2 for the 2-compartment and JWL model are the same. As defined in Eq. (19.9), the influx rate constant, K_1, is the flow extraction efficiency product. Since the two-compartment model estimates K_1, it cannot be equated to F unless $E=1.0$ or the value of E is known a priori. The value for E is dependent on the relative magnitude of PS and F. When PS>>F (flow limited case of contrast distribution in tissue), E≈1.0 and K_1≈F; when PS<<F (diffusion limited case, e.g., brain tumor), E ≈ 0.0 and K_1≈PS.This is the disadvantage of the two-compartment model where K_1 can be F, PS, or FE depending on the value of E, whereas JWL model can always estimate F independent of E and can also estimate PS (or E) together with F. Figure 19.3 compares $R_F^{2C}(t)$ and $R_F^{\text{JWL}}(t)$; it is seen that:

$$\lim_{W\to 0} R_F^{\text{JWL}}(t)=R_F^{2C}(t)$$

In practical terms, when the sampling interval, Δt, of the time-density curves, $C_a(t)$ and $Q(t)$, is much larger than W, then $R_F^{\text{JWL}}(t)\to R_F^{2C}(t)$. In other words, when Δt becomes larger than W, then the estimate of F approaches that of FE instead.

No Contrast Efflux from Interstitial Space: Patlak Model

A special case arises for the two-compartment and JWL model when there is no efflux of contrast from the interstitial compartment back into

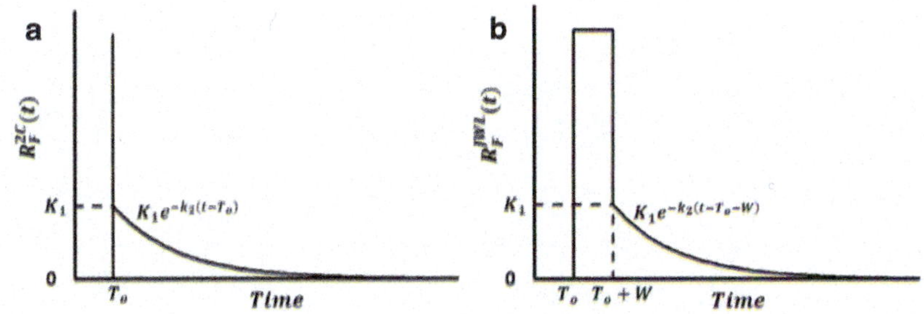

Fig. 19.3 Comparison of (**a**) $R_F^{2C}(t)$ and $R_F^{\text{JWL}}(t)$

the vessels ($k_2 = 0$). From Eq. (19.10), under the condition of no efflux, we have for $t \geq T_o + W$:

$$Q(t) \cong V_b C_a(t) + K_1 \int_0^t C_a(u)\,\mathrm{du}$$

which can be rearranged as:

$$\frac{Q(t)}{C_a(t)} \cong V_b + \frac{K_1 \int_0^t C_a(u)\,du}{C_a(t)} \quad (19.11)$$

Eq. (19.11) is the basis of the Patlak model [26] where $Q(t)/C_a(t)$ vs $K_1 \int_0^t C_a(u)\,\mathrm{du} / C_a(t)$ for $t \geq T_o + W$ is a straight line with intercept equal to vascular volume (V_b), and the slope is the influx rate constant (K_1). The advantage of this model is that the Patlak plot, Eq. (19.11), is simple to implement. One important limitation is the condition of no contrast efflux that may only be satisfied for a very brief time after $T_o + W$. After that time, the Patlak plot deviates from linearity because of contrast efflux into blood vessels and clearance by blood flow leading to a decrease in $Q(t)$. Note that as shown by Patlak [27], Eq. (19.11) is valid for more than one tissue compartment, in fact for many compartments in any arbitrary configuration, provided there is one compartment in which contrast accumulates and never leaves.

Numerical Deconvolution Techniques

Here numerical methods/algorithms to solve for the flow-scaled IRF, $R_F(t)$, from Eq. (19.3) are discussed. Since the equation involves a convolution, the solution for $R_F(t)$ given measured $C_a(t)$ and $Q(t)$ is the inverse of convolution or deconvolution. As in the theory of contrast distribution in tissue, the methods can be grouped into model-independent (black box) and model-based deconvolution.

Model-Independent (Black Box) Deconvolution

A starting point is to write Eq. (19.3) explicitly in integral form:

$$Q(T) = \int_0^T C_a(T-t) R_F(t)\,\mathrm{dt}$$

Discretizing the above equation at time interval, Δt, and if $T = N\Delta t$ and $Q(t)$ and $C_a(t)$ are measured in the interval – $[0,T]$:

$$Q(n) = \Delta t \sum_{i=0}^{n} C_a(n-i) R_F(i),\ n = 0,1,\cdots,N \quad (19.3a)$$

where $t = n\Delta t \in [0,T]$ and $C_a(i)$ and $R_F(i)$ are the values of $C_a(t)$ and $Q(t)$ at $t = i\Delta t$. Equation (19.3a) can be rewritten as a matrix equation:

$$\begin{pmatrix} Q(0) \\ Q(1) \\ \vdots \\ Q(N) \end{pmatrix} = \Delta t \begin{pmatrix} C_a(0) & \cdots & 0 \\ C_a(1) & \ddots & 0 \\ \vdots & & \vdots \\ C_a(N) & \cdots & C_a(0) \end{pmatrix} \cdot \begin{pmatrix} R_F(0) \\ R_F(1) \\ \vdots \\ R_F(N) \end{pmatrix}$$

or

$$\bar{Q} = \widetilde{C_a}\,\overline{R_F} \quad (19.12)$$

where $\bar{Q} = (Q(0), Q(1), \cdots, Q(N))^T$,

$\overline{R_F} = (R_F(0), R_F(1), \cdots, R_F(N))^T$, and

$$\widetilde{C_a} = \Delta t \begin{pmatrix} C_a(0) & \cdots & 0 \\ C_a(1) & \ddots & 0 \\ \vdots & & \vdots \\ C_a(N) & \cdots & C_a(0) \end{pmatrix} \quad (19.13)$$

Solution for $\overline{R_F}$ from Eq. (19.4) amounts to finding the inverse matrix, $\widetilde{C_a}^{-1}$ of $\widetilde{C_a}$ as $\overline{R_F} = \widetilde{C_a}^{-1} \bar{Q}$. One popular matrix inversion method is singular value decomposition (SVD) [28] where $\widetilde{C_a}$ is decomposed into a product of orthogonal matrices $\tilde{U}$ and $\tilde{V}$ and a diagonal matrix, $\tilde{S}$, of singular values: $\widetilde{C_a} = \tilde{U}\tilde{S}\tilde{V}^T$.

Noting that the inverse of an orthogonal matrix is its transpose,

$$\overline{R_F} = \widetilde{C_a}^{-1}\overline{Q} = \tilde{V}\tilde{S}^{-1}\tilde{U}^T\overline{Q} \tag{19.14}$$

Since the diagonal elements of $\tilde{S}^{-1}$ are reciprocals of the singular values of $\widetilde{C_a}$, Eq. (19.14) shows that small singular values result in very unstable estimates of $\overline{R_F}$ [29, 30]. Small singular values arise when some rows of $\widetilde{C_a}$ can be approximated by linear combinations of other rows [28]. As can be seen from its definition in Eq. (19.13), each successive row of the artery matrix $\widetilde{C_a}$ is obtained by shifting the arterial time-density curve one element (time interval) to the right. The linear dependence condition for small singular values is invariably satisfied when the artery time-density curve is changing very slowly in time as would be the case following the first pass phase, and this condition is accentuated with the presence of noise. A simple method to stabilize deconvolution is to set a threshold value, and in the calculation of $\overline{R_F}$ according to Eq. (19.14), the reciprocals of singular values smaller than the threshold are set to zero [31]. This strategy has been widely adopted by investigators. However, the truncation of small singular values can only achieve partial success in stabilizing deconvolution against noise as there are still residual oscillations in $\overline{R_F}$ [32]. One method to reduce oscillations is to set a threshold on the norm of the second derivative of $\overline{R_F}$ (oscillations) and increase the threshold of small singular values to be discarded until this norm is not exceeded [33]. A more effective approach is to cast the deconvolution as an augmented optimization problem (minimizing the sum of squared deviation of the fitted from the measured $Q(t)$) subject to a certain smoothness criterion (e.g., the second derivation of $R_F(t)$) via the Lagrangian multiplier method [28]. Discussion of this approach is outside the scope of this chapter; interested reader is referred to [34].

Since $C_a(t) = 0$ for $t < 0$, $Q(t)$ would always lag behind $C_a(t)$, that is, Eq. [19.3] enforces time causality as would be expected of realizable physiological conditions in tissue. In practice, especially in stroke, when $C_a(t)$ is selected from the ischemic territory, then it may lag behind $Q(t)$ from non-ischemic region. Under this condition, deconvolving $C_a(t)$ from $Q(t)$ would overestimate the peak height of $R_F(t)$ hence blood flow [35]. Discussion on the circulant deconvolution method to deal with this special case is outside the scope of this chapter; the interested reader is referred to the work of Wu et al. [33]. However, there exists a simpler method than circulant SVD to deal with this case. We can shift the tissue curve until it lags the artery curve, and methods in the previous section that deals with lagging tissue curve can then be applied [36].

The practice of measuring the arterial time-density curve from a large vessel to minimize its underestimation from partial volume averaging would result in the tissue time-density curve lagging behind the arterial curve by a finite time shift, T_o. This is especially true in stroke where the T_o for ischemic tissue relative to the arterial time-density curve measured in a large extra- or intra-cranial blood vessel on the unaffected side can exceed 10 s . From Eq. (19.3a), $R_F = 0$ for $t \le T_o$ in this case. However, singular value deconvolution does not enforce this causality condition, and the estimated $\overline{R_F}$ could start before T_o leading to error in estimating the (peak) height of $\overline{R_F}$ or blood flow. Ibaraki et al. [37] proposed a pre-processing step whereby T_o is determined by fitting the front slope of tissue curve and then shift the arterial curve by the determined T_o before performing the singular value deconvolution. The disadvantage with this method is that the separately determined T_o from fitting the front slope of the tissue curve may not be optimal in fitting the entire tissue curve. A method incorporating the estimation of T_o together with R_F using SVD in the framework of constrained optimization of fitting to measured tissue curve is discussed in a US Patent [38]. Because of this problem, in the application of CTP, it is important to use a delay insensitive deconvolution algorithm/method to calculate blood flow.

Model-Based Deconvolution

Model-independent deconvolution is conceptually simpler than model-based one as it treats the tissue as a "black box" obviating the user from proposing an appropriate model to describe the transport of contrast in tissue. The disadvantage is that only blood flow, blood volume, and vascular mean transit time (contrast remains intravascular) or distribution volume and tissue mean transit time (contrast extravasates) can be calculated as the peak height, area, and area over height of the estimated $\overline{R_F}$, respectively. On the other hand, with model (two-compartment or JWL model)-based deconvolution, parameters related to the function of the endothelial barrier – E, FE, and PS – can be derived from the estimated $\overline{R_F}$. These parameters are useful for predicting hemorrhage in stroke [39] and assessing cancer-associated angiogenesis and its response to treatment [18].

Estimation of model parameters in model-based deconvolution is an optimizing problem where the parameters are iteratively changed to minimize the sum of squared deviations (SSD) of the fitted from the measured tissue time-density curve according to the underlying (two-compartment or JWL in the discussion here) model. As the flow-scaled IRF, R_F^{2C} and R_F^{JWL}, involves exponential function of the contrast efflux rate constant, k_2, the deconvolution

becomes a nonlinear optimization problem. There are many high-quality nonlinear optimization software packages that can be used including NAG Numerical Libraries, IMSL Numerical Libraries, and others. However, for rapid prototyping, the "fmincon" function in MATLAB can be used. An issue about nonlinear optimization is that the algorithm can be trapped in a local minimum, so the estimated model parameters are dependent on the initial values used. It is advisable to repeat the estimation with widely different initial values and accept the set of estimated parameters that result in the smallest cost function (SSD of the fitted from the measured tissue curve).

Comparison of Deconvolution Methods for CTP

To illustrate how the discussed deconvolution methods perform in CTP, a simulation study was carried out. An artery time-density curve was obtained from a CTP study of the brain (Fig. 19.4 h inset). It is convolved with a "true" flow-scaled IRF (Fig. 19.4b) to generate the "true" tissue time-density curve to which Gaussian noise with a standard deviation of 5 HU to get the simulated noisy tissue curve (Fig. 19.4a). The standard deviation of 5 HU was chosen so that the signal-to-noise of the simulated noisy tissue curve approximates that of the normal gray matter region curve of a brain CTP study. The "true" flow-scaled IRF had a delay with respect to the arterial curve, a maximum height (F), an area (V_b), and the area/height ($\mathrm{MTT_v}$) of 5 s, 50 mL/min/100 g, 6.3 mL/100 g, and 7.6 s, respectively. Figure 19.4 shows the estimated flow-scaled IRF and the fitted curve for four deconvolution methods discussed above. Figure 19.4a, b shows results from singular value deconvolution with singular values smaller than 15% of maximum truncated. Figure 19.4c, d shows delay corrected singular value deconvolution. The noisy curve was shifted backward in time by 5 s (assuming the pre-processing step [37] determined the true T_o) before singular value deconvolution. In Fig. 19.4c, the noisy and fitted tissue curve are displayed in their original time to facilitate comparison with results from other deconvolution methods. Figure 19.4e, f shows singular value deconvolution subject to non-negativity, monotonicity, and smoothness constraints as formulated in [38]. Figure 19.4g, h shows deconvolution based on the JWL model. Table 19.1 compares the quantitative parameters derived from the estimated flow-scaled impulse residue function by the four deconvolution methods.

In terms of matching the true values of F, V_b, and MTT_v, the order of preference of the deconvolution methods are constrained SVD, JWL model deconvolution, delay-corrected SVD, and SVD. It is also instructive to examine the average SSD of the fitted and true from the noisy curve. All model-independent deconvolution methods (SVD, delay-corrected SVD, and constrained SVD) had an average SSD smaller than that of the true curve suggesting that these methods are overfitting to the noise even though truncation of singular values up to 15% of the

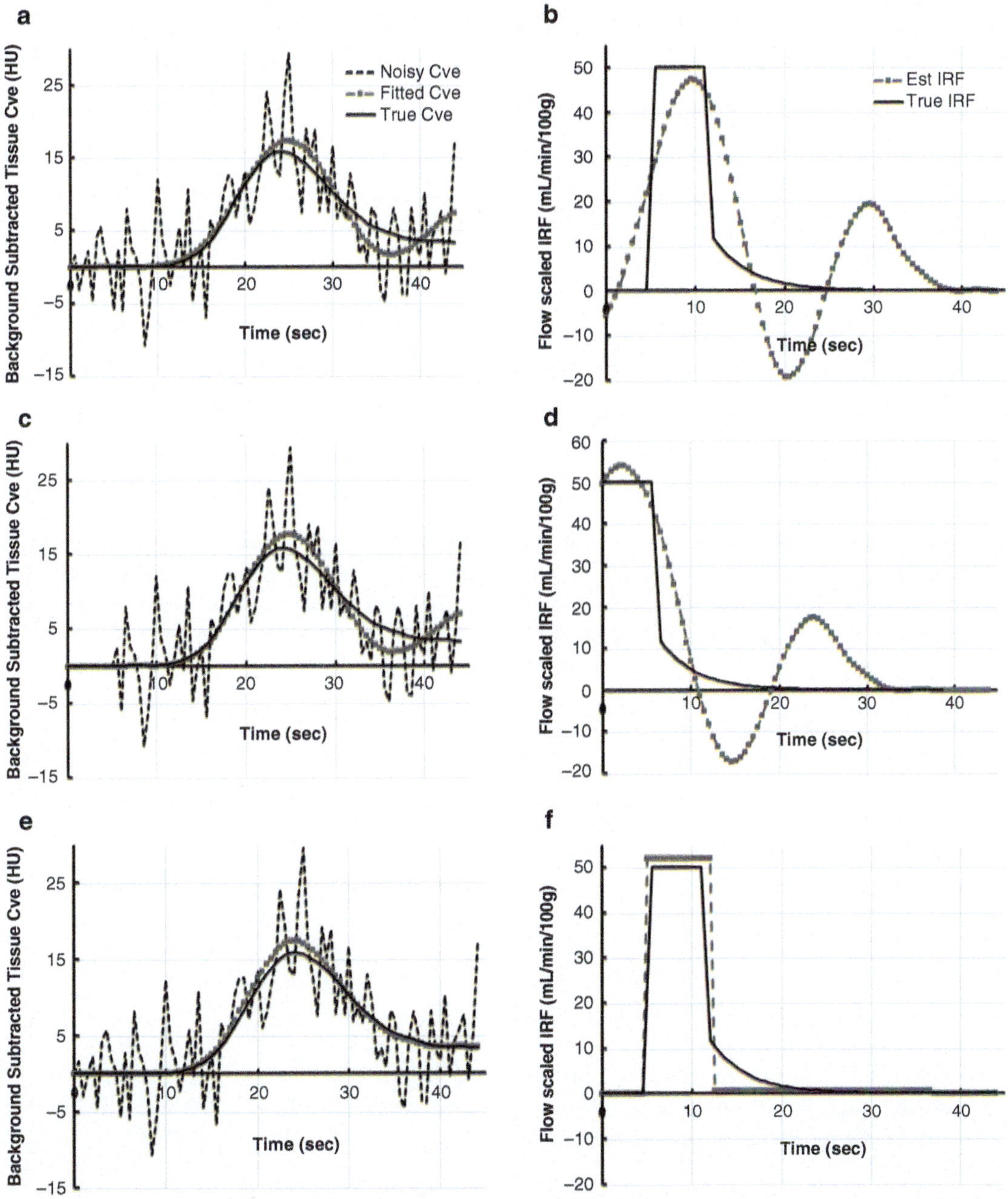

Fig. 19.4 Comparison of four deconvolution methods. Details are provided in the text

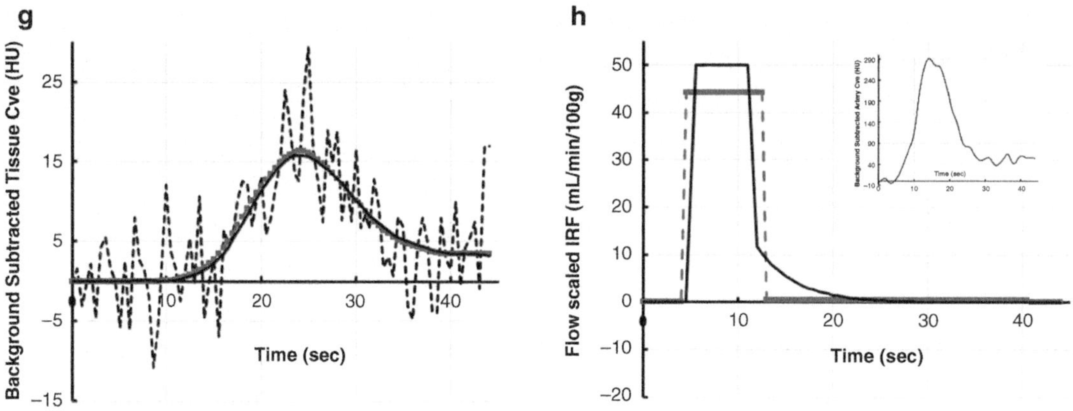

Fig. 19.4 (continued)

Table 19.1 Comparison of quantitative parameters derived from flow-scaled IRF estimated by four deconvolution methods

	True	SVD	Delay-corrected SVD	Constrained SVD	JWL model deconvolution
Height – F (mL/min/100 g)	50.0	47.4	54.1	51.9	44.1
Area – V_b (mL/100 g)	6.3	7.8	7.4	6.7	6.5
Area/height – MTT_v (sec)	7.6	9.9	8.2	7.8	8.9
Delay – T_o (sec)	5.0	0	5	5	4.5
Average SSD	27.1	22.1	24.9	25.7	28.2

maximum had already made the shape of the estimated flow-scaled IRF too smooth (deviating severely from the true shape). The JWL model deconvolution has a larger average SSD than the true average SSD suggesting it is not overfitting the noise and this is corroborated by Fig. 19.4g where the fitted curve almost superimpose on the true tissue curve. Figure 19.4 emphasizes the unstable nature of deconvolution [29, 30], and the fact using SSD of fitted from measured curve as the sole criterion to overcome noise instability is insufficient. As shown in Fig. 19.4, there are many possible solutions for the true flow-scaled IRF; each of them would produce reasonably good fit to the tissue curve. Additional a priori criteria such as constraints of non-negativity, monotonicity, and smoothness [38] or a physiological model, for example, the JWL model [23], are required to select the optimal flow-scaled IRF from the set of infinitely many possible solutions.

The JWL model was introduced above to describe contrast that extravasates into the interstitial space (Fig. 19.2). However, by adopting a different interpretation of the model parameters as discussed in [40], it can apply to CTP studies of stroke where contrast remains intravascular. In essence, T_o remains as the delay between the arrival of contrast at the artery and local tissue time-density curve; W, the width of initial plateau of $R_F^{\mathrm{JWL}}(t)$, is the minimum transit time through a tissue region; (1-E) is the fraction of contrast that has the transit time equal to the minimum transit time (W); and E is the fraction of tracer that has transit times longer than the minimum transit time as described by the "tail" of $R_F^{\mathrm{JWL}}(t)$ which is an exponential decay function with a rate constant of k_2. The mean transit time of this (E) fraction of contrast is $W + {}^{1}\!/_{k_2}$. With this alternative interpretation of the JWL model for stroke studies, the plug (non-dispersive) flow in vessels is also relaxed. The parameters E and k_2 can be used to investigate heterogeneity in vascular transit time (MTT_v) in neurodegeneration [41] and head trauma [42].

CTP Scanning Protocols, Effective Dose, and Image Reconstruction

Two important factors to be considered in the design of scanning protocols for CTP studies of stroke and cancer are image time interval and effective dose (kV, mAs, volume of tissue covered, and duration of acquisition). As discussed in §2.2.2, the image time interval, at least in the first (vascular) phase of the acquisition, has to be less than the minimum transit time, W, through the tissue such that F instead of FE is estimated. Based on this requirement, the image time interval for the vascular phase in most protocols has been set to 1–3 s to cover the vascular peak of the tissue curve, $Q(t)$, typically 40–60 s. Data in the interstitial phase beyond the first (vascular) phase is required for estimation of K_1 (PS) and k_2 (V_e) in tissues where contrast extravasation is expected to occur. This includes all organs except the brain, but even in the latter case, interstitial phase data is required for investigation of blood-brain barrier disruption. Unlike in the vascular phase, there is no theoretical requirement for the image time interval to be not longer than 3–4 s; most protocols use 10–15 s. The acquisition duration in the interstitial phase is usually set to be 90–120 s. To reduce effective dose for CTP study of AIS, there is a strong incentive to reduce the vascular phase acquisition time to as short as possible. However, the ischemic tissue time-density curve may be truncated with a short acquisition time leading to underestimation of blood volume; this could result in the paradoxical reversal of a very low blood volume defect (infarct) [43]. Since it is difficult to predict for individual AIS patients the optimum vascular phase acquisition time required, our recommendation is to add the interstitial phase to AIS CTP studies as discussed above. Besides avoiding the data truncation problem, this has the added advantage that it is possible then to investigate blood-barrier disruption which can be a marker for potential hemorrhagic transformation (see §5.1).

The effective dose of a CTP study is dependent on the volume of tissue irradiated and number of times images of the volume are acquired, while the dose from image acquisition of a single volume is dependent on kV and mAs used. The signal-to-noise of the arterial and tissue time-density curve determines the quality with which the flow-scaled IRF can be estimated with deconvolution in a CTP study. The signal is the arterial and tissue contrast enhancement detected by a CT scanner. Since all CT contrast agents are iodinated compounds, the main process contributing to contrast enhancement is photoelectric absorption of X-ray photons at the energy of the K-edge of iodine or 33.2 keV. A low kV X-ray beam would increase signal (enhancement) and decrease effective dose but at the expense of noise. As demonstrated with a brain size phantom complete with a bone ring to simulate the skull, increasing kV from 80 to 120 but keeping the mAs the same increases the signal-to-noise ratio by 11% but increases radiation dose by over 300% [44]. Thus, when signal-to-noise performance is normalized with respect to radiation dose, 80 kV is better than 120 kV for CT perfusion studies. Essentially the same conclusion is reached in studies by Wintermark et al. and Hirata et al. [45, 46] in which patients were scanned at both 80 and 120 kV and signal-to-noise as well as radiation dose were compared. Huda et al. reached the same conclusion using a body-sized phantom signal-to-noise ratio increased by less than 1.2 times, while radiation dose increased by over 3 times when mAs was kept the same but kV increased from 80 to 120 kV [47]. Thus, 80 kV is the optimal kV to be used in CT tumor perfusion studies regardless of whether tumor is located in the brain or abdominal organs. Recently commercial CT scanners have lowered their available kV to 70; Li et al. showed that compared to 80 kV, 70 kV reduced radiation dose without compromising quality of the perfusion maps in brain CTP studies [48]. Whether the same is true for body CTP studies is currently unknown.

For a fixed kV at either 70 or 80, the signal-to-noise of the artery and tissue time-density curve is determined by the mAs used in acquiring images. Noise insensitive deconvolution algorithms as discussed in §3 can cope with signal-to-noise as low as that shown in Fig. 19.4 which is less than 2:1 to produce reasonable estimates of blood flow and volume and mean transit time as shown in Table 19.1. In our experience, a mAs of 80–150 mAs at 80 kV would produce tissue curves with a signal-to-noise of ~2:1 in both brain and body CTP studies.

Typical effective dose at our institution for a brain CTP study which covers a 10 cm volume of the brain using 80 kV and 80 mAs per volume and acquires 28 volumes over 150 s is 2.8 mSv, while that for body CTP study using the same scan parameters except increasing the mAs from 80 to 120 is 11.6 mSv. The higher effective dose for a body CTP study is due to the increased mAs used to compensate for increased attenuation as well as the presence of more radiation sensitive tissues in the body. Newer iterative image reconstruction algorithms from CT scanner vendors can reduce effective dose but maintain quality of conventional high-resolution anatomical image [49]. One such algorithm (ASIR, GE Healthcare) has been investigated if effective dose can be reduced for brain CTP studies without affecting quality of CTP maps [50]. This study on 37 brain tumor patients showed that the mAs per image acquisition can be reduced from 100 to 50, resulting in a 50% decrease in effective dose without affecting CTP measurements. The vendor-provided iterative image reconstruction algorithms are optimized for high-resolution anatomical imaging which requires ~1000 projections for the reconstruction. CTP imaging is different where high spatial resolution can be traded for signal-to-noise to reduce radiation dose. One effective strategy is to reduce the number of projections (sparse view) for each image acquisition while keeping the dose for each projection the same and compensate for viewing aliasing artifact with compressed sensing reconstruction [51, 52]. Enjilela et al. showed that for liver and cardiac CTP studies, the number of projections, hence radiation dose, can be reduced by three times [51, 52].

Applications in Stroke and Cancer

Hemorrhage Transformation in Stroke

Hemorrhagic transformation (HT) of acute ischemic stroke (AIS) is an undesirable complication that occurs in 2.2%–44.0% of clinical cases [53, 54] and in up to 70% of pathology cases [55]. Among clinical parameters, baseline stroke severity [56], time to reperfusion [57], and tissue plasminogen activator (tPA) treatment [58] are associated with HT. These factors are even more critical now with the positive results from WAKE-UP and EXTEND trial on treating acute ischemic stroke with tPA more than 9 h after symptom onset [59, 60]. However, both trials showed that the rate of symptomatic hemorrhage in the treated (tPA) group was five to seven times higher than the control (placebo) [59, 60]. Disruption of the blood-brain barrier (BBB) integrity, considered focal to the development of HT, has been demonstrated in animal models [61] as an increase in the permeability–surface area product (PS). Furthermore in a pilot trial involving 41 AIS patients within 3 h of symptom onset, we showed that PS derived from admission CTP was able to predict HT at follow-up MRI or CT imaging with 77% sensitivity and 94% specificity using a threshold of 0.23 mL/min/100 g [39]. Figure 19.5 shows the example of one patient study from [39]; all the maps were derived using JWL model deconvolution. The CTP was acquired at 1.0 s image intervals for 45 s in the vascular phase and then at 15.0 s intervals for 90 s in the interstitial phase. The measured artery curve is shown in Fig. 19.5a together with the vein curve from the transverse sinus for partial volume correction of the former [34]. Figure 19.5b is the high signal-to-noise average map obtained by averaging all the images of the same slice in the CTP study together; the gray and white matter are clearly differentiated. Figure 19.5c, d shows the blood flow and volume map in quantitative scale of 0–100 mL/min/100 g and 0–10 mL/100 g. There was ischemia in the right middle cerebral artery

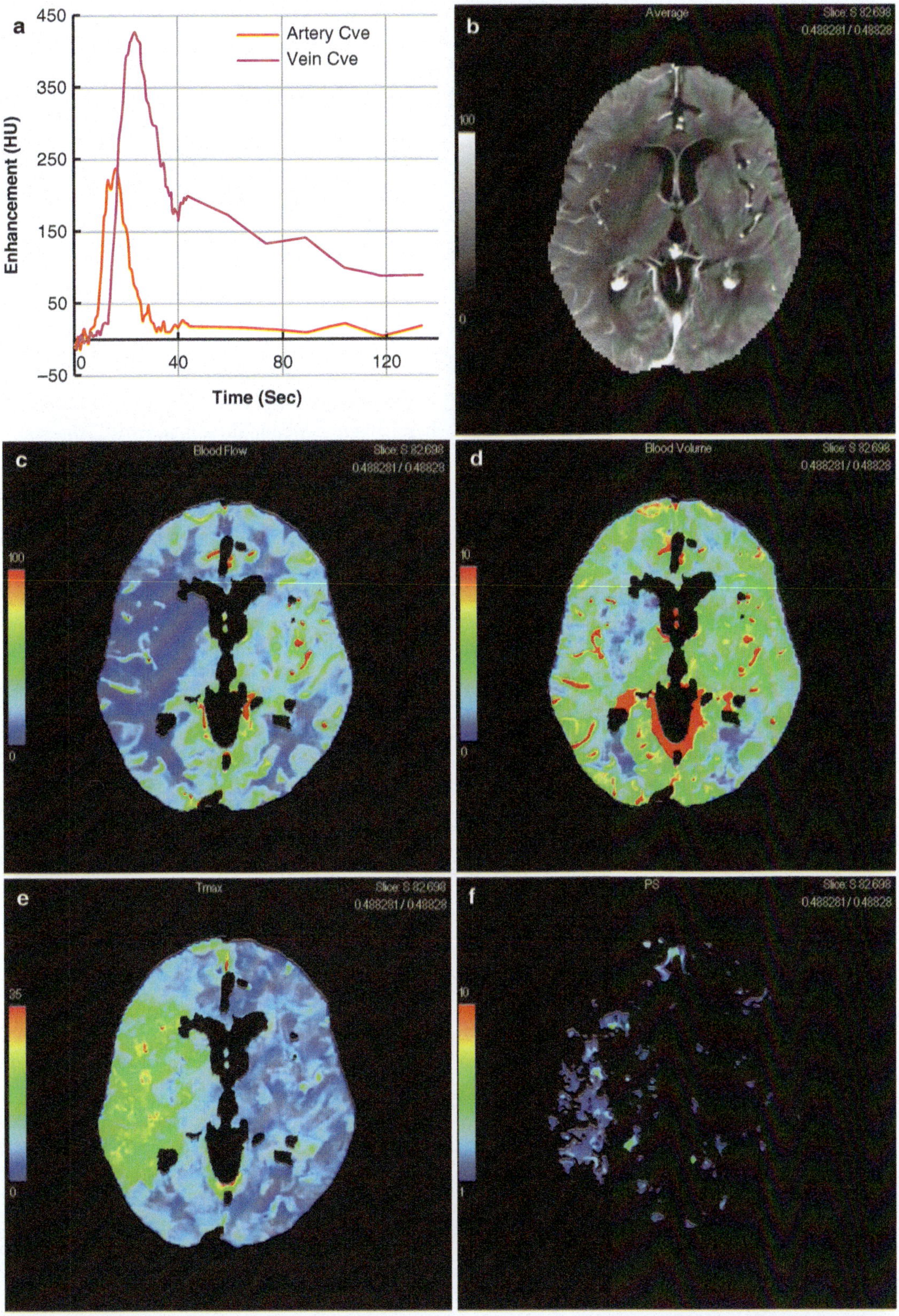

Fig. 19.5 CTP study of an acute ischemic stroke patient with blood-brain barrier disruption and hemorrhagic transformation at follow-up imaging. Details are provided in the text

territory, but blood volume was maintained at close to normal level (cf. the unaffected contralateral (left) hemisphere) except for the basal ganglia. This is usually seen in AIS at early hours after symptom onset, when the ischemic tissue is able to mount autoregulation to rescue itself by dilating blood vessels (hence increase in blood volume) to maintain blood flow above infarction threshold [62]. *T*max in one definition is the time to maximum of the flow-scaled impulse residue function [63], but this ignores the delay (T_o) in contrast arrival at ischemic tissue via collateral pathways. To account for abnormal T_o in ischemic tissue, we proposed [40] a new definition: $T_{\max} = T_o + 0.5\mathrm{MTT}_v$. $T_{\max}$ thus defined will evaluate both collateral circulation and perfusion pressure (inversely proportional to MTT_v [64] at the ischemic tissue. Figure 19.5e is the $T_{\max}$ map according to this alternative definition. Figure 19.5f is the PS map which shows blood-brain barrier disruption in the ischemic region.

Segmentation of Penumbra and Infarct in Stroke

As discussed above, the DEFUSE 3 [16] and EXTEND trial [60] have established the use of CTP for selecting patients for thrombectomy of large vessel occlusion and thrombolysis in extended time window after AIS symptom onset. Based on admission CTP maps, both trials used blood flow <30% of the unaffected hemisphere to define infarct and a $\mathrm{T}_{\max}$ threshold >6 s to define ischemic tissue outside of infarct as penumbra. Figure 19.6 illustrates this method of segmentation for penumbra and infarct based

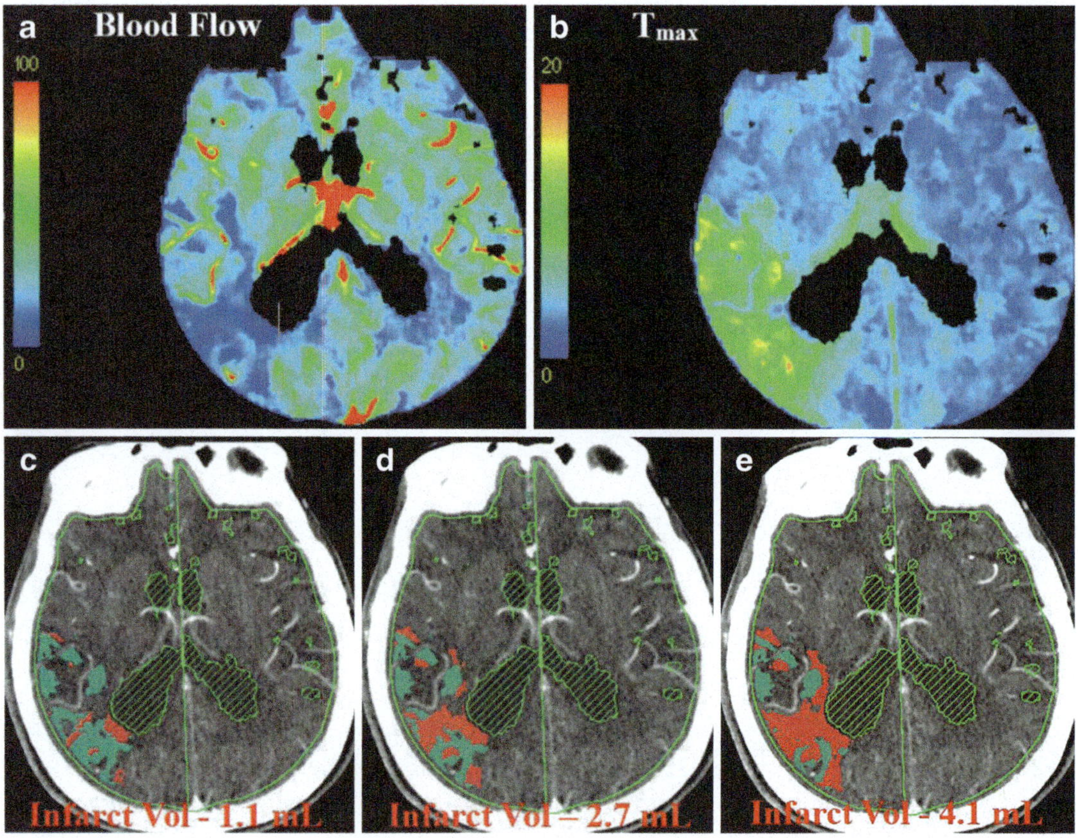

Fig. 19.6 Segmentation of penumbra and infarct based on the CTP blood flow (**a**) and (**b**) $T_{\max}$ map of an AIS patient. Details are provided in the text

on blood flow (Fig. 19.6a) and T_{max} (Fig. 19.6b) map calculated with JWL model deconvolution. Figure 19.6c shows the segmented penumbra (green) and infarct (red) using a blood flow threshold of 9 mL/min/10 g and a T_{max} threshold of 10 s. The blood flow and T_{max} threshold were obtained from a previous study [40]. Note that because the alternative definition to the DEFUSE 3 one was used in [40], the T_{max} threshold was higher (10 vs 6 s).

In AIS caused by large vessel occlusion, the patient has to be transferred from primary stroke centers which lack the equipment and expertise to perform thrombectomy to comprehensive stroke centers for the procedure to be performed. During the transfer time, the infarct could grow at the expense of the penumbra so that the patient may no longer be suitable for thrombectomy according to the DEFUSE 3 criteria. The "futile" transfer would be wasteful on resources. We have determined the time-dependent blood flow threshold for infarction [40]. For 90–190 min after admission, the blood flow threshold increased to 12 mL/min/100 g, and as shown in Fig. 19.6d, the infarct volume increased from 1.1 mL at admission (Fig. 19.6c) to 2.7 mL. For more than 3 h after admission, the blood flow threshold was 15 mL/min/100 g, and the infarct volume further increased to 4.1 mL.

Monitoring Response to Transarterial Chemoembolization of Liver Tumor

Hepatocellular carcinoma (HCC) is the fifth most common solid tumor in the world and accounts for ~500,000 deaths each year [65]. Although the most effective way of treating liver cancer is surgical resection, about two-thirds of liver cancer patients have non-resectable tumor at diagnosis either because of the size or location of the tumor or because the tumor has grown into the blood vessels. For these patients, transarterial chemoembolization (TACE) [66] is one treatment option. However, relying on the conventional RECIST criteria to assess the result of TACE may delay detection of treatment failure and deny patient the opportunity of alternative focal ablative therapy (e.g., radiofrequency ablation [67] or microwave ablation [68]) which may better succeed in tumor control than TACE. In normal liver parenchyma, approximately 75% of the blood supply is via the portal vein; only 25% is via the hepatic artery [69]. In liver cancer, tumor-associated angiogenesis leads to a reversal; a greater proportion of blood supply is coming from the arterial than the (portal) venous route. Therefore, the TACE treatment is successful if arterial blood flow post treatment is significantly reduced compared to before treatment.

The dual blood supply of the liver requires the theory for the measurement of blood flow presented in §2 to be modified as discussed in [16]. The hepatic artery curve, $C_h(t)$, can be approximated by the aortic curve, while the portal vein curve, $C_p(t)$, can be directly measured. If α is the fraction of total liver blood flow that arises from the hepatic artery, then $C_a(t)$ in Eq. (19.3) can be expressed as the weighted sum of $C_h(t)$ and $C_p(t)$:

$$C_a(t) = \alpha C_h(t) + (1-\alpha) C_p(t)$$

With this modification of the artery (input) curve, deconvolution, in particular JWL model deconvolution, can proceed as before to determine total liver blood flow (F) and arterial and portal blood flow as αF and (1-α)F.

Figure 19.7a, b shows the JWL model deconvolution results for a responder and non-responder to TACE. For the responder (Fig. 19.7a), arterial blood flow decreased significantly following TACE and remained low out to 4-week post procedure. Portal blood flow remained largely unchanged from baseline at 2- and 4-week post TACE. For the non-responder (Fig. 19.7b), arterial blood flow was reduced in posterior portion of the tumor at 2-week post TACE but started to be re-established by 4-week post. The anterior portion of the tumor remained unchanged from baseline at 2-week post but increased at 4-week post. Portal blood flow of the whole tumor remained largely unchanged.

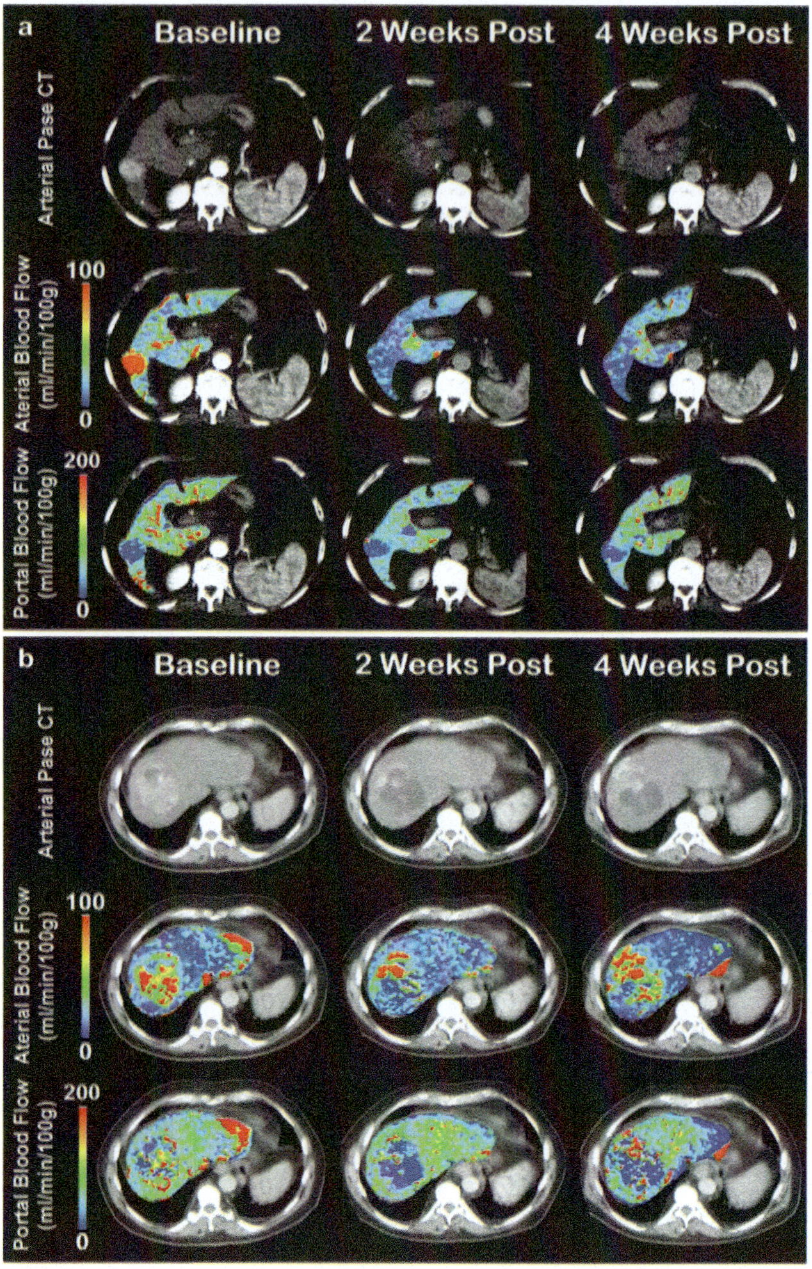

Fig. 19.7 Liver CTP study before and at 2-week and 4-week post TACE for (**a**) responder and (**b**) non-responder

Conclusion

Based on technical and numerical algorithm developments described above in the past two decades, CTP has become a useful clinical tool in the investigation of AIS and cancer. Its advantages include around-the-clock availability in most hospitals throughout the world and short study time of a couple of minutes without the need to ascertain the absence of metallic objects in the patient's body. For emergent situations, like AIS, the door-to-imaging time can be shortened to minutes, and with automatic processing software, the result whether the patient is a candidate for thrombectomy or thrombolysis can be available within minutes after the study is completed. For ambulatory cancer cases, because CT is the "workhorse" in follow-up imaging of cancer patients and because CTP scanning protocol is easy to standardize and implement [19], its use in monitoring treatment response will increase with time. However, if CTP is to continue being relevant in real world clinical situations into the future, it has to overcome two critical hurdles. The first being radiation dose, at the present dose level, CTP cannot be repeated as frequently as demanded by the clinical needs of monitoring treatment response of AIS and cancer. A target effective dose level would be ~1 mSv per CTP study of the whole organ. This can only be achieved by developing new iterative image reconstruction, such as sparse view described above [51, 52], and persuading CT scanner vendors, who for now are still only interested in high-resolution anatomical imaging, to adopt them so they can be used routinely in clinical environments rather than research settings. The second hurdle is standardization. Although it is possible to standardize CT scanning protocols on different scanner platforms [19], currently there are diverse models and methods in the post-processing of CTP studies to generate the different functional maps. There is urgent need for professional societies to convene harmonization workshops and conferences among stakeholders to established uniform post-processing procedures so that equivalent CTP functional maps are routinely produced at all clinical sites around the world.

References

1. Johnson W, Onuma O, Owolabi M, Sachdev S. Stroke: a global response is needed. Bull World Health Organ. 2016;94(9):634A–5A.
2. Koton S, Schneider ALC, Rosamond WD, et al. Stroke incidence and mortality trends in US communities, 1987 to 2011. JAMA – J Am Med Assoc. 2014;312(3):259–68.
3. Yang Q, Botto LD, Erickson JD, et al. Improvement in stroke mortality in Canada and the United States, 1990 to 2002. Circulation. 2006;113(10):1335–43.
4. Lakshminarayan K, Berger AK, Fuller CC, et al. Trends in 10-year survival of patients with stroke hospitalized between 1980 and 2000: the Minnesota stroke survey. Stroke. 2014;45(9):2575–81.
5. Howard G, Goff DC. Population shifts and the future of stroke: forecasts of the future burden of stroke. Ann N Y Acad Sci. 2012;1268:14–20.
6. Hankey GJ, Jamrozik K, Broadhurst RJ, Forbes S, Anderson CS. Long-term disability after first-ever stroke and related prognostic factors in the Perth Community Stroke Study, 1989–1990. Stroke. 2002;33(4):1034–40.
7. Krueger H, Koot J, Hall RE, O'Callaghan C, Bayley M, Corbett D. Prevalence of individuals experiencing the effects of stroke in Canada: trends and projections. Stroke. 2015;46(8):2226–31.
8. Gloede TD, Halbach SM, Thrift AG, Dewey HM, Pfaff H, Cadilhac DA. Long-term costs of stroke using 10-year longitudinal data from the north East Melbourne stroke incidence study. Stroke. 2014;45(11):3389–94.
9. Miles K, Eastwood JD, Konig M, editors. Multidetector computed tomography in cerebrovascular disease: CT perfusion imaging. Abingdon: Informa Healthcare; 2007.
10. Miles K, Charnsangavei C, Cuenod CA, editors. Multidetector computed tomography in oncology: CT perfusion imaging. Abingdon: Informa Healthcare; 2007.
11. Saver JL, Goyal M, Bonafe A, et al. Stent-retriever thrombectomy after intravenous t-PA vs. t-PA alone in stroke. N Engl J Med. 2015;372(24):2285–95.
12. Goyal M, Demchuk AM, Menon BK, et al. Randomized assessment of rapid endovascular treatment of ischemic stroke. N Engl J Med. 2015;372(11):1019–30.
13. Campbell BCV, Mitchell PJ, Kleinig TJ, et al. Endovascular therapy for ischemic stroke with perfusion-imaging selection. N Engl J Med. 2015;372(11):1009–18.
14. Berkhemer OA, Fransen PSS, Beumer D, et al. A randomized trial of intraarterial treatment for acute ischemic stroke. N Engl J Med. 2015;372(1):11–20.
15. Jovin TG, Chamorro A, Cobo E, et al. Thrombectomy within 8 hours after symptom onset in ischemic stroke. N Engl J Med. 2015;372(24):2296–306.
16. Albers GW, Marks MP, Kemp S, et al. Thrombectomy for stroke at 6 to 16 hours with selection by perfusion imaging. N Engl J Med. 2018;378(8):708–18.
17. Lee TY, Purdie TG, Stewart E. CT imaging of angiogenesis. Q J Nucl Med. 2003;47:171–87.
18. García-Figueiras R, Goh VJ, Padhani AR, Baleato-González S, Garrido M, León L, Gómez-Caamaño A. CT perfusion in oncologic imaging: a useful tool? AJR Am J Roentgenol. 2013;200:8–19.
19. Ng CS, Zhang Z, Lee SI, Marques HS, Burgers K, Lee TY, et al. CT perfusion as an early biomarker of treatment efficacy in advanced ovarian cancer: an ACRIN and GOG study. Clin Cancer Res. 2017;23:3684–91.
20. Meier P, Zierler KL. On the theory of the indicator-dilution method for measurement of blood flow and volume. J Appl Physiol. 1954;6:731–44.

21. Robert GW, Larson KB, Spaeth EE. The interpretation of mean transit time measurements for multiphase tissue systems. J Theor Biol. 1973;39:447–75.
22. Klotz E, König M. Perfusion measurements of the brain: using dynamic CT for the quantitative assessment of cerebral ischemia in acute stroke. Eur J Radiol. 1999;30(3):170–84.
23. St Lawrence K, Lee T-Y. An adiabatic approximation to the tissue homogeneity model for water exchange in the brain I. Theoretical derivation. J Cereb Blood Flow Metab. 1998;18:1365–77.
24. Crone C. The permeability of capillaries in various organs as determined by use of the 'indicator diffusion' method. Acta Phsyiol Scand. 1963;58:292–305.
25. Rapoport SI. Blood-brain barrier in physiology and medicine. New York: Raven Press; 1976. p. 20.
26. Patlak CS, Blasberg RG, Fenstermacher JD. Graphical evaluation of blood-to-brain transfer constants from multiple-time uptake data. J Cereb Blood Metab. 1983;3:1–7.
27. Patlak CS, Blasberg RG. Graphical evaluation of blood-to-brain transfer constants from multiple-time uptake data. Generalizations. J Cereb Blood Metab. 1985;5:584–90.
28. Gill PE, Murray W, Wright MH. Practical optimization. London: Academic; 1982.
29. Philips DL. A technique for the numerical solution of certain integral equations of the first kind. J Assoc Comp Math. 1962;9:84–90.
30. Tikhonov AN. Regularizations of uncorrectly posed problems. Soviet Math. 1963;4:1624–9.
31. Østergaard L, Weisskoff RM, Chesler DA, Gyldensted C, Rosen BR. High resolution measurement of cerebral blood flow using intravascular tracer bolus passages. Part I: mathematical approach and statistical analysis. Magn Reson Med. 1996;36:715–25.
32. Calamante F, Gadian DG, Alan Connelly A. Quanti. cation of bolus-tracking MRI: improved characterization of the tissue residue function using Tikhonov regularization. Mag Res Med. 2003;50: 1237–47.
33. Wu O, Østergaard L, Weisskoff RM, Benner T, Rosen BR, Sorensen AG. Tracer arrival timing-insensitive technique for estimating flow in MR perfusion-weighted imaging using singular value decomposition with a block-circulant deconvolution matrix. Magn Reson Med. 2003;50(1):164–74.
34. Lee TY, Murphy B. Implementing deconvolution analysis for perfusion CT. In: Miles K, Charnsangavei C, Cuenod CA, editors. Multidetector computed tomography in oncology: CT perfusion imaging. Abingdon: Informa Healthcare; 2007.
35. Wu O, Østergaard L, Koroshetz WJ, Schwamm LH, O'Donnell J, Schaefer PW, Rosen BR, Weisskoff RM, Sorensen AG. Effects of tracer arrival time on flow estimates in MR perfusion-weighted imaging. Magn Res Med. 2003;50:856–64.
36. Smith MR, Lu H, Trochet S, Frayne R. Removing the effect of SVD algorithmic artifacts present in quantitative MR perfusion studies. Magn Res Med. 2004;51:631–4.
37. Ibaraki M, Shimosegawa E, Toyoshima H, Takahashi K, Miura S, Kanno I. Tracer delay correction of cerebral blood flow with dynamic susceptibility contrast-enhanced MRI. J Cereb Blood Flow Metab. 2005;25:378–90.
38. Lee TY. Method and apparatus for calculating blood flow parameters. US Patent Office. 2005. 6898453.
39. Aviv RI, d'Esterre CD, Murphy BD, Hopyan JJ, Buck B, Mallia G, Li V, Zhang L, Symons SP, Lee TY. Hemorrhagic transformation of ischemic stroke: prediction with CT perfusion. Radiology. 2009;250(3):867–77.
40. d'Esterre CD, Boesen ME, Ahn SH, Pordeli P, Najm M, et al. Time-dependent computed tomographic perfusion thresholds for patients with acute ischemic stroke. Stroke. 2015;46(12):3390–7.
41. Eskildsen SF, Gyldensted L, Nagenthiraja K, Nielsen RB, Hansen MB, Dalby RB, et al. Increased cortical capillary transit time heterogeneity in Alzheimer's disease: a DSC-MRI perfusion study. Neurobiol Aging. 2017;50:107–18.
42. Østergaard L, Engedal TS, Aamand R, Mikkelsen R, Iversen NK, Anzabi M, et al. Capillary transit time heterogeneity and flow-metabolism coupling after traumatic brain injury. J Cereb Blood Flow Metab. 2014;34(10):1585–98.
43. d'Esterre CD, Aviv RI, Lee TY. The evolution of the cerebral blood volume abnormality in patients with ischemic stroke: a CT perfusion study. Acta Radiol. 2012;53(4):461–7.
44. Lee TY, Ellis RJ, Dunscombe PB, McClarty B, Hodson DI, Kroeker MA, et al. Quantitative computed tomography of the brain with xenon enhancement: a phantom study with the GE9800 scanner. Phys Med Biol. 1990;35:925–35.
45. Wintermark M, Maeder P, Verdun FR, Thiran JP, Valley JF, Schnyder P, et al. Using 80 kVp versus 120 kVp in perfusion CT measurement of regional cerebral blood flow. AJNR Am J Neuroradiol. 2000;21:1881–4.
46. Hirata M, Sugawara Y, Fukutomi Y, Oomoto K, Murase K, Miki H, et al. Measurement of radiation dose in cerebral CT perfusion study. Radiat Med. 2005;23:97–103.
47. Huda W, Scalzetti EM, Levin G. Technique factors and image quality as functions of patient weight at abdominal CT. Radiology. 2000;217:430–5.
48. Li ZL, Li H, Zhang K, Li WJ, Chen X, Wu B, et al. Improvement of image quality and radiation dose of CT perfusion of the brain by means of low-tube voltage (70 KV). Eur Radiol. 2014;24(8):1906–13.
49. Marin D, Nelson RC, Schindera ST, Richard S, Youngblood RS, Yoshizumi TT, et al. Low-tube-voltage, high-tube-current multidetector abdominal CT: improved image quality and decreased radiation dose with adaptive statistical iterative reconstruction algorithm--initial clinical experience. Radiology. 2010;254(1):145–53.
50. Murphy A, So A, Lee TY, Symons S, Jakubovic R, Zhang L, Aviv RI. Low dose CT perfusion in acute ischemic stroke. Neuroradiology. 2014;56(12):1055–62.

51. Enjilela E, Lee TY, Hsieh J, Murjoomdar A, Stewart E, Dekaban M, Su F, So A. Ultra-low-dose sparse-view quantitative CT liver perfusion imaging. Tomography. 2017;3(4):175–9.
52. Enjilela E, Lee TY, Hsieh J, Wisenberg G, Teefy P, Yadegari A, Bagur R, Islam A, Branch K, So A. Ultra-low dose quantitative CT myocardial perfusion imaging with sparse-view dynamic acquisition and image reconstruction: a feasibility study. Int J Cardiol. 2018;254:272–81.
53. National Institute of Neurological Disorders and Stroke rt-PA Stroke Study Group. Tissue plasminogen activator for acute ischemic stroke. N Engl J Med. 1995;333:1581–7.
54. Hacke W, Kaste M, Fieschi C, et al. Intravenous thrombolysis with recombinant tissue plasminogen activator for acute hemispheric stroke: the European Cooperative Acute Stroke Study (ECASS). JAMA. 1995;274:1017–25.
55. Fisher M, Adams RD. Observations on brain embolism with special reference to the mechanism of hemorrhagic infarction. J Neuropathol Exp Neurol. 1951;10:92–4.
56. Larrue V, von Kummer R, del Zoppo G, Bluhmki E. Hemorrhagic transformation in acute ischemic stroke: potential contributing factors in the European Cooperative Acute Stroke Study. Stroke. 1997;28:957–60.
57. Molina CA, Alvarez-Sabin J, Montaner J, et al. Thrombolysis-related hemorrhagic infarction: a marker of early reperfusion, reduced infarct size, and improved outcome in patients with proximal middle cerebral artery occlusion. Stroke. 2002;33:1551–6.
58. Larrue V, von Kummer RR, Muller A, Bluhmki E. Risk factors for severe hemorrhagic transformation in ischemic stroke patients treated with recombinant tissue plasminogen activator: a secondary analysis of the European-Australasian Acute Stroke Study (ECASS II). Stroke. 2001;32:438–41.
59. Thomalla G, Simonsen CZ, Boutitie F, Andersen G, Berthezene Y, Cheng B, WAKE-UP Investigators et al, et al. MRI-guided thrombolysis for stroke with unknown time of onset. N Engl J Med. 2018;379(7):611–22.
60. Ma H, Campbell BCV, Parsons MW, Churilov L, Levi CR, Hsu C, the EXTEND Investigators, et al. Thrombolysis guided by perfusion imaging up to 9 hours after onset of stroke. N Engl J Med. 2019;380(19):1795–803.
61. Neumann-Haefelin C, Brinker G, Uhlenkuken U, Pillekamp F, Hossmann KA, Hoehn M. Prediction of hemorrhagic transformation after thrombolytic therapy of clot embolism: an MRI investigation in rat brain. Stroke. 2002;33:1392–8.
62. Jordan JD, Powers WJ. Cerebral autoregulation and acute ischemic stroke. Am J Hypertens. 2012;25(9):946–50.
63. Davis SM, Donnan GA, Parsons MW, Levi C, Butcher KS, Peeters A, EPITHET investigators, et al. Effects of alteplase beyond 3 h after stroke in the Echoplanar Imaging Thrombolytic Evaluation Trial (EPITHET): a placebo-controlled randomised trial. Lancet Neurol. 2008;7(4):299–309.
64. Murphy MJ, Tichauer KM, Sun L, Chen X, Lee TY. Mean transit time as an index of cerebral perfusion pressure in experimental systemic hypotension. Physiol Meas. 2011;32(4):395–405.
65. Parkin DM, Bray F, Ferlay J, Pisani P. Estimating the world cancer burden: Globocan 2000. Int J Cancer. 2001;94:153–6.
66. Biolato M, Marrone G, Racco S, Di Stasi C, Miele L, Gasbarrini G, et al. Transarterial chemoembolization (tace) for unresectable HCC: a new life begins? Eur Rev Med Pharmacol Sci. 2010;14:356–62.
67. Laeseke PF, Frey TM, Brace CL, Sampson LA, Winter TC 3rd, Ketzler JR, et al. Multiple-electrode radiofrequency ablation of hepatic malignancies: initial clinical experience. AJR Am J Roentgenol. 2007;188:1485–94.
68. Liang P, Wang Y. Microwave ablation of hepatocellular carcinoma. Oncology. 2007;72(Suppl 1): 124–31.
69. Chiandussi L, Greco F, Sardi G, Vaccarino A, Ferraris CM, Curti B. Estimation of hepatic arterial and portal venous blood flow by direct catheterization of the vena porta through the umbilical cord in man: preliminary results. Acta Hepatosplenol. 1968;15:166–71.

20 CT Myocardial Perfusion Imaging

Aaron So

Introduction

The use of dynamic contrast-enhanced (DCE) CT for assessment of tissue blood flow (perfusion) was first demonstrated 40 years ago [1]. Perfusion imaging greatly enhances the capability of computed tomography (CT) as a one-stop shop for anatomical and functional diagnosis of many diseases and tissue injuries including stroke [2–4], soft tissue cancers [5–8], and coronary artery disease (CAD) [9–12]. In particular, recent advances in CT technologies including larger acquisition coverage with more detector rows [13, 14] and higher image temporal resolution with faster gantry rotation speed [15] have made the application of CT Perfusion (CTP) more clinical feasible for functional assessment of CAD through measurement of myocardial perfusion.

All the current CTP techniques developed for myocardial perfusion assessment require an intravenous injection of a bolus of iodine-based contrast agent followed by imaging of the heart at a single time or multiple times to monitor the temporal change(s) of signal intensity in the myocardium with respect to the supplying arteries. Theoretically, multiple acquisitions after contrast administration provide us with more dynamic information regarding the kinetics of perfusion tracers in the myocardium, from which a more accurate functional assessment can be achieved. The first-pass perfusion analysis techniques are based on one of the three theories: indicator-dilution, Fick principle, and deconvolution. This chapter reviews the fundamental basis of each of these theories. The technical considerations for the implementation of CTP for myocardial perfusion imaging are also discussed.

Fundamental Physiological Parameters

For ease of discussion, let us first consider the schematic in Fig. 20.1a which represents a unit mass of myocardial tissue. The inlet and outlet orifices represent an input artery (arteriole) and a draining vein (venule) of the tissue. *Blood flow* (F) through the tissue, or perfusion, is defined as the volume of blood that is moving through the vasculature of the tissue per unit time. It is usually expressed in unit of $mL \cdot min^{-1} \cdot g^{-1}$. In CTP, tissue blood flow is usually modeled as a plug of fluid (plug flow) moving through the microvasculature, in which the flow velocity profile across the cross-section of the vessels is constant. Additionally, *blood volume* (V) is defined as the volume of blood within the microvasculature of the tissue that is flowing (non-static). It is usually expressed in unit of $mL \cdot g^{-1}$. In reality, there are numerous small capillaries interconnecting with

A. So (✉)
Imaging Program, Lawson Health Research Institute, London, ON, Canada
e-mail: aso@robarts.ca

© Springer Nature Switzerland AG 2020

E. Samei, N. J. Pelc (eds.), *Computed Tomography*, https://doi.org/10.1007/978-3-030-26957-9_20

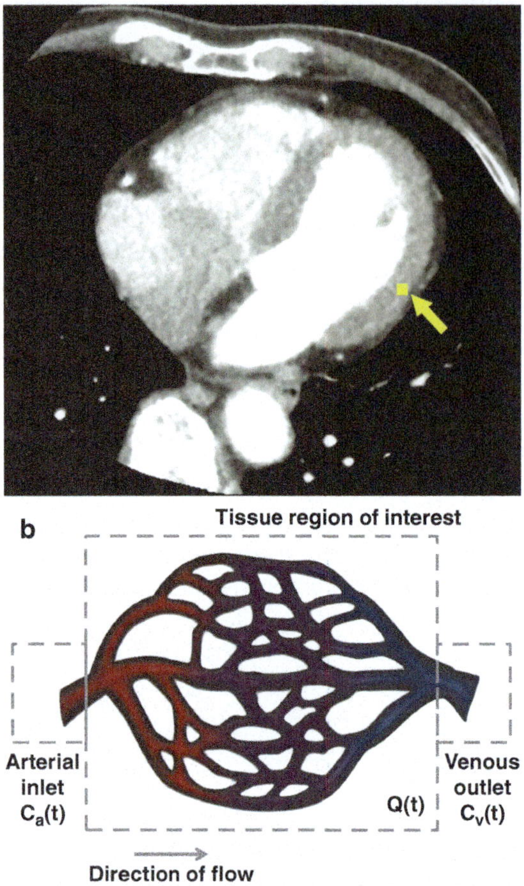

Fig. 20.1 (**a**) Contrast-enhanced CT image of a patient's heart. A voxel of interest in the myocardium is represented by a small yellow box marked with the yellow arrow. (**b**) Schematic of the vasculature of a tissue within the voxel of interest in (**a**). The red arrow denotes the direction of blood flow through the capillaries from arteriole (arterial inlet) to venule (venous outlet). A simple model representing the vasculature is overlaid for illustration. The relationship between the concentration of contrast medium in the input artery (Ca(t)) and draining vein (Cv(t)) and the mass of contrast in tissue (Q(t)) is governed by the Fick principle. The exchange of contrast between the intravascular and interstitial spaces is described by the tracer kinetic models shown in Figs. 20.5 and 20.6

each other rather than a single capillary tube in the tissue (Figs. 20.1b). Thus, upon arrival at the arterial inlet, contrast solutes can take different paths to reach the venous exit. As such, there exists a distribution of transit times, which can be described by a frequency or probability density function of transit time through a vascular bed, *h(t)*, as shown in Fig. 20.2a. The integral of the probability density function, *H(t)*, describes the fraction of contrast solutes that has left the tissue at time *t* (Fig. 20.2b). The total amount of contrast solutes that has left the tissue should increase with time and eventually reach the plateau at unity. This can be explained by the fact that all contrast solutes introduced into the tissue will eventually leave the tissue in due time, and the total amount of contrast leaving the tissue cannot exceed the amount that is introduced into the tissue. It follows that the residual function, *R(t)*, which describes the fraction of contrast solutes remains in the tissue at time *t*, is equal to $1 - H(t)$ (Fig. 20.2c), with the area under curve (AUC) of *R(t)* equals the *mean transit time* – the average time required for the contrast solutes to travel from the arterial inlet to the venous outlet of the tissue (Fig. 20.2d) [16, 17].

During a single capillary transit, contrast materials can diffuse across the permeable endothelium (consists of a single cell layer) to the interstitial (extravascular) space. One exception is the healthy brain tissue, where the blood-brain barrier, consisting of tight junctions between endothelial cells, surrounding basement membrane and astrocytic foot processes, restricts most of the diffusions taking place [18]. The transport of contrast solutes from the intravascular to interstitial space is driven entirely by passive diffusion (concentration gradient between the two spaces). The *extraction fraction*, *E*, describes the fraction of contrast materials diffused from the intravascular to interstitial space during a single passage from the arterial inlet to venous outlet of the capillaries [19]. *E* can be represented by the following equation:

$$E = 1 - e^{-\frac{\mathrm{PS}}{F}} \tag{20.1}$$

where PS is *permeability surface area product* – the product of permeability and the total surface area of capillary endothelium in a unit mass of tissue and hence is the total diffusional flux across all capillaries [19]. It is measured in units of $\mathrm{mL \cdot min^{-1} \cdot g^{-1}}$.

After the introduction of a bolus of iodinated contrast material, repeated rapid CT scanning are

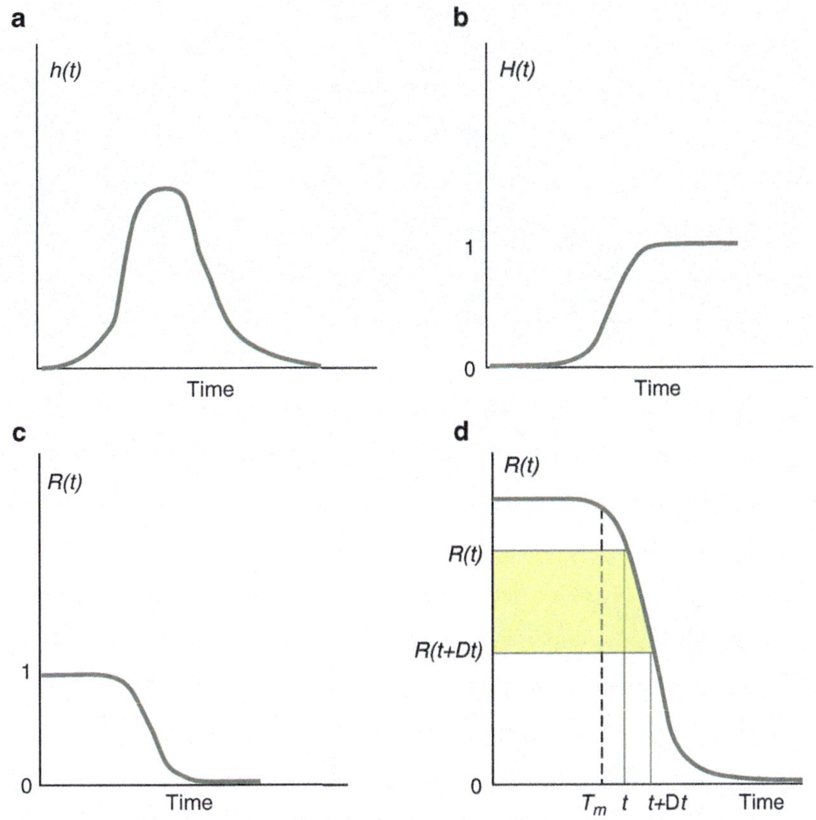

Fig. 20.2 (**a**) The frequency function, h(t), describes the distribution of transit time through a vasculature bed in tissue after a bolus injection of contrast. (**b**) Integral of the frequency function in **a**, $H(t)$, describes the fraction of contrast that has left the system as a function of time. (**c**) The total amount of contrast remains in the tissue as a function of time is given by $1 - H(t)$ or $R(t)$. (**d**) Beyond the minimum transit time, Tm, the fraction of contrast that leaves the tissue between t and $t + \Delta t$ is equal to the difference of $R(t + \Delta t)$ and $R(t)$ (yellow section). This fraction of contrast medium has a transit time of Δt. It follows that the total area under R(t) is equivalent to the mean transit time (MTT)

acquired at the same location to allow determination of time-enhancement curves (TEC). Figure 20.3 illustrates the typical shape of arterial ($C_a(t)$) and tissue ($Q(t)$) TECs acquired from DCE CT scanning. Several methods that are commonly used for analyzing these TECs to derive perfusion values are reviewed in the following sections.

Indicator-Dilution Method

Indicator-dilution method was initially proposed for measurement of blood flow (circulation time) and cardiac output [20]. It was later shown that this technique could also be used to measure tissue blood flow (perfusion) [16, 21]. This technique is based on the fact that, after administration into the circulation, the degree of which tracer molecules (e.g., CT contrast medium) mixed with blood (i.e., dilution) is dependent on blood flow. The indicator-dilution method has since been modified to measure blood flow in tissue using dynamic CT scanning [1, 22]. The basis of the method is briefly reviewed here. If a voxel of interest in a CT image is devoid of major blood vessels, the concentration of contrast medium in the tissue in this voxel at time t, $C_t(t)$, should be lower than that in the vascular space, $C_a(t)$, by the fraction f:

$$C_t(t) = f \cdot C_a(t) \tag{20.2}$$

where f is defined as:

$$f = \frac{V_b}{V_b + V_e + V_{\text{cell}}} \tag{20.3}$$

with V_b, V_e, and V_{cell} being the distribution volumes of contrast medium in the vascular space, interstitial space, and cell(s), respectively. Equations (20.2) and (20.3) suggest that f is essentially the blood volume in tissue which can be estimated by dividing the area under

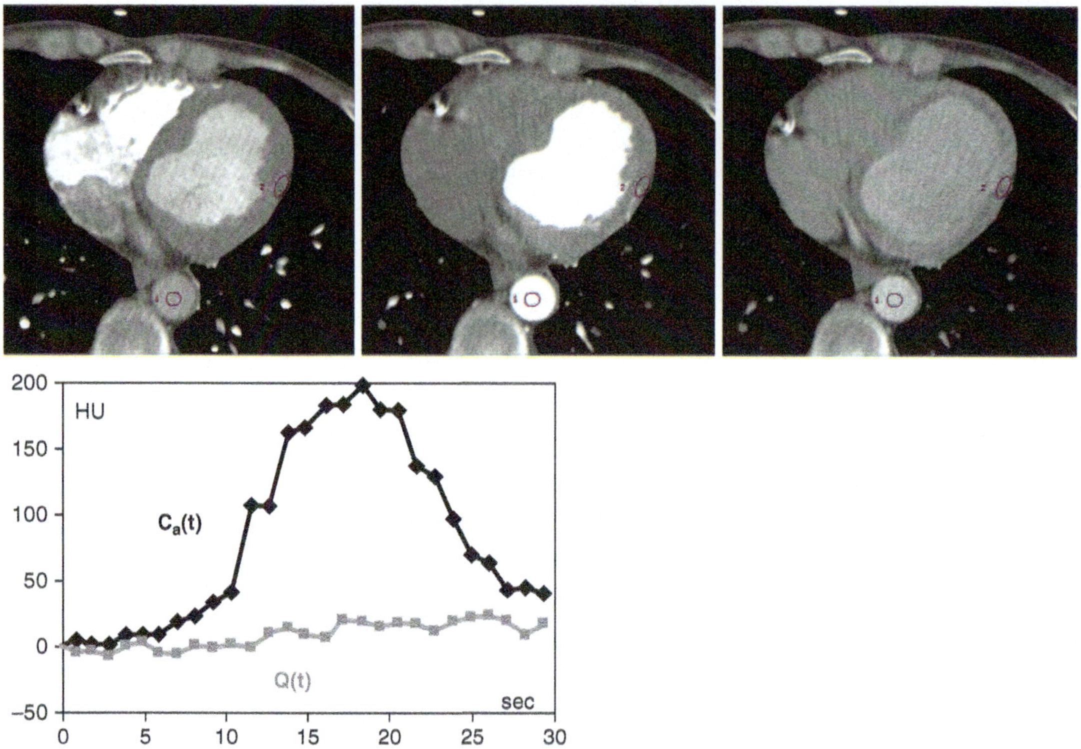

Fig. 20.3 (**a**) DCE CT images of the same patient's heart at different time points. Iodinated contrast medium circulated in the heart chambers and aorta during the time of imaging. (**b**) The arterial and myocardial TEC measured from the same set of DCE CT images

curve (AUC) of the tissue TEC to the AUC of the arterial TEC:

$$V = \frac{\mathrm{AUC}_{\mathrm{tissue}}}{\mathrm{AUC}_{\mathrm{artery}}} \tag{20.4a}$$

$$\mathrm{AUC}_{\mathrm{tissue}} = \int_0^T C_t(t)\,\mathrm{dt} \tag{20.4b}$$

$$\mathrm{AUC}_{\mathrm{artery}} = \int_0^T C_a(t)\,\mathrm{dt} \tag{20.4c}$$

Once the blood volume in tissue is determined, perfusion can be calculated as the ratio of V to the mean transit time (*MTT*) according to the central volume principle [16]:

$$F = \frac{V}{\mathrm{MTT}} \tag{20.5}$$

MTT cannot be measured directly but can be estimated from either deconvolution [23] or the center of gravity [22] of the arterial and tissue TECs:

$$\mathrm{MTT} = C \cdot \left[\langle \mathrm{tissue} \rangle - \langle \mathrm{artery} \rangle\right] \tag{20.6a}$$

$$= C \cdot \left[\frac{\int_0^T t \cdot C_t(t)\,\mathrm{dt}}{\int_0^T C_t(t)\,\mathrm{dt}} - \frac{\int_0^T t \cdot C_a(t)\,\mathrm{dt}}{\int_0^T C_a(t)\,\mathrm{dt}} \right] \tag{20.6b}$$

where <tissue> and <artery> represent the centers of gravity of these two TECs and the center of gravity of each curve is calculated as the first moment of the curve (which can be viewed as a quantitative measure of the shape of the curve) as in Eq. (20.6b); C is a combined correction factor to account for the difference between large vessel (vein or artery) and small vessel (tissue) hematocrit, the difference between contrast arrival times at the measured artery (true input artery to the ROI) and tissue, and the variations in transit times through the ROI to the difference in the first moments of tissue and artery TECs (<tissue> – <artery>) [22]. Although the indicator-dilution method is mathematically more simple than the deconvolution method, this technique has a few major limitations. First, the method relies heavily on the accuracy of blood volume estimate. For healthy brain tissue, contrast medium remains in the intravascular space throughout the capillary transit. However, in abnormal brain tissue where the blood-brain barrier is no longer intact [24, 25] and in other tissues such as the heart and liver [19], extravascular leakage of contrast may occur which will lead to overestimation of blood volume and hence blood flow. Second, the correction factor, C, assumes a certain geometry/topology of the vasculature (or transit time distribution) that makes the method model dependent after all.

Maximum Slope Method

The relationship among tissue blood flow, mass of contrast medium in unit mass of tissue, and concentration of contrast medium in the feeding artery and draining vein can be described using the Fick principle. If we denote $C_a(t)$ and $C_v(t)$ as the contrast concentration at the arterial inlet and venous outlet of the tissue at time t, respectively, and F is the tissue blood flow (perfusion), the influx and efflux rates of contrast are given by $F{\cdot}C_a(t)$ and $F{\cdot}C_v(t)$, respectively. Under the assumption of conservation of mass, the following relationship holds:

$$\frac{\mathrm{dQ}(t)}{\mathrm{dt}} = F \cdot C_a(t) - F \cdot C_v(t) \qquad (20.7)$$

where $Q(t)$ is the mass of contrast in the tissue at time t. Equation (20.7) states that the time rate of change of the mass of contrast in the tissue is equal to the difference in the influx and efflux rates of contrast. Integrating Eq. (20.7) yields:

$$Q(t) = F \cdot \int_0^T \left[C_a(t) - C_v(t)\right] \cdot \mathrm{dt} \qquad (20.8)$$

Equation (20.8) states that the accumulated mass of contrast in the tissue over time (from t = 0 to t = T) is equal to the product of tissue blood flow and the time integral of the difference in the arterial and venous concentration of contrast. One simplification that would make solving Eq. (20.8) easier is to assume no venous outflow of contrast in the tissue (i.e., $C_v(t) = 0$) during the time of study. If the assumption of no venous outflow is valid, Eq. (20.8) can be then simplified to [26]:

$$Q(t) = F \cdot \int_0^T C_a(t) \cdot dt \qquad (20.9)$$

Taking the differentiation on both sides of Eq. (20.9) yields:

$$\frac{dQ(t)}{dt} = F \cdot C_a(t) \qquad (20.10)$$

Equation (20.10) suggests that the rate of contrast accumulation in tissue is maximal when the arterial concentration of contrast reaches the maximum:

$$\left.\frac{\mathrm{dQ}(t)}{\mathrm{dt}}\right|_{\mathrm{max}} = F \cdot C_a(t)\big|_{\mathrm{max}}$$
$$F = \left.\frac{\frac{\mathrm{dQ}(t)}{\mathrm{dt}}}{C_a(t)}\right|_{\mathrm{max}} \qquad (20.11)$$

It follows that F (tissue blood flow) can be estimated by dividing the maximum time rate of change of Q by the maximum arterial concentration of contrast. In DCE CT, the maximum time rate of change of Q can be estimated by measuring the maximum upslope of myocardial TEC. As such, this approach is known as the maximum slope method. The slope of TEC has a unit of Hounsfield unit (HU)/second, which can be converted into (milligram of iodine) (gram of tissue)$^{-1}$/second with a conversion factor provided that the CT scanner is properly calibrated. Similarly, the maximum arterial concentration of contrast can be determined from the peak enhancement in the supplying artery expressed in HU, which can be converted into (millimole of iodine) (milliliter)$^{-1}$. After converting millimole to milligram of iodine with the molar mass of iodine, the tissue blood flow (F) calculated from Eq. (20.11) has a unit of (mL·s^{-1}) per gram of tissue.

The advantage of the maximum slope method is its computation simplicity. Additionally, as only the upslope of myocardial TEC is used for perfusion analysis, acquisition of the entire myocardial TEC covering both the washin and washout phases of contrast is not required, which can reduce the patient radiation dose. However, the maximum slope method is based on the assumptions that there are no venous outflow of contrast and no contrast leakage from the intravascular to interstitial spaces within the tissue during the imaging session. To properly sample the upslope of tissue curve and peak arterial enhancement, the acquisition should be long enough to cover from the non-enhanced phase to peak-enhanced phase, which may take about 10 s or longer (Figure 20.7).

As such, the assumption could be violated in real-world clinical applications which may lead to significant underestimation of the true perfusion value, as suggested by recent simulation and patient studies [27, 28]. Furthermore, signal fluctuation in the myocardial TECs measured with DCE CT can result in over- or underestimation of the maximum upslope of the curves. To overcome this limitation, using a model-based deconvolution to smooth the measured myocardial curves first before applying the maximum slope method to estimate tissue blood flow is proposed. This approach is discussed in more detail in the next section.

Deconvolution Method

The deconvolution method takes a different approach and handles the enhancement in the tissue/organ of interest after contrast administration as a time-invariant linear system problem. For reference, let us first review the characteristics of such a system.

Figure 20.4 illustrates an output signal in response to an impulse signal presented to an

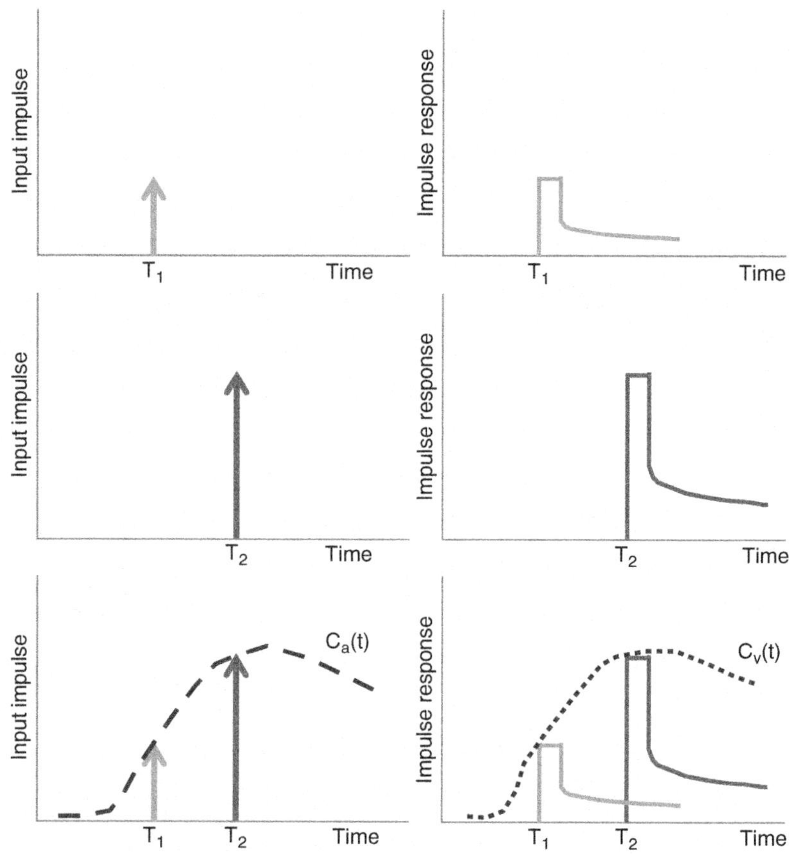

Fig. 20.4 (**a**) An impulse signal to a time-invariant linear system and (**b**) the corresponding IRF. (**c**) A second impulse signal with twice the magnitude as the first impulse introduced to the system at a later time and (**d**) the corresponding IRF to the second impulse. (**e**) An arterial TDC measured from DCE CT scanning can be interpreted as a superimposition of sequential impulses with different magnitudes at different times. (**f**) The corresponding tissue TDC can be viewed as a superimposition of the IRFs scaled by the magnitude and shifted in time to match those of the impulse signals

ideal time-invariant linear system. Both the input and output signals are plotted as arbitrary signal intensity versus time. An impulse signal is instantaneous and transient and can be represented by a Dirac delta function, which is a generalized function with an area of unity (integral over the entire real line is equal to one) (Fig. 20.4a). The output signal consists of a single step of finite width followed by an exponential tail (Fig. 20.4b). The step has the same height as the impulse signal, providing there is no signal lost in the linear system. Here, the width of the step corresponds to the minimum time required by the contrast to pass through the microvasculature in the tissue, whereas the exponential tail describes the gradual decline of the signal over time from the washout of contrast in the tissue region (for intravascular contrast it would be washout from the vasculature). When a second impulse with twice the magnitude as the first impulse is introduced at a later time, the corresponding output signal would have a step that is twice as high as the first output signal and is delayed with respect to the first output signal by the time interval between the two input impulses (Fig. 20.4c, d).

The output signal of a system in response to an impulse input signal is called the impulse response function (IRF), which provides useful information about the characteristic of the system and allows one to infer how the system responds to different inputs. In CTP studies, an arterial TEC, $C_a(t)$, acquired from DCE CT images can be viewed as a superimposition of sequential impulse input signals with different magnitudes (Fig. 20.4e). The corresponding tissue TEC, $Q(t)$, is a superimposition of the IRFs (equivalent to $R(t)$ defined in Fig. 20.2) scaled by the magnitude of corresponding impulse input signal and shift in time to match that of the impulse signal, both of these information are provided by the arterial TEC (Fig. 20.4f). The superimposition of the same IRF using information from the arterial TEC as described above is equivalent to the mathematical operation of convolution between the IRF and $C_a(t)$. Thus, the concentration of contrast medium in tissue at a given time t is controlled by three factors: local blood flow (F), concentration of contrast material in the input artery ($C_a(t)$), and the physiological properties of local vasculature (i.e., blood volume and permeability) as encapsulated in the IRF. The mathematical expression of this statement is [16]:

$$\begin{aligned} Q(t) &= F\cdot C_a(t)\otimes R(t) \\ &= C_a(t)\otimes F\cdot R(t) \\ &= \int_0^t C_a(\tau)\cdot\left[F\cdot R(t-\tau)\right]d\tau \end{aligned} \tag{20.12}$$

where $\otimes$ is the convolution integral. Deconvolution is the opposite mathematical operation to convolution and can be used to "remove" the effect of arterial concentration of contrast on the tissue TEC to arrive at the flow-scaled IRF, $F{\cdot}R(t)$, the height of which is equal to perfusion as $R(t)$ has a height of unity by definition.

Deconvolution can be executed using a number of algorithms, one of which is singular value decomposition (SVD) [29, 30]. SVD formulates the convolution integrals in Eq. (20.12) in algebraic matrix notation:

$$\begin{bmatrix} C_a(t_1) & 0 & \cdots & 0 \\ C_a(t_2) & C_a(t_1) & \cdots & 0 \\ \vdots & \vdots & \vdots & 0 \\ C_a(t_n) & C_a(t_{n-1}) & \cdots & C_a(t_1) \end{bmatrix} \cdot \begin{bmatrix} R(t_1) \\ R(t_2) \\ \vdots \\ R(t_n) \end{bmatrix} = \begin{bmatrix} C_e(t_1) \\ C_e(t_2) \\ \vdots \\ C_e(t_n) \end{bmatrix} \tag{20.13}$$

The first matrix on the left side of Eq. (20.13) represents the arterial concentration of contrast at different times (from $t = 1$ to n seconds); the second matrix on the left side of the equation represents the corresponding IRFs from t_1 to t_n; the matrix on the right side of the equation denotes the corresponding contrast concentration in tissue from t_1 to t_n. $C_a(t)$, and $C_e(t)$ can be measured directly from the aorta and myocardium in DCE CT images of the heart, provided that a correct factor is used to convert Hounsfield unit into contrast concentration in milligram of iodine per milliliter (mg/mL). At 100 kV tube voltage, every 1 mg/mL of iodine concentration results in roughly 25 HU of enhancement (increase in voxel intensity from baseline) in a CT image [31]. If we use A to represent the first matrix on the left side of Eq. (20.13), then the singular values of A can be derived from the square roots of the nonzero eigenvalues of $A^T \cdot A$, where A^T is the transpose of A, and sequentially the least squares solution of $R(t)$ can be computed from $(A^T \cdot A)^{-1} \cdot A^T$, where $(A^T \cdot A)^{-1}$ is the inverse of A^T.

Deconvolution can be performed without prior assumption of the form of IRF. However, the deconvolution process is unstable and highly sensitive to signal fluctuation in the arterial and myocardial TECs measured from DCE CT images [32, 33], which could lead to inaccurate estimation of the IRF and perfusion in presence of excessive image noise. As such, it is recommended to perform a model-based deconvolution where the estimated IRF is constrained to certain forms that have realistic physiological meaning, by using a proper tracer kinetic model to simulate the exchange of contrast medium between vascular and interstitial spaces within the tissue of interest.

In the next sections, the tracer kinetic models that are commonly used in model-based deconvolution are briefly reviewed. The complexity of each model depends on the degree of assumption made to facilitate the solving of the governing mathematical equations of the model. It should be noted that regardless of the choice of model, there is always a compromise between mathematical complexity of the model and the practical limits set by the data (i.e., limited temporal and spatial resolution and signal-to-noise ratio).

Tracer Kinetic Models

Two-Compartment Exchange Model

As x-ray contrast agents are hydrophilic and metabolically inert, they are excluded from the intracellular space and not metabolized within the intravascular and interstitial spaces under normal condition. As such, a two-compartment exchange model can be used to describe the intravascular-interstitial exchange of contrast solutes through the permeable capillary endothelium [34–37]. This model assumes instantaneous mixing of contrast solutes upon arrival in the intravascular and interstitial spaces in the tissue. In other words, the contrast concentration within each compartment changes only temporally not spatially. The rate of change of the mass of contrast solutes in the interstitial compartment can be described by the following equation:

$$V_e \frac{\mathrm{d}C_e(t)}{\mathrm{d}t} = k_1 \cdot C_b(t) - k_2 \cdot C_e(t) \quad (20.13a)$$

where V_e is the distribution volume of contrast solutes in the interstitial space and $C_e(t)$ and $C_b(t)$ are the concentration of contrast solutes in the interstitial and intravascular spaces, respectively. As contrast is assumed to be mixed instantaneously upon arrival, $C_b(t)$ is essentially equal to $C_a(t)$ as defined above. k_1 is the forward transfer constant of contrast solutes from the intravascular to interstitial space and has a unit of min^{-1} and, similarly, k_2 is the backward transfer constant in min^{-1} from the interstitial to intravascular space. Both k_1 and k_2 are equal to the product of flow and extraction fraction of the contrast solutes or $F \cdot E$ [38]. A schematic of this model is provided in Fig. 20.5. It should be emphasized that the intravascular space represents a combination of all capillaries, while the interstitial space represents the total extravascular space outside the capillaries within a tissue. Equation (20.13a) can be rewritten as:

$$\frac{\mathrm{d}C_e(t)}{dt} = \frac{FE}{V_e}\left[C_a(t) - C_e(t)\right] \quad (20.13b)$$

The solution to Eq. (20.13b) is given by:

$$C_e(t) = \frac{FE}{V_e} \cdot \int_0^t C_a(u) \cdot e^{-\frac{FE}{V_e} \cdot (t-u)} \mathrm{d}u \quad (20.14)$$

Because the mass of contrast solutes in tissue $Q(t)$ measured with DCE CT is contributed by both the contrast in the interstitial and intravascular spaces, therefore:

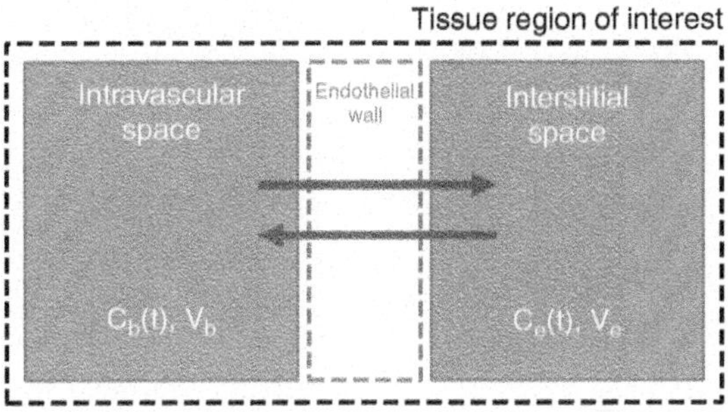

Fig. 20.5 Diagram of a two-compartment exchange model used to describe the tracer kinetics in a tissue. The model assumes instantaneous mixing of contrast solutes upon arrival in blood and interstitium. Therefore, the concentration of contrast in the blood, C_b, and interstitium, C_e, are dependent on time t only. The governing rate constants of the forward and backward diffusion of contrast medium between these spaces are $F \cdot E$

$$\begin{aligned} Q(t) &= C_e(t)\cdot V_e + C_a(t)\cdot V_b \\ &= \mathrm{FE}\int_0^t C_a(u)\cdot e^{\frac{\mathrm{FE}}{\mathrm{Ve}}(t-u)}\mathrm{d}u + C_a(t)\cdot V_b \end{aligned} \quad (20.15)$$

where V_b is the distribution volume of contrast in the intravascular space. According to the definition of convolution, Eq. (20.15) can be rewritten as follows:

$$Q(t) = C_a(t)\otimes\left[FE\cdot e^{-\frac{\mathrm{FE}}{V_e}\cdot t} + V_b\cdot\delta(t)\right] \quad (20.16)$$

where $\delta(t)$ is the Dirac delta function defined above. The convolution of $C_a(t)$ with $\delta(t)$ yields $C_a(t)$, as the integration of $\delta(t)$ is equal to unity. By comparing Eqs. (20.12) and (20.16), the flow-scaled IRF ($F{\cdot}R(t)$) of the two-compartment model has the following form:

$$F\cdot R(t) = V_b \text{ when } t = 0 \quad (20.17a)$$

$$= F\cdot E\cdot e^{-\frac{\mathrm{FE}}{V_e}\cdot t} \text{ when } t > 0 \quad (20.17b)$$

Given the DCE CT measurements of $C_a(t)$ and $Q(t)$, the parameters $F{\cdot}E$, V_b, and V_e can be estimated using nonlinear regression methods [39]. The advantage of compartmental modeling is its mathematical simplicity. The main drawback of this approach is that F and E cannot be estimated separately, as they are determined together as a transport constant (k_1 and k_2). By assuming both the intravascular and interstitial spaces are well-stirred compartments, all the information relating to the convective transport of contrast solutes along the capillaries is lost. To estimate F, a constant value of E has to be assumed. This is a limitation as E is likely to be different among different tissue types (e.g., normal vs. ischemic vs. infarcted).

Patlak Model

The Patlak model or graphical analysis is based on the two-compartment exchange model with an additional assumption that the efflux of contrast solutes from the interstitial space back to the intravascular space is negligible [36, 37]. This assumption implies the contrast distribution volume in the interstitial space (V_e) is very large so that the ratio of $F{\cdot}E$ to V_e is close to zero and the exponential term in Eq. (20.16), $e^{-FE/Ve}$, is roughly equal to unity. Under this assumption, the flow-scaled IRF, $F{\cdot}R(t)$, becomes:

$$F\cdot R(t) = F\cdot E\cdot H(t) + V_b\cdot\delta(t) \quad (20.18)$$

where $H(t)$ is the Heaviside unit step function and is equal to zero at $t \leq 0$ and unity at $t > 0$. The unit step function, which by definition is zero at $t = 0$, is added in this equation to ensure the diffusion process, as governed by the forward transfer rate constant ($k_1 = F{\cdot}E$), and does not start before the arrival of contrast solutes. Equation (20.15) then becomes:

$$Q(t) = F \cdot E \int_0^t C_a(u)\,\mathrm{du} + C_a(t) \cdot V_b \quad (20.19)$$

By dividing both sides by $C_a(t)$, Eq. 20.19 can be rewritten as:

$$\frac{Q(t)}{C_a(t)} = F \cdot E \cdot \frac{\int_0^t C_a(u)\,\mathrm{du}}{C_a(t)} + V_b \quad (20.10)$$

Equation (20.10) is a linear equation in the form of $y = mx + b$, where m and b are the slope and intercept, respectively. Thus, if $\frac{Q(t)}{C_a(t)}$ is plotted against $\frac{\int_0^t C_a(u)\,\mathrm{du}}{C_a(t)}$, a straight line is produced with its slope equals $F \cdot E$ and intercept equals V_b. This method is known as the Patlak graphical plot. This approach can be interpreted as a mathematical transformation to "stretch" the measured tissue TEC into a straight-line plot. Unfortunately, the limitation of the two-compartment exchange model also applies to the Patlak model, which is the fact that F and E cannot be determined separately. Another problem with the Patlak graphical method is that the no backward diffusion assumption may not be applicable in all situations.

Tissue Homogeneity Model

Compared to the two-compartment exchange model, the tissue homogeneity model is a more realistic model to describe the kinetic behavior of contrast solutes in a single capillary transit. The tissue homogeneity model assumes a spatially nonuniform concentration gradient from the arterial to venous ends in the intravascular space to account for the potential loss of contrast solutes in blood via diffusion through the capillary endothelium [40]. Radial gradient of contrast concentration within the capillaries is assumed to be negligible because convective (blood flow) transport of contrast in the axial direction (from arterial inlet to venous outlet) is much larger than radial diffusion. In contrast to the intravascular space, the surrounding interstitial space is considered as a compartment. This assumption is reasonable because capillaries in tissue are randomly oriented; therefore contrast solutes essentially diffuse from all directions into the interstitial space, which mimics a well-mixed interstitial compartment. From conservation of the mass of tracers (contrast) in both the intravascular and interstitial spaces, the tissue homogeneity model leads to the following two equations describing the tracer transports during a single capillary transit:

$$\pi r^2 \frac{\partial C_b(x,t)}{\partial t} + \pi r^2 v \frac{\partial C_b(x,t)}{\partial x} = 2\pi r P\left(C_e(t) - C_b(x,t)\right) \quad (20.21a)$$

$$V_e \frac{\partial C_e(t)}{\partial t} = \int_0^l 2\pi r P\left(C_b(x,t) - C_e(x,t)\right)\mathrm{dx} \quad (20.21b)$$

where r is the radius of the capillary; $C_b(x,t)$ is the concentration of contrast material within the capillary at time t and distance x relative to the arterial inlet; $C_e(t)$ is the concentration within the interstitial space at time t; v is the flow velocity of tracer; P is the permeability coefficient of the endothelial wall to the contrast; V_e is the distribution volume of contrast in the interstitial space; and l is the axial length of the capillary. A schematic of the tissue homogeneity model is provided in Fig. 20.6. Equation (20.21a) describes the convective transport in the axial direction, while Eq. (20.21b) describes the diffusive transport of the contrast solutes between capillaries (intravascular) and interstitial space. As the total diffusional flux of contrast solutes is best described using the product of permeability coefficient (P) and the total surface area (S) of capillary endothelium, the above equations can be rewritten as follows:

$$\frac{\partial C_b(x,t)}{\partial t} + \frac{\mathrm{FL}}{V_b}\frac{\partial C_b(x,t)}{\partial x} = \frac{\mathrm{PS}}{V_b}\left[C_e(t) - C_b(x,t)\right] \quad (20.22a)$$

$$V_e \frac{dC_e(t)}{dt} = \frac{\mathrm{PS}}{L}\int_0^L \left[C_b(x,t) - C_e(t)\right]\mathrm{dx} \quad (20.22b)$$

Equations (20.22a) and (20.22b) are subject to the following initial and boundary conditions:

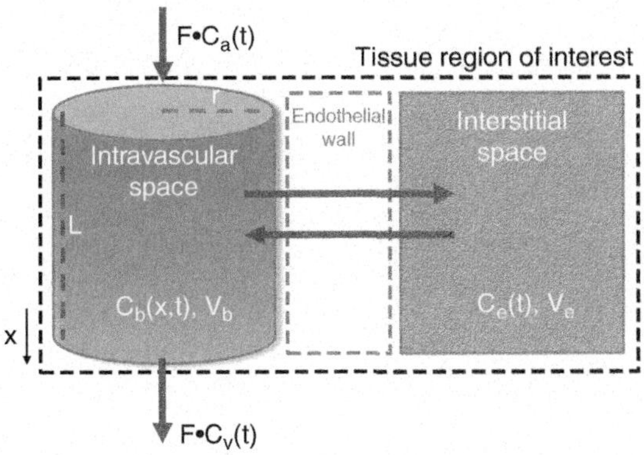

Fig. 20.6 Diagram of a tissue homogeneity model used to describe the tracer kinetics in a tissue. According to the model, there is a concentration gradient of contrast medium in the capillaries along the net flow direction as a result of potential diffusion across the endothelium into the interstitial space. Thus, $C_b(t)$ is a function of both the position in the capillaries (x) and time (t). Diffusion of contrast across the capillary endothelium is governed by PS. The interstitial space is still considered as a compartment where contrast medium is instantaneously mixed within the compartment upon arrival

$$\begin{aligned} C_b(x,t=0) &= C_e(t=0) = 0 \\ C_b(x=0,t>0) &= C_a(t) \end{aligned} \quad (20.23)$$

The above initial and boundary conditions are justified by the fact that contrast concentration at t = 0 should be zero. Additionally, the concentration of contrast at the arterial end of the capillary is equal to the arterial concentration. Given the DCE CT measurements of $C_a(t)$ and $Q(t)$, Laplace transform can be used to determine the solution of these equations which satisfied the above boundary and initial conditions. As such, solutions to these differential equations only exist in the frequency domain which significantly hampers the use of this tracer model [38]. It has been shown that a solution in the time domain can be derived by employing the adiabatic approximation, which assumes a much slower rate of change of contrast concentration in the interstitial space ($C_e(t)$) relative to that in the intravascular space ($C_b(x,t)$) [38]. With this assumption, $C_e(t)$ can be approximated by a sequence of discrete steps where $C_e(t)$ is constant within the duration of each step which is much shorter than the capillary transit time. Within each discrete of $C_e(t)$, $C_b(x,t)$ can be expressed in terms of the constant $C_e(t)$ by solving Eq. (20.22a) [38]. The other details of the adiabatic approximation are outside the scope of this book chapter and are omitted here for brevity. The $F{\cdot}R(t)$ derived from the adiabatic solution has the following form:

$$F \cdot R(t) = \begin{cases} 0 & t<0 \\ F & 0<t<W \\ F \cdot E \cdot e\dfrac{\mathrm{FE}}{\mathrm{Ve}} \cdot (t-\mathrm{Tc}) & t \geq W \end{cases} \quad (20.24)$$

where W is the vascular minimum transit time. According to this model, there exists a finite transit time for contrast solutes to travel from the arterial to venous ends of the capillaries. As such, all contrast solutes should remain in the tissue within the mean transit time and is reflected by the plateau of the flow-scaled residual function. At $t = W$, $F{\cdot}R(t)$ immediately drops to a value of $F{\cdot}E$, as a portion (1–E) of contrast solutes begins to leave the tissue through the venous end, and the fraction (E) diffused into the interstitial space is what remains in the tissue. The extracted contrast in the tissue follows a mono-exponential decay for t > W, corresponding to the slower efflux from interstitial to vascular spaces and subsequent washout by blood flow [38].

Model-Based Maximum Slope Analysis

The method of using the upslope of myocardial TEC for deriving myocardial blood flow is discussed in section "Maximum Slope Method". As the upslope of myocardial TEC can be largely

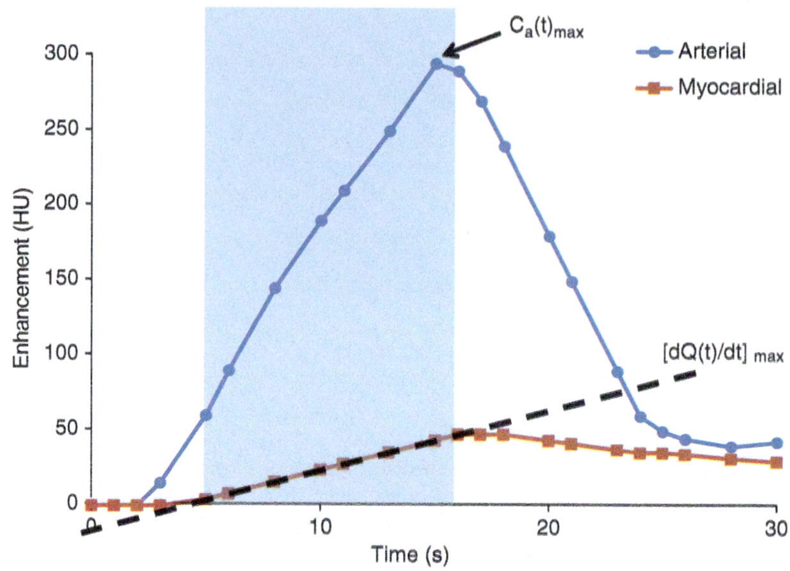

Fig. 20.7 Schematic illustration of the maximum slope method. The section in the graph that is highlighted with blue color represents the amount of dynamic data used for the maximum slope analysis.

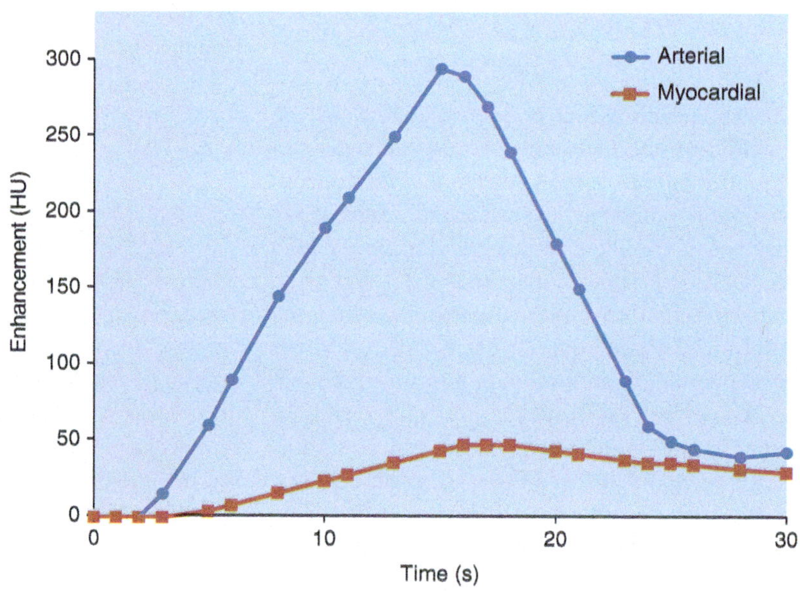

Fig. 20.8 In comparison to Fig. 20.7, this graph illustrates the approximate amount of dynamic data used for a model-based deconvolution analysis

distorted by the noise presented in DCE CT images, a model-based maximum slope analysis technique has been proposed. In this approach, each myocardial TEC acquired from DCE CT images is first "smoothed" with a model-based deconvolution analysis. The upslope of each "smoothed" myocardial TEC is then used to derive myocardial blood flow as described in section "Maximum Slope Method" (Figs. 20.7 and 20.8). While the model-based maximum slope analysis technique is theoretically more reliable than the analysis method described in section "Maximum Slope Method", it has been demonstrated that the absolute myocardial blood flow value derived with this approach is still significantly underestimated. In this section, the adiabatic approximation of the tissue homogeneity model is used to illustrate how the maximum slope method leads to underestimation of myocardial blood flow.

For soft tissue where contrast exchanges bidirectionally between vascular and extravascular spaces, the blood flow-scaled impulse residue function, $R_F(t)$, is given by the adiabatic approximation of the tissue homogeneity model as:

$$R_F(t)=\begin{cases}0 & t<0\\ F & 0\le t<W\\ FEe^{-k(t-W)} & t\ge W\end{cases} \quad (20.25)$$

where F is the tissue blood flow; E is the tracer extraction efficiency in tissue; k is the transfer rate constant; and W is the minimum transit time of tracer in tissue. The tissue residual curve, $Q(t)$, is given by:

$$Q(t)=C_a(t)*R_F(t) \quad (20.26)$$

where $C_a(t)$ is the arterial blood concentration of tracer and $*$ is the convolution operator. The Heaviside step function, $H(t)$, is defined as:

$$H(t)=\begin{cases}0 t<0\\ 1 t\ge 0\end{cases} \quad (20.27)$$

Using the Heaviside function, $R_F(t)$ in Eq. (20.25) can be expressed as:

$$\begin{aligned}R_F(t)&=\mathrm{FH}(t)-\mathrm{FH}(t-W)\\ &+\mathrm{FEe}^{-k(t-W)}H(t-W)\end{aligned} \quad (20.28)$$

Taking derivative of (20.26) yields:

$$\begin{aligned}\frac{\mathrm{dQ}(t)}{\mathrm{dt}}&=\frac{d}{\mathrm{dt}}\left(C_a(t)*R_F(t)\right)\\ &=C_a(t)*\frac{\mathrm{dR}_F(t)}{\mathrm{dt}}\end{aligned} \quad (20.29)$$

Substitute (20.28) into (20.29), the derivative of $R_F(t)$ in the above equation can be expressed as:

$$\frac{\mathrm{dR}_F(t)}{\mathrm{dt}}=\frac{d}{\mathrm{dt}}\left(\mathrm{FH}(t)-\mathrm{FH}(t-W)+\mathrm{FEe}^{-k(t-W)}H(t-W)\right) \quad (20.30)$$

For time less than the minimum transit time or $0\le t<W$:

$$\frac{\mathrm{dR}_F(t)}{\mathrm{dt}}=\frac{d}{\mathrm{dt}}\left(\mathrm{FH}(t)\right)=F\delta(t) \quad (20.31)$$

where $\delta(t)$ is the Dirac delta function. Substituting (20.31) into (20.29):

$$\frac{\mathrm{dQ}(t)}{\mathrm{dt}}=C_a(t)*F\delta(t)=FC_a(t)$$

or

$$\frac{\mathrm{dQ}(t)}{\mathrm{dt}}/C_a(t)=F \quad (20.32)$$

For time equals or longer than the minimum transit time, or $t\ge W$:

$$\begin{aligned}\frac{\mathrm{dR}_F(t)}{\mathrm{dt}}&=\frac{d}{\mathrm{dt}}\left(\mathrm{FH}(t)-\mathrm{FH}(t-W)+\mathrm{FEe}^{-k(t-W)}H(t-W)\right)\\ &=F\delta(t)-F\delta(t-W)+\mathrm{FE}\frac{d}{\mathrm{dt}}\left(e^{-k(t-W)}H(t-W)\right)\\ &=F\delta(t)-F\delta(t-W)+\mathrm{FEe}^{-k(t-W)}\delta(t-W)-\mathrm{FEke}^{-k(t-W)}H(t-W)\end{aligned} \quad (20.33)$$

Substituting (20.33) into (20.29):

$$\frac{dQ(t)}{dt} = C_a(t) * \left(F\delta(t) - F\delta(t-W) + \mathrm{FEe}^{-k(t-W)}\delta(t-W) - \mathrm{FEke}^{-k(t-W)}H(t-W)\right)$$
$$= \mathrm{FC}_a(t) - \mathrm{FC}_a(t-W) + \mathrm{FEC}_a(t) * \left(e^{-k(t-W)}\delta(t-W)\right) - \mathrm{FEkC}_a(t) * \left(e^{-k(t-W)}H(t-W)\right) \quad (20.34)$$

The first convolution term in equation (34) can be simplified to:

$$C_a(t) * \left(e^{-k(t-W)}\delta(t-W)\right) = \int_0^t C_a(t-u)e^{-k(u-W)}\delta(u-W)\mathrm{du} = C_a(t-W)$$
$$C_a(t) * \left(e^{-k(t-W)}\delta(t-W)\right) = \int_0^t C_a(t-u)e^{-k(u-W)}\delta(u-W)\mathrm{du}$$
$$C_a(t) * \left(e^{-k(t-W)}\delta(t-W)\right) = \int_0^t C_a(t-u)e^{-k(u-W)}\delta(u-W)\mathrm{du} \quad (20.35)$$
$$= \int_W^t C_a(t-u)\delta(u-W)\mathrm{du}$$
$$= C_a(t-W)$$

The second convolution term in Eq. (20.34) can be simplified to:

$$C_a(t) * \left(e^{-k(t-W)}H(t-W)\right) = \int_0^t C_a(t-u)e^{-k(u-W)}H(u-W)\mathrm{du}$$
$$= \int_W^t C_a(t-u)e^{-k(u-W)}\mathrm{du} = \int_0^{t-W} C_a(t-W-v)e^{-\mathrm{kv}}\mathrm{dv} \quad (20.36)$$
$$= C_a(t-W) * e^{-k(t-W)}$$

The integral term in (20.36) is rewritten by introducing the term $v = u - W$. Substitute (20.35) and (20.36) into (20.29) yields:

$$\frac{dQ(t)}{dt} = FC_a(t) - FC_a(t-W) + FEC_a(t-W) - FEk\left[C_a(t-W) * e^{-k(t-W)}\right]$$
$$= F\left[C_a(t) - C_a(t-W)\right] + FEC_a(t-W) - FEk\left[C_a(t-W) * e^{-k(t-W)}\right]$$

and

$$\frac{dQ(t)}{dt} / C_a(t) = FE + F(1-E)\frac{C_a(t) - C_a(t-W)}{C_a(t)} - FEk\frac{\left[C_a(t) * e^{-kt}\right]_{t=t-W}}{C_a(t)} \tag{37}$$

Therefore, in tissue where contrast exchanges bidirectionally between blood vessels and interstitial space:

for $0 \leq t < W$

$$\frac{\mathrm{d}Q(t)}{dt} / C_a(t) = F$$

for $t \geq W$

$$\frac{dQ(t)}{dt} / C_a(t) = FE + F(1-E)\frac{C_a(t) - C_a(t-W)}{C_a(t)} - FEk\frac{\left[C_a(t) * e^{-kt}\right]_{t=t-W}}{C_a(t)} \tag{20.38}$$

Equation (20.38) suggested that for time equal to or longer than the mean transit time, the parameter estimated from the maximum slope method is not simply a product of $F{\cdot}E$ and rather a complicated function of F and E.

Practical Issues of Tracer Kinetic Modeling

In CTP studies, the measurement of arterial and tissue TECs may be affected by several factors. The potential effect of each factor on IRF modeling is reviewed in this section.

Recirculation of Contrast Medium

Recirculation refers to the reentry of contrast material to the organ/tissue of interest after previously leaving it and passing through the systematic circulation. Recirculation can occur as soon as 20–25 s after a bolus injection of contrast at 4 mL·s^{-1} (assuming 50 mL of contrast is administered and a normal resting heart rate and cardiac output of the patient). Thus, the effect of recirculation should be addressed in most CT perfusion studies. Let us denote $C_a(t)_{fp}$ and $C_a(t)_r$ as the first-pass and recirculation components of an arterial TEC, respectively. Similarly, $Q(t)_{fp}$ and $Q(t)_r$ are the first-pass and recirculation components of a tissue TEC, respectively. With the above definitions, $C_a(t)$ and $Q(t)$ are the summation of the two respective components:

$$C_a(t) = C_a^{fp}(t) + C_a^{r}(t) \tag{20.39a}$$

$$Q(t) = Q^{fp}(t) + Q^{r}(t) \tag{20.39b}$$

According to the convolution equation in (20.12):

$$Q^{fp}(t) = C_a^{fp}(t) \otimes \left[F \cdot R(t)\right] \tag{20.40a}$$

$$Q^{r}(t) = C_a^{r}(t) \otimes \left[F \cdot R(t)\right] \tag{20.40b}$$

Substituting Eqs. (20.40a) and (20.40b) into (20.39b), and according to the distributive property of convolution, we have:

$$\begin{aligned} Q(t) &= Q^{fp}(t) + Q^{r}(t) \\ &= C_a^{f}p(t) \otimes \left[F \cdot R(t)\right] + C_a^{r}(t) \otimes \left[F \cdot R(t)\right] \\ &= \left[C_a^{f}p(t) + C_a^{r}(t)\right] \otimes \left[F \cdot R(t)\right] \end{aligned} \tag{20.41}$$

The above equation demonstrates that the $F{\cdot}R(t)$ can still be estimated from the measured arterial and tissue TECs, with both containing the first-pass and recirculation phases, using the deconvolution approach. Therefore, there is no need to correct for recirculation in the measured TECs. Although the above derivation can be easily generalized to include more than one recirculation component, the effect of second or third recirculation component is expected to be negligible compared to the first recirculation component.

Dispersion in True Arterial TEC Relative to Measured Arterial TEC

Dispersion refers to the "spreading" of the arterial TEC at the true input site to a tissue region relative to the measurement site. An arterial TEC is normally acquired at a distance upstream to the tissue region to avoid significant partial volume effect owing to the small size of the local input artery (will be discussed in a later section). In the presence of dispersion, the true and measured arterial TEC satisfy the following relationship:

$$C_a(t) = C_a^{m}(t)\cdot h(t) \quad (20.42)$$

where $h(t)$, as introduced in section "Introduction", is the probability function or transit time spectrum that describes the various times required by individual contrast solute to travel from the measurement site to the actual arterial input site following a bolus injection. Substituting Eqs. (20.42) into (20.12), and based on the associative property of convolution, yields:

$$\begin{aligned} Q(t) &= \left[C_a^{m}(t)\otimes h(t)\right]\otimes F\cdot R(t) \\ &= C_a^{m}(t)\otimes\left[h(t)\otimes F\cdot R(t)\right] \end{aligned} \quad (20.43)$$

Equation (20.43) states that deconvolution of the measured arterial and tissue TECs returns a flow-scaled residual function convolved with the arterial dispersion transit time spectrum. Previous phantom experiments suggested that the arterial TEC has negligible dispersion effect input curve if the measurement site is within 90 cm of the input site [38]. Thus, $h(t)$ can be approximated by a Dirac delta function, and Eq. (20.43) is essentially identical to (20.12). Hence, no dispersion correction is required for the arterial TEC as long as the measurement site is reasonably close to the true input site.

Delay of Tissue TEC Relative to Measured Arterial TEC

Because an arterial TEC is measured at a distance from the actual input site to a tissue region, there is a slight time delay in the arrival of contrast in tissue relative to the measured arterial TEC. Such delay can be accounted for by making modifications to the equation for the IRF of each kinetics model. Let us denote $C_a^{m}(t)$ as the measured arterial TEC and T_o is the delay time relative to the measurement site.

$$C_a(t) = C_a^{m}(t - T_o) \quad (20.44)$$

Note that $(t - T_o)$ results in a positive time shift of the measured arterial TEC (as the true arterial TEC should lag behind the measured arterial TEC). Substituting Eq. (20.44) into (20.12) yields:

$$\begin{aligned} Q(t) &= C_a(t)\otimes F\cdot R(t) = C_a^{m}(t-T_o)\otimes F\cdot R(t) \\ &= F\cdot\int_0^t C_a(t-T_o)\cdot R(t-\tau)\,d\tau \\ &= F\cdot\int_0^t C_a(t)\cdot R(t-T_o-\tau)\,d\tau \\ &= C_a^{m}(t)\otimes F\cdot R(t-T_o) \end{aligned} \quad (20.45)$$

Equation (20.45) confirms that if there is a time delay between the measured and true arterial input curve, the arrival of contrast in the tissue region will be delayed by the same amount of time. As such, the flow-scaled residual function for each of the above models can be modified accordingly to account for the delayed arrival of contrast in the tissue region relative to the measured arterial TEC.

For the two-compartment model, $F\cdot R(t)$ in Eq. (17) is modified to:

$$F\cdot R(t-T_o) = F\cdot E\cdot e^{-\frac{FE}{V_e}(t-T_o)} + V_b\cdot\delta(t-T_o) \quad (20.46)$$

For the Patlak model, $F\cdot R(t)$ in Eq. (20.18) is modified to:

$$F\cdot R(t-T_o) = F\cdot E\cdot H(t-T_o) + V_b\cdot\delta(t-T_o) \quad (20.47)$$

For the adiabatic approximation of the tissue homogeneity model, $F\cdot R(t)$ in Eq. (20.24) is changed to:

$$F\cdot R(t-T_o) = \begin{cases} 0 & 0 \le t < T_o \\ F & T_o \le t \le T_o + W \\ F\cdot E\cdot e^{-\frac{FE}{V_e}(t-T_o-W)} & t > T_o + W \end{cases} \quad (20.48)$$

Implementations

An overview of the technical issues for the implementation of CTP for measurement of myocardial perfusion is provided in this section.

Contrast Administration

Contrast Materials

Commonly used nonionic radiographic contrast agents for CTP imaging of the heart include iodixanol, iohexol, and isovue [41–43]. The molecular weight of these iodine-based contrast agents is about 760 g·mol^{-1} (Dalton). The osmolality (solute concentration) of these contrast agents is considered to be low (290–796 mOsm·kg^{-1}). Iodine concentration is available in the range of 140–370 mg of iodine per milliliter, and ~320 mgI/mL is recommended for most cardiac CTP studies to ensure good image quality and contrast (see 2.1.3.). As the viscosity of these contrast agents is lower at higher temperatures, it is recommended that these contrast agents should be warmed to match the patient body temperature (~37 °C) before injection.

Contrast Injection Rate

Contrast agent is usually injected into an antecubital vein with an automated injection pump through an 18-gauge cannula. At a fixed volume of contrast solution, a faster injection rate increases the rate of delivery which leads to a larger degree of accumulation of contrast material and sequentially a higher peak enhancement in the region of interest [44]. A faster injection rate also shortens the time required to reach the peak enhancement. The typical bolus injection rate of contrast agent for CT perfusion is between 4 and 7 mL·s^{-1} [10, 11, 45–47]. Injection rate greater than 10 mL·s^{-1} is not likely to improve the enhancement further owing to the inherent mixing of contrast medium in the blood and retrograde reflux which restricts fast propagation of contrast to the target region [48, 49]. If a dual injector is used, saline flush can be applied immediately after contrast injection to reduce the dispersion of contrast during the passage in vasculature and to improve the bolus geometry and level of contrast enhancement [50], [48, 51].

Contrast Concentration

At a fixed contrast injection rate and volume, a higher iodine concentration results in a higher level of peak enhancement [44], which improves the signal-to-noise ratio of the arterial and myocardial TECs. However, a higher iodine concentration also leads to a larger beam-hardening effect, which particularly affects CT myocardial perfusion imaging due to the presence of substantial amount of contrast material in the heart chambers during the first-pass circulation. The root causes of beam hardening are the polychromatic nature of the x-rays used in clinical CT scanners and the energy dependence of x-ray attenuation in materials [52]. If not corrected, the beam-hardening effect can induce unpredictable shift in CT number, leading to tissue enhancement that is unrelated to the perfusion level and sequentially misdiagnosis of myocardial ischemia [52]. Furthermore, a higher iodine concentration may also lead to more intense streak artifacts emanating from the right heart chamber during the first pass of contrast material, which may distort the myocardial TECs in the interventricular septal wall [53]. Iodine concentration of ~320 mgI/mL is recommended for most cardiac CTP studies to ensure good image contrast with minimal artifacts that may affect the TEC measurement in the myocardium.

Contrast Volume

After intravenous injection, contrast agent is diluted by the blood on route to the targeted organ/tissue of interest. Such dilution occurs to a greater extent in patients with larger body sizes due to the proportionally larger blood volumes. Thus, the volume of contrast agent used in a CTP study should be tailored to the patient body weight to ensure the TECs sampled at the targeted regions have good signal-to-noise ratio. The recommended contrast volume for each CTP acquisition is 0.7 mL·kg^{-1} up to a maximum of 60–70 mL. For a rest and stress cardiac CTP protocol, the total contrast volume is between 120 and 140 mL.

Acquisition Settings

The acquisition settings for DCE CT cardiac imaging should be carefully selected to achieve optimal balance between image quality and patient radiation dose. Some of the most important settings are reviewed in this section.

Tube Voltage

Generally speaking, DCE CT with iodine-based contrast agent should be performed at a lower tube voltage (such as 80 kilovolts or kV) so that the mean x-ray photon energy is closer to the K-edge of iodine (~33 kiloelectron volts or keV) to maximize the probability of photoelectric interactions [54] and the signal-to-noise ratio of arterial and tissue TECs. Thus, the standard acquisition protocol for neuro perfusion studies uses 80 kV as the tube voltage setting [55, 56]. For thoracic perfusion studies including the heart and liver, a higher tube voltage (100 or 120 kV) is recommended to compensate for the larger degree of x-ray attenuation by the patient body. This is because x-ray photons at lower energies are more preferentially absorbed by the patient body and unable to reach the detectors, which results in larger degree of signal fluctuation in the TECs measured from DCE CT images.

Tube Current

While the tube voltage determines the x-ray photon energies, the tube current controls the x-ray photon flux. The setting of tube current (measured in milliampere or mA) or tube current-second (the product of tube current and exposure time, in mA·s) should be adjusted according to the patient body size and the radiosensitivity of the organ/tissue of interest. Compared to neuro perfusion imaging, a lower mA·s setting should be used for myocardial perfusion imaging due to the relatively higher radiosensitivity of the organs and tissues within the thoracic section of the body [57] (in some cardiac perfusion studies part of the abdominal section is also covered). While radiation dose decreases in proportion to mA·s, image noise increases by about 40% when the mA·s setting is reduced by halves (noise $\propto \frac{1}{\sqrt{mA \cdot s}}$) [58]. As such, the choice of mA·s should be carefully selected to achieve a good balance between diagnostic image quality and radiation dose. There is currently no consensus on the optimal mA·s setting for dynamic myocardial perfusion imaging. Previous clinical myocardial perfusion studies have used a wide range of mA·s settings from 30 to several hundreds [10, 41–43, 59, 60]. Practically, the choice of mA·s is likely dependent on other factors including the number of acquisitions in a dynamic imaging session (ranges from ~15 to 30 acquisitions over ~ 30 s) and the slice thickness (ranges from ~3 to 5 mm; image noise reduces with larger slice thickness) and, perhaps more importantly, the analytic algorithm applied for deriving myocardial blood flow [27].

Gantry Rotation Speed

The temporal resolution of a CT image is largely limited by the gantry rotation speed. CT myocardial perfusion imaging requires excellent temporal resolution to minimize cardiac motion for accurate sampling of myocardial TECs. As such, DCE CT images of the heart should be acquired using the fastest gantry speed available (e.g., ~ 250 ms per full rotation for single-source CT scanners).

Total Acquisition Time

The total acquisition time determines the amount of dynamic data available for analysis and is dependent on the physiological processes to be modeled using the analytic techniques discussed above. Ideally, the acquisition time should be long enough to cover the first pass of contrast material in the myocardium if absolute myocardial blood flow and blood volume are the only parameters to be estimated. With a contrast injection rate of 5–6 mL·s^{-1} and contrast volume of 60–70 mL, the first pass of contrast material in the myocardium can be monitored in about 30 s under rest and stress conditions. The acquisition time may extend to several minutes if vascular permeability and other parameters such as the contrast distribution volume in infarcted myocardium are studied. It is noteworthy to mention that the acquisition time of a single imaging session is limited by the patient's ability of breath-holding to minimize respiratory motion, and therefore multiple sessions of acquisition are required if vascular permeability or contrast distribution volume is studied.

Sampling Frequency

The sampling frequency refers to the time delay between consecutive acquisitions in a single dynamic imaging session. In CT myocardial perfusion imaging, sampling frequency mainly depends on two factors: patient heart rate and axial coverage of the scanner. Most clinical CT scanners have the capability of performing dynamic myocardial perfusion imaging with prospective ECG triggering, in which acquisitions are taken at a single phase (around mid-diastole) of every (or every other) heartbeat [61]. As such, the time interval between successive acquisitions is dependent on the patient heart rate. For scanners with a smaller axial coverage (e.g., 4 or 5 cm), whole-heart perfusion imaging can be performed with a table "goggling" or "shuttling" technique, in which the scanner table moves back and forth between two adjacent positions to double the axial coverage (Fig. 20.9). However, such approach results in suboptimal sampling in each table position as the acquisition time interval at each table position could increase to a few seconds [62]. A larger time gap between successive acquisitions at each slice location increases the risk of missing the peak of TECs. It has been previously shown that cerebral blood flow was overestimated when the sampling interval exceeded 4 s [45, 63]. The sampling interval should be shorter than the time sales of the physiological processes that are to be modeled. As the vascular transit time of the contrast material during its single transit is in the order of few seconds, it is recommended that the sampling interval should be no more than 2 s to minimize errors in blood flow modeling, which is equivalent to sampling every one to two heartbeats at heart rates between 60 and 80 bpm.

Image Reconstruction

Image reconstruction plays a crucial role in the diagnostic quality of CT images by which the accuracy of CT perfusion measurement is influenced. This section discusses several aspects of image reconstruction that are relevant to the cardiac application of CT perfusion.

CT myocardial perfusion imaging is challenged by several spectral artifacts arising from beam hardening, wide cone-beam geometry, and partial-scan reconstruction. These artifacts can significantly distort the linear relationship between signal intensity and mass of contrast material in each voxel, leading to inaccurate myocardial perfusion measurement with the analytic algorithms described in sections "Indicator-Dilution Method", "Maximum Slope Method", "Deconvolution Method", and "Tracer Kinetic Models". Beam hardening arises from the inconsistent x-ray attenuation among different path lengths through the patient body that leads to large differences in effective x-ray energy at different views. As the linear attenuation coefficients that are to be reconstructed along each path length from the projections at different views are dependent on x-ray energies, errors in image reconstruction occur that lead to unpredictable changes in CT number in image voxels [52].

Newer CT scanners are equipped with large detector panels that facilitate whole-heart coverage in a single gantry rotation. This feature is particularly useful for acquiring coronary CT angiography and CT myocardial perfusion imaging with a single bolus contrast injection. However, the wide cone-beam geometry causes insufficient sampling in some regions within the scan field of view per circular trajectory for exact cone-beam reconstruction, leading to shading and streaking artifacts in CT images when standard image reconstruction techniques are used.

Cardiac CT images are reconstructed from a subset of projections acquired over 360° (partial-scan reconstruction) to optimize the image temporal resolution needed for freezing cardiac motion [64, 65]. In dynamic CT myocardial perfusion imaging, multiple acquisitions of the heart are taken after contrast administration with each acquisition triggered based on the patient's ECG signals. As such, the views spanned by each acquisition are likely different from others. Coupled with the rapid circulation of contrast

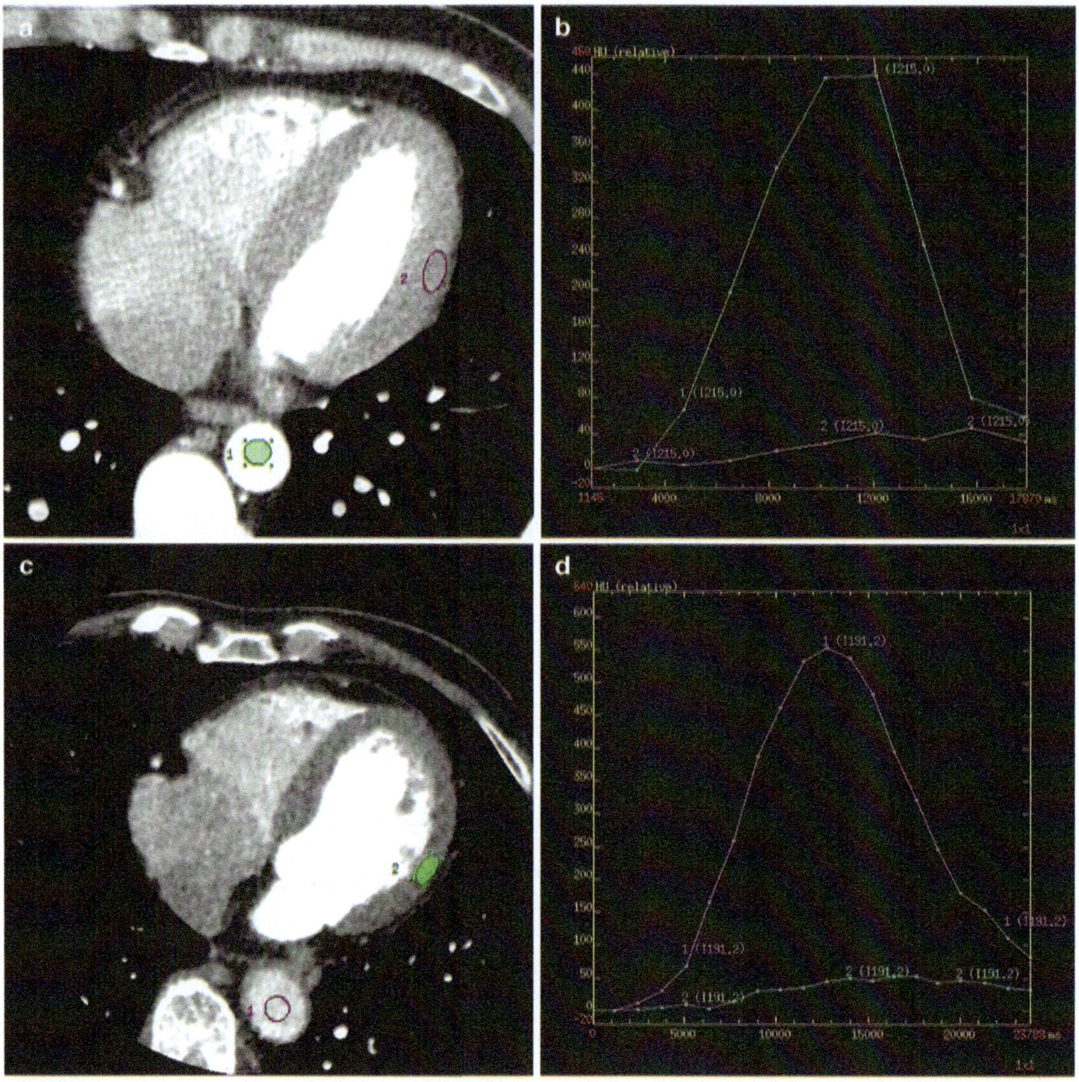

Fig. 20.9 (**a**) Contrast-enhanced cardiac CT image and (**b**) the corresponding arterial and myocardial time-enhancement curves acquired with a CT scanner with limited axial coverage (4 cm). The CTP study was performed with an axial shuttling technique where the sampling frequency in each slice is about 2 s. (**c**) Contrast-enhanced cardiac CT image of another patient with similar heart rate to that shown in (**a**) acquired with a large-coverage CT scanner (12 cm). (**d**) The corresponding arterial and myocardial time-enhancement curves were sampled at a higher frequency (~1.2 s)

material in the heart chambers during the entire dynamic imaging session, the partial-scan reconstruction can induce inconsistent shifts in CT number from one DCE heart image to another and sequentially large signal fluctuations in the arterial and myocardial TECs. Thus, DCE heart images acquired for myocardial perfusion imaging have traditionally been reconstructed with full-scan (360°) projections which leads to insufficient temporal resolution to freeze cardiac motion at higher heart rates [64].

Advanced image reconstruction algorithms are implemented in newer CT systems, to tackle these spectral artifacts to facilitate whole-heart myocardial perfusion measurement. Quality assurance testing with dedicated phantoms [31] should be regularly performed by the scanner users to ensure these spectral artifacts are minimized for accurate and reproducible perfusion assessment.

Reconstruction Filter

Reconstruction kernel is the "filter" applied to the measured projections in the backprojection process. The sharper (high-pass) filters that preserve higher spatial frequencies result in higher image noise compared to the smoother (low-pass) filters [66]. In CT myocardial perfusion imaging, the primary objective is to maximize low-contrast resolution in the soft tissue (myocardium), and therefore a sharp kernel is not recommended because high image noise deteriorates image contrast. Generally speaking, a "standard" or "soft" filter available on the scanner console can smooth away noises while preserving sharp edges, thus providing a fine balance between image contrast and resolution for CT myocardial perfusion measurement. It should be noticed that the cutoff frequency of the reconstruction kernel is also dependent on the field of view (FOV). When a small FOV is used (as in the case of targeted reconstruction), the limiting factor is the CT system geometry such as the detector cell size and focal spot size. Conversely, the limiting factor is the image pixel size when a large FOV is used.

Statistical-Based Iterative Reconstruction

Iterative image reconstruction algorithms are more computationally intensive than the conventional filtered backprojection (FBP) algorithm, and therefore their applications in real-world clinical CT studies were limited in early years. With significant improvements in computer processing speed and developments of GPU-based algorithms for image reconstruction [67–69], iterative reconstruction (IR) is increasingly used in the past decade for many low-dose CT applications including coronary angiography and myocardial perfusion imaging. It has been shown in numerous studies that IR permits radiation dose reduction while retaining excellent diagnostic image quality. Compared to FBP, the merit of IR is that modeling of x-ray photon statistics can be incorporated into the reconstruction process to correct for the signal fluctuation in the projections arising from low-dose acquisition, from which image quality can be maintained. While modeling of the CT system optics and geometry can also be incorporated to improve image spatial resolution, the predominant use of IR in low-dose dynamic CT myocardial perfusion imaging is for image noise reduction. All major CT vendors have developed their own IR algorithms [70]. Although each of these algorithms is slightly different from the others, preliminary results have suggested that these algorithms are equally effective in reducing image noise. In order to address the fact that the "look" of IR images is different from that of conventional FBP images, stepwise implementation of IR that permits the blending of IR and FBP images may be considered. However, the main objective in quantitative CT myocardial perfusion measurement is to optimize low-contrast resolution in presence of noise, and therefore it is recommended to use the full strength (100%) of IR to generate the source images for perfusion analysis.

Sparse-View Reconstruction

Besides IR, another attractive option for radiation dose reduction in dynamic CT myocardial perfusion imaging is sparse-view image reconstruction, which is currently not available on most clinical CT systems yet. Quantitative CT myocardial perfusion imaging requires multiple acquisitions over a short duration of time (~30 s) after contrast administration to monitor the first pass of contrast in the myocardium. In addition to the option of lowering the tube current setting for acquisition, one approach for radiation dose reduction is to decrease the number of projections acquired in each full gantry rotation, but the resulting aliasing artifacts in the images reconstructed with FBP could lead to large signal variation in the TECs and inaccurate myocardial perfusion measurement. In recent years, compressed sensing (CS), a signal processing technique that was initially proposed for sparse signal recovery [71, 72] has been used to reconstruct CT images from much fewer projections than what the Nyquist-Shannon theorem dictates for FBP [73, 74]. Preliminary results have suggested that CS-based image reconstruction can minimize the artifacts in DCE CT heart images arising from projection undersampling, and myocardial perfusion measurement can be performed with at least 50% less projections than the full projection set without affecting the perfusion measurement [75, 76]. Current efforts have been devoted to investigate whether concomitant use of low tube current and sparse-view acquisition could potentially reduce the radiation dose of whole-heart CT myocardial perfusion study to sub-milli-Sieverts while preserving the diagnostic quality.

Clinical Applications

Coronary CT angiography (CCTA) has become routinely used for anatomic assessment of coronary artery disease (CAD) in symptomatic patients by direct visualization of stenosis similar to invasive coronary angiography but without the complications associated with catheterization [77, 78]. Although numerous studies have demonstrated the high sensitivity and negative predictive value of CCTA for detecting high-grade stenosis, identification of high-grade lesion with CCTA alone is not a reliable indicator of physiological ischemia. In clinical settings, cardiac CTP is predominantly used for functional assessment of CAD through measurement of myocardial blood flow downstream of epicardial coronary arteries. A recent meta-analysis has shown that dynamic cardiac CTP has a pooled sensitivity and specificity of about 90% and 75%, respectively, for assessing functionally significant coronary artery lesions against different reference standards [79, 80]. Previous studies have collectively suggested that dynamic CTP provides useful incremental value to CCTA to improve the overall diagnostic performance of cardiac computed tomography for comprehensive assessment of CAD.

Two examples of dynamic CTP for functional assessment of coronary artery lesions are provided in Figs. 20.10 and 20.11 for illustration. In **Fig. 20.10**, the patient had a single-vessel CAD, in which the obtuse marginal branch of the left circumflex artery (LCx) was occluded as revealed by invasive coronary angiography. The polar maps of the single-photon emission computed tomography (SPECT) perfusion maps acquired at rest and dipyridamole stress showed absence in uptake of perfusion tracers (technetium-99 m sestamibi) in the lateral myocardium in different short-axis slices, indicating that the perfusion level in the myocardium supplied by the LCx was lower than that in the adjacent myocardium perfused by other non-stenosed coronary arteries. The corresponding CT myocardial perfusion maps acquired at dipyridamole stress in three short-axis slices are also shown in the figure. These maps were generated with a model-based deconvolution algorithm using the adiabatic approximation to the tissue homogeneity model described in section "Deconvolution Method" and "Tracer Kinetic Models". Ischemia in the lateral myocardium depicted in the stress CT myocardial perfusion maps agreed with the finding of SPECT myocardial perfusion maps. The results of this study suggest that CTP is a good alternative tool to SPECT for myocardial perfusion assessment in patients with CAD. Figure 20.11 shows another patient who had a single-vessel CAD, in which the left anterior descending artery (LAD) had a complex proximal calcified and non-calcified plaque followed by an implanted stent as revealed by CCTA. The stented coronary lumen could not be visualized clearly due to the blooming artifacts. The stress CT myo-

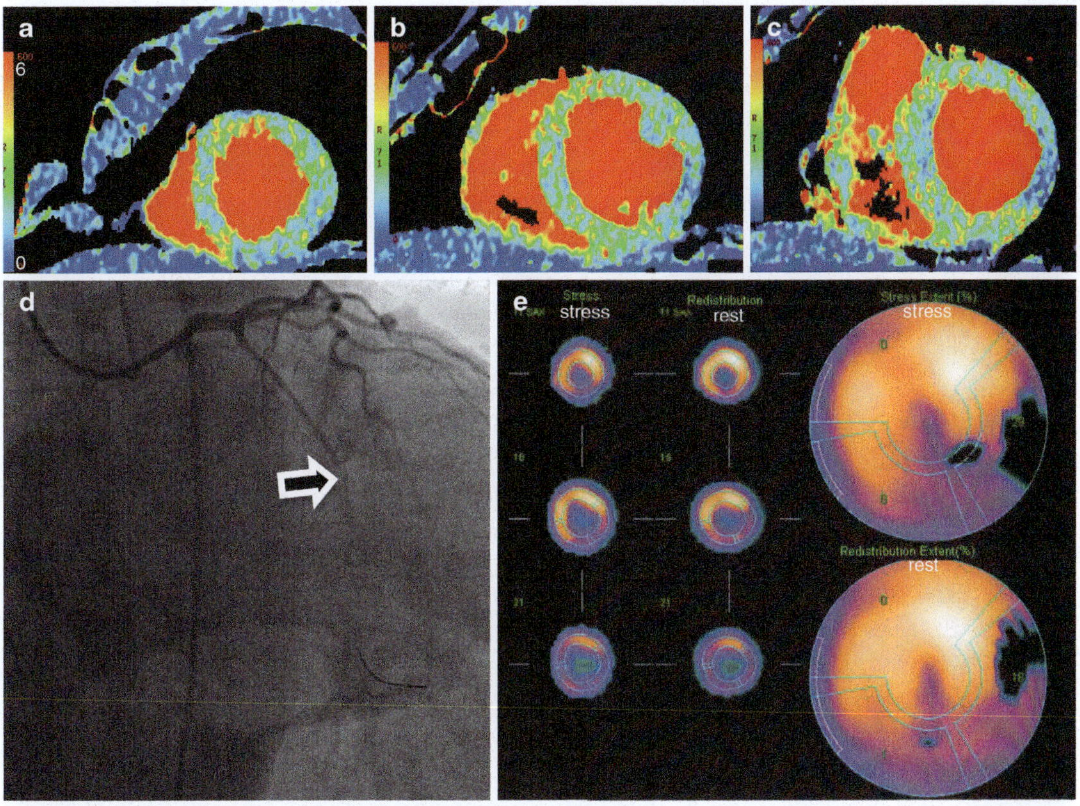

Fig. 20.10 (**a–c**) Stress CT myocardial perfusion maps in the apical, mid, and basal short-axis slices, respectively. The color scale of the CT perfusion maps ranges from 0 (blue) to 6 (red) mL/min/g. (**d**) Invasive coronary angiography revealed a totally occluded obtuse marginal branch of the left circumflex artery (black arrow). (**e**) The SPECT perfusion maps in the short-axis and polar view revealed a perfusion defect in the basal and mid-lateral wall (LCx territory). The CT stress perfusion maps in three short-axis slices (i–iii) also revealed ischemia in the lateral wall in the basal and mid-slices.

cardial perfusion maps reveal functional ischemia in the downstream apical-septal wall that was perfused by the LAD, indicating that the LAD lesions was functionally significant (flow limiting).

While the current clinical applications of cardiac CTP are largely focused on functional assessment of coronary artery lesions, CT measurement of myocardial perfusion can also provide useful diagnostic information regarding the viability status of ischemic myocardium [81–83]. Absence of increase in myocardial blood flow from rest during maximal vasodilatory stress indicates the presence of microvascular obstruction which is a hallmark of tissue infarction [84]. The superior spatial resolution of CTP allows accurate delineation of the myocardial infarct size, which is related to the short- and long-term mortality risk of acute myocardial infarction [85, 86].

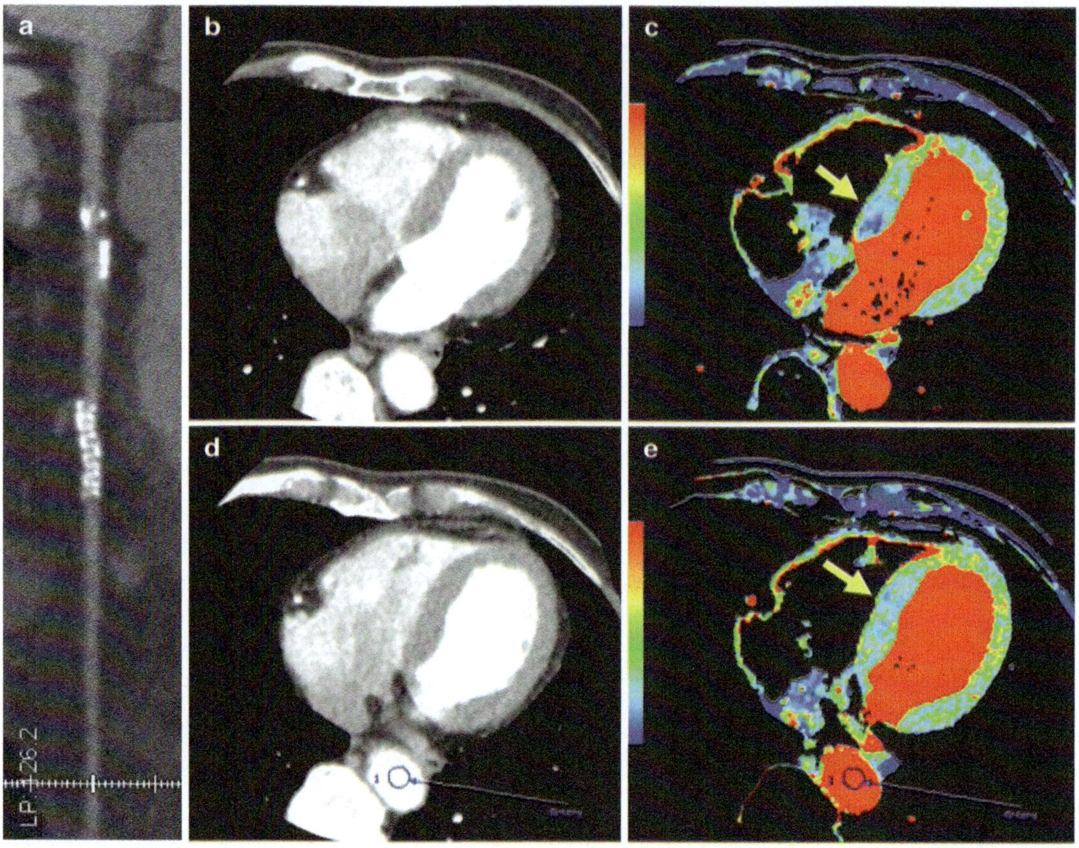

Fig. 20.11 (**a**) Reformatted view of the left anterior descending artery (LAD). (**b**, **d**) Contrast-enhanced CT images in two axial slice locations acquired during maximal pharmacological stress with adenosine infusion. (**c**, **e**) Corresponding stress myocardial perfusion maps. The color scale of these maps ranges from 0 to 3.5 mL/min/g. The stress CT perfusion maps revealed ischemia in the apical-lateral wall of the myocardium (yellow arrows)

Conclusion

This chapter reviews the theoretical basis of dynamic CTP for quantitative myocardial perfusion measurement and the technical issues for clinical implementation of dynamic CTP for functional assessment of coronary artery disease.

References

1. Axel L. Cerebral blood flow determination by rapid-sequence computed tomography: theoretical analysis. Radiology. 1980;137(3):679–86.
2. Obach V, et al. Multimodal CT-assisted thrombolysis in patients with acute stroke: a cohort study. Stroke. 2011;42(4):1129–31.
3. Silvennoinen HM, et al. CT perfusion identifies increased salvage of tissue in patients receiving intravenous recombinant tissue plasminogen activator within 3 hours of stroke onset. AJNR Am J Neuroradiol. 2008;29(6):1118–23.
4. Aviv RI, et al. Alberta stroke program early CT scoring of CT perfusion in early stroke visualization and assessment. AJNR Am J Neuroradiol. 2007;28(10):1975–80.
5. Jain R, et al. First-pass perfusion computed tomography: initial experience in differentiating recurrent brain tumors from radiation effects and radiation necrosis. Neurosurgery. 2007;61(4):778–86; discussion 786–7.
6. Nakashige A, et al. Quantitative measurement of hepatic portal perfusion by multidetector row CT with compensation for respiratory misregistration. Br J Radiol. 2004;77(921):728–34.
7. Meijerink MR, et al. The use of perfusion CT for the evaluation of therapy combining AZD2171 with gefitinib in cancer patients. Eur Radiol. 2007;17(7):1700–13.

8. Jiang T, et al. Monitoring response to antiangiogenic treatment and predicting outcomes in advanced hepatocellular carcinoma using image biomarkers, CT perfusion, tumor density, and tumor size (RECIST). Investig Radiol. 2012;47(1):11–7.
9. George RT, et al. Diagnostic performance of combined noninvasive coronary angiography and myocardial perfusion imaging using 320-MDCT: the CT angiography and perfusion methods of the CORE320 multicenter multinational diagnostic study. AJR Am J Roentgenol. 2011;197(4):829–37.
10. So A, et al. Non-invasive assessment of functionally relevant coronary artery stenoses with quantitative CT perfusion: preliminary clinical experiences. Eur Radiol. 2012;22(1):39–50.
11. Bastarrika G, et al. Adenosine-stress dynamic myocardial CT perfusion imaging: initial clinical experience. Investig Radiol. 2010;45(6):306–13.
12. Ho KT, et al. Stress and rest dynamic myocardial perfusion imaging by evaluation of complete time-attenuation curves with dual-source CT. JACC Cardiovasc Imaging. 2010;3(8):811–20.
13. Prokop M. New challenges in MDCT. Eur Radiol. 2005;15(Suppl 5):E35–45.
14. Page M, et al. Comparison of 4 cm Z-axis and 16 cm Z-axis multidetector CT perfusion. Eur Radiol. 2010;20(6):1508–14.
15. Flohr TG, Raupach R, Bruder H. Cardiac CT: how much can temporal resolution, spatial resolution, and volume coverage be improved? J Cardiovasc Comput Tomogr. 2009;3(3):143–52.
16. Meier P, Zierler KL. On the theory of the indicator-dilution method for measurement of blood flow and volume. J Appl Physiol. 1954;6(12):731–44.
17. Bassingthwaighte JB, Knopp TJ, Anderson DU. Flow estimation by indicator dilution (bolus injection). Circ Res. 1970;27(2):277–91.
18. Pardridge WM, et al. Blood-brain barrier: interface between internal medicine and the brain. Ann Intern Med. 1986;105(1):82–95.
19. Crone C. The permeability of capillaries in various organs as determined by use of the 'indicator diffusion' method. Acta Physiol Scand. 1963;58:292–305.
20. Hamilton WFM, Moore JW, Kinsman JM, Spurling RG. Simultaneous determination of the pulmonary and systemic circulation times in man and of a figure related to cardiac output. Am J Phys. 1928;84:338–44.
21. Stephenson JL. Theory of the measurement of blood flow by the dilution of an indicator. Bull Math Biophys. 1948;10(3):117–21.
22. Gobbel GT, Cann CE, Fike JR. Measurement of regional cerebral blood flow using ultrafast computed tomography. Theoretical aspects. Stroke. 1991;22(6):768–71.
23. Axel L. Tissue mean transit time from dynamic computed tomography by a simple deconvolution technique. Invest Radiol. 1983;18(1):94–9.
24. Yang Y, Rosenberg GA. Blood-brain barrier breakdown in acute and chronic cerebrovascular disease. Stroke. 2011;42(11):3323–8.
25. de Vries HE, et al. The blood-brain barrier in neuroinflammatory diseases. Pharmacol Rev. 1997;49(2):143–55.
26. Mullani NA, Gould KL. First-pass measurements of regional blood flow with external detectors. J Nucl Med. 1983;24(7):577–81.
27. Bindschadler M, et al. Comparison of blood flow models and acquisitions for quantitative myocardial perfusion estimation from dynamic CT. Phys Med Biol. 2014;59(7):1533–56.
28. Ishida M, et al. Underestimation of myocardial blood flow by dynamic perfusion CT: explanations by two-compartment model analysis and limited temporal sampling of dynamic CT. J Cardiovasc Comput Tomogr. 2016;10(3):207–14.
29. Ostergaard L, et al. High resolution measurement of cerebral blood flow using intravascular tracer bolus passages. Part I: mathematical approach and statistical analysis. Magn Reson Med. 1996;36(5):715–25.
30. Wintermark M, et al. Simultaneous measurement of regional cerebral blood flow by perfusion CT and stable xenon CT: a validation study. AJNR Am J Neuroradiol. 2001;22(5):905–14.
31. So A, et al. Technical note: evaluation of a 160-mm/256-row CT scanner for whole-heart quantitative myocardial perfusion imaging. Med Phys. 2016;43(8):4821.
32. Gamel J, et al. Pitfalls in digital computation of the impulse response of vascular beds from indicator-dilution curves. Circ Res. 1973;32(4):516–23.
33. Ostergaard L, et al. High resolution measurement of cerebral blood flow using intravascular tracer bolus passages. Part II: experimental comparison and preliminary results. Magn Reson Med. 1996;36(5):726–36.
34. Groothuis DR, et al. A method to quantitatively measure transcapillary transport of iodinated compounds in canine brain tumors with computed tomography. J Cereb Blood Flow Metab. 1991;11(6):939–48.
35. Groothuis DR, et al. Quantitative measurements of capillary transport in human brain tumors by computed tomography. Ann Neurol. 1991;30(4):581–8.
36. Patlak CS, Blasberg RG, Fenstermacher JD. Graphical evaluation of blood-to-brain transfer constants from multiple-time uptake data. J Cereb Blood Flow Metab. 1983;3(1):1–7.
37. Patlak CS, Blasberg RG. Graphical evaluation of blood-to-brain transfer constants from multiple-time uptake data. Generalizations. J Cereb Blood Flow Metab. 1985;5(4):584–90.
38. St Lawrence KS, Lee TY. An adiabatic approximation to the tissue homogeneity model for water exchange in the brain: I. theoretical derivation. J Cereb Blood Flow Metab. 1998;18(12):1365–77.
39. Gill PE, Murray W, Wright MH. Practical optimization. London: Academic; 1981.
40. Johnson JA, Wilson TA. A model for capillary exchange. Am J Phys. 1966;210(6):1299–303.
41. Ho KT, et al. Dynamic CT myocardial perfusion measurements of resting and hyperaemic blood flow in

low-risk subjects with 128-slice dual-source CT. Eur Heart J Cardiovasc Imaging. 2015;16(3):300–6.
42. Pontone G, et al. Incremental diagnostic value of stress computed tomography myocardial perfusion with whole-heart coverage CT scanner in intermediate- to high-risk symptomatic patients suspected of coronary artery disease. JACC Cardiovasc Imaging. 2019;12(2):338–49.
43. George RT, et al. Computed tomography myocardial perfusion imaging with 320-row detector computed tomography accurately detects myocardial ischemia in patients with obstructive coronary artery disease. Circ Cardiovasc Imaging. 2012;5(3):333–40.
44. Bae KT. Intravenous contrast medium administration and scan timing at CT: considerations and approaches. Radiology. 2010;256(1):32–61.
45. Wintermark M, et al. Dynamic perfusion CT: optimizing the temporal resolution and contrast volume for calculation of perfusion CT parameters in stroke patients. AJNR Am J Neuroradiol. 2004;25(5):720–9.
46. Sahani DV, et al. Advanced hepatocellular carcinoma: CT perfusion of liver and tumor tissue--initial experience. Radiology. 2007;243(3):736–43.
47. Ippolito D, et al. Hepatocellular carcinoma treated with transarterial chemoembolization: dynamic perfusion-CT in the assessment of residual tumor. World J Gastroenterol. 2010;16(47):5993–6000.
48. Claussen CD, et al. Bolus geometry and dynamics after intravenous contrast medium injection. Radiology. 1984;153(2):365–8.
49. Miles KA. Perfusion CT for the assessment of tumour vascularity: which protocol? Br J Radiol. 2003;76(Spec 1):S36–42.
50. Schoellnast H, et al. Aortoiliac enhancement during computed tomography angiography with reduced contrast material dose and saline solution flush: influence on magnitude and uniformity of the contrast column. Investig Radiol. 2004;39(1):20–6.
51. Hopper KD, et al. Thoracic spiral CT: delivery of contrast material pushed with injectable saline solution in a power injector. Radiology. 1997;205(1):269–71.
52. Brooks RA, Di Chiro G. Beam hardening in x-ray reconstructive tomography. Phys Med Biol. 1976;21(3):390–8.
53. Haage P, et al. Reduction of contrast material dose and artifacts by a saline flush using a double power injector in helical CT of the thorax. AJR Am J Roentgenol. 2000;174(4):1049–53.
54. Coursey CA, et al. Dual-energy multidetector CT: how does it work, what can it tell us, and when can we use it in abdominopelvic imaging? Radiographics. 2010;30(4):1037–55.
55. Wintermark M, et al. Using 80 kVp versus 120 kVp in perfusion CT measurement of regional cerebral blood flow. AJNR Am J Neuroradiol. 2000;21(10):1881–4.
56. Shankar JJ, Lum C, Sharma M. Whole-brain perfusion imaging with 320-MDCT scanner: reducing radiation dose by increasing sampling interval. AJR Am J Roentgenol. 2010;195(5):1183–6.
57. McNitt-Gray MF. AAPM/RSNA physics tutorial for residents: topics in CT. Radiation dose in CT. Radiographics. 2002;22(6):1541–53.
58. McCollough CH, Zink FE. Performance evaluation of a multi-slice CT system. Med Phys. 1999;26(11):2223–30.
59. Bamberg F, et al. Accuracy of dynamic computed tomography adenosine stress myocardial perfusion imaging in estimating myocardial blood flow at various degrees of coronary artery stenosis using a porcine animal model. Investig Radiol. 2012;47(1):71–7.
60. Greif M, et al. CT stress perfusion imaging for detection of haemodynamically relevant coronary stenosis as defined by FFR. Heart. 2013;99(14):1004–11.
61. Lee TY, Chhem RK. Impact of new technologies on dose reduction in CT. Eur J Radiol. 2010;76(1):28–35.
62. Roberts HC, et al. Multisection dynamic CT perfusion for acute cerebral ischemia: the "toggling-table" technique. AJNR Am J Neuroradiol. 2001;22(6):1077–80.
63. Wiesmann M, et al. Dose reduction in dynamic perfusion CT of the brain: effects of the scan frequency on measurements of cerebral blood flow, cerebral blood volume, and mean transit time. Eur Radiol. 2008;18(12):2967–74.
64. Primak AN, et al. A technical solution to avoid partial scan artifacts in cardiac MDCT. Med Phys. 2007;34(12):4726–37.
65. Meinel JA, et al. Reduction of half-scan shading artifact based on full-scan correction. Acad Radiol. 2006;13(1):55–62.
66. Eldevik K, Nordhoy W, Skretting A. Relationship between sharpness and noise in CT images reconstructed with different kernels. Radiat Prot Dosim. 2010;139(1–3):430–3.
67. Jia X, et al. GPU-based fast low-dose cone beam CT reconstruction via total variation. J Xray Sci Technol. 2011;19(2):139–54.
68. Chou CY, et al. A fast forward projection using multithreads for multirays on GPUs in medical image reconstruction. Med Phys. 2011;38(7):4052–65.
69. Yan H, et al. Towards the clinical implementation of iterative low-dose cone-beam CT reconstruction in image-guided radiation therapy: cone/ring artifact correction and multiple GPU implementation. Med Phys. 2014;41(11):111912.
70. Thibault JB, et al. A three-dimensional statistical approach to improved image quality for multislice helical CT. Med Phys. 2007;34(11):4526–44.
71. Candes EJ, Romberg J, Tao T. Robust uncertainty principles: exact signal reconstruction from highly incomplete frequency information. Inform Theor IEEE Trans. 2006;52(2):489–509.
72. Donoho DL. Compressed sensing. Inform Theor IEEE Trans. 2006;52(4):1289–306.
73. Lauzier PT, Tang J, Chen GH. Prior image constrained compressed sensing: implementation and performance evaluation. Med Phys. 2012;39(1):66–80.
74. LaRoque SJ, Sidky EY, Pan X. Accurate image reconstruction from few-view and limited-angle data in dif-

fraction tomography. J Opt Soc Am A Opt Image Sci Vis. 2008;25(7):1772–82.
75. Enjilela E, et al. Ultra-low dose quantitative CT myocardial perfusion imaging with sparse-view dynamic acquisition and image reconstruction: a feasibility study. Int J Cardiol. 2018;254:272–81.
76. Chen GH, Tang J, Leng S. Prior image constrained compressed sensing (PICCS): a method to accurately reconstruct dynamic CT images from highly undersampled projection data sets. Med Phys. 2008;35(2):660–3.
77. Budoff MJ, et al. Diagnostic performance of 64-multidetector row coronary computed tomographic angiography for evaluation of coronary artery stenosis in individuals without known coronary artery disease: results from the prospective multicenter ACCURACY (assessment by coronary computed tomographic angiography of individuals undergoing invasive coronary angiography) trial. J Am Coll Cardiol. 2008;52(21):1724–32.
78. Meijboom WB, et al. Diagnostic accuracy of 64-slice computed tomography coronary angiography: a prospective, multicenter, multivendor study. J Am Coll Cardiol. 2008;52(25):2135–44.
79. van Werkhoven JM, et al. Prognostic value of multislice computed tomography and gated single-photon emission computed tomography in patients with suspected coronary artery disease. J Am Coll Cardiol. 2009;53(7):623–32.
80. Gould KL. Does coronary flow trump coronary anatomy? JACC Cardiovasc Imaging. 2009;2(8):1009–23.
81. Hoffmann U, et al. Acute myocardial infarction: contrast-enhanced multi-detector row CT in a porcine model. Radiology. 2004;231(3):697–701.
82. Rogers IS, et al. Comparison of postprocessing techniques for the detection of perfusion defects by cardiac computed tomography in patients presenting with acute ST-segment elevation myocardial infarction. J Cardiovasc Comput Tomogr. 2010;4(4):258–66.
83. Camici PG, Rimoldi OE. The clinical value of myocardial blood flow measurement. J Nucl Med. 2009;50(7):1076–87.
84. Orn S, et al. Microvascular obstruction is a major determinant of infarct healing and subsequent left ventricular remodelling following primary percutaneous coronary intervention. Eur Heart J. 2009;30(16):1978–85.
85. Miller TD, et al. Infarct size after acute myocardial infarction measured by quantitative tomographic 99mTc sestamibi imaging predicts subsequent mortality. Circulation. 1995;92(3):334–41.
86. Burns RJ, et al. The relationships of left ventricular ejection fraction, end-systolic volume index and infarct size to six-month mortality after hospital discharge following myocardial infarction treated by thrombolysis. J Am Coll Cardiol. 2002;39(1):30–6.

Part VII

Special Purpose CT

CT in Musculoskeletal Applications 21

Wojciech B. Zbijewski

Role of Radiography and CT in Musculoskeletal Radiology

Musculoskeletal (MSK) radiology is concerned with a wide variety of pathologies, including trauma, deformity and malalignment, and chronic disease, in particular osteoporosis and various forms of arthritis. The burden of musculoskeletal disease is significant, and likely to rise given the aging of the population and the increasing rates of obesity. For example, there are approximately 5.6 million fractures per year in the USA, and as many as 10% of them show protracted healing [1], often requiring multiple surgeries and leading to prolonged disability. The prevalence of osteoporosis (OP) in the US population is estimated at ~10 million cases [2], approximately 30 million US adults are suffering from osteoarthritis (OA), 1.5 million have rheumatoid arthritis (RA), and ~8 million are suffering from gout. Across the whole spectrum of MSK disease, there is still a need for new biomarkers for early detection and treatment monitoring. Improved imaging technologies are likely to be essential in the development of such new biomarkers, enhancing the already substantial role that radiology plays in the current MSK standard of care.

W. B. Zbijewski (✉)
Department of Biomedical Engineering, Johns Hopkins University, Baltimore, MD, USA
e-mail: wzbijewski@jhu.edu

MSK diagnosis involves all major imaging modalities, with conventional CT and MRI used predominately in more complex pathologies. Projectional x-ray radiography remains the mainstay of MSK radiology, especially for first-order assessment [3]. The advantages of radiography in this setting include simplified logistics, high spatial resolution (although limited by tissue superposition), and the ability to image under weight-bearing and in stress positions. The latter two features are extremely valuable, considering that one of the primary roles of the MSK system is locomotion. Radiography thus provides an important functional imaging capability that is not readily available with conventional multidetector CT (MDCT) or MRI.

The need to provide functional information, involving weight-bearing, stress, or even motion, is one of the unique considerations for development of MSK imaging technologies. Another important aspect of MSK radiology is its quantitative character. The measurements of interest extend from macroscopic metrics of bone and joint morphology to quantification of trabecular and cortical microstructure and bone composition. Examples of morphological measurements include a variety of anatomical metrics of the knee (e.g., tibial slopes, static alignment) and the foot (e.g., calcaneal inclination angle) [4]. Many of those metrics have originally been defined using radiographs but are now being translated to volumetric imaging due to the increasing access

© Springer Nature Switzerland AG 2020

E. Samei, N. J. Pelc (eds.), *Computed Tomography*, https://doi.org/10.1007/978-3-030-26957-9_21

to 3D modalities and the obvious benefit of avoiding anatomical overlap [5].

Among the microscopic and compositional measurements, bone mineral density (BMD) is well recognized in assessment of bone loss in, e.g., osteoporosis. BMD can be obtained either as aerial BMD, (aBMD) from projectional dual-energy x-ray absorptiometry, or as volumetric BMD (vBMD) from quantitative CT (qCT). Here again, the lack of anatomical overlap is a significant advantage of CT, mitigating biases due to bone size (integrated thickness) and providing the capability to separately analyze the cortical and trabecular compartments [6]. The extent to which vBMD improves prediction of fractures compared to aBMD remains a subject of clinical studies, with current evidence pointing to superior performance in vertebral fractures, but potentially no significant benefit in hip fractures [6]. Independent of whether aBMD or vBMD is used, it is estimated that only approximately 70% of variation in bone strength can be explained using those metrics [7]. The likely reason is that BMD is a cumulative measurement that combines bone quantity, i.e., the amount of mineralized tissue in a macroscopic region of interest (ROI), and bone quality. The latter term encompasses mineralization and microstructure of the bone inside the ROI. However, direct in vivo evaluation of cortical and trabecular microarchitecture is challenging because of the small size of the features of interest – e.g., the average thickness of the trabeculae is approximately 100–150 μm [8], 2–3× smaller than the spatial resolution of conventional CT. A specialized investigational high-resolution peripheral quantitative CT (HR-pQCT) scanner (XtremeCT, Scanco Medical AG) has been developed to enable measurements of bone microarchitecture in humans [9]. By incorporating a similar imaging chain as in μCT (low-power microfocus x-ray source and a CCD detector), the newest generation of HR-pQCT achieves approximately 60 μm spatial resolution [10]. The primary drawback of this design is that the low-power tube and small detector pixels lead to noise considerations that limit size of the object that can be imaged. HR-pQCT is thus restricted to the peripheral skeleton.

The overview of MSK applications of x-ray imaging modalities points to complementary roles of radiography and MDCT. Advantages of radiography include low cost, easy access, and the capability for examination under weight-bearing. The first two benefits are not only valuable in prompt assessment of MSK trauma but also greatly simplify the logistics of longitudinal follow-up in, e.g., fracture healing. Weight-bearing imaging is routinely used in assessment of malalignment and in evaluation of joint space width in OA [11]. Slowing of radiographically determined joint space narrowing is an FDA-recommended structural outcome measure for clinical trials of OA treatments [12].

Conventional MDCT lacks the capability for weight-bearing imaging and is associated with higher cost and more complex logistics than radiography. Benefits of CT include soft-tissue contrast and the lack of anatomical overlap. Volumetric imaging improves detection of subtle abnormalities, reduces the impact of patient positioning, and has the potential to yield more accurate quantification of joint alignment, bone morphology, and bone quality, as discussed above.

Considering the important role of weight-bearing examination in MSK radiology, there is a compelling case for the development of a system that combines 3D assessment provided by CT with weight-bearing imaging. This objective has been realized with the introduction of a variety of musculoskeletal flat-panel detector (FPD) cone-beam CT (CBCT) scanners. As with dedicated CBCT for other diagnostic applications (dental, otolaryngology [13], breast [14]), the benefits of MSK CBCT extend beyond weight-bearing acquisitions and include relatively low-cost, small-footprint, and low-power requirements compatible with in-office use, as well as lower imaging dose and higher spatial resolution than current conventional CT. In the remainder of this chapter, we will discuss the design, imaging performance, clinical applications, and new diagnostic capabilities provided by weight-bearing MSK CBCT. We will focus on CBCT scanners for extremity imaging, which have enjoyed a significant growth over the past decade. For other aspects of CBCT, see Chap. 2. The last subsection will provide an overview of other emerging technologies in MSK CT: CBCT for weight-bearing imaging of spine and hips and ultra-high resolution MDCT.

Development of Specialized Cone-Beam CT for Musculoskeletal Extremities

Early efforts to reduce the effects of anatomical overlap in weight-bearing x-ray examinations of the extremities involved the application of tomosynthesis [15], followed by implementation of fully 3D imaging using appropriately adapted radiographic/fluoroscopic C-arms [16]. The latter line of research continues using robotic interventional C-arms [17] and ceiling-mounted robotic x-ray systems [18]. In parallel with the work employing general purpose C-arms, CBCT systems designed specifically for weight-bearing extremity imaging were being introduced. Current reports of clinical applications of such extremity CBCT scanners are predominately based on three scanner configurations: Planmed Verity (Planmed Oy, Helsinki, Finland) [19, 20], Carestream OnSight3D (Fig. 21.1, Carestream Health, Rochester NY) [21, 22], and CurveBeam PedCat (CurveBeam, Hatfield PA) [23, 24]. Below, we review the major aspects of those three designs.

All three extremity CBCT systems utilize an FPD and a relatively compact gantry. The relatively low weight (approximately 5 kg for a 25 × 30 cm panel) and small form factor of FPD (thickness of 50–100 mm) were crucial in enabling imaging in a weight-bearing configuration. The Planmed Verity and Carestream OnSight3D systems feature a tilting gantry that can be configured either in a horizontal orientation for upright imaging or in a vertical orientation for unloaded scans of lower and upper extremities. The OnSight gantry enables weight-bearing acquisitions in a natural standing stance (both feet on the ground, approximately 35 cm

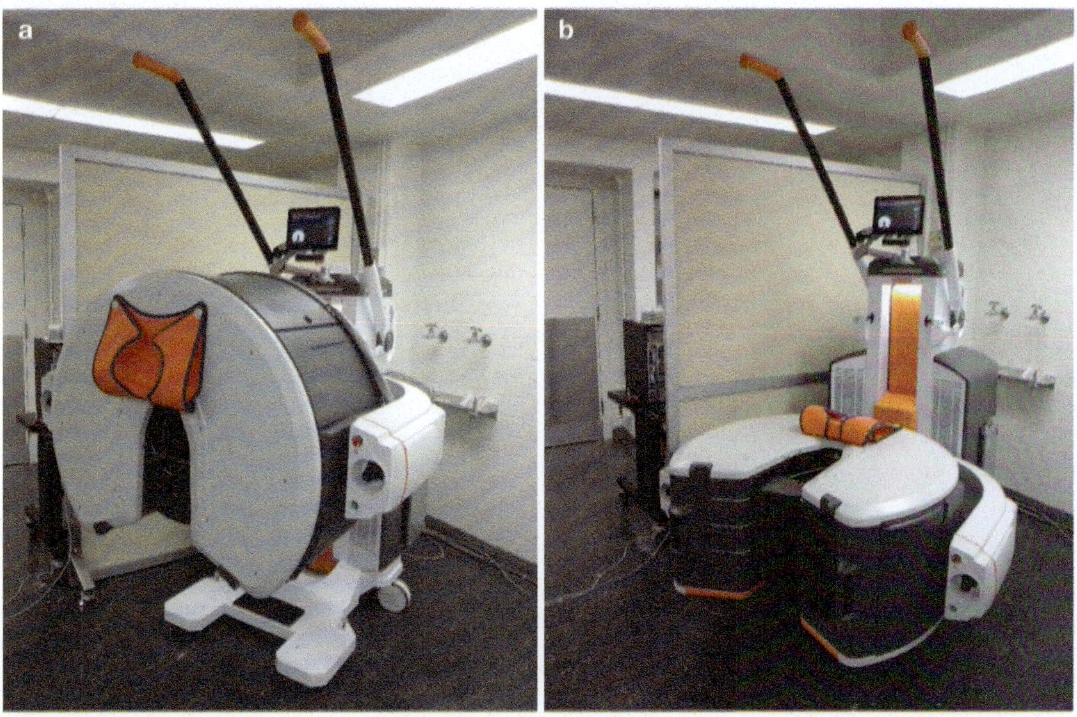

Fig. 21.1 Extremity CBCT (Carestream OnSight3D) in a sitting configuration for imaging of non-weight-bearing upper and lower extremity (**a**) and in a standing configuration for weight-bearing scans (**b**)

distance between the centers of the knees), whereas in the Verity system, the contralateral leg is resting on the gantry. The OnSight3D and Verity scanners can be applied to both the lower and upper extremities but permit only unilateral scans. In contrast, the PedCat was designed for bilateral acquisitions, but only of the feet (recently, CurveBeam has introduced a new system with knee imaging capability). Despite all those differences, extremity CBCT systems share many common engineering solutions and deliver comparable image quality. The following discussion of technical implementation of extremity CBCT will be based on the OnSight scanner (Fig. 21.1).

The imaging chain of OnSight extremity CBCT consists of a compact fixed-anode x-ray source with 0.5 mm nominal focal spot and a 25×30 cm amorphous silicon (aSi) FPD with an approximately 600-μm-thick CsI scintillator. The native detector pixel size is 139 μm, but the acquisitions are typically performed in a 2×2 binned mode for speed and x-ray detection efficiency. Because a fixed-anode source is used, the x-ray power is limited to approximately 1 kW. The tube is typically operated in a pulsed mode, synchronized with detector readout. The scanner geometry involved approximately 55 cm source-detector distance and magnification factor of approximately 1.3, resulting in almost equal balance between the effects of source and detector blur [21].

A sickle-shaped arm supports the source and detector. During the tomographic acquisition, the arm rotates on a mechanical track inside the scanner bore. Patient setup is performed with the scanner arm positioned so that its opening coincides with an opening in the bore, providing an entry into the gantry. After the patient inserts the extremity into the gantry, a door is closed to isolate the rotating parts during the scan. For a lower-extremity scan, the subject is thus straddling the door while maintaining a natural weight-bearing stance. This scan setup is made possible by the relatively narrow envelope of the FPD, which allows it to slide between patient legs during the rotation of the arm. Conventional fixed-anode x-ray sources are typically too wide to fit in the same manner, and thus the rotation is limited to the short scan range of approximately 220°. The scan time is approximately 20 s and the reconstructed field of view is on the order of $20 \times 20 \times 20$ cm^3. Gantry covers are lined with lead to provide self-shielding, simplifying radiation protection requirements for the scanner room.

The radiation dose delivered by extremity CBCT is typically lower than MDCT operating an extremity imaging protocol. This is partly due to the cone-beam geometry, permitting volumetric coverage without beam overlap often present in helical MDCT. In a series of comprehensive studies using MOSFET dosimeters embedded in anthropomorphic phantoms [25, 26], Koivisto et al. found effective doses of ~20 μSv for MDCT, 6 μSv for Verity extremity CBCT, and approximately 1 μSv for radiography in foot and ankle imaging. For the knee, the results were 27–48 μSv for MDCT, 13 μSv for Verity CBCT, and also approximately 1 μSv for radiography. Even though the absolute dose values reported for various extremity CBCT embodiments differ depending on the imaging technique and measurement protocols, the general trend toward 2–3x lower radiation exposure with CBCT is well established [20–22, 25, 27]. However, results of such comparative studies should be interpreted in caution. First, the imaging dose of MDCT protocols for extremity imaging can likely be decreased with further task-based optimization of x-ray techniques and model-based reconstruction. Second, even in situations where higher dose might be desirable from the diagnostic perspective, CBCT is restricted by inherent limitations of the imaging chain: the use of the low-power x-ray tubes and the compact system geometry that may lead to detector saturation at higher x-ray outputs. Third, the differences in beam shape, scan coverage (e.g., unilateral vs. bilateral imaging), and acquisition orbit (e.g., short vs. full rotation) between different models of extremity CBCT and between CBCT and MDCT make direct comparisons of various indices of imaging dose difficult. One example of challenges in achieving standardized CBCT dosimetry is the highly nonuniform, asymmetric dose distribution for the 220°

scanning arc of the OnSight system, with almost 8× higher local dose at peripheral sites close to the midpoint of the orbit compared to locations near scanner door [22]. Finally, it needs to be noted that distal extremities are not considered highly radiosensitive, with an organ-specific weighting factor of 0.0005 mSv/mGy cm [28]. While any examination involving radiation must be performed in a manner that minimizes patient exposure to the lowest acceptable level for the diagnostic task, the relatively low radiosensitivity of the extremities might permit development of CBCT protocols with somewhat higher doses than those discussed above. This might be necessary to support new applications of extremity CBCT, such as high-resolution imaging of bone microstructure.

Technical assessment of image quality in extremity CBCT revealed two general characteristics of this technology: somewhat better spatial resolution than MDCT and somewhat worse (but still sufficient for diagnosis) contrast resolution. The improved spatial resolution is largely due to the use of an FPD with 100–250 μm pixels. Minimal resolvable line-pair frequency of 17 lp/cm for the native detector pixel readout and 15 lp/cm for 2×2 binned readout have been reported for the OnSight system [22]. Clinical imaging protocols typically employ 2×2 binning because of the approximately 2× faster scan time compared to a full-resolution acquisition (40–60 s for a 1×1 scan compared to 20 s for a 2×2 scan).

The technical factors that affect contrast resolution of extremity CBCT include the limited x-ray output of the compact, low-power sources typical in those systems, and the quantum efficiency and electronic noise of the FPDs. Nevertheless, optimized x-ray techniques were found to deliver signal difference-to-noise ratios (SDNRs) of approximately three for differentiation of water and adipose [22]. As discussed below, such optimized protocols also provide adequate visualization of tendons.

Observer studies of CBCT image quality in clinical tasks confirm the performance characteristics discussed above. Extremity CBCT is generally found to deliver better bone visualization than MDCT, owing to the improved spatial resolution. In soft-tissue imaging, CBCT is somewhat inferior to MDCT but still satisfactory for typical diagnostic tasks. An expert observer study with 20 cadavers (10 hands and 10 knees) has been reported for the OnSight3D system [27]. Performance was evaluated for tendon, cartilage, muscle, and fat visualization (soft-tissue tasks) and for assessment of medullary bone, cortical bone, and fracture (bone tasks). MDCT and CBCT were compared using a five-point diagnostic satisfaction scale, obtained individually for each modality, and a five-point preference scale in side-by-side comparisons. In terms of diagnostic satisfaction, CBCT was rated "excellent" for bone visualization and "good" to "adequate" for soft tissues. MDCT satisfaction was "excellent" for both types of tasks. Preference tests indicated slight preference for MDCT in soft tissues and a tendency toward higher preference for CBCT in the bone (although the median score across all tasks was "no preference" for either modality). As mentioned earlier, the slightly lower performance of CBCT in low-contrast tasks can be at least partly attributed to inherent dose limitations; MDCT was operated at 2–3× higher dose than the power limit of CBCT. Similar findings were reported in a study of 50 human subjects using the Verity extremity CBCT [20]. Two readers found CBCT to deliver greater bone detail than MDCT in the majority of examined cases. In one case, CBCT revealed a fracture line that was not visible in MDCT. Soft-tissue image quality was somewhat better in MDCT, but the difference in low-contrast performance did not affect the diagnosis.

Artifacts and Corrections in Extremity CBCT

Extremity CBCT is prone to the same imaging artifacts as other CBCT scanner configurations. Among the most deleterious factors is x-ray scatter, which leads to loss of contrast and image nonuniformity in the form of cupping and streaks. Furthermore, scatter-induced artifacts affect quantitative accuracy of the reconstructed attenuation values, which diminishes the feasibility of using CBCT for BMD measurements. However, recent progress in scatter correction methods resulted in a variety of approaches that yield a robust and nearly complete removal of the artifacts and incur only modest costs in processing time.

Among the algorithmic methods that do not require any hardware modifications, application of accelerated Monte Carlo (MC) scatter correction to extremity CBCT has been reported [29, 30]. Here, a scatter estimate is obtained from a MC simulation performed using a first-pass reconstruction. To reduce the computational burden of MC, a GPU implementation with variance reduction techniques is used [31, 32]. Furthermore, scatter is estimated only for a subset of projections (every 5–10°), and only a relatively low number of photons (on the order of 10^5) is tracked per projection. Since MC obeys Poisson statistics, the outcome of such a low-count simulation is noisy. Kernel denoising is thus applied to yield the final noiseless estimates which are interpolated for the missing projections. This approach has been shown to yield robust scatter correction in a variety of CBCT applications, with typical runtimes of 10 min or less per scan (for three iterations of MC estimation), with further acceleration possible using multiple GPU configurations [33]. In extremity CBCT, the MC-based approach was shown to reduce shading artifacts and restore soft-tissue contrast to a level similar to a reference image obtained with thin collimation and thus minimized scatter [30].

A number of other algorithmic scatter correction methods have been proposed for CBCT, including kernel-based estimation [34], fast analytical solvers of the Boltzmann transport equation [35], and the use of deep convolutional neural networks to predict scatter projections [36]. All those previously published and validated algorithms are likely applicable to extremity CBCT. Overall, while scatter is still a significant image degradation factor, its effects can be managed fairly efficiently with recent advances in correction and mitigation strategies.

Considering other sources of artifacts, two effects deserve a more detailed discussion in the context of extremity CBCT: cone-beam artifacts and patient motion. Because of the incompleteness of the circular CBCT scan orbit, the structures that are perpendicular to the axis of rotation and located off the central plane suffer from streaking and shading known as a cone-beam artifact. In extremity imaging, the articular surfaces are typically arranged in this unfavorable manner. This leads to degraded image quality around the joint spaces, which are often the primary target for examination using extremity CBCT [22]. In an effort to mitigate such artifacts, one of the commercially available scanners (OnSight3D) implements a custom-designed multi-source x-ray tube [37]. Three x-ray sources are arranged axially (along the longitudinal direction) with approximately 13 cm spacing between them. Each of the sources provides an axial region of adequate 3D sampling centered on its central ray (the ray that is perpendicular to the axis of rotation). By combining the data from the three x-ray beams, areas of poor sampling of one source are compensated by the improved sampling of the same region provided by an adjacent beam [37]. This leads to appreciable reduction in streaking artifacts, improved visualization of the joint spaces, and extended axial field-of-view compared to a single-source design. Following up on our earlier discussion of CBCT dosimetry, it needs to be noted that the multi-source configuration yields a fairly complex, nonuniform dose distribution, underscoring the need for development of new dosimetric standards and indices for CBCT imaging.

Extremity CBCT is susceptible to motion artifacts because the data are acquired in a weight-bearing patient configuration, and the scan times are relatively slow (20–30 s) [20]. In clinical practice, cushions and other light immobilization are frequently deployed inside the scanner bore to minimize patient motion. This preventive approach is often adequate: we found moderate-to-severe motion artifacts in less than 10% of extremity CBCT scans out of a sample of almost 300 weight-bearing and non-weight-bearing datasets [38]. When considering only weight-bearing acquisitions, the incidence of motion artifacts was 14%. However, in cases when motion is present, the resulting degradation in image quality is often severe enough to warrant a re-scan. In such cases, algorithmic compensation strategies are desirable to avoid additional imaging. Other scenarios that might benefit from motion compensation include extremity imaging on open-gantry C-arm systems, where immobilization is more challenging than in closed-bore extremity CBCT, and in applications requiring very high spatial resolution, where even minor motions might be detrimental.

Motion compensation in extremity CBCT has been demonstrated using algorithms based on (a) skin fiducials [39, 40], (b) 3D-2D registration of a motion-free prior image [17], (c) Fourier consistency conditions [41], and (d) autofocus methods [38, 42]. The latter approach involves using a metric of regional image sharpness as an objective function for motion estimation under the assumption that motion causes blur. All algorithms described above were shown to be capable of achieving some degree of compensation in the setting of extremity imaging. However, only the Fourier consistency-based algorithm and the autofocus approach do not require any modifications to the workflow such as fiducials or prior scans. The autofocus method confers the advantage of being directly applicable to regional correction, i.e., it can be used to compensate local motion in an ROI. This capability is useful for cases involving joint flexion or extension, where global correction might require a complex deformable motion model. It is unclear whether Fourier consistency conditions can also be used for regional correction.

In summary, extremity CBCT images affected by motion can often be restored to diagnostic quality by means of a compensation algorithm. For example, in a study of motion-contaminated scans acquired on the OnSight scanner, we found that the fraction of cases scored better than "fair" on a diagnostic satisfaction scale increased from less than 10% prior to autofocus compensation to 40–70% (depending on the visualization task) after the compensation [38].

Overall, recent developments in artifact correction algorithms have resulted in tremendous progress in CBCT image quality. Extremity CBCT has benefitted from those technical advances, which are now enabling a host of new clinical applications.

Current and Emerging Clinical Applications of Extremity CBCT

Extremity CBCT is a new imaging modality that still requires careful clinical studies to establish its diagnostic performance in orthopedic medicine. Recent years have seen a significant growth in such studies, in particular evaluating the benefits of volumetric weight-bearing imaging for various conditions in the knee and foot and ankle. Increasing interest in this topic among the clinical community led to the formation of the International Weight-Bearing CT Society [43].

Early clinical studies of extremity CBCT provided comparisons with radiography, which remains the mainstay of orthopedic radiology. The primary goal here was to understand the benefits of 3D information in settings which traditionally relied on projectional imaging. The focus of those comparisons was in assessment of fracture. CBCT was found to achieve 2× improved identification of complex fractures compared to radiography [44]. In another study, the Verity extremity CBCT system was deemed superior to radiography in 50% of hand fractures and 30% of ankle fractures, as well as in over 50% of fractures with hardware (irrespective of the site) [20]. Improved diagnostic satisfaction in assessment of fracture healing in the presence of metal was also shown using the OnSight3D scanner and visual grading characteristics analysis [45].

In the recent years, there has been an increasing number of studies investigating various applications of volumetric weight-bearing imaging enabled by extremity CBCT. Most of the activity is concentrated in diagnosis of the foot and ankle [46, 47]. Because extremity CBCT is a new modality, there is still a need for standardization of anatomical measurements used to evaluate joint alignment using volumetric weight-bearing data. Currently, most of the metrics are directly adapted from radiography, but 3D-specific measurements are being proposed [48, 49]. Normal and pathological ranges and reference values for the anatomical parameters need to be established [50, 51] before the metrics can be used diagnostically. Another active area of research involves identification of joint alignment parameters that show significant difference between weight-bearing and non-weight-bearing and investigation of whether those differences might correlate with disease. Such efforts have been reported both in the knee [52, 53] and in foot and ankle studies [54–58]. Other examples of potential value of weight-bearing include conditions were the difference in certain anatomical features between control and disease groups becomes more apparent under load than in non-weight-bearing, as in evaluation of hallux valgus [59] and meniscal extrusion in knee OA [60, 61]. In OA, extremity CBCT has also been shown to yield better sensitivity and specificity in detection of cysts and osteophytes compared to radiography [62].

The clinical publications summarized above illustrate the breadth of activity associated with updating current diagnostic standards to utilize the newly available volumetric information provided by extremity CBCT. This effort will surely continue in the years to come, since long-term follow-up of large patient cohorts is often essential to establishing the clinical value of new metrics and procedures. We will now turn our attention to recent technical developments that aim to further expand the range of applications of extremity CBCT. The discussion below will focus on two areas: automated image analysis to support orthopedic diagnosis and quantitative imaging of bone microstructure and composition.

The three-dimensional information provided by extremity CBCT may enhance the accuracy of various anatomical measurements by removing the effects of tissue superposition associated with radiography. At the same time, analysis of CBCT images places additional burden on the operator, who must now contend with larger and much more complex search space when looking for features of interest. This might affect the inter- and intra-reader variability of anatomical metrics, which often rely on manually identified landmarks (see Fig. 21.2a) for an example of a landmark-based tibial slope measurement that was directly adapted from radiography to 3D imaging). Consequently, there is a need for automatic systems to perform the measurements. One way to achieve this goal is to automatically local-

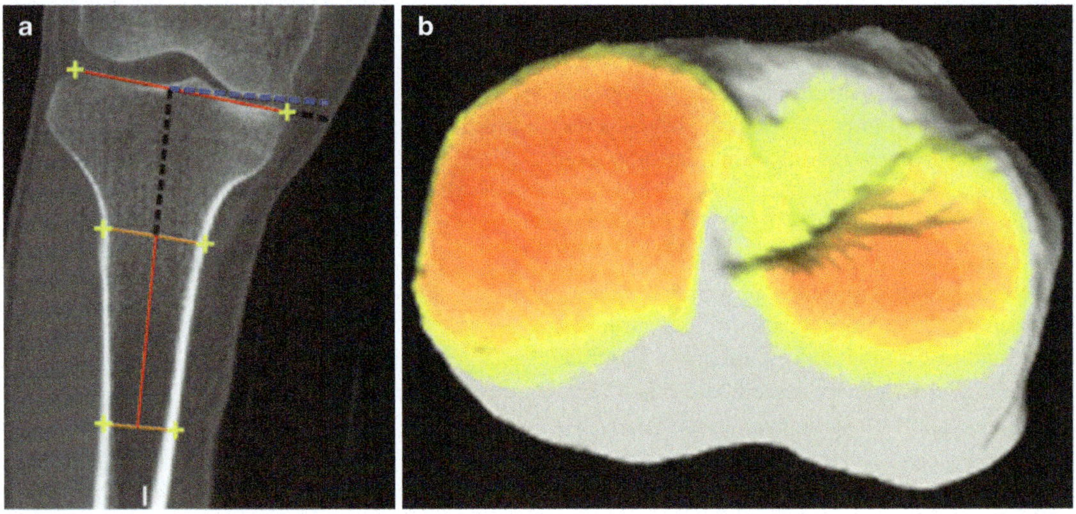

Fig. 21.2 The emergence of specialized extremity CBCT systems motivates interest in development of anatomical measurements for quantitative assessment of joint alignment in 3D weight-bearing images. (**a**) A landmark-based measurement of tibial slope that was directly translated from 2D radiography. (**b**) A joint space map designed specifically to take advantage of the rich 3D information provided by musculoskeletal CBCT

ize the landmarks required by the measurements. This can be done by using geometric feature detection [63, 64] or by employing an atlas set of training images that have been annotated by expert readers. The expert landmarks are then transferred from the atlas set onto the target image using image registration [65, 66]. In application to extremity CBCT, high correlations with expert users were found for metrics of the tibiofemoral joint using atlas-based automatic measurements [66].

Another application of extremity CBCT that might benefit from application of advanced image analysis is assessment of joint space width in OA. As described earlier in the chapter, weight-bearing radiography is conventionally used to evaluate joint space narrowing. This approach is somewhat susceptible to biases due to tissue overlap that make identification of the corresponding regions on the opposing articular surfaces difficult. Weight-bearing CBCT provides the opportunity to examine local variations in joint space width across the entire articular surface. To fully benefit from this new 3D information, it is desirable to develop solutions for statistical examination of spatial patterns of joint space narrowing (as opposed to reducing the complex 3D data to a few local or regional measurements). To this end, maps of local distance between the articular surfaces need to be first created. However, a variety of definitions of this local distance are possible. For example, Segal et al. created joint space maps (JSMs) of the knee from extremity CBCT data by finding the shortest distance to the femur for each point on the surface of the tibia [67, 68]. Using this approach, they demonstrated that projectional measurements systematically underestimate joint space width in any sagittal plane through the medial tibial plateau [67]. However, such closest point measurement is not necessarily unique (multiple points on the tibia might be mapped onto the same point on the femur) or symmetric (JSMs might depend on whether they were computed from tibia to femur or vice versa). To overcome such limitations, an algorithm based on an electrostatic model of the joint was proposed [69]. Here, a unique and symmetric mapping is obtained by considering the two articular surfaces as two plates of a capacitor and measuring the length of the field lines between them (see Fig. 21.2b) for an example of an JSM created using this approach). By combining this approach with Principal Component Analysis of the resulting JSMs and a Support Vector Machines classifier, improved detection of OA was achieved in extremity CBCT data compared to a simple point measurement (namely, the closest tibiofemoral distance in the medial joint compartment).

The applications discussed above were primarily concerned with bone and joint macrostructure. Along the same lines, in imaging of bone microstructure, extremity CBCT provides a compelling platform for development of new clinical capabilities. As discussed earlier in the chapter, such analysis is typically performed using specialized high-resolution peripheral CT systems developed specifically for research applications. Conventionally, the data obtained from such devices is first segmented (binarized) into bone voxels and surrounding tissue. The binary images of the bone are then subject to mathematical processing to obtain maps of local indices of microstructure, e.g., trabecular thickness (Tb.Th), trabecular spacing (Tb.Sp), and bone volume/total volume fraction (BV/TV). The accuracy of such measurements depends on the quality of the initial binarization, which requires high spatial resolution. The improved resolution of FPDs compared to MDCT detectors spurred interest in examining the performance of extremity CBCT in imaging of bone microstructure. While absolute agreement with gold standard micro-CT (which delivers resolution on the order of 10 μm, but is only available for ex vivo samples and small animals) could not be achieved, correlations of 0.93 for BV/TV, 0.89 for Tb.Th, and 0.91 for Tb.Sp were reported using a CBCT binarization algorithm that combined local segmentation and pre-thresholding [70].

To further advance spatial resolution of extremity CBCT and enable improved quantification of bone microstructure, recent studies have proposed replacing the FPD with a CMOS detector. Due to the use of crystalline silicon and active pixel design with on-pixel amplification,

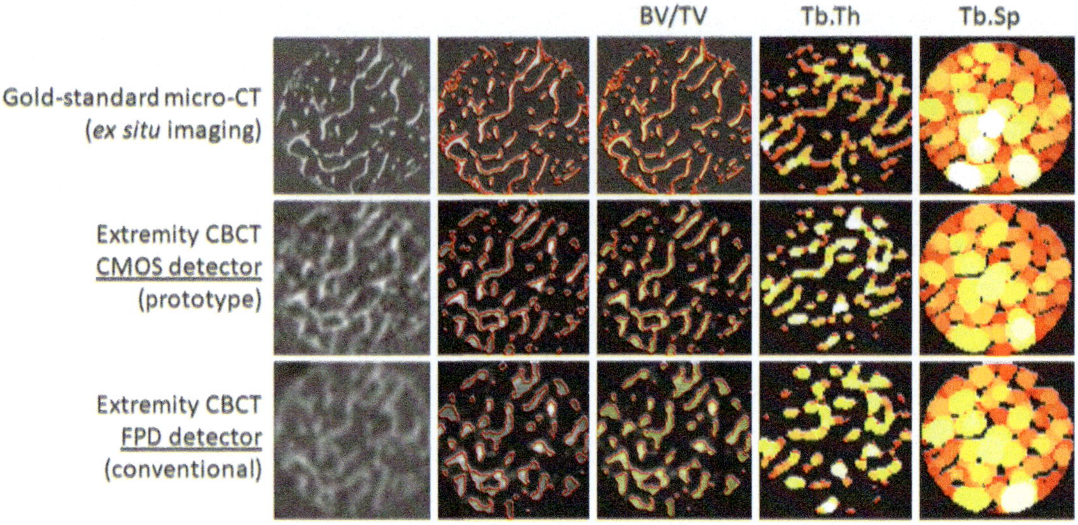

Fig. 21.3 The application of a CMOS detector in a prototype high-resolution extremity CBCT (center row) enhanced the visualization of cancellous bone compared to conventional CBCT with an FPD detector (bottom row). This enabled more accurate segmentation of the trabeculae (red overlays). Color maps of local bone volume fraction (BV/TV), trabecular thickness (Tb.Th), and spacing (Tb. Sp) are compared for the three modalities in the right panel, illustrating the improved agreement in quantitative indices of bone microstructure obtained by CMOS-CBCT

CMOS x-ray detectors provide 5×–10× lower electronic noise, approximately 4× faster readout speeds, and smaller pixels than FPDs. All those characteristics are beneficial for high-resolution imaging. Recently, an extremity CBCT prototype equipped with a 30 × 30 cm CMOS detector with 100 μm pixels was reported [71]. The system was built on the OnSight3D gantry. The thickness of the CsI scintillator on the CMOS detector was optimized for high-resolution bone imaging tasks; the optimal thickness was found to be 400 μm compared to the standard 600 μm layer [72]. The CMOS-based CBCT (CMOS-CBCT) showed promising performance in preliminary studies of bone imaging applications. Figure 21.3 illustrates the benefits of CMOS-CBCT in microstructural evaluation of the bone. In comparison with FPD-based CBCT, CMOS-CBCT achieved approximately 15% improved correlation with micro-CT for the measurement of Tb.Th and 6% improvement for Tb.Sp [73]. CMOS-CBCT maintains similar soft-tissue imaging performance as FPD-CBCT, making it a promising platform for comprehensive examination of micro- and macroscopic aspects of orthopedic health.

New Directions in Musculoskeletal CT

Extremity CBCT is not the only recent development in orthopedic applications of CT. Continuing the trend toward functional, weight-bearing imaging, new devices enabling upright imaging of the entire skeleton have been proposed. For example, this capability can be implemented using a twin-robotic x-ray system (Siemens Multitom RAX), where the source and detector are mounted on two robotic arms that enable flexible motion patterns around the patient [18, 74, 75]. Another area of interest is in applications of CT to quantify bone microstructure and assess fracture risk. While the resolution of current-generation CT is typically too low to reliably segment the trabeculae, some studies have shown prediction of osteoporotic fracture using apparent microstructural parameters derived from conventional CT, even under low-dose conditions [76]. Finite element models derived from CT scans provide another promising avenue for fracture risk assessment [6]. Most importantly, recent advances in CT technology have resulted in new scanners, such as Siemens Somatom Force and Canon Aquilion Precision, with 1.5–2× improved spatial resolution compared to earlier systems [77, 78]. The Precision system has been demonstrated to visualize details down to 150 μm size, potentially enabling more precise assessment of bone microstructure throughout the entire skeleton, in particular in the spine and hips. Extensive validation studies are needed to establish the benefits of such high-resolution CT in bone imaging.

References

1. Grigoryan M, Lynch JA, Fierlinger AL, Guermazi A, Fan B, MacLean DB, et al. Quantitative and qualitative assessment of closed fracture healing using computed tomography and conventional radiography. Acad Radiol. 2003;10(11):1267–73.
2. Burge R, Dawson-Hughes B, Solomon DH, Wong JB, King A, Tosteson A. Incidence and economic burden of osteoporosis-related fractures in the United States, 2005-2025. J Bone Miner Res. 2007;22(3):465–75.
3. McKinnis LN. Fundamentals of musculoskeletal imaging. 4th ed. Philadelphia: F.A. Davis; 2014.
4. Waldt S, Woertler K. Measurements and classifications in musculoskeletal radiology. Stuttgart: Thieme; 2013.
5. Hashemi J, Chandrashekar N, Gill B, Beynnon BD, Slauterbeck JR, Schutt RC, et al. The geometry of the tibial plateau and its influence on the biomechanics of the tibiofemoral joint. J Bone Joint Surg Am. 2008;90(12):2724–34.
6. Johannesdottir F, Allaire B, Bouxsein ML. Fracture prediction by computed tomography and finite element analysis: current and future perspectives. Curr Osteoporos Rep Curr Osteoporosis Rep. 2018;16(4):411–22.
7. Ammann P, Rizzoli R. Bone strength and its determinants. Osteoporos Int [Internet]. 2003;14(S3):13–8. Available from: http://link.springer.com/10.1007/s00198-002-1345-4.
8. Burghardt AJ, Link TM, Majumdar S. High-resolution computed tomography for clinical imaging of bone microarchitecture. Clin Orthop Relat Res [Internet]. 2011;469(8):2179–93. Available from: http://link.springer.com/10.1007/s11999-010-1766-x.
9. Boutroy S, Bouxsein ML, Munoz F, Delmas PD. In vivo assessment of trabecular bone microarchitecture by high-resolution peripheral quantitative computed tomography. J Clin Endocrinol Metab. 2005;90(12):6508–15.
10. Scanco XtremeCT [Internet]. Available from: http://www.scanco.ch/en/systems-solutions/clinical-microct/xtremect1.html.
11. Hayashi D, Roemer FW, Jarraya M, Guermazi A. Imaging of osteoarthritis. Geriatr Imaging [Internet]. Elsevier Inc. 2013;55(5):93–121. Available from: https://doi.org/10.1016/j.rcl.2017.04.012.
12. Conaghan PG, Hunter DJ, Maillefert JF, Reichmann WM, Losina E. Summary and recommendations of the OARSI FDA osteoarthritis assessment of structural change working group. Osteoarthr Cartil [Internet]. 2011;19(5):606–10. Available from: https://linkinghub.elsevier.com/retrieve/pii/S1063458411000756.
13. Zoumalan RA, Lebowitz RA, Wang E, Yung K, Babb JS, Jacobs JB. Flat panel cone beam computed tomography of the sinuses. Otolaryngol –Head Neck Surg [Internet]. 2009;140(6):841–4. Available from: http://oto.sagepub.com/content/140/6/841.abstract.
14. Lindfors KK, Boone JM, Nelson TR, Yang K, Kwan ALC, Miller DF. Dedicated breast CT: initial clinical experience. Radiology [Internet]. 2008/01/16. 2008;246(3):725–33. Available from: http://radiology.rsna.org/content/246/3/725.abstract.
15. Flynn MJ, McGee R, Blechinger J. Spatial resolution of x-ray tomosynthesis in relation to computed tomography for coronal/sagittal images of the knee. Hsieh J, Flynn MJ, Medical imaging 2007: physics of medical imaging [Internet]. 1st San Diego: SPIE; 2007 [cited 2013 Jul 8]. 65100D–651009. Available from: http://link.aip.org/link/?PSI/6510/65100D/1.
16. Ellis SJ, Deyer T, Williams BR, Yu JC, Lehto S, Maderazo A, et al. Assessment of lateral hindfoot pain in acquired flatfoot deformity using weightbearing multiplanar imaging. Foot Ankle Int [Internet]. 2010 [cited 2013 Jul 7];31(5):361–71. Available from: http://www.ncbi.nlm.nih.gov/pubmed/20460061.
17. Berger M, Müller K, Aichert A, Unberath M, Thies J, Choi J-H, et al. Marker-free motion correction in weight-bearing cone-beam CT of the knee joint. Med Phys [Internet]. 2016;43(3):1235–48. Available from: https://doi.org/10.1118/1.4941012
18. Fieselmann A, Steinbrener J, Jerebko AK, Voigt JM, Scholz R, Ritschl L, et al. Twin robotic x-ray system for 2D radiographic and 3D cone-beam CT imaging. Proc SPIE 9783, Medical Imaging 2016: Physics of Medical Imaging, 97830G (22 March 2016).
19. Tuominen EKJ, Kankare J, Koskinen SK, Mattila KT. Weight-bearing CT imaging of the lower extremity. Am J Roentgenol. 2013;200(1):146–8.
20. Huang AJ, Chang CY, Thomas BJ, MacMahon PJ, Palmer WE. Using cone-beam CT as a low-dose 3D imaging technique for the extremities: initial experience in 50 subjects. Skeletal Radiol [Internet]. 2015;6–8. Available from: http://link.springer.com/10.1007/s00256-015-2105-9.
21. Zbijewski W, De Jean P, Prakash P, Ding Y, Stayman JW, Packard N, et al. A dedicated cone-beam CT system for musculoskeletal extremities imaging: design, optimization, and initial performance characterization. Norbert JP, Ehsan S, Robert MN, editors. Med Phys [Internet]. 2011/09/21. SPIE. 2011;38(8):4700. Available from: http://link.aip.org/link/?PSI/7961/796104/1.
22. Carrino JA, Al Muhit A, Zbijewski W, Thawait GK, Stayman JW, Packard N, et al. Dedicated

cone-beam CT system for extremity imaging. Radiology [Internet]. 2014;270(3):816–24. Available from: http://pubs.rsna.org/doi/abs/10.1148/radiol.13130225.

23. Richter M, Zech S, Hahn S, Naef I, Merschin D. Combination of pedCAT® for 3D imaging in standing position with pedography shows no statistical correlation of bone position with force/pressure distribution. J Foot Ankle Surg [Internet]. Elsevier Ltd. 2016;55(2):240–246. Available from: https://doi.org/10.1053/j.jfas.2015.10.004
24. Richter M, Seidl B, Zech S, Hahn S. PedCAT for 3D-imaging in standing position allows for more accurate bone position (angle) measurement than radiographs or CT. Foot Ankle Surg [Internet]. 2014;20(3):201–7. Available from: https://linkinghub.elsevier.com/retrieve/pii/S1268773114000617.
25. Koivisto J, Kiljunen T, Wolff J, Kortesniemi M. Assessment of effective radiation dose ofan extremity cbct, msctand conventional x ray for knee area using mosfet dosemeters. Radiat Prot Dosim. 2013;157(4):515–24.
26. Koivisto J, Kiljunen T, Kadesjö N, Shi X-Q, Wolff J. Effective radiation dose of a MSCT, two CBCT and one conventional radiography device in the ankle region. J Foot Ankle Res [Internet]. 2015;8(1):8. Available from: http://www.jfootankleres.com/content/8/1/8.
27. Demehri S, Muhit A, Zbijewski W, Stayman JW, Yorkston J, Packard N, et al. Assessment of image quality in soft tissue and bone visualization tasks for a dedicated extremity cone-beam CT system. Eur Radiol [Internet]. 2015;25(6):1742–51. Available from: http://link.springer.com/10.1007/s00330-014-3546-6.
28. Joemai RMS, Zweers D, Obermann WR, Geleijns J. Assessment of patient and occupational dose in established and new applications of MDCT fluoroscopy. Am J Roentgenol [Internet]. 2009 [cited 2013 Jun 9];192(4):881–6. Available from: http://www.ncbi.nlm.nih.gov/pubmed/19304690.
29. Cao Q, Sisniega A, Stayman JW, Yorkston J, Siewerdsen JH, Zbijewski W. Quantitative cone-beam CT of bone mineral density using model-based reconstruction. In: Bosmans H, Chen G-H, Gilat Schmidt T, editors. Medical Imaging 2019: Physics of Medical Imaging [Internet]. SPIE; 2019. p. 33. Available from: https://www.spiedigitallibrary.org/conference-proceedings-of-spie/10948/2513216/Quantitative-cone-beam-CT-of-bone-mineral-density-using-model/10.1117/12.2513216.full.
30. Zbijewski W, Sisniega A, Stayman JW, Muhit A, Thawait G, Packard N, et al. High-performance soft-tissue imaging in extremity cone-beam CT. In: Whiting BR, Hoeschen C, editors. SPIE medical imaging [Internet]. 2014. p. 903329. Available from: http://proceedings.spiedigitallibrary.org/proceeding.aspx?doi=10.1117/12.2043463.
31. Badal A, Badano A. Monte Carlo simulation of X-ray imaging using a graphics processing unit. 2009 IEEE Nucl Sci Symp Conf Rec [Internet]. Ieee; 2009 Oct;(3):4081–4. Available from: http://ieeexplore.ieee.org/lpdocs/epic03/wrapper.htm?arnumber=5402382.
32. Sisniega A, Zbijewski W, Badal A, Kyprianou IS, Stayman JW, Vaquero JJ, et al. Monte Carlo study of the effects of system geometry and antiscatter grids on cone-beam CT scatter distributions. Med Phys [Internet]. 2013 [cited 2013 May 22];40(5):051915. Available from: http://www.pubmedcentral.nih.gov/articlerender.fcgi?artid=3651212&tool=pmcentrez&rendertype=abstract.
33. Sisniega A, Zbijewski W, Xu J, Dang H, Stayman JW, Yorkston J, et al. High-fidelity artifact correction for cone-beam CT imaging of the brain. Phys Med Biol [Internet]. 2015;60(4):1415–39. Available from: http://stacks.iop.org/0031-9155/60/i=4/a=1415?key=crossref.ff5c134a2a7a4263e696e19c9cdf4241.
34. Sun M, Star-Lack JM. Improved scatter correction using adaptive scatter kernel superposition. Phys Med Biol [Internet]. 2010 [cited 2013 Jul 8];55(22):6695–720. Available from: http://www.ncbi.nlm.nih.gov/pubmed/21030750.
35. Wang A, Maslowski A, Wareing T, Star-Lack J, Schmidt TG. A fast, linear Boltzmann transport equation solver for computed tomography dose calculation (Acuros CTD). Med Phys [Internet]. 2019;46(2):925–33. Available from: http://doi.wiley.com/10.1002/mp.13305.
36. Maier J, Eulig E, Vöth T, Knaup M, Kuntz J, Sawall S, et al. Real-time scatter estimation for medical CT using the deep scatter estimation: method and robustness analysis with respect to different anatomies, dose levels, tube voltages, and data truncation. Med Phys [Internet]. 2019;46(1):238–49. Available from: http://doi.wiley.com/10.1002/mp.13274.
37. Gang GJ, Zbijewski W, Mahesh M, Thawait G, Packard N, Yorkston J, Demehri S, Siewerdsen JH. Image quality and dose for a multisource cone-beam CT extremity scanner. Med Phys. 2018;45:144–55. https://doi.org/10.1002/mp.12659.
38. Sisniega A, Thawait G, Shakoor D, Siewerdsena JH, Demehri S, Zbijewski W. Motion compensation in extremity cone-beam computed tomography. Skeletal Radiol. 2019;Under revi. 2019. https://doi.org/10.1007/s00256-019-03241-w. [Epub ahead of print]
39. Choi J-H, Fahrig R, Keil A, Besier TF, Pal S, McWalter EJ, et al. Fiducial marker-based correction for involuntary motion in weight-bearing C-arm CT scanning of knees. Part I. Numerical model-based optimization. Med Phys [Internet]. 2013 ;40(9):091905. Available from: https://doi.org/10.1118/1.4817476.
40. Choi J-H, Maier A, Keil A, Pal S, McWalter EJ, Beaupré GS, et al. Fiducial marker-based correction for involuntary motion in weight-bearing C-arm CT scanning of knees. II. Experiment. Med Phys [Internet]. 2014;41(6Part1):061902. Available from:. https://doi.org/10.1118/1.4873675.

41. Berger M, Xia Y, Aichinger W, Mentl K, Unberath M, Aichert A, et al. Motion compensation for cone-beam CT using Fourier consistency conditions. Phys Med Biol IOP Publishing. 2017;62(17):7181.
42. Sisniega A, Stayman JW, Yorkston J, Siewerdsen JH, Zbijewski W. Motion compensation in extremity cone-beam CT using a penalized image sharpness criterion. Phys Med Biol [Internet]. 2017;62(9):3712–34. Available from: http://stacks.iop.org/0031-9155/62/i=9/a=3712?key=crossref.84caaff65ba9b2a3f6da8ee49365aca7.
43. International WBCT Society [Internet]. Available from: https://www.wbctsociety.org/.
44. De Smet E, De Praeter G, Verstraete KL, Wouters K, De Beuckeleer L, Vanhoenacker FMHM. Direct comparison of conventional radiography and cone-beam CT in small bone and joint trauma. Skeletal Radiol [Internet]. 2015;i:12–6. Available from: https://doi.org/10.1007/s00256-015-2127-3.
45. Osgood GM, Thawait GK, Hafezi-nejad N, Shaner A, Yorkston J, Zbijewski WB, et al. Image quality of cone beam computed tomography for evaluation of extremity fractures in the presence of metal hardware : visual grading characteristics analysis. Br J Radiol. 2017;90:20160539.
46. Barg A, Bailey T, Richter M, de Cesar NC, Lintz F, Burssens A, et al. Weightbearing computed tomography of the foot and ankle: emerging technology topical review. Foot Ankle Int. 2018;39(3):376–86.
47. Lintz F, Cesar Netto C, de Barg A, Burssens A, Richter M. Weight bearing CT international Stu. Weight-bearing cone beam CT scans in the foot and ankle. EFORT Open Rev. 2018;3(5):278–86.
48. Burssens A, Peeters J, Buedts K, Victor J, Vandeputte G. Measuring hindfoot alignment in weight bearing CT: a novel clinical relevant measurement method. Foot Ankle Surg [Internet]. European Foot and Ankle Society. 2016;22(4):233–238. Available from: https://doi.org/10.1016/j.fas.2015.10.002.
49. Lintz F, Welck M, Bernasconi A, Thornton J, Cullen NP, Singh D, et al. 3D biometrics for hindfoot alignment using weightbearing CT. Foot Ankle Int [Internet]. 2017;38(6):684–9. Available from: http://journals.sagepub.com/doi/10.1177/1071100717690806.
50. Lepojärvi S, Niinimäki J, Pakarinen H, Leskelä H-V. Rotational dynamics of the Normal distal tibiofibular joint with weight-bearing computed tomography. Foot Ankle Int [Internet]. 2016;37(6):627–35. Available from: http://journals.sagepub.com/doi/10.1177/1071100716634757.
51. Lepojarvi S, Niinim J, Pakarinen H, Koskela L, Leskel H. Rotational dynamics of the talus in a normal. J Bone Joint Surg Am. 2016;98:568–75.
52. Hirschmann A, Buck FM, Fucentese SF, Pfirrmann CWA. Upright CT of the knee: the effect of weight-bearing on joint alignment. Eur Radiol. 2015;25(11):3398–404.
53. Marzo J, Kluczynski M, Notino A, Bisson L. Comparison of a novel weightbearing cone beam computed tomography scanner versus a conventional computed tomography scanner for measuring patellar instability. Orthop J Sport Med [Internet]. 2016;4(12):1–7. Available from: http://ojs.sagepub.com/lookup/doi/10.1177/2325967116673560.
54. Hirschmann A, Pfirrmann CWA, Klammer G, Espinosa N, Buck FM. Upright cone CT of the hindfoot: comparison of the non-weight-bearing with the upright weight-bearing position. Eur Radiol. 2014;24(3):553–8.
55. Netto CC, Demehri S, Dein EJ, Thawait GK, Zhang H, Fonseca LF, et al. Flexible adult acquired flatfoot deformity: comparison between weightbearing and nonweightbearing cone-beam CT examinations. In: AOFAS annual meeting. 2016.
56. Shakoor D, Osgood GM, Brehler M, Zbijewski WB, de Cesar Netto C, Shafiq B, et al. Cone-beam CT measurements of distal tibio-fibular syndesmosis in asymptomatic uninjured ankles: does weight-bearing matter? Skeletal Radiol [Internet] 2019;48(4):583–94. Available from: https://doi.org/10.1007/s00256-018-3074-6.
57. Malhotra K, Welck M, Cullen N, Singh D, Goldberg AJ. The effects of weight bearing on the distal tibiofibular syndesmosis: a study comparing weight bearing-CT with conventional CT. Foot Ankle Surg [Internet]. 2018. Available from: https://linkinghub.elsevier.com/retrieve/pii/S1268773118301140.
58. Lawlor MC, Kluczynski MA, Marzo JM. Weight-bearing cone-beam CT scan assessment of stability of supination external rotation ankle fractures in a cadaver model. Foot Ankle Int [Internet] 2018;39(7):850–7. Available from: https://doi.org/10.1177/1071100718761035.
59. Collan L, Kankare JA, Mattila K. The biomechanics of the first metatarsal bone in hallux valgus: a preliminary study utilizing a weight bearing extremity CT. Foot Ankle Surg [Internet]. European Foot and Ankle Society. 2013;19(3):155–161. Available from: https://doi.org/10.1016/j.fas.2013.01.003.
60. Muhit AA, Arora S, Ogawa M, Ding Y, Zbijewski W, Stayman JW, et al. Peripheral quantitative CT (pQCT) using a dedicated extremity cone-beam CT scanner. Weaver JB, Molthen RC, editors. Proc SPIE [Internet]. 2013 [cited 2013 Jul 12];8672:867203–867203-7. Available from: http://proceedings.spiedigitallibrary.org/proceeding.aspx?doi=10.1117/12.2006939.
61. Thawait GK, Demehri S, AlMuhit A, Zbijweski W, Yorkston J, Del Grande F, et al. Extremity cone-beam CT for evaluation of medial tibiofemoral osteoarthritis: initial experience in imaging of the weight-bearing and non-weight-bearing knee. Eur J Radiol [Internet]. 2015;84(12):2564–70. Available from: https://linkinghub.elsevier.com/retrieve/pii/S0720048X15300954.
62. Segal NA, Nevitt MC, Lynch JA, Niu J, Torner JC, Guermazi A. Diagnostic performance of 3D standing CT imaging for detection of knee osteoarthritis features. Phys Sportsmed [Internet]. 2015;43(3):213–20.

Available from: http://www.tandfonline.com/doi/full/10.1080/00913847.2015.1074854.

63. AmerinatanziA, SummersR, AhmadiK, GoelV, Hewett T, Nyman E. Automated measurement of patient-specific tibial slopes from MRI. Bioengineering [Internet]. 2017;4(3):69. Available from: http://www.mdpi.com/2306-5354/4/3/69.
64. Subburaj K, Ravi B, Agarwal M. Automated identification of anatomical landmarks on 3D bone models reconstructed from CT scan images. Comput Med Imaging Graph. 2009;33(5):359–68.
65. Jacinto H, Valette S, Prost R. Multi-atlas automatic positioning of anatomical landmarks. J Vis Commun Image Represent [Internet]. Elsevier. 2018;50(November 2017):167–177. Available from: https://doi.org/10.1016/j.jvcir.2017.11.015.
66. Brehler M, Thawait G, Shyr W, Ramsay J, Siewerdsen JH, Zbijewski W. Atlas-based automatic measurements of the morphology of the tibiofemoral joint. In: Krol A, Gimi B, editors. 2017. p. 101370E. Available from: http://proceedings.spiedigitallibrary.org/proceeding.aspx?doi=10.1117/12.2255566.
67. Segal N A, Frick E, Duryea J, Nevitt MC, Niu J, Torner JC, et al. Comparison of tibiofemoral joint space width measurements from standing CT and fixed flexion radiography. J Orthop Res. 2017;35(7):1388–95. https://doi.org/10.1002/jor.23387.
68. Segal NA, Bergin J, Findlay C, Anderson DD. Test-retest reliability of tibiofemoral joint space width measurements using low-dose standing CT. Osteoarthr Cartil [Internet]. Skelet Radiol. 2015;23:A230–1. Available from: http://ovidsp.ovid.com/ovidweb.cgi?T=JS&CSC=Y&NEWS=N&PAGE=fulltext&D=emed13&AN=71906931%5Cn http://bifrost.bib.sdu.dk:9003/sfx_local?sid=OVID:embase&id=pmid:&id=doi:&issn=1063-4584&isbn=&volume=23&issue=&spage=A230&pages=A230-A231&date=2015&title=Osteoarth.
69. Cao Q, Thawait G, Gang GJ, Zbijewski W, Reigel T, Brown T, et al. Characterization of 3D joint space morphology using an electrostatic model (with application to osteoarthritis). Phys Med Biol [Internet]. IOP Publishing. 2015;60(3):947–60. Available from: http://stacks.iop.org/0031-9155/60/i=3/a=947.
70. Brehler M, Cao Q, Moseley KF, Osgood GM, Morris CD, Demehri S, et al. Robust quantitative assessment of trabecular microarchitecture in extremity cone-beam CT using optimized segmentation algorithms. In: SPIE Med Im accepted. 2018.
71. Cao Q, Brehler M, Sisniega A, Stayman JW, Yorkston J, Siewerdsen J, et al. High-resolution extremity cone-beam CT with a CMOS detector: task-based optimization of scintillator thickness. SPIE Med Imaging. 2017;10132:1–6.
72. Cao Q, Sisniega A, Brehler M, Stayman JW, Yorkston J, Siewerdsen JH, et al. Modeling and evaluation of a high-resolution CMOS detector for cone-beam CT of the extremities. Med Phys [Internet]. 2018;45(1):114–30. Available from: http://doi.wiley.com/10.1002/mp.12654.
73. Subramanian S, Brehler M, Cao Q, Quevedo-Gonzalez FJ, Breighner RE, Carrino JA, et al. Quantitative evaluation of bone microstructure using high-resolution extremity cone-beam CT with a CMOS detector. In: SPIE Medical Imaging 2019. 2019.
74. Benz RM, Harder D, Amsler F, Voigt J, Fieselmann A, Falkowski AL, et al. Initial assessment of a prototype 3D cone-beam computed tomography system for imaging of the lumbar spine, evaluating human cadaveric specimens in the upright position. Invest Radiol [Internet]. 2018;53(12):714–9. Available from: http://insights.ovid.com/crossref?an=00004424-201812000-00002.
75. Noo F, Oktay MB, Ritschl L, Vogt S, Fieselmann A, Herbst M, et al. X-ray cone-beam imaging of the entire spine in the weight-bearing position. In: Chen G-H, Lo JY, Gilat Schmidt T, editors. Medical Imaging 2018: Physics of Medical Imaging [Internet]. SPIE; 2018. p. 27. Available from: https://www.spiedigitallibrary.org/conference-proceedings-of-spie/10573/2293579/X-ray-cone-beam-imaging-of-the-entire-spine-in/10.1117/12.2293579.full.
76. Mei K, Kopp FK, Bippus R, Köhler T, Schwaiger BJ, Gersing AS, et al. Is multidetector CT-based bone mineral density and quantitative bone microstructure assessment at the spine still feasible using ultra-low tube current and sparse sampling? Eur Radiol Eur Radiol. 2017;27(12):5261–71.
77. Chen C, Zhang X, Guo J, Jin D, Letuchy EM, Burns TL, et al. Quantitative imaging of peripheral trabecular bone micro-architecture Using MDCT. Med Phys. 2018;45(1):236–49.
78. Yanagawa M, Hata A, Honda O, Kikuchi N, Miyata T, Uranishi A. Subjective and objective comparisons of image quality between ultra-high-resolution CT and conventional area detector CT in phantoms and cadaveric human lungs. Eur Radiol. 2018:5060–8.

Utility of CBCT in Neurovascular Diagnosis and Interventions

22

Charles M. Strother and Sebastian Schafer

Introduction

Rotational angiographic acquisitions with 3D reconstructions originally were developed as a tool for improving the ability to characterize vascular abnormalities [1]. It rapidly became apparent; however, these images also improved the ability to better understand not only these complex vascular pathologies but also their anatomical relationships to important adjacent structures. In contrast to MDCT detector arrays, flat panel detector pixel arrays have homogenous side length. The resulting ability to obtain multiplanar high spatial resolution images having true isotropic resolution is an inherent and significant advantage of flat panel CBCT [2, 3]. Having this capability in the angiography suite adds potential value in diagnosis, treatment planning, and guidance and in the evaluation of treatment outcomes. In this chapter, we describe and illustrate the utilities of C-arm cone-beam CT (CBCT) technology for diagnosis, treatment planning, and intervention in diseases of the CNS.

C. M. Strother (✉)
Department of Radiology, University of Wisconsin School of Medicine and Public Health, Madison, WI, USA
e-mail: Cstrother@uwhealth.org

S. Schafer
Siemens Healthineers, Advanced Therapies, Madison, WI, USA

Treatment Planning and Guidance

The endovascular treatment of intracranial aneurysms is now, for many aneurysms, the treatment of choice. The primary method of endovascular treatment of intracranial aneurysms is the use of a variety of techniques in which detachable coils are placed into the aneurysm lumen. Typically, 3D-DSA is used along with 2D-DSA for treatment planning, while fluoroscopy and 2D-DSA acquisitions are used to judge the degree of aneurysm occlusion achieved by the treatment. This application for 3D-DSA is discussed later in the section on flat panel DSA. Because of the severe streaking artifacts, caused by the platinum alloy used to make the detachable coils, CBCT has been, until recently, not helpful in these cases. However, software is now available which significantly reduces the severity of these artifacts [4].

Although the availability and utility of detachable coils revolutionized the treatment of intracranial aneurysms, there were still many aneurysms that, because of their size or morphology, could not be safely and effectively treated with these coils. To address this limitation, alternatives to detachable coils were developed. The first attempts involved the use of a balloon or stent to perform balloon or stent-assisted coiling. These techniques involved first placing one microcatheter through which coils could be delivered into an aneurysm. Then, another microcatheter was used to place a balloon or stent

© Springer Nature Switzerland AG 2020

E. Samei, N. J. Pelc (eds.), *Computed Tomography*, https://doi.org/10.1007/978-3-030-26957-9_22

across the aneurysm's ostium. Using these techniques it was possible to treat an aneurysm with a neck (ostium) so large that, without the presence of a balloon or stent, coils would herniate out of the aneurysm and thereby compromise blood flow in the parent artery and/or adjacent branches. More recently, a type of stent designated as a flow diverter has become available. These flow diverters fall into two categories: (a) intrasaccular (placed into an aneurysm's sac) and (b) intraluminal (placed into the parent artery lumen, across an aneurysm's ostium). They are designed to hinder blood flow into and out of an aneurysm, thereby causing stagnation to a degree that thrombosis and thereby obliteration of the aneurysm occur [5]. Because these new devices are made from nitinol alloys, the ability to visualize them fluoroscopically is very limited. Although their design includes radiopaque markers positioned so an operator can visualize their ends and relationship to a delivery catheter, this information is not sufficient for one to accurately determine aspects such as the degree of vessel wall apposition or the completeness of device deployment, i.e., opening. These features are important because they may influence further treatment decisions, e.g., balloon dilation and posttreatment anticoagulation. They are also important in predicting the likelihood of posttreatment aneurysm occlusion [6, 7].

A CBCT done in conjunction with injection of contrast medium has proven to be extremely useful in visualizing stents and flow diverters used for aneurysm treatment [8, 9] (Fig. 22.1). In theory, there could be value added to the safe and effective use of flow diverters by using a workflow in which multiple CBCTs were acquired at various stages of a procedure, e.g., at the time of positioning, after deployment, and just prior to final detachment. The radiation dose from such an exam, approximately twice that of a conventional MDCT scan of the head, is, however, prohibitive for use of this approach [10]. A variety of methods have previously been used trying to reduce this dose to acceptable levels. Until recently, however, none of these provided adequate image quality [11, 12]. A recent "volume-of-interest" technique in which the x-ray beam is collimated vertically and laterally to a ROI which provides an image field of view of either 12% or 28% results in both excellent image quality and a dramatic reduction in x-ray exposure [13] (Fig. 22.2).

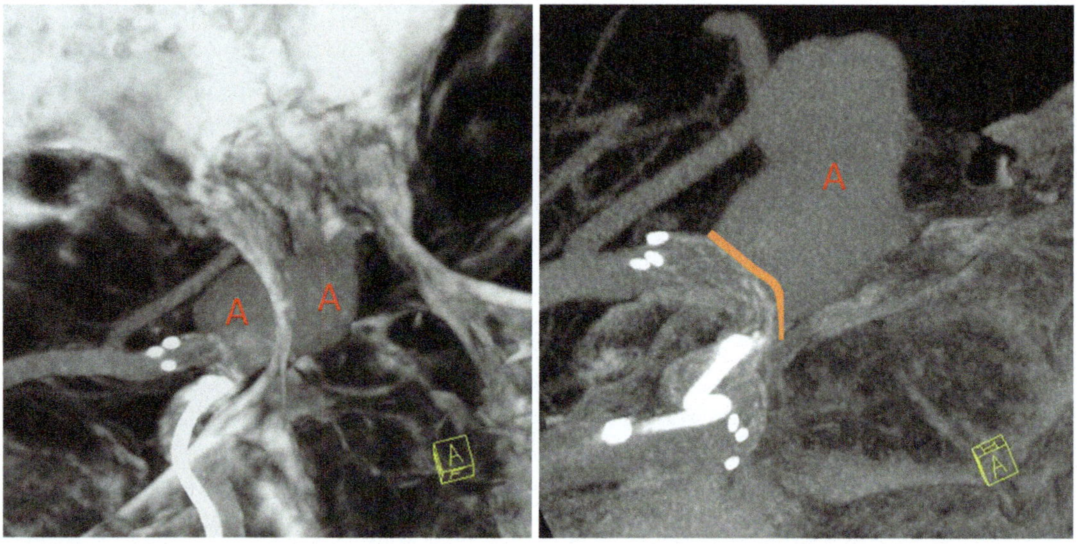

Fig. 22.1 Two views from a CBCT done in conjunction with the intra-arterial injection of dilute contrast medium. A stent has been placed across the ostium (orange line) of a large internal carotid artery aneurysm (red As). A microcatheter is inside of the stent (solid line marks the microcatheter). The image shows that the ostium is covered by the stent, making it safe to position detachable coils into the aneurysm

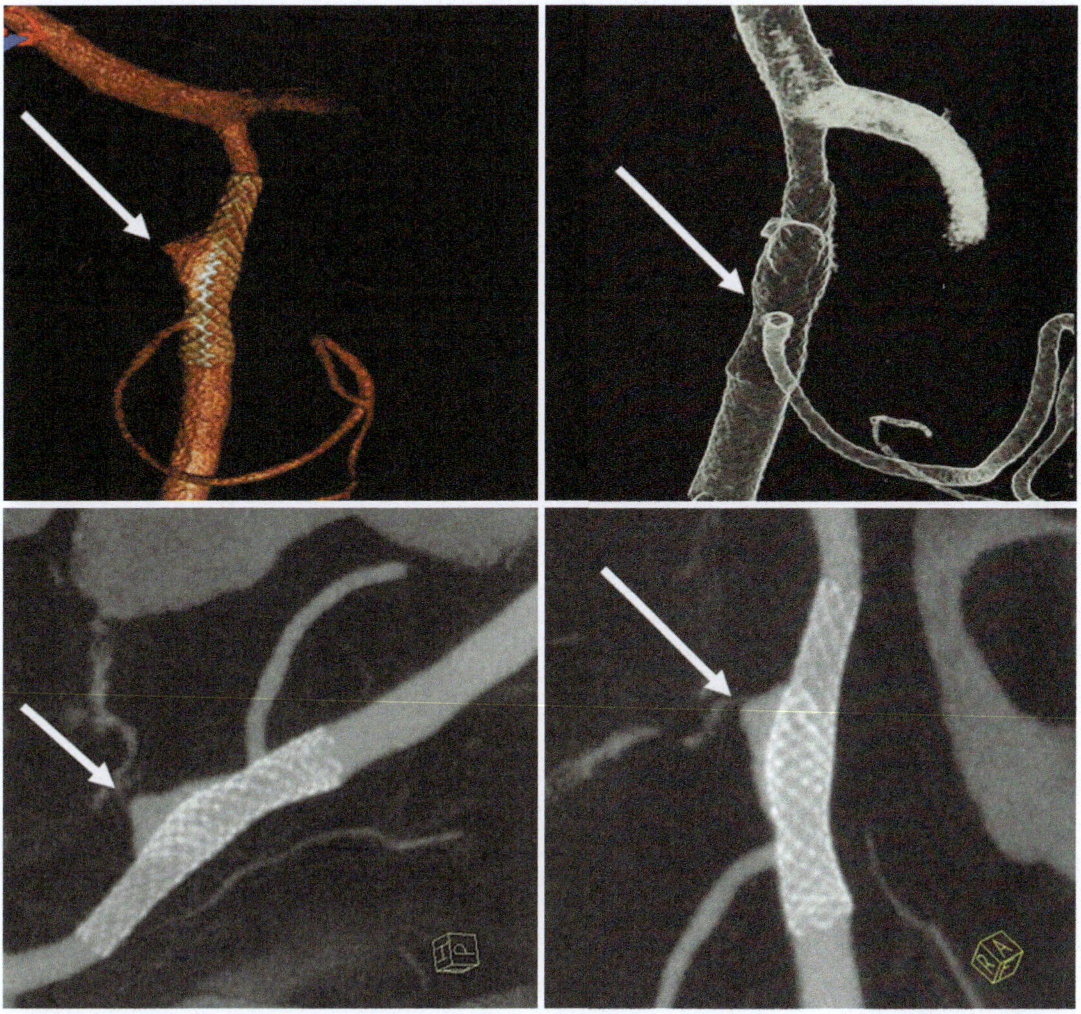

Fig. 22.2 Montage of views from a CBCT done in conjunction with the intra-arterial injection of contrast medium. A flow diverter has been placed across the ostium of a dissecting aneurysm (red arrow) of the left vertebral artery. The device is fully open, and there is excellent wall apposition

The availability of CBCT in the angiography suite greatly enhances the capacity to rapidly and effectively determine if there has been vessel or aneurysm perforation during an endovascular intervention. While most such hemorrhages will be manifest either by changes in a patient's vital signs and/or evidence of contrast medium extravasation, some small hemorrhages may be occult. These, while initially clinically occult, may have significant impact on posttreatment management, i.e., anticoagulation. Because of this, in some practices, a non-contrast CBCT is acquired at the end of any case where there has been guide-wire and catheter manipulation in the intracranial vasculature.

Although the planning and monitoring of aneurysm treatment was the first area where CBCT became widely used in the neuroangiographic suite, there are a variety of other CNS diseases where the use of CBCT has also been shown to add value in treatment planning and guidance. These include preoperative embolization of highly vascular intracranial tumors, e.g., hemangioblastomas and meningiomas [14, 15], and, perhaps most importantly, acute ischemic stroke.

While 2D-DSA can be used to obtain detailed images of a tumor's blood supply, these images often do not provide clear definition of the relationships of feeding arteries and draining veins to either the tumor itself or to adjacent parenchymal and osseous structures. A CBCT done in conjunction with the intra-arterial injection of contrast medium can clearly display these relationships (Fig. 22.3).

Often, during performance of a percutaneous or an interventional treatment, it is difficult to be certain of the precise relationship of a microcatheter or needle to the parenchyma and skull. In order to perform safe embolization, drug delivery, or ablation, it is essential for an operator to know what parenchymal structures might be affected by an intervention. In such instances, the uncertainty can be resolved

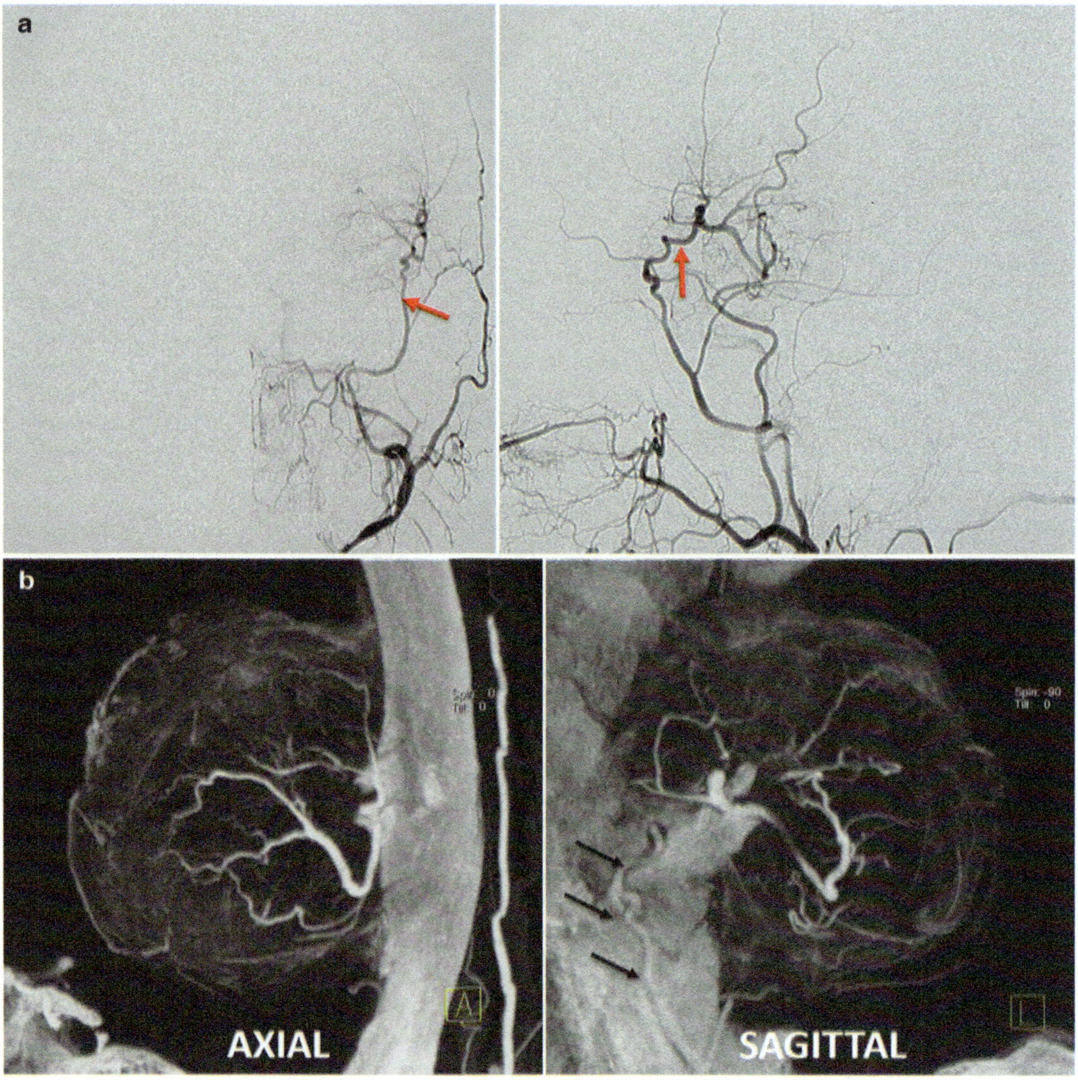

Fig. 22.3 (**a**) AP (left) and lateral (right) 2D-DSA projections of an external carotid artery arteriogram showing the vasculature to a left frontal meningioma. The blood supply, derived from the middle meningeal artery (red arrow), is clearly seen as a series of tiny arteries radiating into the tumor. (**b**) Multi-planar [axial (left) and parasagittal (right)] reconstructions from a CBCT done in conjunction with contrast injection into the middle meningeal artery. On the axial view, the arterial supply is seen entering the base of the tumor at the point where the middle meningeal artery passes through the skull. On the parasagittal view, the middle meningeal artery is seen as it passes though the skull and into the tumor (black arrows)

by acquiring a CBCT in conjunction with contrast injection though an upstream guiding catheter. Reconstructing the projections using a native kernel will show the parenchyma, the catheter, and the opacified vascular structures [16] (Fig. 22.4).

Finally, there is increasing interest in the use of stereotactic radiosurgery for the treatment of arteriovenous malformations (AVMs) involving the brain [17]. A key to achieving treatment success (AVM obliteration) as well as limiting adverse effects from stereotactic radiosurgery is accurate identification of the AVM nidus at the time of treatment planning. This allows avoidance of radiation injury to parenchyma, feeding arteries, and draining veins that lie adjacent to the AVM nidus. The superior spatial resolution and good high-contrast resolution of CBCT makes it an ideal modality to use to define an AVM nidus. Use of CBCT

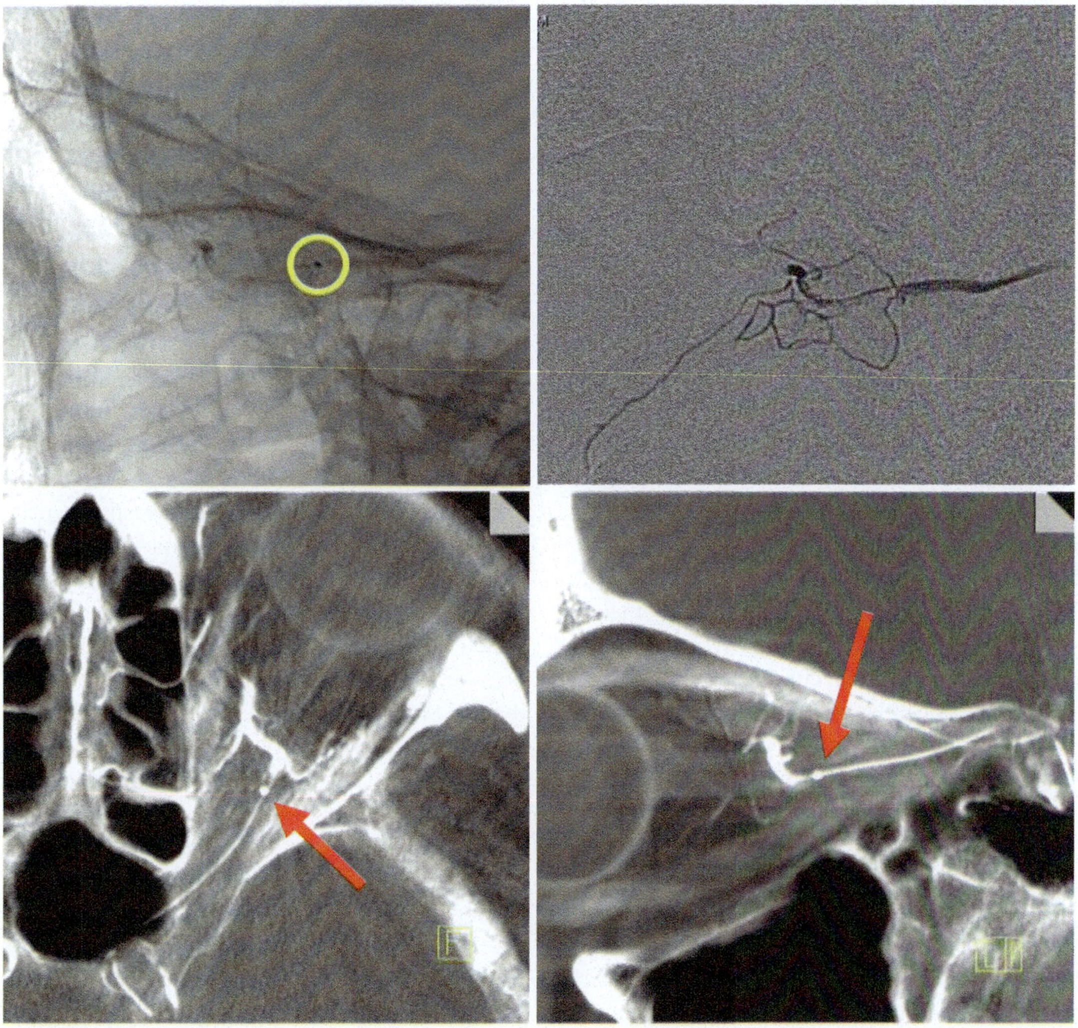

Fig. 22.4 (**a**) A montage of un-subtracted (left) and subtracted (right) 2D-DSA images of a selective ophthalmic artery injection. The patient had an acute ophthalmic artery occlusion. The goal of the intervention was to inject thrombolytic drug into the artery supplying the retina. The tip of the catheter is clearly seen because of a platinum tip marker (yellow circle). There is no blood supply to the retina seen. From these images it is not evident whether the catheter is proximal or distal to the origin the retinal blood supply. (**b**) Multi-planar axial (left) and sagittal (right) reconstructions of a CBCT done in conjunction with contrast injection into the ophthalmic artery. The blood supply to the retina originates as the artery passes over (superior) to the optic nerve (red arrow). The position of the contrast-filled catheter in relationship to the optic nerve and thus to the retina's blood supply is clearly seen

for this task has been shown to result in alteration of the nidal definition as defined by MRA [18].

Acute Ischemic Stroke

Rapidly accumulating evidence shows that many patients with acute ischemic stroke (AIS) benefit from treatment with a combination of IV thrombolysis and mechanical thrombectomy [19–21]. Critical to optimizing the likelihood of a good outcome in these patients is minimizing the time from stroke onset to revascularization [22]. Comprehensive Stroke Center (CSC) guidelines require that patients with AIS have CT imaging started within 15 min and image interpretation available in less than 45 min from the time of hospital arrival [23]. Depending upon the views of the treating physician as well as the resources available, e.g., MRI, there is great variation in the imaging workflow for these patients. Although comprehensive imaging, i.e., non-contrast CT, CTA, and CTP, can be done quickly, there is often considerable delay between imaging and groin puncture, i.e., the picture-to-puncture (p2p) time [24].

There is compelling evidence for a profound effect from shortening the time from hospital arrival to reperfusion on clinical outcomes; in the HERMES study, every 15-min improvement in this time resulted in less disability in 39 patients [25]. This observation combined with the tiny percentage of patients (4%), in which groin puncture was achieved within 30 min of MDCT, suggests that, for patients with clinical signs of an acute anterior circulation stroke and a large vessel occlusion (LVO), i.e., NIHSS ≥8, that, if feasible, it would save precious time if all pretreatment imaging was performed at the point of treatment, i.e., in the angiographic suite.

Motivated by the knowledge of the large potential benefit of shortening the interval between hospital arrival and reperfusion, efforts have been made to develop a "one-stop-shop" approach where, after initial clinical evaluation, AIS patients suspected of having a LVO would bypass conventional CT or MR imaging and, instead, be taken directly to the angiographic suite for triage imaging. For such a workflow to be feasible, three requirements must be provided by angiographic C-arm CBCT. First, the exclusion of intracranial bleeding; second, determining the amount of tissue in the area of ischemia that is salvageable, i.e., penumbra, and the tissue that has been irreversibly injured, i.e., ischemic core; and third, assessing the presence and extent of collateral blood supply and thrombus burden.

Good evidence exists that, for supratentorial hemorrhages, a high-quality non-contrast CBCT has adequate sensitivity for the first task [26, 27]. Ongoing improvement in pre-and post-processing algorithms will, in the foreseeable future, further enhance this ability. Until quite recently, the low-contrast resolution of C-arm CBCT was not adequate to adequately detect the early ischemic changes that are used for judging the extent and degree of ischemic injury. This limited the utility of C-arm CBCT for triage of AIS patients because visualization of these changes is the basis of the ASPECTS score, the principal CT method used to estimate penumbra and ischemic core [28]. Now, the latest generation angiography equipment is equipped with 16-bit flat panel detectors. This, combined with a series of new pre-and post-processing algorithms, greatly increases the low-contrast resolution of new angiographic systems. Initial studies indicate that this advance has resulted in an ability to detect early ischemic changes with C-arm CBCT comparable to that of MDCT [29]. Penumbra may also be distinguished from ischemic core by perfusion imaging. Most often, this has been done using MDCT which provides dynamic maps of rCBV, rCBF, MTT, and TTP (or T_{max}). The temporal resolution and temporal sampling density of MDCT is 0.5 s. Acquiring dynamic perfusion maps with an angiographic C-arm requires a multi-rotational acquisition typically consisting of a ten back and forth movements. Each rotation takes 4.3 s, and there is a pause of just over 1 s between rotations. The combination of this lower temporal resolution and temporal sampling compromises the ability to accurately follow a contrast bolus as it passes through the brain. To address this challenge, a variety of novel image reconstruction methods using model-based reconstructions, temporal under sampling, sub-scan reconstructions with undersampling artifact removal, and reconstruction of differences between baseline and contrast-enhanced scans have resulted in the ability to derive, from a multi-rotational rotation CBCT acquisition, dynamic perfusion maps that are not inferior to ones obtained using conventional MDCT [30–35] (Fig. 22.5).

The presence and robustness of collaterals is a critical determinant of the survival of downstream tissue after a large vessel occlusion. A series of collateral scores has been developed largely based on a comparison of the presence and distribution of opacified arteries in the normal and abnormal cerebral hemispheres as seen on a contrast-enhanced CT scan. Uncertainty in bolus timing, abnormalities in cardiac output and the inability to determine whether filling is retrograde or antegrade have all hampered the ability to accurately determine collateral status using this approach. The use of contrast-enhanced multiphase MDCT studies has decreased but has not eliminated these problems [36]. Fully time-resolved CTAs can be derived from data contained in a multi-rotational CBCT perfusion acquisition. These have been shown to have accuracy in identifying the site of a LVO, in identifying collaterals, and in determining thrombus burden [37, 38] (Fig. 22.6).

Initial results indicate that, using a variety of imaging protocols, the one-stop-shop workflow can be used safely and effectively to shorten the interval between hospital arrival and revascular-

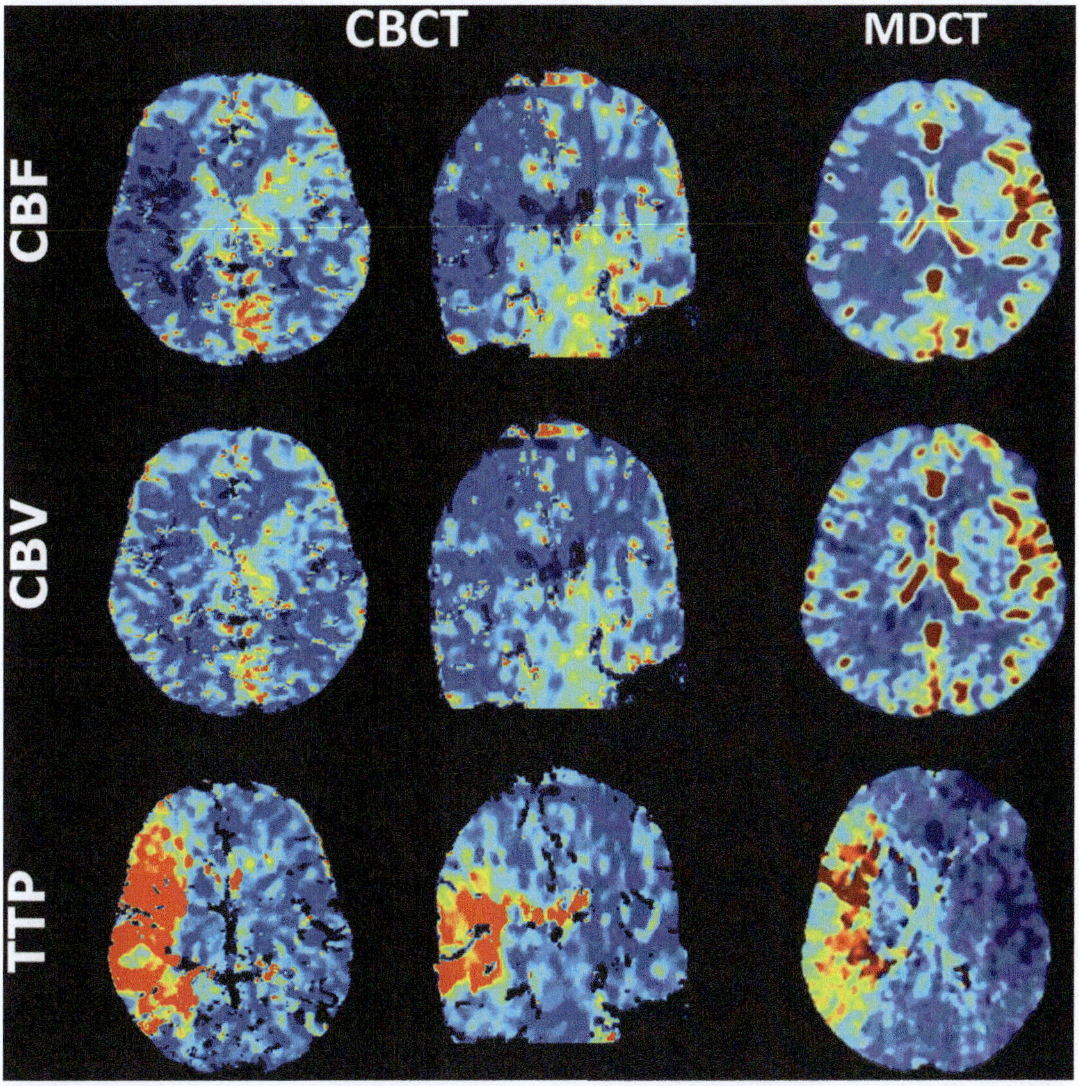

Fig. 22.5 CBCTP and MDCTP maps showing perfusion abnormalities due to occlusion of the M1 segment of the right middle cerebral artery. There is a mismatch between the CBF and CBV maps showing that there is a significant volume of potentially salvageable parenchyma. Note that the CBCTP are reconstructed in orthogonal planes

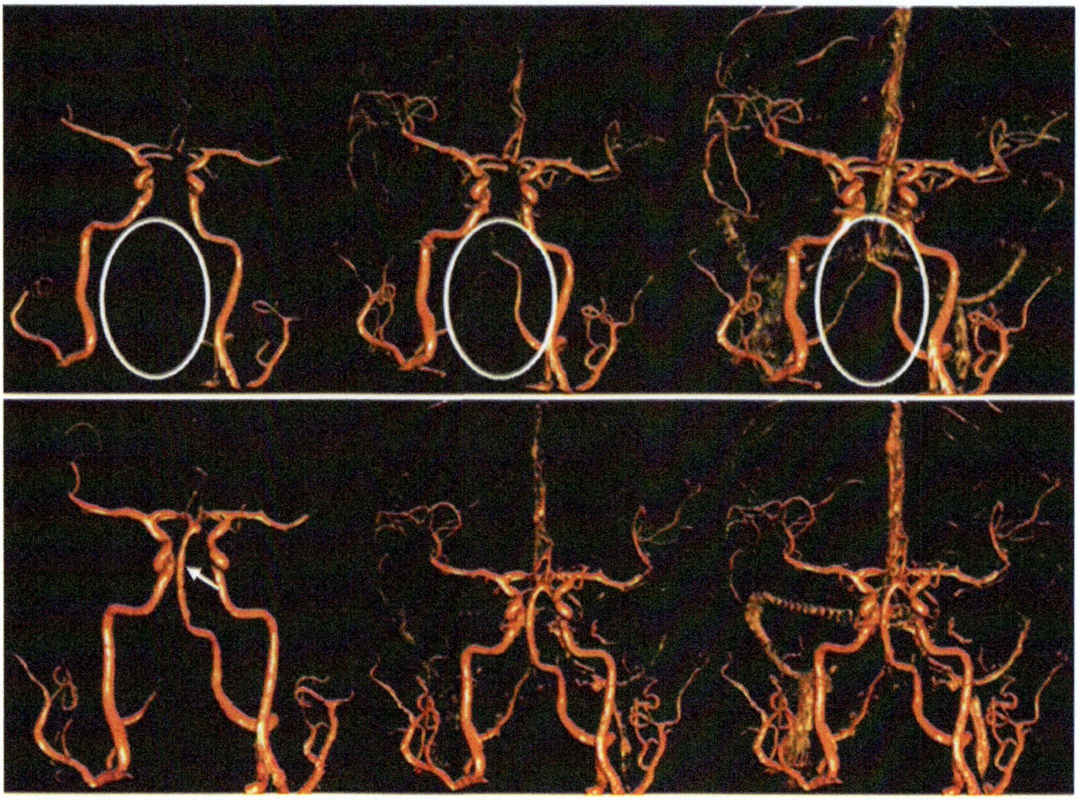

Fig. 22.6 Time-resolved CBCTA images before (top row) and after endovascular treatment of an acute ischemic stroke. There is an occlusion of the basilar artery with slow filling of a dominant left vertebral artery (white ellipse). After treatment the basilar artery fills normally (white arrows)

ization [39, 40]. Because a CBCT perfusion acquisition can be done at a very low radiation and contrast medium dose (4 mSv and 60 cc, respectively), acquiring dynamic perfusion maps before, during, and after an intervention could likely add value in patient selection, determining when to stop an intervention and in improving the ability to optimally manage AIS patients in the period immediately following an intervention [41].

Flat Detector Digital Subtraction Angiography

Although multi-detector CT angiography (CTA) and magnetic resonance angiography (MRA) are adequate for many indications, DSA remains the technique offering the best spatial and temporal resolution [42, 43]. For these reasons, it is the technique most often chosen for treatment planning and procedure guidance involving complex vascular abnormalities. The intracranial vessels that are most germane to this topic range in size between 4 and 5 mm (internal carotid artery) to less than a millimeter (2nd division branches of the middle cerebral artery). They are also tortuous and lie in such close proximity to one another that they often overlap in many viewing projections. Because of this, accurate depiction of pathologic changes using MR or MDCT methods is often quite challenging.

New biplane angiography systems allow simultaneous two-view high frame rate (15 fps) 2D acquisitions. Single-plane rotational acquisitions acquire high frame rate (30 fps or 60 fps) acquisitions with varying rotation times (2–20s) and image/degree increments (0.4–1.5°), as well as detector element binning (1 × 1 to 4 × 4). For both 2D and rotational acquisitions, the spatial resolution of the acquired images depends on the employed detector. The latest detector generations have pixel element side lengths of 0.154 mm.

Parametric Color-Coded 2D-DSA

The primary uses of DSA today are either the evaluation of vascular abnormalities, e.g., aneurysms or arterial venous malformations (AVMs), or the monitoring and guidance of endovascular interventions. Because of the vasculature's structural complexity and the rapid velocity of blood flow, it is often difficult or impossible using 2D-DSA to clearly define the exact sequence of filling and emptying of some abnormalities.

The value of adding color to visual tasks requiring search (identification) and recognition (categorization) has been well established [44, 45]. The application of a color- and intensity-coded algorithm to 2D images is one way that blood flow information can be displayed in a way that improves the ability to characterize flow dynamics [3]. This technique creates a single image which displays the full "history" of a contrast bolus as it passes through the vasculature. While this image contains no "new" information, it does contain information that is impossible to visualize without application of the algorithm, e.g., time to peak (TTP) or half time to wash out (HTWO) (Fig. 22.7).

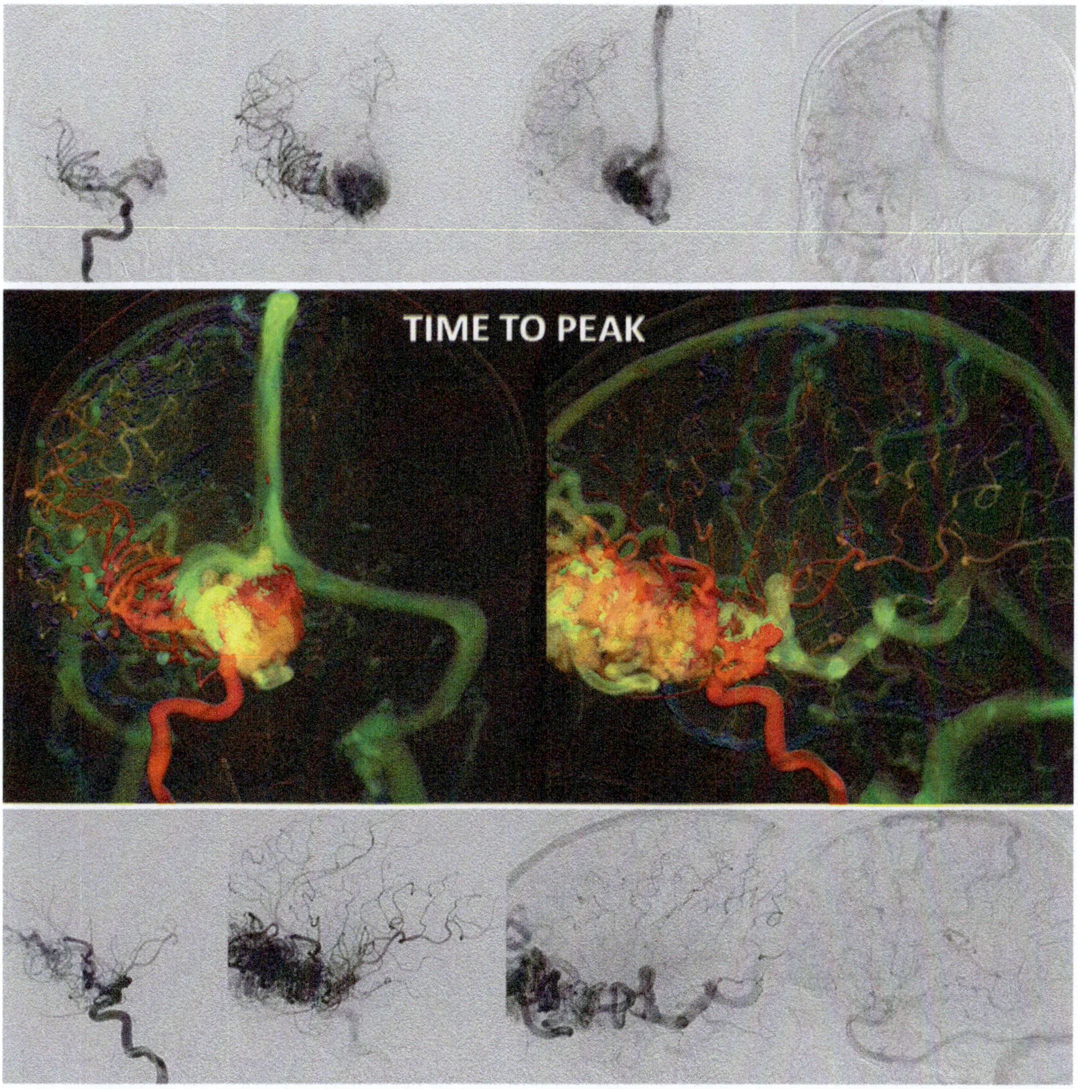

Fig. 22.7 Right internal carotid AP and lateral DSA sequences (top and bottom rows) of an AVM. The color-coded composite images derived from these 2D sequences (middle row) allow easier determination of the pattern of nidal filling and venous drainage than dose the 2D-DSA sequence

In a variety of disease states, the application of such an algorithm to a 2D-DSA sequence has been shown to add value in treatment planning, in judging the result of an intervention, and in diagnosis [3] (Fig. 22.8). This has been shown to be true for both inexperienced and experienced observers [46]. Recently, there has been effort to derive further information from the underlying parenchyma, especially in the case of stroke. Commonly, a vessel suppression algorithm is

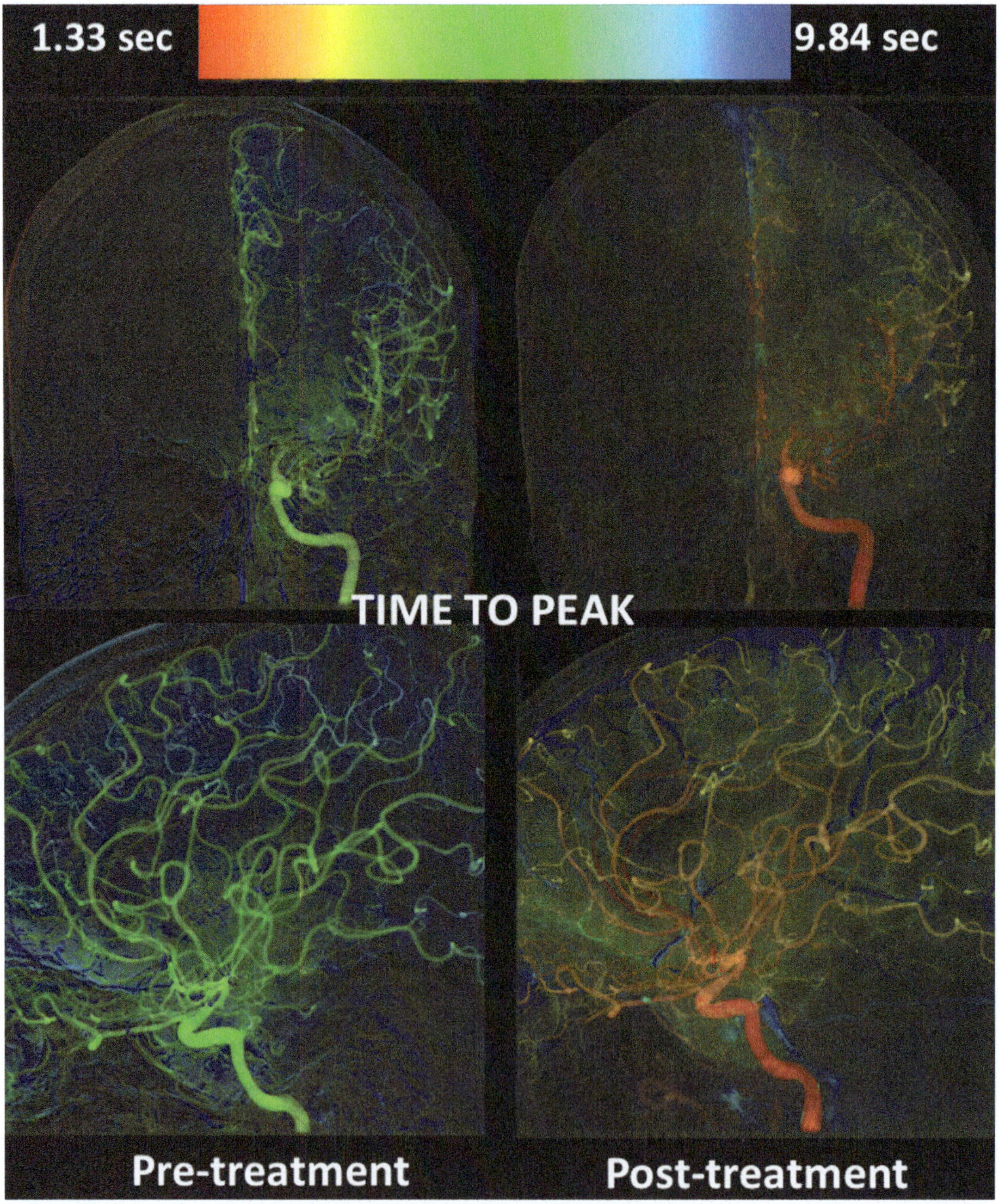

Fig. 22.8 Composite colored-coded images before and after treatment of post subarachnoid hemorrhage. Vasospasm. The color-coded images make it much easier to see the change in blood flow than was possible on the 2D images from which the composite were derived

employed that allows the physician to better delineate the affected parenchyma pre-intervention and the treatment effect post-intervention [47].

3D-DSA and Time-Resolved 3D-DSA (4D-DSA)

In 1997, Fahrig and colleagues showed the feasibility of using the projections from a rotational DSA acquisition (one rotation to acquire a mask followed by a second rotation done in conjunction with injection of contrast medium, i.e., fill rotation) to create a single 3D vascular volume [48, 49]. Rapidly, the utility of 3D-DSA became evident, and 3D-DSA became a key component in the diagnosis and treatment planning of complex vascular abnormalities. The ability to view an abnormality from any desired angle combined with post-processing capabilities that allow display as either a surface-rendered volume or as multi-planar images offers obvious advantages over two-dimensional projections. 3D-DSA has been found to be particularly useful in imaging aneurysms and complex vascular abnormalities such as arteriovenous malformations (AVMs) [50–52]. Even with 3D-DSA, however, it is often difficult or impossible both to obtain unobstructed views of critical structures and determine the sequence of blood flow entering and leaving an abnormality (Fig. 22.9). Because of this most studies are now done using combinations of 2D and 3D acquisitions; for complex abnormalities it is not uncommon for a study to include one or more 3Ds and as many as 10–15 2D acquisitions.

Analogous to MDCT image reconstructions, a user can choose a 3D-DSA reconstruction kernel that will optimize the display of a particular element of the data, e.g., vascular anatomy or Hounsfield units. Within these two subgroups, image characteristics can be selected ranging from smooth to sharp. For example, when the primary purpose of the examination is diagnosing vascular abnormalities, a vessel enhancement filter with a neutral image impression would be appropriate. This provides an image with sharp delineation of the vasculature through with a tradeoff between image noise and optimal spatial resolution. If a structure, such as a coil mass, or a device, such as a stent, is contained within the 3D-DSA volume, a dual-volume reconstruction can be performed. For this application, a reconstruction of only the vasculature is made along with a second reconstruction of the device (this is done using data from the mask acquisition); for

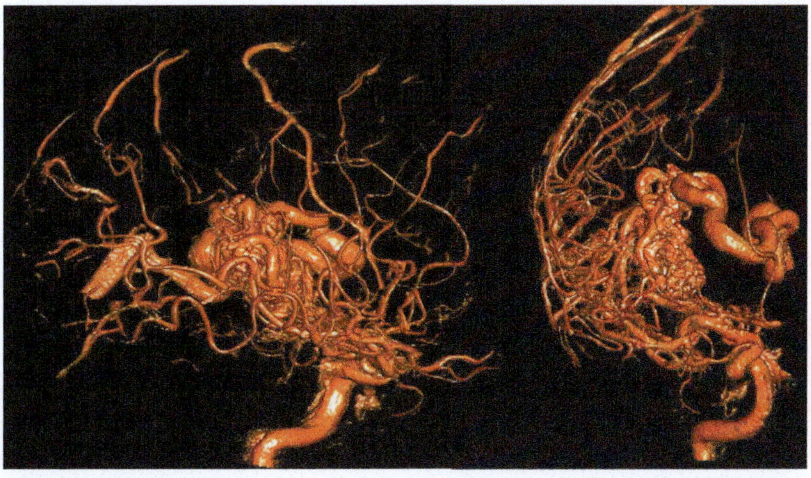

Fig. 22.9 3D-DSA showing three views of an AVM. While the images clearly show the AVM, it is not possible to ascertain the sequence of filling and emptying, the detailed structure of the nidus, or details about the arterial supply or venous drainage

this purpose, a sharp image impression and a Hounsfield unit kernel would be appropriate. Both datasets are fused in the image viewer, thereby allowing a viewer to see the relationship of the device to the opacified vasculature. These may be displayed surface rendered or multiplanar images.

In 2012, Davis and colleagues described a technique whereby a series of fully time-resolved vascular volumes can be obtained using the projections from a conventional 3D-DSA rotational acquisition [53]. Application of this algorithm to a rotational 3D-DSA acquisition generates a fully time-resolved 4D-DSA. A 4D-DSA volume cannot only be viewed at any desired angle but may also be viewed at any desired time during a contrast bolus' passage through the vasculature (Fig. 22.10). This is achieved using the same x-ray and contrast medium dose that is required to create a single 3D-DSA volume.

The steps in a 4D-DSA reconstruction can be described as follows: (a) C-arm rotational acquisitions without (mask) and following contrast injection (fill) are performed. (b) A conventional 3D-DSA volume is reconstructed and, through thresholding, is optimized for viewing. This volume is then used as a constraint volume, (c) for each projection image, the constraint volume is forward projected into the 2D domain and a ratio image is generated, and (d) the generated ratio image is then back projected, and each foreground voxel within the constraint volume is corrected by a function based on the ray-dependent ratio. This process generates "N" 3D-DSA volumes, where N represents the number of projection images. Error sources in the process include in-plane vessel overlap. Different methods have been suggested for correction [54, 55].

3D-DSAs are used largely to evaluate anatomical details and to make measurements of vascular dimensions. Optimal reconstruction of geometrical features requires a consistent distribution of the contrast medium during a rotational acquisition. 4D-DSAs are intended to be used primarily to visualize the angioarchitecture of an abnormality, e.g., AVM nidus, the sequences of blood flow into and out of a vascular abnormality, and for blood flow quantification. For these tasks it is important to capture the inflow of the contrast medium during the fill acquisition. The contrast injection protocols for a 3D and a 4D acquisition are thus somewhat different. These differences are discussed in the section "Injection and Acquisition Protocols."

Studies have shown the utility of 4D-DSA in the evaluation of AVMs and AVFs and in radiosurgical planning [56–59]. In each of these applications, the ability to visualize, at any desired view and any desired time in bolus passage, is added to the understanding of anatomy and flow dynamics.

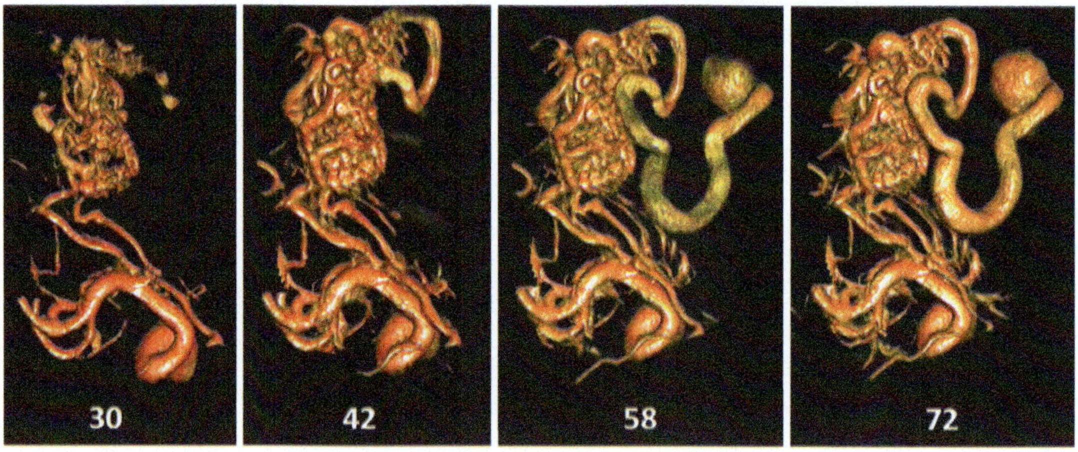

Fig. 22.10 4D-DSA showing an AVM. Four time frames surface rendered. The details of filling, nidal angioarchitecture, and venous drainage are clearly displayed. These images may be viewed at any desired angle at any time of contrast bolus passage

In theory, this combination of excellent spatial and temporal resolution and the ability to view at any angle and at any time means that the availability of a 4D-DSA could obviate the need to obtain both 3D and 2D acquisitions. This would result in a reduction in radiation and contrast medium dose needed for many studies. Initial reports have shown that, in fact, the information content contained in a 4D-DSA is largely equivalent to that of a combination of 2D- and 3D-DSAs [4, 5].

The temporal information contained in a 4D-DSA is sufficient to quantify blood flow velocity [6, 7]. This, combined with the ability to measure vessel lengths and diameters using a surface-rendered reconstruction, allows quantification of blood flow. Flow derivation in volume is based on identifying the contrast bolus movement captured within the 4D-DSA time frames. Each voxel contains a time–concentration curve (TCC) that depicts the inflow of the bolus, a steady state, and the outflow of the bolus. As the bolus moves through the vasculature, with every cardiac cycle, there is an oscillation in the ratio of contrast medium to non-opacified blood. This is seen in the TCCs as quasi-sine wave pulsatility. Investigating the TCCs shows a position-dependent temporal shift between the contrast arrival time and the phase of the contained quasi-sine curve. Two methods have been suggested to exploit these phenomena to delineate volumetric flow: shifting of the time curves in each vascular segment with respect to each other to delineate the temporal difference and using the phase shift of the sine curve to delineate the temporal shift. Combining the temporal shift with distance and diameter measurements allows flow derivation for a given vascular segment. Both methods have shown good results for the proximal intracranial arteries [59, 60]. Evaluation of these techniques in more distal arteries is ongoing.

Acquisition and Contrast Injection Protocols

Depending on the imaging task, the optimal acquisition and injection protocols vary considerably. For all 3D-/4D-DSAs and CBCT acquisitions, it is recommended that contrast be injected by a power injector. Power injectors with dual syringes offer a real advantage over single syringe injectors as they allow both easy modifications of the contrast medium concentration and improved bolus integrity through use of a saline chase when IV injections are appropriate. While commonly available in most countries, dual-head power injectors were only introduced for the angiographic market in the United States in 2018.

For most 3D-/4D-DSA studies, it is recommended that 100% contrast be used with a volume and rate of injection appropriate for the vasculature being studied. In cases where there is fast flow, e.g., AVMs, some increase in contrast volume and injection rate over that used when flow is normal is usually indicated. CBCT 3D acquisition protocols vary by vendor and system generation. The main technical factors impacting these protocols are the maximal rotation speed of the C-arm and the flat panel detector read-out speed. In general, shorter acquisitions require less contrast, and may be useful in minimizing patient motion; they are usually adequate when blood flow is normal or when there is an AVM or AVF. Longer acquisitions allow a more complete reconstruction of the vasculature, i.e., arteries and veins, are more likely to capture vasculature in which flow is slow, and provide more temporal data for time-resolved 3D-DSA (4D DSA) reconstructions. Volumetric reconstruction theory dictates complete sampling of the structures of interest across at least 180 degrees plus the cone angle for CBCT. To satisfy this, angiographic 3D acquisitions make use of an x-ray delay (delayed start of image data acquisition) to allow enough time between the injection of contrast and the start of image acquisition for the vasculature to fill. The injection continues throughout the data acquisition. In instances when time-resolved 3D images are desired, i.e., 4D-DSA, the contrast injection should either coincide with the start of the image data acquisition or to be certain that the inflow of the contrast is captured; a very short injection delay (~0.5 s) should be programed into the power injector. In order to satisfy the image reconstruction requirements, if a time resolved 3D is desired, the C-arm rotation arc is extended up to 260°.

CBCT studies are usually done either as part of an intervention in order to allow simultaneous visualization of vasculature, parenchyma, and/or devices or to measure perfusion. For CBCT studies done in order to depict the relationships of vasculature, parenchyma, and devices, an intra-arterial injection is usually done. These studies are often viewed as multi-planar reconstructions. To reduce high-contrast streaking artifacts, contrast is diluted to, e.g., 50%; when the goal is also device visualization, the contrast dilution should be greater than, e.g., 20%, to avoid obscuring the device. Timing of the injection should be programed so that there will be full opacification of the vasculature throughout the acquisition.

For perfusion measurements, an IV injection is used with injection of 100% contrast medium followed by a saline chase. Current multi-rotational acquisitions start the data acquisition simultaneously with the contrast injection. Because of time delay, as the bolus passes through the veins and lungs, data from the first two C-arm rotations will not contain contrast medium; these data can be used to reconstruct masks which can be used to create subtracted images from the subsequent rotations. In general, perfusion imaging uses a multi-rotational (10×) acquisition covering about 60 s. This time window allows the capture of the contrast bolus arrival, passage through the parenchyma, and venous washout.

References

1. Fahrig R, Fox AJ, Lownie S, Holdsworth DW. Use of a C-arm system to generate true three-dimensional computed rotational angiograms: preliminary in vitro and in vivo results. AJNR. 1997;18:1507–14.
2. Baba R, Konno Y, Ueda K, Ikeda S. Comparison of flat-panel detector and image-intensifier detector for cone-beam CT. Comput Med Imaging Graph. 2002;26:153–8.
3. Akpek S, Bruner T, Benndorf G, Strother C. Three-dimensional imaging and cone beam volume CT in C-arm angiography with flat panel detector. Diagn Interv Radiolo. 2005;11:10–3.
4. Enomoto Y, Yamachi K, Takahiko A, et al. Effect of metal artifact reduction software on image quality of C-arm cone-beam computed tomography during intracranial aneurysm treatment. Interv Neuroradiol. 2018;24(3):303–8.
5. Goubergrits L, Schaller J, Kertzscher U, et al. Hemodynamic impact of cerebral aneurysm endovascular treatment devices: coils and flow diverters. Expert Rev Med Devices. 2014;11(4):361–73.
6. Aquarius R, deKorte A, Smits D, et al. The importance of wall apposition in flow diverters. Neurosurgery. 2018;82(4):804–10.
7. Richter G, Engelhorn T, Struffert T, et al. Flat panel detector angiographic CT for stent-assisted coil embolization of broad-based cerebral aneurysms. AJNR. 2007;28:1902–8.
8. Richter G, Engelhorn T, Struffert T, et al. Detector angiographic CT for stent-assisted coil embolization of broad-based cerebral aneurysms. AJNR Am J Neuroradiol. 2007;28:1902–8.
9. Kizilkilic O, Kocer N, Metaxas GE, et al. Utility of VasoCT in the treatment of intracranial aneurysm with flow-diverter stents. J Neurosurg. 2012;117:45–9.
10. Struffert T, Hauer M, Banckwitz R, et al. Effective dose to patient measurements in flat-detector and multi-slice computed tomography: a comparison of applications in neuroradiology. Eur Radiol. 2014;24:1257–65.. CrossRef Medline
11. Xia Y, Dennerlein F, Bauer S, et al. Scaling calibration in region of interest reconstruction with the 1D and 2D ATRACT algorithm. Int J Comput Assist Radiol Surg. 2014;9:345–56.
12. Dennerlein F, Maier A. Approximate truncation robust computed tomography: ATRACT. Phys Med Boil. 2013;58:6133–48.
13. Yang P, Ahmed A, Schafer S, et al. Low-dose volume-of-interest C-arm CT imaging of intracranial stents and flow diverters. AJNR. 2016;37:648–54.
14. Gore P, Theodore N, Brasiliense L, et al. The utility of onyx for preoperative embolization of cranial and spinal tumors. Neurosurgery. 2008;62:1204–11.
15. Ahmed S, Hassan T, Hisham AE, et al. The value of preoperative embolization in large and giant solid cerebellar hemangioblastomas. Interv Neuroradiol. 2016;22:482–8.
16. Liu A, Liu J, Zenghui Q, et al. Onyx embolization of cavernous sinus dural arteriovenous fistulas via direct transorbital puncture under the guidance of three-dimensional reconstructed skull images. Acta Neurochir. 2014;156:897–900.
17. Friedman WA, Bova FJ. Radiosurgery for arteriovenous malformations. Neurol Res. 2011;33:803–19.
18. Kang J, Huang J, Gilloud P, et al. Planning evaluation of C-arm cone beam CT angiography for target delineation in stereotactic radiation surgery of bran AVMs. Radiat Oncol. 2014;90:430–7.
19. McMeekin P, White P, James MA, et al. Estimating the number of UK stroke patients eligible for endovascular thrombectomy. Eur Stroke J. 2017;2(4):319–26.
20. Forlivesi S, Bonetti B, Cappellari M. Number of ischemic strokes potentially eligible for revascularization treatments in an Italian comprehensive stroke center:

a modeling study. J Thromb Thrombolysis. 2018; https://doi.org/10.1007/s11239-018-1712-4.
21. Jadhav AP, Desai SM, Kenmuir CL, al e. Eligibility for endovascular trial enrollment in the 6-to 24 hour time window: analysis of a single comprehensive stroke center. Stroke. 2018;49(4):1015–7.
22. Mulder MJHL, Jansen IGH, Goldhoom RB, et al. Time to endovascular treatment and outcome in acute ischemic stroke: MR CLEAN registry results. Circulation. 2018;138(3):232–40.
23. Jauch EC, Saver JL, Adams HP, et al. Guidelines for the early management of patients with acute ischemic stroke: a guideline for healthcare professionals from the American Heart Association/American Stroke Association. Stroke. 2013;44:870–947.
24. Ribo M, Molina CA, Cobo E, et al. Association between time to reperfusion and outcome is primarily driven by the time from imaging to reperfusion. Stroke. 2016;47:999–1004.
25. Saver JL, Goyal M, van der Lugt A, et al. HERMES collaborators. Time to treatment with endovascular thrombectomy and outcomes from ischemic stroke: a meta-analysis. JAMA. 2016;316:1279–88.
26. Leyhe JR, Tsogkas I, Hesse AC, et al. Latest generation of flat detector CT as a peri-interventional diagnostic tool: a comparative study with multidetector CT. J Neurointerv Surg. 2017;9:1253–5.
27. AM F'l, Buhk JH, Fiehler J, et al. Voxel-based sensitivity of flat panel CT for the detection of intracranial hemorrhage: comparison to multi-detector CT. PLoS One. 2016;11:e0165794.
28. Barber PA, Demchuk AM, Zang J, Buchan AM. Validity and reliability of a quantitative computed tomography score in predicting outcome of hyperacute stroke before thrombolytic therapy. ASPECTS study group. Alberta stroke Programme early CT score. Lancet. 2000;355(9216):1670–4.
29. Msier IL, Leyhe JR, Tsogkas I, et al. Diagnosing early ischemic changes with the latest-generation flat detector CT: a comparative study with multidetector CT JNR. Am J Neuroradiol. 2018;39:881–86 May.
30. Wagner M, Deuerling-Zheng Y, Mohlenbrunch B, et al. A model based algorithm for perfusion estimation in interventional C-arm CT systems. Med Phys. 2013;40(3):031916.
31. Ganguly A, Fieselmann A, Boese J, et al. In vitro evaluation of the imaging accuracy of C-arm conebeam CT in cerebral perfusion imaging. Med Phys. 2012;39(11):6652–9.
32. Fieselmann A, Ganguly A. Deuerling-Zheng y, et al. interventional 4-D C-arm CT perfusion imaging using interleaved scanning and partial reconstruction interpolation. IEEE Trans Med Imaging. 2012;31(4):892–906.
33. Chen GH, Li Y. Synchronized multiartifact reduction with tomographic reconstruction (SMART-RECON): a statistical model based iterative image reconstruction method to eliminate limited-view artifacts and to mitigate the temporal-average artifacts in time-resolved CT. Med Phys. 2015;42(8):4698–707.
34. Niu K, Yang P, Wu Y, et al. C-arm conebeam CT perfusion imaging in the angiographic suite: a comparison with multidetector CT perfusion imaging. AJNR. 2016;37(7):1303–9.
35. Mow M, Zbijewski W, Sisniega A, Xu J, Dang H, Stayman JW, Wang X et al. Brain perfusion imaging using a Reconstruction-of-Difference (RoD) approach for cone-beam computed tomography. In Medical imaging 2017: physics of medical imaging, vol. 10132, p. 1013212. International Society for Optics and Photonics, 2017.
36. Shin NY, Kim KE, Park M, et al. Dual-phase CT collateral score: a predictor of clinical outcome in patients with acute ischemic stroke. PLoS One. 2014;9(9):e107379.
37. Yang P, Niu K, Wu Y, et al. Evaluation of collaterals and clot burden using time-resolved c-arm conebeam CT angiography in the angiography suite: a feasibility study. AJNR. 2017;38(4):747–52.
38. Yang P, Niu K, Wu Y, et al. Time-resolved C0arm computed tomographic angiography derived from computed tomographic perfusion acquisition: new capability for one-stop-shop acute ischemic stroke treatment in the Angiosuite. Stroke. 2015;46(12):3383–9.
39. Psychogios MN, Behme D, Schregel K, et al. One-stop management of acute stroke patients: minimizing door-to-reperfusion times. Stroke. 2017;48:3152–5.
40. Psychogios MN, Buhk JH, Schramm P, et al. Feasibility of angiographic CT in peri-interventional diagnostic imaging: a comparative study with multidetector CT. AJNR. 2010;31:1226–31.
41. Kallmes DF, Rabinstein AA, Gounis M. To be or not 2b? To see or not 2c? Alas, the clock is ticking on TICI. JSNIS. 2018;10:323–4.
42. Veldhoen S, Schollchen M, Hanken H, et al. Performance of cone-beam computed tomography and multidetector computed tomography in diagnostic imaging of the midface: a comparative study on phantom and cadaver head scans. Eur Radiol. 2017;27:790–800.
43. Vertinsky AT, Schwartz NE, Fischbein NJ, et al. Comparison of multidetector CT angiography and MR imaging of cervical artery dissection. AJNR. 2008;29:1753–60.
44. Cole BL, Maddocks JD, Sharpe K. Visual search and the conspicuity of coloured targets for colour vision normal and colour vision deficient observers. Clin Exp Optom. 2004;87:294–304.
45. D'Zmura M. Color in visual search. Vis Res. 1991;31:951–66.
46. Strother CM, Bender F, Deuerling-Zheng Y, et al. Parametric color coding of digital subtraction angiography. AJNR. 2010;31:919–24.
47. Elsaid N, Saied A, Joshi K, Nelson J, Baumgart J, Lopes D. 2D parametric parenchymal blood flow as a predictor of the hemorrhagic events after endovascular treatment of acute ischemic stroke: a single-center retrospective study. Interv Neurol. 2018;7:522–53.48.

48. Fahrig R, Fox AJ, Lownie S, et al. Use of a C-arm system to generate true three-dimensional computed rotational angiograms: preliminary preliminary in vitro and in vivo results. AJNR. 1997;18:1507–14.
49. Fahrig R, Moreau M, Holdsworth DW. Three-dimensional computed tomographic reconstruction using a C-arm mounted XRII: correction of image intensifier distortion. Med Phys. 1997;24:1097–1.
50. Anxionnat R, Bracard S, Ducrocq X, et al. Intracranial aneurysms: clinical value of 3D digital subtraction angiography in the therapeutic decision and endovascular treatment. Radiology. 2001;218:799–808.
51. Van Rooij WJ, Sprengers ME, de Gast AN, et al. 3D rotational angiography: the new gold standard in the detection of additional intracranial aneurysms. AJNR. 2009;29:976–7952.. Van Rooij W J, Peluso J P P, Sluzewski M, Beute G N. Additional Value of 3D Rotational Angiography in Angiographically Negative Aneurysmal Subarachnoid Hemorrhage: How Negative is Negative. AJNR 2008; 29: 962-66
52. Davis B, Royalty K, Kowarschik M, et al. 4D digital subtraction angiography: implementation and demonstration of feasibility. AJNR. 2013;34:1914–21.
53. Copeland AD, Mangoubi RS, Mukund ND, et al. Temporal data fusion for 3D+T image reconstruction in cerebral angiography. IEEE Trans Med. 2010;29:1238–51.
54. Waechter I, Bredno J, Hermans R, et al. Model-based flow quantification from rotational angiography. Med Image Anal. 2008;12:586–602.
55. Lescher S, Gehrisch S, Klein S, Berkefeld J. Time-resolved 3D angiography; display of detailed neurovascular anatomy in patients with intracranial vascular malformations. J Neurounterv Surg. 2017;9:887–94.
56. Chen KK, Guo WY, Yang HC, et al. Application of time-resolved 3D digital subtraction angiography to plan cerebral arteriovenous malformation radiosurgery. AJNR. 2017;38:740–6.
57. Sandoval-Garcia C, Royalty K, Yang P, et al. 4D-DSA a new technique for arteriovenous malformation evaluation: a feasibility study. J Neurointerv Surg. 2016;8:300–4.
58. Sandoval-Garcia C, Yang P, Schubert T, et al. Comparison of the Diagnostic utility of 4D-DSA with conventional 2D and 3D-DSA in the diagnosis of cerebrovascular abnormalities. AJNR. 2017;38:729–34.
59. Wu Y, Shaughnessy G, Hoffman CA, et al. Quantification of blood velocity with 4D DSA using the shifted least-squares method. AJNR. 2018;39:1871–7.. [Epub ahead of print]
60. Shaughnessy G, Schafer S, Speidel MA, Strother CM, Mistretta CA. Measuring blood velocity using 4D-DSA: a feasibility study. Med Phys 2018. 2018;45:4510–8.. [Epub ahead of print]

CT in Cardiac Applications

23

Arya Iranmanesh and Geoffrey D. Rubin

The Heart

The mechanical action of the heart may be simplified to that of a pump having two discrete chambers, the right and left heart. In the normal state, these chambers do not directly communicate; the right heart receives and pumps deoxygenated blood to the lungs (pulmonary circulation) where it is oxygenated and returned to the left heart and then pumped throughout the much larger network of blood vessels throughout the body (systemic circulation). Because it must deliver blood through the higher-pressure systemic circulation, the left heart forms much of the cardiac mass of the heart.

The muscular portions of the heart which are responsible for the propulsion of blood through the pulmonary and systemic circulations are referred to as the ventricles. These form two of the four major chambers of the heart. The remaining two chambers are the atria and sit atop each ventricle and are significantly smaller in size and have thinner walls. The right and left atria serve as intermediary chambers that continuously receive blood flow back to the heart, subsequently "preloading" the ventricles with a small but forceful contraction prior to the end of diastole (which has been described as the "resting" or "filling" phase). The right atrium receives deoxygenated venous blood from the superior vena cava (SVC), which drains venous blood from the head and much of the thorax, and the inferior vena cava (IVC), which prior to coursing through the liver and into the heart, receives blood from the abdomen, pelvis, and lower extremity veins.

The mechanical action of the heart is governed by electrical signals which travel through the cardiac conducting system resulting in a progressive wave of depolarization and associated myocardial contraction. The normal rhythm of the heart is generated by the sinoatrial node, often referred to as the "pacemaker" of the heart. This rhythmic electrical signal originates from the right atrium and travels through the left atrium to the "atrioventricular" node, which serves as a "gatekeeper" to regulate electrical activity reaching the ventricular myocardium.

Anatomy

The heart is a complex structure in both its normal and abnormal states. The following anatomic discussion is limited to anatomy relevant to common cardiac CT applications.

Aorta and Coronary Artery Origins

The portion of the aorta that directly receives the left ventricular outflow is the "aortic root." Although forming only a short segment of the

A. Iranmanesh · G. D. Rubin (✉)
Duke University School of Medicine, Department of Radiology, Durham, NC, USA
e-mail: arya.iranmanesh@duke.edu; grubin@duke.edu

© Springer Nature Switzerland AG 2020

E. Samei, N. J. Pelc (eds.), *Computed Tomography*, https://doi.org/10.1007/978-3-030-26957-9_23

aorta, the aortic root is the site of significant pathology. It extends from the aortic annulus, formed by the basal attachment of the leaflets of the aortic valve, includes the entirety of the aortic valve and the three sinuses of Valsalva, and terminates at the sinotubular junction, where the aortic profile transitions from the three bulging sinuses to a cylindrical form with circular cross sections [1]. The left and right main coronary arteries arise from two of three sinuses of Valsalva, referred to as left, right, and noncoronary sinuses. Although anatomic variations exist (some of which are pathologic), the right and left coronary arteries typically arise from the respectively named aortic sinus. The caliber of the ascending aorta subsequently narrows slightly at the sinotubular junction. The "tubular" ascending aorta forms the bulk of the ascending aorta and is so named due to both the morphologic appearance and lack of branch vessels. The transverse aorta, also referred to as the aortic arch, gives rise to the great vessels, the first of which, the "innominate artery" (also referred to as the "brachiocephalic artery"), delineates the proximal boundary of the arch. Most commonly, three vessels arise from the arch, with the left common carotid and the left subclavian artery origins, respectively, following the innominate artery origin. At the distal aspect of the transverse aorta, approximately 2 cm beyond the origin of the left subclavian artery origin, the aorta narrows slightly at the aortic "isthmus". The remainder of the thoracic aorta following the aortic isthmus is referred to as the "descending aorta."

Coronary Arteries

Similar to other arteries throughout the body, a normal coronary artery is composed of three distinct layers. The intima is a single layer of endothelial cells which form the innermost layer of the vessel. The media forms the central layer and is primarily composed of smooth muscle cells, which relax and contract to regulate flow through altered luminal dimensions. Finally, the adventitia, which provides a significant portion of the tensile strength of larger arteries, is composed largely of collagen to form the outermost layer.

Modern MDCT allows for visualization of the major coronary arteries and their second-order branches (with variable visualization of smaller branches). Arterial blood supply to the heart muscle is via three major coronary arteries: the right (RCA), left anterior descending (LAD), and left circumflex (LCx) coronary arteries. Arising from the left sinus of Valsalva, the left coronary artery (referred to as the "left main" prior to bifurcation) after a short, 1–15 mm distance gives rise to two of the three major coronaries: the left anterior descending (LAD) artery and the left circumflex artery (LCx). In a significant minority of patients, a trifurcation of the left main is present, with a third "ramus intermedius" branch present in the middle.

The left main supplies much of the left ventricle (LV) of the heart, colloquially named the "widow maker," as occlusions are often fatal. The LAD courses anterolaterally in the interventricular sulcus obliquely toward the LV apex [2, 3]. The LAD gives rise to diagonal and septal branches. Commonly labeled D1, D2, etc., the diagonal branches follow a lateral course across the anterior LV myocardium to supply the anterior portions of the LV free wall. Smaller "septal perforator" branches course medially to supply the mid and distal interventricular septum and, in conjunction with the right coronary artery, much of the basal septum as well [3].

The LCx is the second major branch of the left coronary artery, with proximal course in the left atrioventricular groove (coronary sulcus) with branch vessels termed "obtuse marginals" (OM1, OM2, etc.). The lateral LV free wall is supplied by the LCx and the OM branches [2].

The right coronary artery aptly arises from the right coronary sinus and, despite substantial variations in proximal branching patterns, serves to supply the right heart (both atrium and ventricle). Specifically, the distribution most commonly also supplies the interatrial septum, with resultant supply to both the sinoatrial (SA) and atrioventricular (AV) nodes.

The coronary tree is defined as being either right dominant (90%), left dominant (5%), or codominant (5%), depending upon the source of blood supply to the inferior intraventricular septum and posterolateral wall of the left ventricle via the posterior descending coronary and posterolateral coronary arteries, respectively.

Coronary Veins

In contrast to the arterial system of the heart, the venous system of the heart is infrequently the site of significant pathology, but mapping of the coronary venous system with CT has been used to guide placement of and assess ventricular pacing leads. The small veins of the heart often demonstrate significant normal variability in course, with only the larger proximal epicardial portions identified by name in routine evaluation.

The cardiac veins can be anatomically separated into the "greater" and "lesser" venous systems. The greater venous system is formed by the larger veins of the heart which course along the epicardial surface, the proximal portions of which are typically identifiable on cardiac CT. The majority of these veins coalesce centrally into the coronary sinus, a prominent (but short) venous channel which courses in the atrioventricular (coronary) groove prior to draining into the right atrium. Drainage of the left ventricle is almost exclusively through tributaries of the coronary sinus, the largest of which is the great coronary vein [4]. Coronary veins of the right ventricle, in contrast, are infrequently tributaries of the coronary sinus, instead most commonly draining directly into the right atrium.

Pericardium

The pericardium, composed of a fibrous parietal and a serous visceral layer, encases both the right and left cardiac chambers and the proximal portion of their respective outflow tracts. The thin inner visceral layer, separated from the epicardium by a variable amount of epicardial fat, appears as the lining of the heart on gross examination [5]. Pericardial layers are separated by a potential space containing a trace amount (15–50 mL) of "lubricating" serous fluid derived from plasma. Formed by dense collagen fibers, the outer "parietal" pericardium serves to anchor and stabilize the heart through fibrotendinous attachments to surrounding structures, including the sternum anteriorly and diaphragm inferiorly.

Physiology

Unlike imaging of other organ systems, the dynamic nature of the heart necessitates comprehension not only of the target anatomy but also of the fundamentals of cardiac physiology – knowledge of which allows for optimization of scanner design to both compensate and accommodate for the complexities of the cardiac cycle. The most obvious challenge in generating static images of the beating heart lies in effectively "freezing" myocardial motion to capture diagnostic images free of motion degradation. Such a task necessitates recording of the electrical impulses resulting in cardiac contraction through an electrocardiogram acquired during scanning, allowing for "synchronization" of imaging with cardiac motion [6]. Furthermore, knowledge of normal cardiac rhythm and potential aberrations is necessary to attempt to mitigate potential pitfalls which may result in nondiagnostic acquisitions.

Cardiac Cycle

The cardiac cycle consists of coordinated electrical and mechanical events which in the normal physiologic state result in sinus rhythm with atrial then ventricular contractions followed by refilling and a brief period of relaxation. The cardiac cycle may be grossly simplified into two phases, systole and diastole. During systole, the ventricles contract with associated mechanical action rapidly decreasing the cavity size and forcefully ejecting blood into the pulmonary circulation from the right ventricle and into the systemic circulation from the left ventricle. During the subsequent diastolic phase, the ventricles are in a relaxed state to allow for filling. The right and left atria are the site of inflow into the heart, with the pulmonary veins carrying recently oxygenated blood draining into left atrium and systemic veins (the inferior and superior vena cava) draining deoxygenated blood into the right atrium. During the latter portion of diastole, the atria contract ("atrial kick") to contribute a final but significant (~20%) bolus of blood into the ventricles to assist in achieving maximal preload. At end of diastole, the ventricles are maximally dilated. End diastolic volume is a common measurement to evaluate for ventricular dilation in the pathologic state. At the onset of systole, rapid rises in intraventricular pressure result from coordinated and near synchronous contraction of the right and left ventricular myocardium. This increased pressure, once above that of atrial pressures, causes abrupt closure of the valves positioned between the ventricles and atria (mitral valve on the left and tricuspid valve on the right), preventing retrograde movement of blood flow.

The aorta serves as the outflow tract of the left ventricle and supplies oxygenated blood to the tissues of the body, while outflow of the right ventricle delivers deoxygenated blood into the pulmonary circulation via the main pulmonary artery. Valves also separate the outflow tracts from the ventricles, with the valves named according to the respective outflow vessel (the aortic valve on the left and pulmonic valve on the right). These valves are closed in diastole. In early systole as intraventricular pressures rise to exceed the diastolic pressure in their outflow vessels, the outflow valves open to allow egress of blood into the pulmonary and systemic circulations.

In the normal state, the ventricles eject slightly more than half of the blood volume achieved at end systole. The percentage of blood ejected from each ventricle is termed the "ejection fraction" (calculated as the difference between the end diastolic volume and end systolic volume divided by the end diastolic volume). The ejection fraction normally ranges from 55% to 65% and is the most commonly used value to determine ventricular health/function, with both decreased and increased values indicative of underlying pathology. At end systole, the ventricles are in the most contracted state, with corresponding maximal reduction in cavity size. With ventricular blood volume at the lowest point in the cardiac cycle, intracavitary pressures decline below those of the aorta and pulmonary arteries, closing the ventricular outflow valves and preventing blood from regurgitating back into the ventricles. This marks the beginning of diastole. Relaxation of the ventricles causes their intracavitary pressures to rapidly decline below that of the atria, resulting in reopening of the mitral and tricuspid valves and allowing the ventricles to refill.

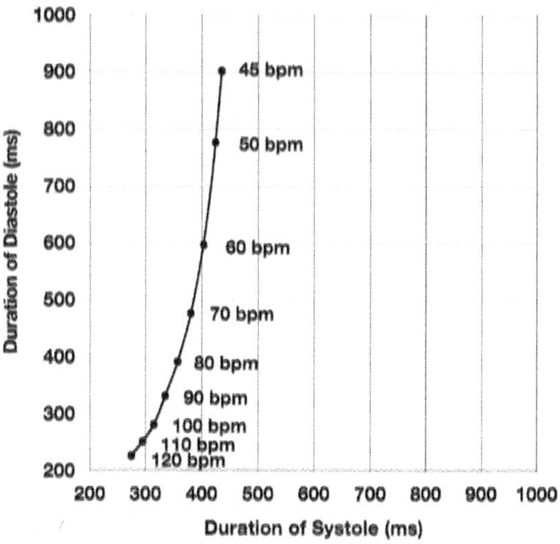

Fig. 23.1 Plot illustrates the substantial variation in duration of diastole as a function of heart rate, a >4-fold change from 45 to 120 bpm. Variation in systole is approximately 1/5th that of diastole. (Data from Bazan and Ortiz [74])

The cardiac period is the duration of a single cardiac cycle and is determined as the sum of the durations of systole and diastole. The relative contribution of each varies significantly by heart rate with an approximately fivefold greater range in diastolic duration relative to systole (Fig. 23.1, adapted from [7, 8]). The mid portion of diastole, termed "diastasis", is the time of least myocardial motion. Although the entirety of the diastolic phase is free of active ventricular contraction, the volume of the heart increases most quickly during early diastole, the "rapid filling" phase, and increases again in late diastole following atrial contraction. Based on the premise that high-quality CT scanning necessitates imaging of the heart when it is most quiescent, the ideal time window corresponds to diastasis. However, diastasis only occurs with heart rates less than 80 bpm (Fig. 23.2, adapted from [8]).

The Electrocardiogram and Cardiac Rhythms

The coordinated rhythmic contraction of the heart is a result of propagation of depolarizing

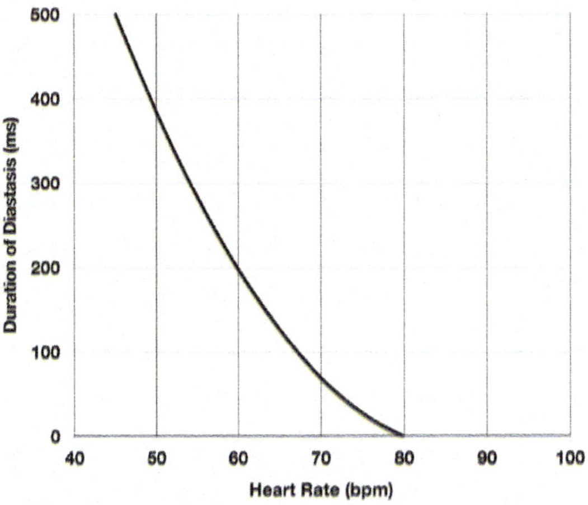

Fig. 23.2 Diastasis, the period when the heart is motionless in diastole, does not exist for heart rates greater than 80 bpm. In order to acquire a CT scan when the heart is completely motionless, the scan window should be less than or equal to the duration of diastasis. Lower heart rates provide a larger target for scanning when the heart is motion-free. (Derived from data in Chung et al. [8])

electrical signals through a network of specialized conductive myocardial cells, the electrical signature of which is visualized on an electrocardiogram (ECG). In sinus rhythm, the electrical signal initiating the cascade of events culminating in a heartbeat originates in the sinoatrial (SA) node, self-excitatory cells located superiorly in the right atrium, near the superior cavoatrial junction. Through internodal pathways, the electrical signal is propagated through both the right and left atria, resulting in atrial depolarization and subsequent contraction. The electrical signal next reaches the atrioventricular node, located in the inferior portion of the right atrium. A brief physiologic delay of the electrical signal at this node not only serves to regulate conduction of aberrant rapid signals to the ventricles in the pathologic state, but in the normal state allows time for enhanced preload from the atrial kick. The electrical impulse is then transmitted into the bundle of His, forking into the right and left bundle branches which course in parallel along the interventricular septum prior to further subdividing and ultimately the Purkinje fibers, which carry the depolarizing current through the ventricular myocardium resulting in ventricular contraction.

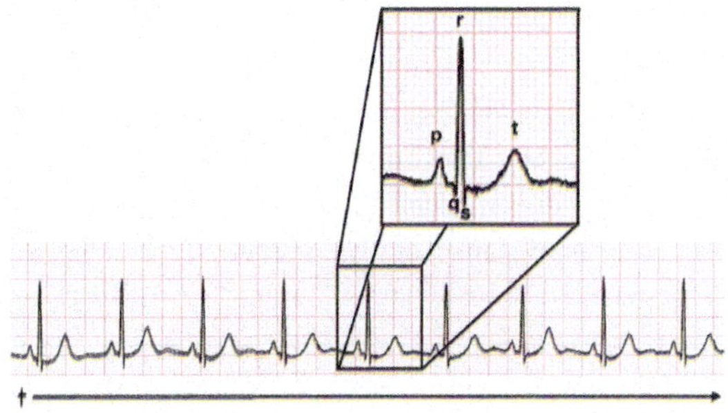

Fig. 23.3 Electrocardiogram (ECG) tracing. Time is indicated on the horizontal axis and voltage on the vertical axis. The labeled waves include (p) atrial depolarization, (qrs) ventricular depolarization, and (t) repolarization. Mechanical systole begins at the approximate moment of R-wave and lasts approximately 100 ms

This propagating wave of depolarization is appreciated on the ECG as a series of distinct upward and downward deflections with direction of deflections indicating the vector of electrical activity with respect to the recording lead (Fig. 23.3). The first wave, a small upward deflection termed the "P"-wave, marks the atrial contraction occurring in late diastole, with the subsequent lack of visible electrical activity correlating with the brief delay at the AV node. The most pronounced waveform in the EKG is formed by ventricular depolarization and is termed the qrs complex. Of particular importance in cardiac CT, the R-wave is a large discernible wave which corresponds to depolarization of the bulk of the left ventricular mass.

When functioning normally, the cardiac conduction system produces "normal sinus rhythm," which is associated with a mostly steady heart rate, although beat-to-beat variability in the cardiac cycle length is a normal physiological phenomenon with many influences. Arrhythmia represents a variation from normal sinus rhythm and usually indicates an underlying cardiac abnormality. A comprehensive discussion of cardiac arrhythmia and its influence on CT imaging is beyond the scope of this chapter. A brief introduction of the most commonly encountered stable arrhythmias is presented herein.

Sinus tachycardia represents a sinus rhythm with an abnormally high rate of >100 beats per minute (bpm). Sinus tachycardia is best managed pharmacologically to lower heart rate into an acceptable range. Atrial fibrillation occurs due to a constant state of disorganized electrical activity in the atria resulting in intermittent initiation of ventricular depolarization at the AV node and is associated with an irregularly irregular heart rate. Uncontrolled heart rate in atrial fibrillation is often tachycardic. Among the more challenging arrhythmias to image with CT, rate control is needed to reduce the cardiac period to an acceptable duration, and single-beat imaging (using a wide-area detector CT system) prevents inter-beat misregistration that will occur with multi-beat imaging. Premature atrial contractions and premature ventricular contractions (PACs and PVCs) originate from the atria or the ventricles, respectively. PACs are typically idiopathic isolated phenomena, but also occur in association with caffeine use as well as certain medications. PVCs may also be idiopathic and benign, but when occuring frequently usually indicate underlying cardiac disease and may be isolated or repeating. When PVCs repeatedly occur between two normal beats, it is termed trigeminy, while when they occur on every other beat basis, they are termed bigeminy. All forms of premature contractions disrupt the regular cardiac rhythm and almost always result in misregistration of the cardiac volume when encompassed within a multi-beat CT acquisition. Increasing frequency or multifocality of PVCs is associated with instability, with a risk of degeneration into malignant cardiac rhythms.

Evolution of Cardiac CT

Despite the prevalence and morbidity associated with heart disease, particularly atherosclerosis of the coronary arteries, CT has only recently become a clinically important tool in the setting of suspected cardiac pathology. Beyond the use of stress scintigraphy in evaluating of possible ischemia in intermediate- to high-risk patients without known coronary disease [9], invasive coronary angiography has long been considered the only definitive means for coronary artery evaluation. Furthermore, echocardiography, despite many known limitations, long represented the only readily available modality for dynamic evaluation of myocardial/valvular morphology and function. CT and MRI, although both considered routine in the evaluation of extracardiac pathology, were for many years limited by the unique challenge of evaluating the beating heart – due to limitations in both spatial and temporal resolution [10]. However, following the advent of spiral/helical technology and subsequently the introduction of multidetector CT scanners near the turn of the century, rapid increases in scanner speed and temporal resolution have allowed for CT to generate volumetric images of subcentimeter structures. These advances ultimately not only allowed for diagnostic imaging of the heart but also placed cardiac CTA in the unique position to provide a noninvasive alternative to conventional angiography in the evaluation of coronary artery disease. Cardiac CT also has shown additional benefit with respect to potential simultaneous high-resolution dynamic cardiac imaging and three-dimensional anatomic delineation of both cardiac structures and adjacent extracardiac structures that is essentially unrivaled in other imaging modalities [11].

Early Designs

Modern CT scanners utilize a continuously rotating X-ray tube with simultaneously rotating multirow detector systems to achieve what is referred to as a "spiral" or "helical" acquisition. This is in contrast to traditional sequential "step-and-shoot" techniques, which was imposed in the pre-slip ring era by the need to unwind cabling (necessary in communication of electrical signals and data between the stationary and the rotating portion of the gantry) following each rotation. With the widespread introduction of slip ring interfaces in the early 1990s [12], helical acquisition techniques were enabled, allowing for continuous gantry rotation. This technology, together with the subsequent introduction of multidetector row geometry revolutionized the application of CT to the arterial system [13].

Electron Beam CT

One noteworthy precursor to this technology development that in its day provided unparalleled volumetric cardiac imaging was electron beam computed tomography (EBCT). EBCT positioned an electron source at the head of the patient and electromagnetically steered its output utilized onto four fixed 210-degree tungsten anode targets. In this historical design, only the electron beam moves, sweeping across the tungsten anode to generate a "fan beam" of X-ray which then passes through the patient to strike a fixed detector array [12]. Electrocardiographically gated thin section tomographic images were created with a temporal resolution of 50–100 ms, allowing for quantification of coronary artery calcium and, following injection of intravenous contrast (Fig. 23.4), assessment for high-grade luminal stenosis [14, 15].

Early work with EBCT laid the foundation from which modern multidetector cardiac CT would ultimately flourish. The electron beam design overcame the temporal constraints of conventional CT, providing the first clinically viable demonstration of CT for evaluating the coronary arteries [16]. Prior to quickly falling out of favor with the introduction of MDCT in the latter part of the twentieth century, advancements over several iterations allowed for EBCT temporal resolutions of as little as 33 ms [17], higher than that of even modern-day MDCT. Limitations in spatial resolution, however, with section thickness of 1.5 mm (compared to a 0.5–0.6 mm on modern MDCT), and limited ability to acquire volumetric 3D datasets, ultimately led to abandonment of the technology in favor of multirow helical designs.

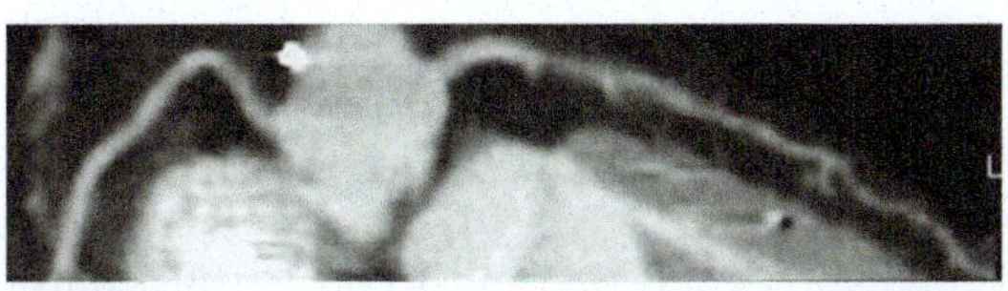

Fig. 23.4 Coronary EBCT scan acquired at Lucile Packard Children's Hospital in May 1997. The configuration of the scanner only allowed imaging of the proximal coronary arteries. Temporal resolution was 100 ms, but spatial resolution was limited, precluding evaluation of more distal, smaller, coronary branches

Multidetector Row CT

Since the late 1990s, multidetector CT (MDCT) has become the dominant CT design and has evolved considerably in ways that greatly benefit imaging of the heart. A detailed description of MDCT geometries and characteristics is presented in Chap. 1; however, we herein highlight key characteristics that enable and refine the unique demands of cardiac imaging.

Detector Width and Row Number

Electrocardiographically gated cardiac CT originated with electron beam CT in 1995 and then became broadly available with 4-row and 8-row MDCT in 1999 and 2000, respectively (Fig. 23.5). Improving with the successive development of wider detector arrays with a greater number of detector rows, it was not until the introduction of 64-slice CT where cardiac

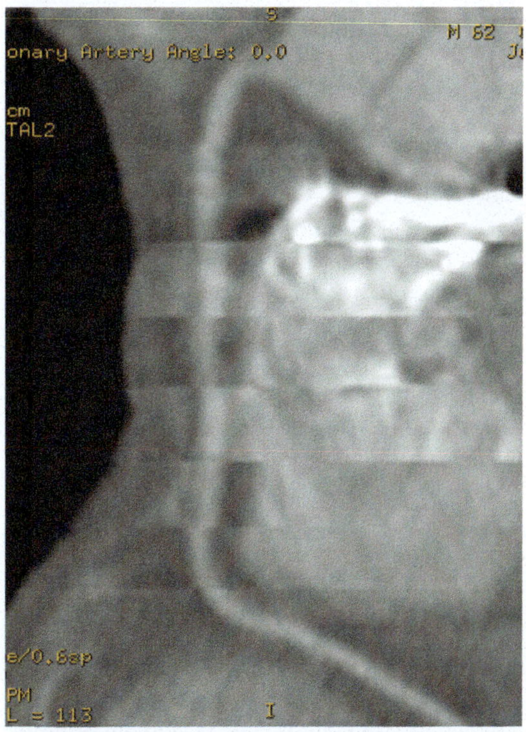

Fig. 23.5 Curved planar reformation through the right coronary artery using an eight-row MDCT scanner from 2000. With a detector width of 10 mm, as many as 16 heartbeats were required to image the entirety of the heart, resulting in misregistration through the longitudinal axis of the scan

CT truly became a clinically viable modality for the assessment of the coronary arteries, which is the most common indication for cardiac CT scanning [18]. The benefit of greater detector widths is the ability to cover greater portion of the heart with each gantry rotation. With a typical detector width of 0.5–0.6 mm, a 64-row MDCT scanner covers between 3.2 and 4.0 cm per rotation. Most hearts require between 12 and 16 cm of longitudinal coverage for complete imaging; thus, for a contiguous nonhelical (conventional) acquisition using 64-row MDCT, between 3 and 5 gantry rotations are required to image the entire heart.

Over the past 5 years, wider detector arrays have been introduced into clinical practice. Currently available configurations include 128×0.6, 256×0.625, and 320×0.5 MDCT scanners with respective coverage of 80, 160, and 160 mm per rotation, respectively. Consequently, the 256- and 320-row scanners are capable of imaging the entirety of the heart within a single rotation. Because conventional scanning of the heart using prospective ECG triggering results in one rotation during every other heartbeat (with movement of the patient through the gantry between beats), the composition of a volumetric image is typically composed of multiple heartbeats. The exception to this occurs with 160 mm detector arrays where the heart can be imaged during a single beat. This is a substantial advantage as there are many reasons why the heart may occupy a slightly different position within the scan volume on successive beats, which results in misregistration between serially acquired regions. The more beats required to image the heart, the more likely it is that misregistration will manifest within the acquired CT volume. The causes of beat-to-beat cardiac positional variability are discussed later in this chapter.

Another advantage of single-beat imaging is that the heart and associated phase of intravenous contrast enhancement is imaged simultaneously, which has been used to determine of the physiologic impact of coronary lesions through analysis of intra-coronary enhancement gradients [19].

Multiple Radiation Sources

Initially introduced in 2007, dual-source CT scanners utilize two X-ray tubes with each having a corresponding detector array [20]. The tubes are offset approximately 90° relative to each other in the gantry assembly. Current implementations include a detector with a full field of view (often 50 cm), with the second detector having a limited field of view (typically on the order of 30 cm due to physical size constraints of the gantry), with the effective field of view limited to overlap of the two projections [21]. The dual-source configuration offers a number of unique imaging approaches and advantages. Most applicable to cardiac imaging is the fact that a dual-source gantry needs to rotate half the distance of a single-source gantry in order to acquire the projections necessary for a given reconstruction strategy, improving the temoral resolution by a factor of two, as will be discussed in greater detail later in the chapter.

Gantry Rotation Time

Gantry rotation time is defined as the duration of time necessary (measured in milliseconds) for the gantry to perform a complete 360-degree rotation and thus acquire a complete set of radial projections. Since the late 1990s, gantry rotation times have fallen from 750 ms to as low as 250 ms. The extent of motion degradation when imaging a moving object is inversely proportional to the rotation time of the gantry (a critical factor in determining the temporal resolution of a scanner, discussed in detail in later sections). Somewhat analogous to the "speed" of photographic film, the gantry rotation time can be likened to the "exposure time" or "shutter speed" in photography. For instance, a scanner with a gantry rotation time of 350 ms acquiring a single section reconstructed with full 360-degree interpolation will ultimately reconstruct an image which reflects a temporal average of the imaged structure over a period of 350 ms. In this example, it should be evident that in the setting of rapid motion, the resultant image may suffer from substantial blurring and artifact formation resulting in a nondiagnostic study.

Cardiac-Specific Considerations for CT Acquisition and Reconstruction

Spatial Resolution

The epicardial coronary arteries, representing the proximal portions of the coronary tree that sits on the surface of the myocardium, generally have diameters between 2 and 6 mm. The ability to resolve the margins of the coronary arteries and in particular the margins of atherosclerotic plaque within the coronary arteries places some of the highest and most consequential spatial resolution demands among all clinical CT applications. Because of their varying orientation to the acquisition planes, cardiac CT scanners need to be capable of near isotropic submillimeter spatial resolution, currently 0.5–0.625 mm. The determinants of transverse and longitudinal spatial resolution are distinct and have been detailed in prior chapters. In brief, transverse spatial resolution depends on factors related to the X-ray source (specifically focal spot size), the matrix size, detector size, and reconstruction kernel. Longitudinal spatial resolution is largely influenced by the detector width, scan pitch, helical interpolation algorithm, and section increment [22].

When compared to catheter angiography, which has a spatial resolution of 0.16 mm, even the most advanced CT scanners are incapable of providing comparatively precise measurements of residual coronary arterial luminal dimensions, where even at a isotropic resolution of 0.5 mm, the lumen of a vessel which is <2 mm may be represented by four voxels or less [23]. It follows that both precise measurement and characterization of submillimeter plaques are limited. Of particular clinical relevance is the presence of calcium or metallic stents within or adjacent to the wall of the coronary artery. Limitations in spatial resolution, manifesting through partial volume averaging, blur the margins of these high attenuation structures, potentially hindering evaluation of the adjacent residual lumen.

Temporal Resolution

Among the many challenges of cardiac imaging, rapid motion of the target structures is perhaps the greatest challenge to acquiring consistently diagnostic images, free of significant motion artifact. While traditionally associated with individual reconstructions, temporal resolution can be considered from two perspectives, individual reconstructions and the entire cardiac volume. Within an individual transverse reconstruction, cardiac motion-based image degradation manifests as blurring and streaking, when there is substantial displacement of cardiac structures within the aquisition time, thereby comprising data collection for that transverse reconstruction. As previously discussed in the section on physiology, these effects are influenced both by resting heart rate and by heart rate variability which occurs on a beat-to-beat basis. When considering the whole cardiac volume, image quality is additionally influenced by the number of heartbeats required to image the entire cardiac volume and, in particular, cardiac, respiratory, or bulk patient motion occurring that time interval.

Contrast Considerations

While native CT imaging is utilized for coronary calcium scoring, which quantifies coronary calcifications for assessment of cardiac risk, cardiac imaging with CT otherwise is exclusively performed following the administration of intravenous iodinated contrast. Iodine, if properly administered, can result in high-contrast resolution between regions with high blood flow (such as the coronary arteries) and surrounding structures [23]. The degree of luminal enhancement following intravenous contrast material administration is dependent on several factors, namely, timing of the contrast bolus (ensuring delivery to desired structures at the time of imaging, without inappropriate contrast washout), the amount of iodine administered per unit time (i.e., iodine flux – related to iodine concentration of injected contrast media and the rate of injection), and X-ray tube voltage (which if lowered closer to the k-edge of iodine results in increased photoelectric absorption and greater tissue contrast) [23]. Details of contrast material delivery strategies are beyond the scope of this chapter.

Image Artifacts

The term "image quality" when used to describe the end product of a radiologic study, although grossly assessed with relative ease by even the most novice of imagers, reflects the result of a complex interaction of multiple factors related to both technical factors of the scanner and method of image acquisition. Additionally quality of imaging depends significantly upon characteristics of the patient (both anatomic and physiologic) and, particularly in the setting of cardiac imaging, the anatomic region of interest [24]. Given that the coronary arteries not only are the most often evaluated cardiac structure on CT examination, but require both high spatial and temporal resolution, much of the discussion of commonly encountered artifacts will focus upon coronary CT angiography. However, the dominant contributors to image quality during coronary artery evaluation, although potentially of greater consequence, are not unique to coronary imaging. In particular, Ghekiere et al. in a 2017 review of coronary CT image quality generalized the multitude of contributing quantitative and qualitative factors contributing to perceived quality into three broad categories: "noise, vascular enhancement, and motion" [24] (Fig. 23.6). Many of the arti-

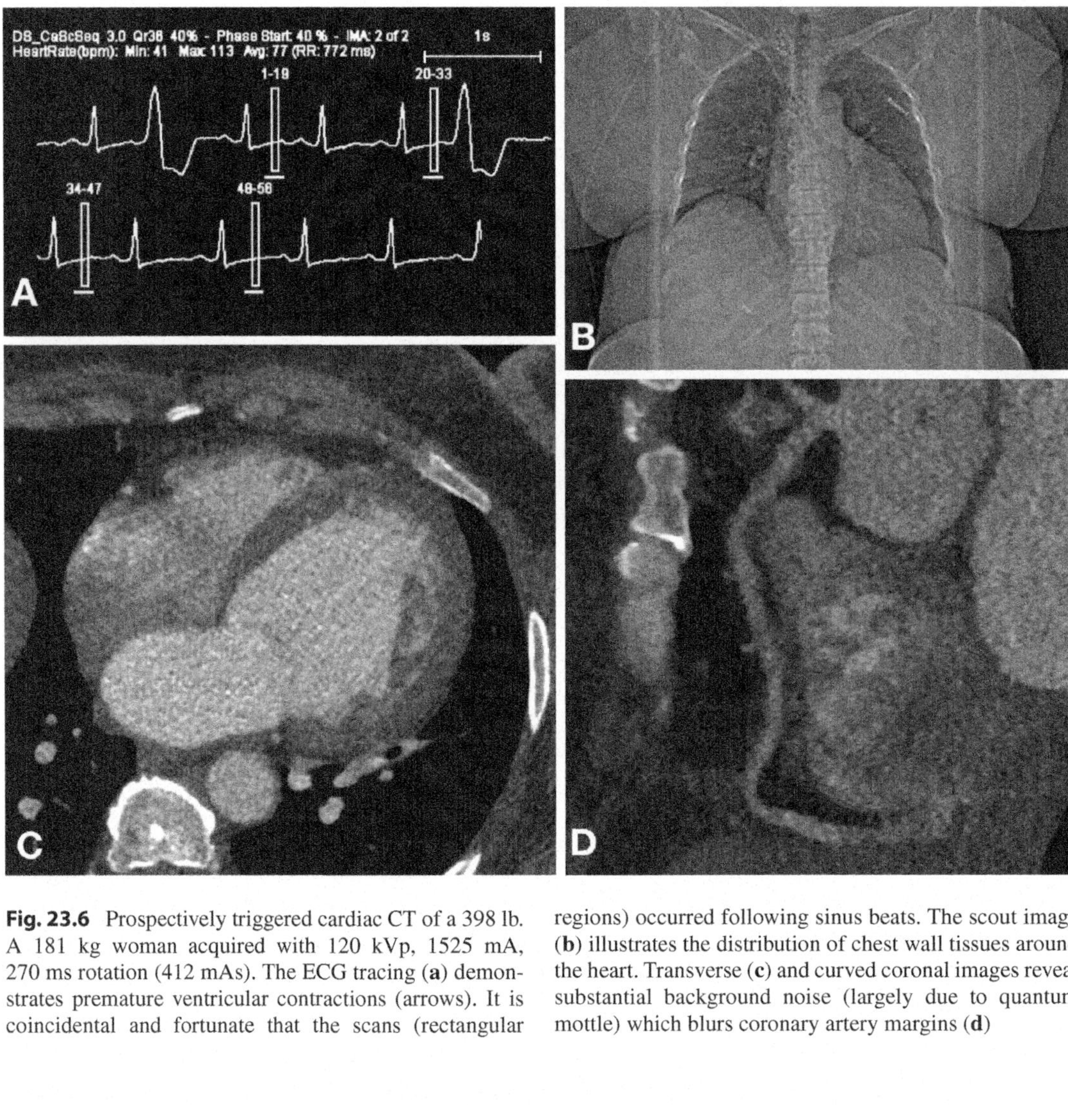

Fig. 23.6 Prospectively triggered cardiac CT of a 398 lb. A 181 kg woman acquired with 120 kVp, 1525 mA, 270 ms rotation (412 mAs). The ECG tracing (**a**) demonstrates premature ventricular contractions (arrows). It is coincidental and fortunate that the scans (rectangular regions) occurred following sinus beats. The scout image (**b**) illustrates the distribution of chest wall tissues around the heart. Transverse (**c**) and curved coronal images reveal substantial background noise (largely due to quantum mottle) which blurs coronary artery margins (**d**)

facts encountered at cardiac CT, most notably quantum mottle, beam hardening, and metal-induced streak, have been discussed in prior chapters. In addition to calcium or metallic cardiac implants or supportive devices, dense contrast in the ventricular cavity may also result in beam hardening not overcome by routine correction algorithms. Such artifacts not only complicate interpretation, rendering some regions nondiagnostic, but may manifest in a more subtle fashion, such as a low attenuation region in the post-contrast myocardium mimicking a perfusion defect characteristic of ischemia [25] or falsely low attenuation of regions of calcified plaque, simulating higher-risk soft plaque or thrombus [26].

Beyond those universal CT artifacts, "motion-related artifacts," while potentially influential on all CT scans, are particularly important for cardiac CT owing to the unique challenge of rapid cardiac motion (with associated rhythmic movement of the coronary arteries). Although image degradation resulting from motion may be readily apparent (Fig. 23.7), in some cases rendering an evaluation (or significant portion therein) nondiagnostic, the interpreting clinician must be aware of the more subtle manifestations of motion artifact, which may be indistinguishable from underlying pathologic conditions. With distal coronary vessels tapering to submillimeter diameters, the entirety of the lumen of a vessel may be depicted by one or two pixels on the interpreted image. In such a case, undetected motion through such a vessel may result in apparent complete effacement of the lumen, potentially resulting in unnecessary invasive testing (angiography) for further evaluation and/or attempted intervention.

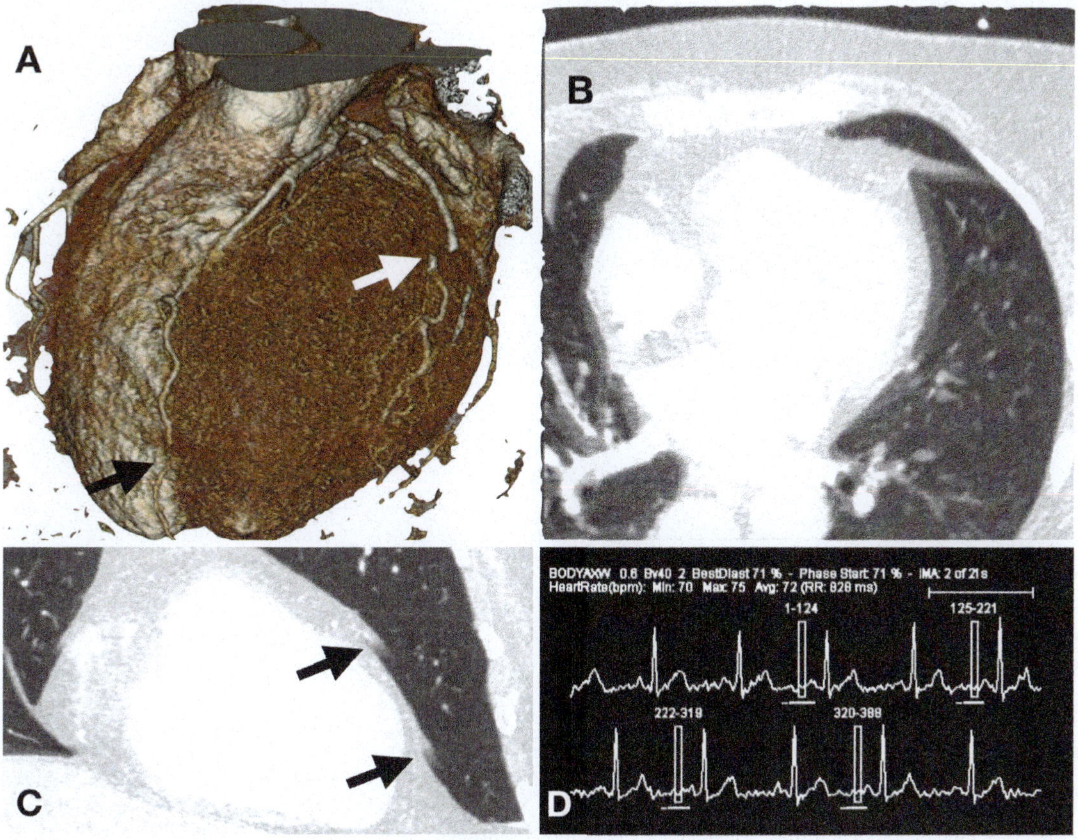

Fig. 23.7 Prospectively triggered CT scan acquired during three heartbeats demonstrates misregistration between the slabs corresponding to the three beats (arrows) on a volume rendering (**a**) and coronal MPR (**b**). The transverse reconstruction in (**c**) is at the level of the lower arrow in (**b**) and demonstrates motion blurring of cardiac and adjacent pulmonary structures. (**d**) ECG tracing acquired during the scan with heart rate varying between 70 and 75 bpm

Display Planes

Unlike other organ systems, which are most commonly evaluated exclusively in the acquired transverse plane or using orthogonal reformations in the sagittal and coronal planes (irrespective of the true axis of the organ), owing to the influence of echocardiography which predates clinical cardiac CT by several decades, the heart is routinely imaged in cardiac-specific planes centered along anatomically defined cardiac axes (Fig. 23.8).

The routine acquisition of isotropic volumetric CT datasets provides the basis for reformatting the CT reconstruction into cardiac-specific planes.

In evaluating left ventricular anatomy and/or function, four standard views are used across imaging modalities, which may be simplified into two broad categories, "long-axis" and "short-axis." The cardiac "short-axis" view most closely resembles the traditional axial plane, providing a cross-sectional view through the left ventricular myocardium, perpendicular to a plane extending from the mitral valve through the left ventricular apex. As with other axial acquisitions, diagnostic evaluation in the short axis requires a "stack" of representative images to provide adequate z-axis coverage. By convention, the left ventricle is evaluated in the short axis in three approximate locations: the base, mid myocardium, and apex. Evaluation in the short axis allows for detailed segmental analysis of myocardial anatomy, pathology, and motion (through use of gated retrospective acquisitions). Additionally, three "long-axis" views are routinely obtained in car-

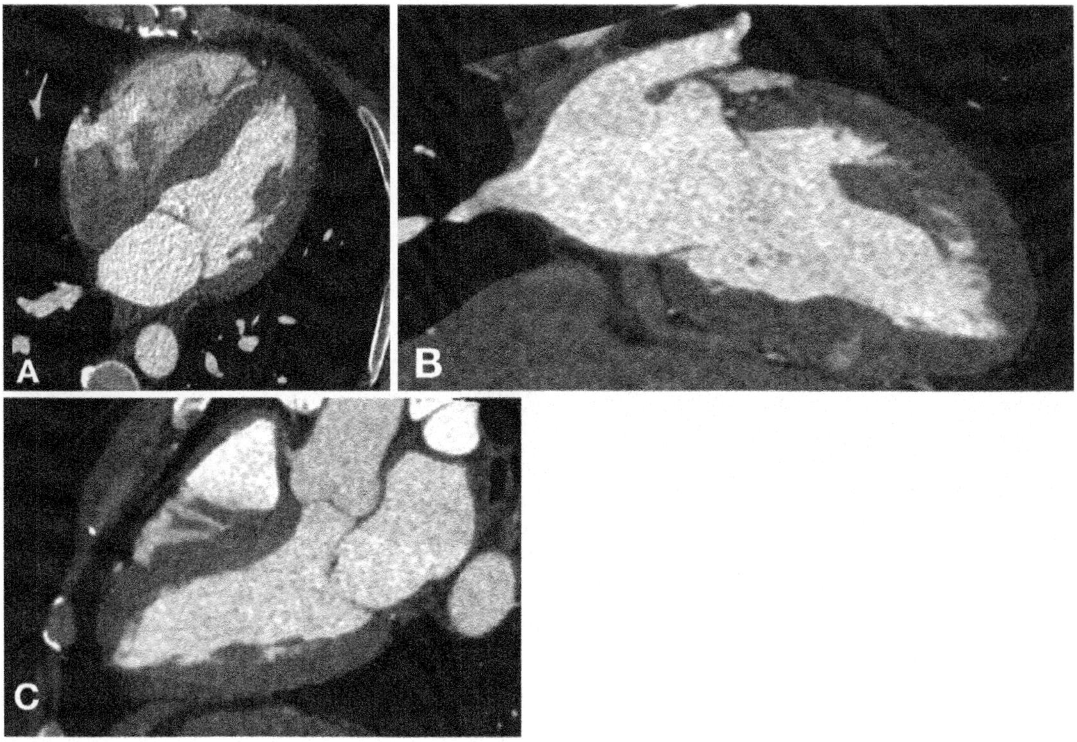

Fig. 23.8 Cardiac display planes, (**a**) four-chamber view. Similar in orientation to the standard axial plane, the four-chamber view is acquired such that the cross-sectional plane is oriented such that all four chambers of the heart are visible. (**b**) Two-chamber view: Useful in evaluating the mitral valve as well as the anterior and inferior walls of the left ventricle, the two-chamber view allows for visualization of the left ventricle and left atrium along their long axis (parallel to the LV septum). (**c**) Three-chamber view: A long-axis view oriented obliquely, the three-chamber view allows for visualization of both left ventricular inflow from the left atrium and outflow into through the aortic root and into the proximal tubular ascending aorta. The mitral and aortic valves are likewise well assessed

diac imaging, which, unlike the short-axis view, evaluates the length of the ventricular myocardium in a single representative view.

Cardiac-Specific Strategies for Patient Preparation, CT Acquisition, and CT Reconstruction

Because the heart contracts, rotates, and translates with each beat, cardiac CT acquisition must accommodate to this motion in order to provide a coherent image of the whole heart volume during a defined portion of the cardiac period. Features implemented in cardiac CT scanners to effectively freeze cardiac motion and allow multiple cardiac phases to be reconstructed include specific strategies for patient preparation, CT acquisition, and image reconstruction.

Managing Heart Rate for Improved Scan Quality

Although continued improvements in MDCT have made imaging across a range of heart rates possible, a regular rhythm less than 60–65 beats per minute remains optimal for consistently diagnostic coronary imaging. Although initially measured during the resting state, several alterations to resting physiology influence heart rate at the time of CT acquisition resulting in an increase on average of 5–10 bpm. Given the potential for positive variation at the time of imaging, a resting heart rate of <60, if attainable, is most often considered optimal. Pharmacologic means, typically beta-adrenergic blockade, are routinely employed to near this target heart rate and blunt physiologically induced beat-to-beat variability. With modern scanners, use of beta-blockade to achieve a rate of 75 bpm or less at the time of imaging most often results in diagnostic imaging (although lower rates remain desirable to consistently prevent motion degradation).

Potential Causes of Heart Rate Elevation or Lability

A large variety of drugs may cause potential abnormalities in rate and rhythm which can degrade the quality of cardiac CT acquisition. Of potentially interfering pharmaceuticals, stimulants are not only the most commonly encountered, but also the class with the most potential for physiologic response resulting in image degradation. Caffeine, being the most frequently encountered stimulant, increases both heart rate and contractile force. As a result, caffeine and other stimulants should be withheld for at least 24 hours prior to cardiac CT scanning.

When the high-flow bolus of iodinated material is administered intravenously, patients can often feel the injection as a cool sensation in his/her arm and are often directly alerted to the injection by the nurse or technologist administering the contrast material. This can induce a transient increase in heart rate owing to activation of the sympathetic nervous system.

Nitroglycerine is commonly administered immediately preceding both invasive coronary angiography and coronary CT angiography as a means of dilating the coronary arteries, improving their visualization and accentuating regions of fixed stenosis due to atherosclerotic plaque. In the body, nitroglycerin is converted to nitric oxide which has a direct relaxation effect in vascular smooth muscle resulting in rapid coronary artery and systemic vasodilation, with associated varying degrees of hypotension and tachycardia.

Beta Blockade to Lower and Stabilize Heart Rate

Although continued improvements in temporal resolution may ultimately obviate the need for pharmacologic reduction of the heart rate, in the absence of contraindications, utilization of beta-blockers remains routine in most centers for patients with resting regular heart rates >60–65 bpm with lower thresholds for those with irregularities of rhythm [27, 28].

Oral or intravenous administration of beta-blockers may be utilized. Oral administration is substantially more effective than intravenous administration, however oral dosing requires at least an hour (preferably several hours) for maximal effect. Depending on resting heart rate, patient size, and patient condition, an oral dose of metoprolol ranging from 25 to 200 mg (higher dose for higher heart rates and larger patients) is given approximately 1 h prior to the study and may be repeated (either orally or intravenously) at the discretion of the physician overseeing the exam. While typically less effective, when expediency is needed, metoprolol may be administered intravenously in 5–10 mg doses. Repeated intravenous doses (as appropriate based on current vital signs) may subsequently administered every 5 min for a maximum of 15–30 mg IV. Decreases in blood pressure, even when administered with nitroglycerin, are typically mild and transient. Expected reductions in heart rate range from 10 to 15 bpm [29], often with the additional benefit of mild improvement in rhythm regularity. Because of the potential profound influence on cardiac physiology, beta-blocker administration should be administered by a nurse under physician guidance or by a physician directly. However, although precautions are necessary, beta-blockers are administered without significant adverse events in the vast majority of patients, with severe adverse events rarely encountered.

Acquisition Modes for Cardiac CT

Multi-beat Acquisition Modes

Depending upon the configuration of the CT scanner, cardiac CT scans are performed across multiple heartbeats or a single heartbeat, with the latter approach being preferable for reasons detailed subsequently. Because the majority of cardiac CT scans performed today use multi-beat lathes, they are presented first.

Prospective Triggering

Prospective triggering utilizes the ECG signal to periodically initiate scanning during the desired phase of the cardiac cycle. Rather than utilizing helical acquisition, prospective acquisition is "step-and-shoot" technique. Although the gantry remains in continuous rotation, the X-ray tube is active intermittently with the patient table stationary during acquisition. The CT acquisition is initiated after either a fixed (millisecond) or relative (percent time to next R-wave) delay after the triggering R-wave. At a minimum, the duration of the acquisition is just long enough to acquire the projections necessary to reconstruct a single cross section. Increases in the time that the radiation source is on result in "padding" which provides flexibility of reconstruction within an enlarged temporal window. Padding typically varies between 20% and 50% of the R-R interval. Once the first set of sections are acquired, during the subsequent heartbeat, the table is advanced to the next position a distance equal to one detector array width with the radiation source. This cycle repeats until the entire volume of interest has been imaged (Fig. 23.9a–c).

Prospective triggering is most effective when the heart rate is slow and regular. Beat-to-beat variations in the cardiac period can result in mis-

Fig. 23.9 ECG compensated scan modes illustrated. ECG tracings represent time on the horizontal axis. All plots include the ECG tracing with scan acquisition indicated by colored rectangles. The vertical axis encodes table position (z) for all parts of the figure except (**e**) where it denotes tube current. (**a**) Prospective triggered acquisition with a 4 cm detector requires four heartbeats to image the entirety of a 16-cm-long heart. Gantry rotation period of 300 ms results in a 150 ms temporal resolution (rectangle width) when reconstructed with half-scan interpolation. (**b**) Same scan mode and detector width as in (**a**), except dual-source configuration results in higher temporal resolution (one quarter of the gantry rotation period) indicated by narrower rectangles. Note that whole temporal resolution of the reconstructed CT sections is much improved compared to (**a**), although the temporal resolution of the volume is the same, requiring seven beats to occur in order to acquire the full cardiac volume. (**c**) Same scan as in (**b**) with the addition of padding. The temporal resolution is the same, but there is now flexibility for reconstruction at any time window within the rectangular regions. (**d**) Retrospective gating results in a continuous helical acquisition. While seven beats are also required for this scan, in contrast to prospective triggering (A–C), the X-ray source is on throughout the acquisition resulting in substantially greater radiation exposure but allowing reconstruction at any position within the cardiac period. Tube current modulation (**e**) maximizes exposure in mid diastole while reducing the dose by 80% during the rest of the cardiac cycle. (**f**) Prospective triggering with a wide (16 cm) detector allows the heart to be imaged with in a single heartbeat, while the table is stationary. (**g**) Prospectively triggered high-pitch helical scan using a dual-source CT scanner also images the entire heart during a single beat. The high table speed associated with this acquisition results in relatively brief exposure to each region of the heart resulting in very low radiation dose. This acquisition mode precludes the use of padding, so it has the lowest tolerance of irregular or high heart rates

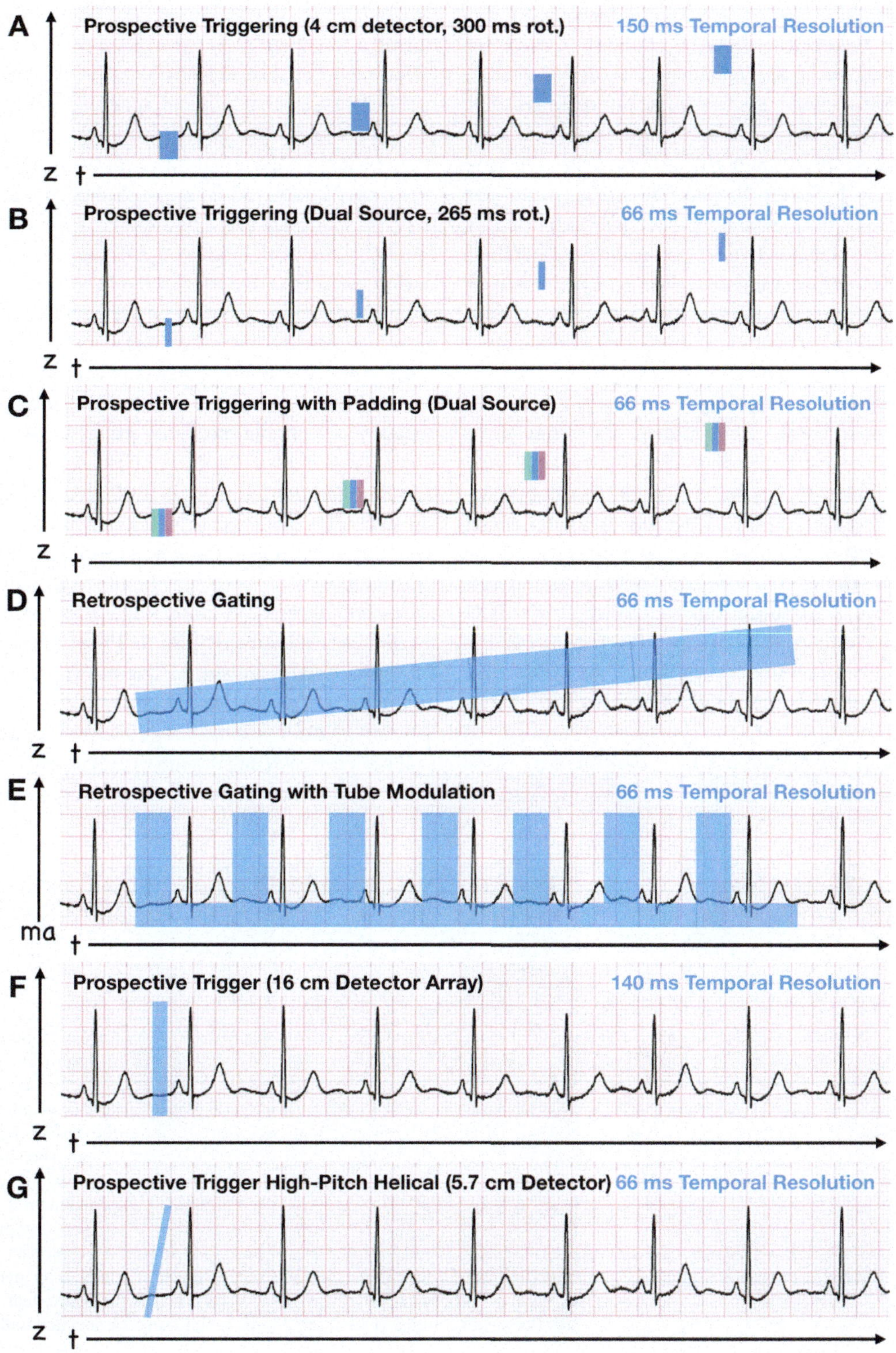
A
Prospective Triggering (4 cm detector, 300 ms rot.)
150 ms Temporal Resolution
z
t
B
Prospective Triggering (Dual Source, 265 ms rot.)
66 ms Temporal Resolution
z
t
C
Prospective Triggering with Padding (Dual Source)
66 ms Temporal Resolution
z
t
D
Retrospective Gating
66 ms Temporal Resolution
z
t
E
Retrospective Gating with Tube Modulation
66 ms Temporal Resolution
ma
t
F
Prospective Trigger (16 cm Detector Array)
140 ms Temporal Resolution
z
t
G
Prospective Trigger High-Pitch Helical (5.7 cm Detector)
66 ms Temporal Resolution
z
t

registration between sections acquired during different heartbeats. Padding provides a basis for creating multiple volume reconstructions in an effort to create the most motion-free images. However, when heart rates and beat-to-beat variability are high, the utility of approaches utilizing padding becomes limited [30]. The heart rate threshold over which prospective triggering is considered ineffective for demanding applications (such as coronary angiography) is dependent upon the temporal resolution of the CT scanner and usually ranges between 65 and 75 beats per minute.

Retrospective Gating

Retrospectively gated cardiac CT relies on a continuous helical acquisition with a relatively slow table speed resulting in a pitch of approximately 0.2–0.4 (Fig. 23.10). The low pitch value is necessary to assure that the entirety of the heart is imaged across the duration of the cardiac cycle. Simultaneous recording of the ECG tracing allows for retrospective reconstruction of the heart at any point throughout the cardiac cycle and provides the data necessary for functional evaluation of the myocardium and valves through generation of multiplanar cine sequences (Fig. 23.9d).

Continuous activation of the X-ray source during a low pitch scan can expose the patient to radiation doses that are substantially greater than essentially all other clinical scanning strategies regardless of body region (with the exception of the repeated CT acquisitions required to measure organ perfusion) [18]. These high exposure levels may be moderated by ECG-based tube current modulation, which reduces the X-ray tube output during portions of the cardiac cycle considered to be of less importance (or at least tolerant of greater levels of imaging noise) in diagnostic evaluation [31]. Such modulation almost always occurs during systole, when cardiac motion is greatest and optimal coronary arterial visualization is least likely (Fig. 23.9 E). ECG-based tube current modulation reduces radiation exposure substantially. A commonly applied modulation protocol would lower the tube current to 20% of the output for 50% of the acquisition, while a relatively aggressive dose reduction protocol might lower the tube current to 4% of the output for 80% of the acquisition. These two strategies applied to a scan that would otherwise result in a dose of 15 mSv without modulation reduces the radiation dose 9.0 and 3.5 mSv respectively. Such extreme dose reductions come at the expense of

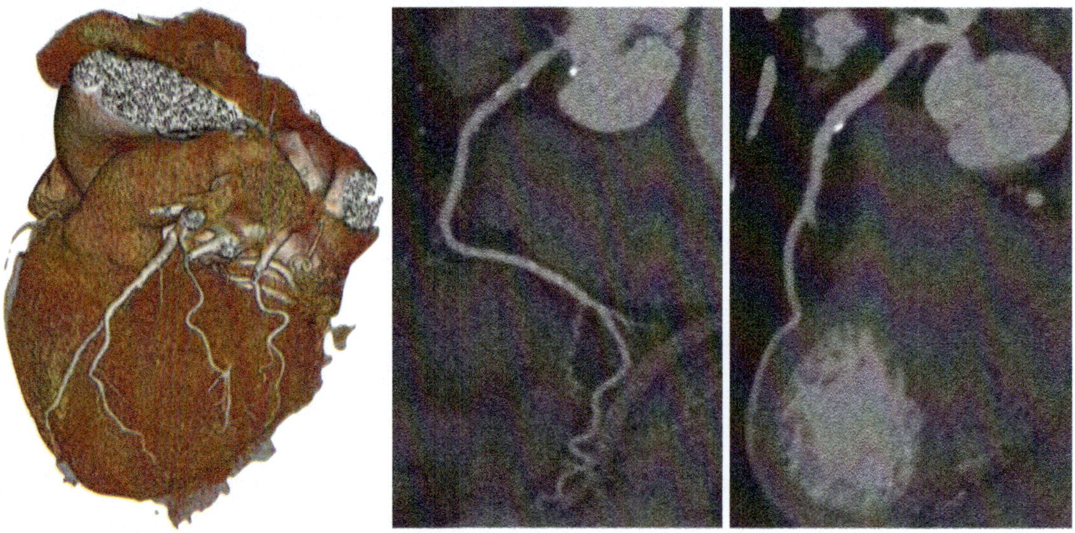

Fig. 23.10 Retrospectively gated coronary CTA illustrated with volume rendering on the left and two curved planar reformations through the LAD on the right and center

markedly reduced image quality with significant increases in noise due to quantum mottle. An additional limitation of this technique lies in the prospective nature of modulation, which is subject to failure in the setting of heart rate irregularity. These challenges have led to development of advanced systems able to react to ectopy and rate variability through recognition of R-R interval variation.

If multi-segment reconstruction is combined with retrospective gating, artifacts encountered from incorporation of segments obtained at the incorrect portion of the cardiac cycle (as may occur in the setting of arrhythmia or premature contraction) may be corrected following completion of image acquisition. Because the radiologist has data from the entirety of the cardiac cycle at his/her disposal, the ECG may be reviewed with selective modifications of the timing of reconstructed phases, potentially limiting significant artifacts without the need for re-scanning.

The relative advantages and disadvantages of prospective triggering and retrospective gating are summarized in Table 23.1.

Single-Beat Acquisition Modes

Introduced earlier in this chapter, wide-area detectors support longitudinal scan coverage that can encompass the entirety of the heart in a single rotation, allowing the heart to be imaged during a single heartbeat and obviating the need for movement of the CT table (Fig. 23.9f). The scan modes used for single-beat imaging with wide-area detectors are directly analogous to multi-beat imaging using prospective triggering with or without padding. Likewise, when functional imaging is indicated, then a mode analogous to retrospective gating (without table movement) provides for reconstruction of the heart during a single or multiple temporal windows positioned at any point within the cardiac cycle.

Table 23.1 Relative advantages of prospective triggering and retrospective gating

Prospective triggering	Retrospective gating
Radiation exposure lower by up to a factor of 3–5, when compared to retrospective gating	Provides functional information, including myocardial motion, valvular motion, and contrast material flow dynamics
Stationary table during acquisition precludes artifacts inherent to helical acquisitions	Greater reconstruction flexibility to mitigate misregistration and cardiac motion-induced artifacts
	Multisector reconstruction provides higher effective temporal resolution when heart rates are high

The unique geometry of dual-source CT scanners allows for the use of a "high-pitch" spiral mode implemented at a pitch value of 3.2 without observable helical artifacts [32]. Using a current third-generation dual-source CT scanner, maximal table speed is 737 mm/s using this mode, which allows a 160 mm scan of the heart to be completed in 220 ms. ECG triggering can be combined with this mode to acquire a single-beat scan; however, padding is not possible, and thus this mode of acquisition is best applied to subjects with particularly low heart rates (<55–60 bpm) and regular rhythms (Figs. 23.9g and 23.11).

Temporal Resolution of CT Sections

The temporal resolution of a CT section is largely a function of the gantry rotation time, with modern scanners having minimum rotation times of approximately 250 ms. While faster gantry rotation speeds are possible, they are challenged by an associated need to engineer the assembly of CT gantry and its sophisticated components to withstand progressively higher G forces [23]. Unlike most clinical CT applications, cardiac CT reconstructions are not created from data acquired across the full 360° of gantry rotation. Instead, half-scan reconstruction is the main mode of reconstruction. Half-scan reconstruction requires data acquired from a 180° rotation which provides projectional data through 180° plus the fan angle of the X-ray beam or approximately 225°.

Half-Scan Reconstruction

Although CT evaluation of most anatomic structures is performed using a full 360-degree rotation of the gantry, temporal resolution may be increased by using partial-scan techniques. That

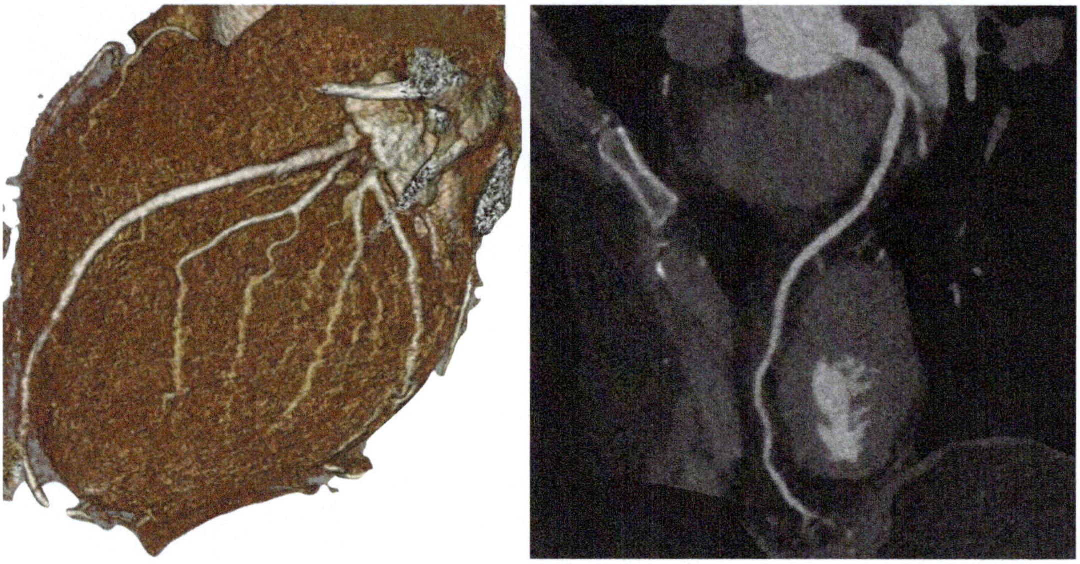

Fig. 23.11 (**a**, **b**) Single-beat high-pitch dual-source CT scan acquired in patient with heart rate of 57 bpm. Image quality is excellent and free from misregistration or motion blurring

is, the full axial image may be reconstructed from only a partial (180°) rotation of the gantry given the knowledge that the second portion of the gantry rotation creates X-ray projections mirroring those generated during the first half of rotation. Limiting the time of acquisition to one half of a scanner rotation results in theoretical 50% reduction in gantry rotation time and associated doubling of temporal resolution. In practice, data required for half-scan reconstruction is slightly greater than 180° due to the need to also image the fan angle of approximately 45°.

Limiting acquisition to projections obtained during partial rotation of the gantry requires the use of reconstruction algorithms which assume rotational symmetry [26]. Specifically, partial-scan techniques are possible due to the inherent redundancy of data acquired in a full 360-degree rotation. Accordingly, various artifacts (referred to generically as "partial-scan artifact") arise from compromise of angular symmetry. Such artifacts may be minimized by attempts to improve symmetry of imaged anatomy by appropriately centering the heart and maintaining the body fully inside of the field of view (most importantly through raising of the arms) [26]. With half-scan reconstruction, a temporal resolution of 125 ms can be attained from a gantry rotation period of 250 ms.

Multi-segment Reconstruction

Beyond the use of half-scan reconstruction, which is applied to all cardiac CT scans, several other methods have been developed to further reduce temporal resolution. The first is multi-segment reconstruction, which collects the necessary data for a half-scan reconstruction across multiple heartbeats. Using "segments" of data from sequential heartbeats, a linear reduction in temporal resolution may be achieved. The acquisition is performed helically with retrospective ECG gating and a pitch sufficiently low such that the scanner is covering a single portion of the heart two or more times (once for each desired segment). The end effect is that the effective temporal resolution becomes a fraction of the nominal value.

For example, a two-segment reconstruction collects data through 90° of rotation for two successive heartbeats, and a three-segment reconstruction collects data through 60° of rotation for three successive heartbeats, resulting in theoretical temporal resolution of 75 and 50 ms, respectively, for a 300 ms gantry rotation period. While a common strategy for cardiac CT during the late 1990s and early 2000s when gantry rotation periods were closer to 400–500 ms, at the time of this writing in 2019, multi-segment reconstruction is rarely used clinically owing to the limitation that even the slightest irregularities in R-R interval or beat-to-beat changes in cardiac position will result in image blurring, because each transverse reconstruction is composed of projections from multiple heartbeats. Another limitation of multi-segment reconstruction is the necessity for substantially lower pitch values required to image each region of the heart through multiple heartbeats, resulting in substantially greater radiation exposure to the patient.

Dual-Source CT

One major advantage of the dual-source system is 180° of projectional data can be acquired with 90° of gantry rotation. Consequently, a temporal resolution of 75 ms is achieved from a 250 ms gantry rotation without the use of multisegment reconstruction. By a substantial margin, this is the best temporal resolution achievable on any current clinical CT scanner where transverse reconstructions are composed of projectional data from one heartbeat (in contrast to multisegment reconstruction which utilizes data from several cardiac cycles).

Anatomically Directed Motion Correction

Yet another approach to motion compensation reconstructs a cross section using information regarding coronary artery and arterial segment trajectories acquired from adjacent cardiac phases within a single cardiac cycle, allowing correction of motion-related effects and essentially compressing the temporal window for reconstruction [33, 34]. Because specialized hardware is not required for this technique, it theoretically could be retrofitted to existing scanners, particularly those with higher gantry rotation speeds, improving image quality and potentially reducing nondiagnostic scans (Fig. 23.12).

Radiation Exposure

Increased use of medical diagnostic imaging utilizing ionizing radiation (with associated increased cumulative patient doses) has resulted in growing concern for the long-term effects of such exposure, particularly neoplasia. Because of potentially high doses (particularly using early CT technology with retrospective gating prior to the availability of ECG-based tube current modulation was standard practice), cardiac CT was once targeted as an examination to be avoided [35]. While it is true that for particularly vulnerable populations (such as infants, children, and adolescents where the risk of radiation are far greater than that of an adult [36]), technology has evolved to a point where radiation exposure from cardiac CT exams is similar to, or less than, that of other cardiac imaging tests - including radionuclide myocardial perfusion imaging and invasive coronary angiography [37].

Dedicated evaluations of patient dose from cardiac CT have focused upon the specific application of coronary CT angiography (CCTA), the most common application of cardiac CT. The Prospective Multicenter Study on Radiation Dose Estimates of Cardiac CT Angiography in Daily Practice I (PROTECTION I) evaluated 1965 patients undergoing predominantly 64-slice CCTA in 2007 at 50 international sites to determine the radiation dose associated with routine coronary CT evaluation [31]. Although there was significant variability among study sites, the study revealed an estimated median effective radiation dose of 12 mSv (median DLP of 885 mGy x cm) [31]. Reporting on 4502 CCTAs from 61 hospitals in 32 countries performed 10 years later in 2017, PROTECTION VI found a 78% reduction in radiation exposure from a median dose length product of 885 to 195 mGy•cm [38]. These approximate radiation dose levels of 18.1 and 4.0 mSv, respectively, using ICRP 103 conversion factor for the chest of 20.4 [39]. Major differences in acquisition characteristics resulting in these significant dose reductions are

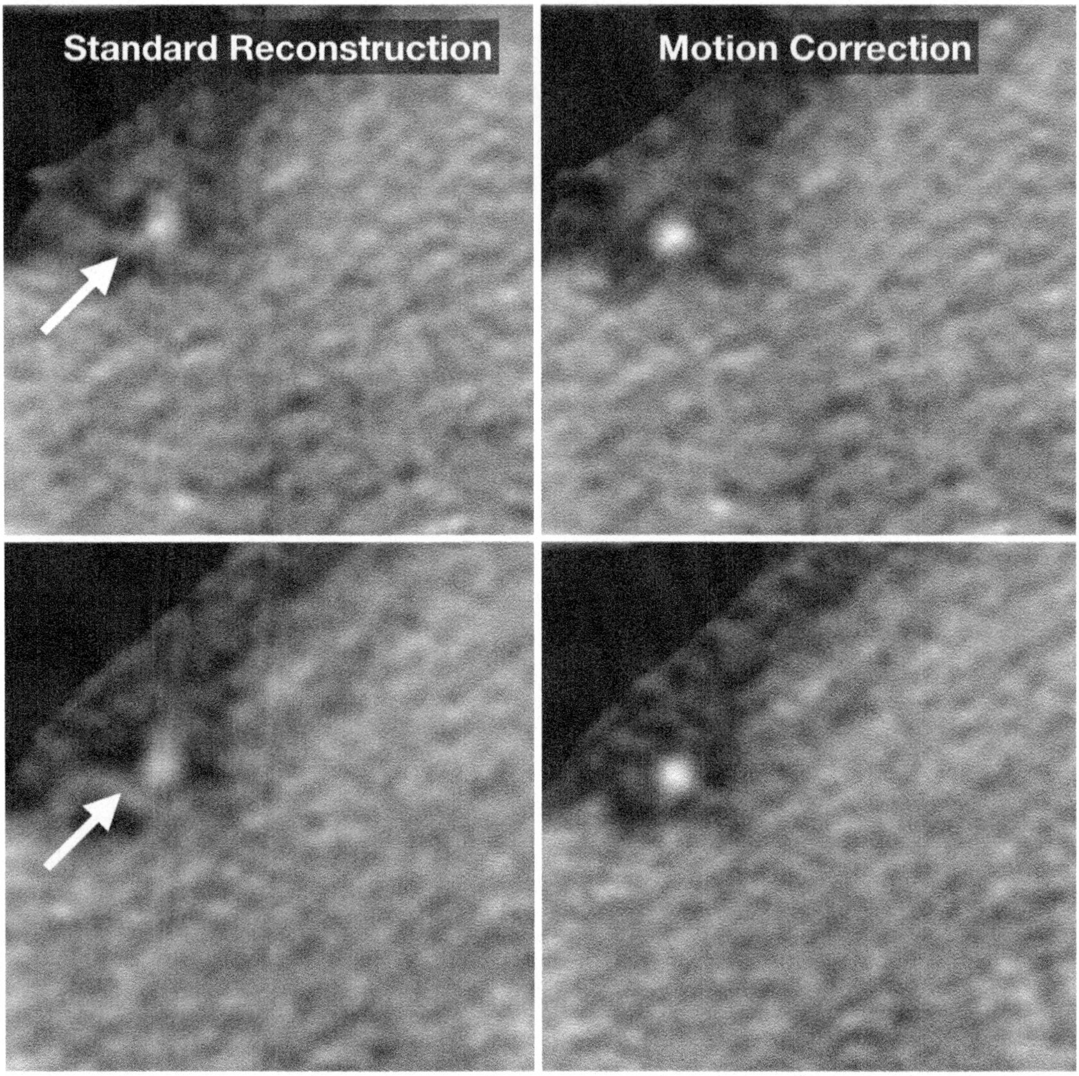

Fig. 23.12 Prospectively triggered coronary CTA using standard iterative reconstruction without motion correction (left) demonstrates blurring of the right coronary artery due to cardiac motion (arrows). Images from the same scan following motion correction (right) result in much sharper coronary artery margins

presented in Table 23.2. The specific impact of some of these strategies is articulated below.

Low kV Imaging

Cardiac CTA has traditionally been performed with a fixed tube voltage of 120 kVp (and 140 kVp or possibly higher in larger/obese patients), similar to standard body imaging. Two factors are most responsible for the transition to voltage levels <120 kVp: higher power sources and iterative reconstruction. The apparent paradox that more powerful X-ray tubes lead to lower dose scans is reconciled when recognizing that higher current is required to maintain the signal-to-noise ratio when tube voltage is reduced, resulting in overall lower radiation dose and higher contrast-to-noise for iodine-enhanced structures. Iterative reconstruction, by producing lower noise images when compared to filtered back projection, also contributes to allow for

Table 23.2 Radiation dose reduction strategies for cardiac CT 2007 versus 2017 [38]

	2007	2017
Median DLP (mGy•cm)	885	195
$CTDI_{vol}$ (mGy)	54	14
Tube potential ≤100 kV, %	5	56
Tube potential <100 kV, %	0	14
Retrospectively ECG-gated helical scan protocol, %	94	11
Retrospectively ECG-gated with ECG-based tube current modulation, %	95	73
Prospectively ECG-triggered axial scan protocol, %	6	78
Prospectively ECG-triggered high-pitch helical scan protocol, %	0	11
Iterative image reconstruction, %	0	83

lower tube voltage usage as well as lower tube current [40]. Lowering tube potential to 100 kVp from 120 kVp can result in average dose reductions of 29–53% without significantly impairing diagnostic quality in nonobese patients [18, 41]. Although increased image noise is inevitable at lower tube potential, this is partially offset by improved contrast resolution on angiography due to increased photoelectric interaction with iodine at lower energies [40, 42].

Scan Mode

The use of prospective ECG-triggered scanning has been shown to reduce radiation exposure by at least 69% when compared to retrospective gating with comparable image quality [41, 43]. This data includes retrospectively gated scanning using ECG-based tube current modulation and highlights the importance of achieving low heart rates (allowing for prospective gating) as means of reducing radiation exposure as well as assuring higher image quality.

Particularly noteworthy is the previously discussed high-pitch mode used with dual-source CT scanners. Although least tolerant of higher heart rates, when usable, prospectively triggered high-pitch dual-source scans provide some of the lowest radiation exposures reported. A recent study of 59 pairs of weight, height, sex, and heart rate-controlled subjects revealed an average effective dose of 1.2 mSv and 4.2 mSv for prospectively triggered high-pitch and prospectively triggered conventional "step-and-shoot" scanning, respectively [44].

Iterative Reconstruction

The characteristics of iterative reconstruction versus filtered back projection and its impact on radiation dose reduction are discussed in a prior chapter. As shown in the PROTECTION VI data, the use of iterative reconstruction has become a key component of cardiac CT in 2017 when compared to its complete absence in the 2007 data from PROTECTION I (Table 23.2) [38].

Clinical Applications

The spectrum of clinical applications for cardiac CT has been the basis for entire books. It is not possible to provide a comprehensive treatment of this topic within the context of a single chapter. Consequently, major applications as they relate to clinical practice on 2019 will be emphasized exclusively. Readers desiring greater depth and breadth of these topics are referred to [45].

Coronary Arteries

The majority of cardiac CT is performed as a noninvasive means of detecting and characterizing coronary artery disease. Coronary artery disease, defined by the presence of atherosclerotic plaque in the coronary tree supplying blood to the heart, represents not only a dominant cause of mortality and morbidity in developed countries but also a challenging disease to effectively treat in order to prevent future events. Although some patients with significant disease on imaging may be essentially asymptomatic, others with relatively mild disease may suffer from angina (chest pain with exertion), develop ischemic cardiomyopathy (heart failure), or have sudden occlusion of a vessel resulting in acute myocardial ischemia with subsequent infarction ("heart attack") and death.

CT plays a role in the assessment of coronary artery disease through risk stratification of asymptomatic individuals using unenhanced CT (coronary calcium "scoring") and intravenous contrast material-enhanced coronary CT angiography for direct visualization of the amount and extent of atherosclerotic plaque and associated narrowing of the coronary artery lumen.

Coronary Calcium Measurement

Calcium is associated with atherosclerosis and is commonly observed in the coronary arteries (Fig. 23.13). The amount of coronary calcium has been utilized as a surrogate for overall extent of atherosclerotic burden, and its quantification has been the basis for the stratification of risk for future cardiovascular events in low to intermediate risk asymptomatic adults [46]. A number of algorithms exist for quantification of coronary artery calcium burden into a reportable score, with the Agatston score among the most commonly used. To attempt to standardize results, a consensus standard was established for CT acquisition in preparation for Agatston scoring as follows [47]:

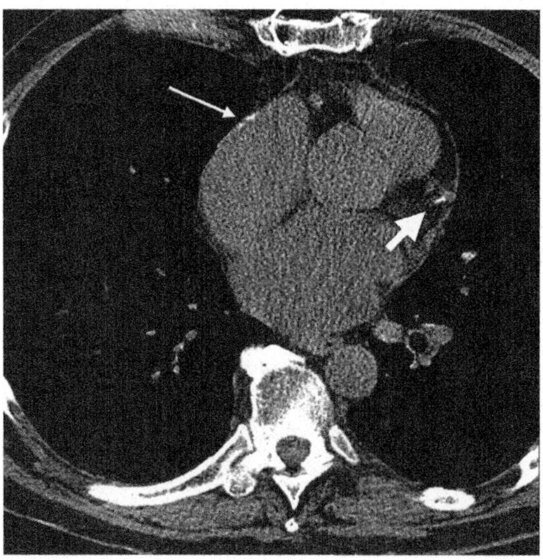

Fig. 23.13 Unenhanced ECG-triggered CT scan demonstrates calcium in the left anterior descending coronary artery (wide arrow). Pericardial calcium is incidentally noted as well (narrow arrow)

- Calcium in the coronary artery is defined as pixels with HU >130.
- MDCT scans should be performed at 120 kVp.
- 3 mm section thickness.
- Non-contrast technique.
- Prospective ECG triggering without padding at 80% of the R-R interval. (Retrospective ECG gating while recommended ion the referenced publication is not appropriate with modern CT scanners)
- Sharp reconstruction kernel (B35f equivalent).

While authors have argued that thinner sections and a lower attenuation threshold would provide greater sensitivity and potentially reproducibility of calcium measurements, the basis of these parameters relates to historical data collected using older-generation CT scanners and the detailed population-based assessments of risk that were performed based upon these standardized techniques. Moreover, although retrospective cardiac gating was recommended in these 2007 guidelines, prospective triggering remains the dominant means for coronary calcium measurement (due to both its historical origins with electron beam CT as well as the substantially lower radiation exposure). Radiation dose becomes a particularly important consideration given that coronary calcium scoring most commonly is utilized in screening of asymptotic individuals. Despite an extensive evidence base that coronary calcium measurement is an independent predictor of cardiac events, its clinical utilization remains limited [48].

Coronary CT Angiography

Today, the principal application for cardiac CT is the detection and characterization of obstructive atherosclerotic plaque by intravenous contrast material-enhanced coronary CT angiography. A major determinant in the diagnostic quality of cardiac CT is the degree of contrast enhancement.

In order to sufficiently opacify the small coronary artery branches, a high-flow injection of high-iodine concentration (370–400 mgI/ml) contrast material is injected into a peripheral vein. To assure that the brief injection results in homogeneously high coronary artery enhancement, the start of the CT acquisition is timed using either a small preliminary test injection or a monitoring phase early during the contrast material injection to determine the timing of contrast arrival into the ascending aorta prior to triggering the volumetric angiographic acquisition. Contrast injection rates used during cardiac CT average 6 mL/s (with rates as low as 4 mL/s and as high as 8 mL/s), necessitating large bore intravenous access (typically 16 or 18 gauge in the antecubital fossa).

Coronary CT angiography should be acquired and reconstructed to produce the narrowest (submillimeter) section thickness available. Reconstruction of overlapping sections can further improve longitudinal resolution. Occasionally thicker (1 mm) sections may be required as a means of mitigating high noise images acquired in patients of particularly high body mass indices. Once appropriately selected contrast medium delivery and X-ray exposure parameters have been selected, the most important determinant of image quality and a diagnostic examination is the minimization of motion-related artifacts, as has been discussed earlier in this chapter.

The use of nitroglycerine is another important component of coronary CT angiography. Multiple studies have demonstrated improved image quality and diagnostic accuracy following nitroglycerine administration, which has been reported to increase coronary artery luminal diameter 6–28% with greatest effect in smaller vessels [49]. Standard doses vary between 0.4 mg and 0.8 μg administered sublingually (with lower doses typically still providing adequate coronary vasodilation with decreased frequency of undesirable effects such as tachycardia and hypotension). Peak effect is achieved within 3–5 min with duration of effects rapidly tapering following the subsequent 5-min half-life following absorption. Undesirable decreases in blood pressure and increases in heart rate have been variably reported, although severe hypotension is uncommon. Male patients should be routinely screened for use of phosphodiesterase-5 inhibitor erectile dysfunction medications within 24 h for short-acting medications (Viagra, Levitra) or 48 h for longer-acting drugs (Cialis) – which when combined with nitrates can potentiate severe rapid decline in blood pressure. Additionally, patients with known severe aortic stenosis should not be administered nitrates because of the risk of severe hypotension (due to the effects of systemic vasodilation in the setting of fixed obstruction at the aortic valve).

Image Analysis

Anatomic evaluation of the coronary arteries is performed utilizing the axial dataset both to interpret the extracardiac findings and to achieve an "overview" of the anatomy. Detailed evaluation and estimation of stenosis are performed using 3D post processing real-time workstation software packages, which allows dynamic multiplanar reformats of the heart as well as curved planar reformatting of the coronary arteries. Such software allows a vessel to be viewed in a virtual plane sampled along a spline coursing through the center of the lumen [45]. Functional evaluation is also performed at the workstation, using software which allows retrospective datasets to play correctly as a "cine". A system for reporting coronary artery lesions, CAD-RADS, has been published as a consensus statement of several professional societies focused on cardiac CT [50].

Application to Assessing Coronary Artery Disease

Using 64-slice MDCT angiography, the 2008 ACCURACY trial confirmed the role of modern cardiac CTA as an effective noninvasive means for exclusion of obstructive coronary artery disease with a 99% negative predictive value, 95% sensitivity, and 83% specificity for determination of ≥70% stenosis compared invasive angiography [51]. Cardiac CT provides the additional benefit of simultaneous high-resolution anatomic evaluation of the heart and surrounding structures and, if acquired with retrospective gating, functional assessment of the myocardium and valves.

Fractional flow reserve (FFR), measured as the ratio of arterial pressure distal to a region of coronary artery stenosis compared to arterial pressure within the aorta obtained during maximal blood flow following an intra-coronary injection of adenosine, has proven efficacious during invasive coronary angiography as a means of predicting the likelihood of severe cardiac events/functional significance of a particular lesion. Therefore, the need to revascularize a particular coronary segment with stent may be reflected by an FFR value of <0.8, with resvascularization of the segment potentially not providing clinical benefit if FFR value is ≥0.8 [52, 53]. Calculated using a catheter-mounted pressure-sensitive transducer during conventional coronary angiography to measure aortic pressure relative to coronary post-stenotic pressure during pharmacologically induced hyperemia, invasive FFR is now considered the reference standard for evaluation of functional significance of a coronary lesion [54].

Recently, mathematical techniques have been described and implemented which, using computed Newtonian fluid dynamics on volumetric reconstructions of the coronary arteries derived from coronary CT angiography, approximate invasive FFR [55]. By combining anatomic CTA analysis of coronary luminal stenosis with computed functional FFR-CT data, the need for potential revascularization is determined more accurately, with the potential of reducing unnecessary invasive coronary techniques [56–58] (Fig. 23.14). This is of particular importance given the known overestimation of luminal narrowing when comparing CT angiography to reference invasive techniques (with positive predictive values reported between 48% and 64% despite negative predictive values of as high as 99%) [51]. The likelihood of overestimating the significance of luminal narrowing when visually assessing CCTA scans is even higher when compared to a reference standard of FFR [59].

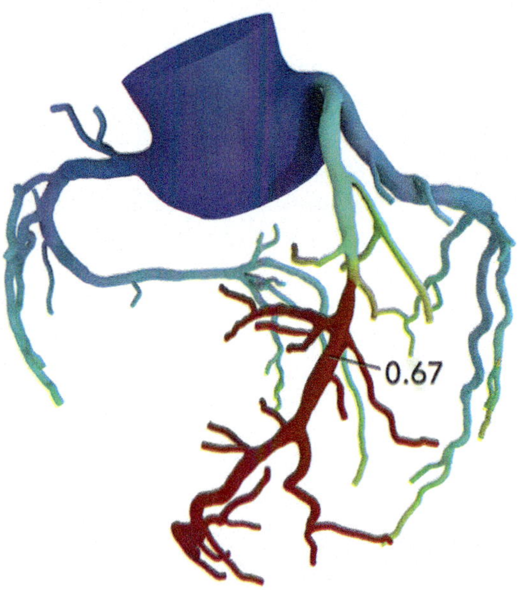

Fig. 23.14 Map of color-coded FFRCT values throughout the coronary tree demonstrates a mid-LAD lesion that results in a flow-limiting stenosis with FFRCT of 0.67. Regions in red indicate FFRCT values <0.80

Anomalous Coronary Artery Course

A form of congenital anomaly affecting the normal branch pattern of the coronary arteries, anomalous course of the coronary arteries is most often noted incidentally on routine imaging. Although many variations are considered benign, a "malignant" course of the coronary arteries follows an inter-arterial path between the aorta and pulmonary artery after arising from the coronary sinus contralateral to the expected normal anatomic origin. Compression caused by the aberrant course can result in angina, syncope, and sudden death [60], with the least common, but most high-risk, variation that of the inter-arterial ("malignant") left coronary artery [61]. Other potentially symptomatic courses include coronary arteries which are partially covered by a portion of the myocardium, called "myocardial bridging." These anomalies, if suspected, are best evaluated with MDCT which depicts the origin and anatomic course of the vessels more clearly than even conventional angiography [60].

Surgical Planning

Owing to the high-resolution three-dimensional maps available from cardiac CT, it is an invaluable tool for planning a variety of cardiac interventions, both transcatheter and through open surgery.

Pulmonary Vein Evaluation

Atrial fibrillation is the most common cardiac arrhythmia. Its symptoms range from palpitations and fatigue to shortness of breath and syncope. Electrical isolation of the pulmonary veins form the left atrium via radiofrequency or cryoablation is a commonly performed procedure for treating atrial

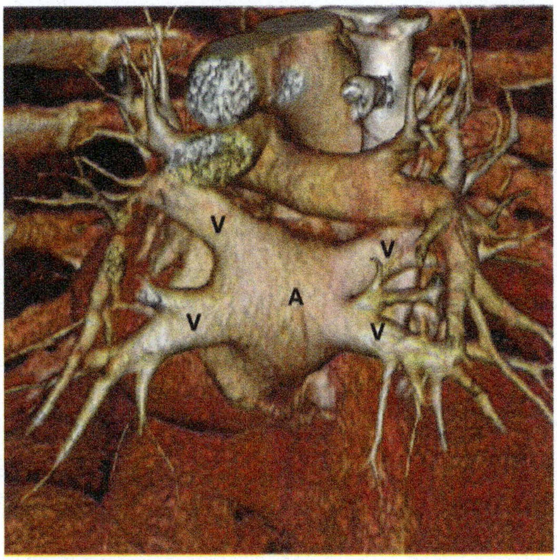

Fig. 23.15 Volume rendering of the left atrium (**a**) and four pulmonary veins (V) viewed posteriorly. Images such as this are invaluable for illustrating the nuances of pulmonary venous origin and branch pattern variation

fibrillation [62]. The procedure is guided using preprocedural mapping of the diameter, length, and position of origin of the pulmonary veins (Fig. 23.15). Also, cardiac CT may be performed following ablation to evaluate for complications such as posttreatment cardiac vein stenosis.

Resynchronization

Biventricular pacing (i.e., "cardioresynchronization therapy"), which utilizes a lead positioned within the coronary sinus to allow delivery of current directly to the left ventricular myocardium for patients with heart failure and dyssynchronous contraction of the left ventricle. Most commonly, dyssynchrony is a result of left bundle branch block, which results in asymmetric progression of depolarization through the functional right bundle and resultant contraction of the septum prior to the lateral left ventricular wall [63]. Uncoordinated contraction disrupts normal dynamics, with potentially precipitous decline in left ventricular function. In contrast to the relatively uncomplicated access of the right heart required for placement of other pacing systems, difficulties arise when attempting to place coronary sinus leads. Variations in normal venous anatomy may present the cardiologist with unfavorable anatomy poorly delineated using intra-procedural fluoroscopy. Complications in such situations range from increased patient discomfort and prolongation of otherwise uneventful procedures to perforation and dissection of the coronary veins, reported in up to 2 and 4% of series, respectively [64]. As a result, cardiac CT is routinely utilized prior to insertion or removal of cardiac pacing leads to detect anomalies and provide a map of coronary venous anatomy to guide the procedure.

Transcatheter Valve Replacement

Aortic stenosis is associated with extremely poor survival rates if left untreated. Classic open surgical techniques for aortic stenosis are complicated by poor surgical candidacy of many patients, due to both the sequela of stenosis itself and age of many of the patients (with up 30% considered too high risk for open approaches to valve replacement [1]). Transcatheter aortic valve replacement (TAVR) has become a routine method of valvular replacement for patients, and has been shown to be non-inferior to traditional open approaches [65]. Moreover, TAVR can be performed using conscious sedation rather than more risky general anesthesia.

TAVR planning studies are performed as a CT angiogram of the chest, abdomen, and pelvis, with additional retrospectively gated cardiac acquisition, which is performed without tube current modulation given the relatively low risk of radiation induced effects in this population (compared to potentially serious complications which may arise from inadequate preprocedural assessment). The most critical portion of the exam is evaluation of the aortic root - measurements from which are used to size the prosthesis. Due to the large caliber of the catheter utilized for deployment, and often advanced patient age with associated high likelihood of significant atherosclerosis, segmental measurements are performed on major arteries of both the lower and upper extremities to evaluate for luminal narrowing that may result in complications during device delivery and cather access/removal.

Re-operative Cardiac Surgery

The potential need for re-operative cardiac surgery, necessitating access into mediastinal structures distorted by one or more prior sternotomies, presents unique challenges to the surgeon with multiple factors resulting in increased morbidity and mortality when compared to primary intervention [66]. Particularly in the setting of prior coronary artery bypass grafting (CABG), variability in postsurgical vascular anatomy may potentially place graft vessels in close proximity to the sternum. Additionally, the surgeon may encounter dense adhesions tethering cardiac and mediastinal structures to the anterior chest well. Presurgical evaluation in patients with planned sternal reentry may reduce the incidence of complication through identification of high-risk findings [66].

Structural Heart Disease

Structural heart disease in the broadest sense refers to non-coronary pathology of the cardiac system [67]. Although echocardiography and cardiac MRI serve as the dominant imaging modalities in evaluation of structural heart disease, cardiac CT has played an increasing role due to accessibility, speed, and high spatial resolution. The volume and wall thickness of the cardiac chambers, particularly the left ventricle, are among the commonly evaluated structural aspects of the heart.

Congenital Heart Disease

Congenital heart disease represents a vast array of malformations of the heart and great vessels. Depending on the complexity of the aberrations of anatomy, multistage surgical corrections may be necessary, with the child or adult likely requiring close follow-up and serial imaging surveillance. Although more common simple abnormalities (such as atrial septal defects) may be diagnosed and followed by echocardiography or MRI, the spatial resolution and anatomic delineation offered by CT are often used to evaluate complex pathology pre- and postoperatively - with MR reserved for routine surveillance to reduce cumulative radiation exposures.

Tumors/Masses

Like all organ systems, the heart is susceptible to neoplasia, with both metastatic and primary cardiac tumors encountered. Primary cardiac tumors are most commonly benign, with myxomas the most frequently encountered benign lesion. Because both thrombus and myxomas are often found in the left atrium and appear low attenuation on CT with occasional calcification, the predilection of thrombus for the atrial appendage as well as the characteristic (but variably appreciable) heterogenous enhancement of myxomas can be used to differentiate these two common cardiac masses. Lipomas are additionally encountered benign cardiac tumors, presenting as circumscribed fat-attenuation masses lacking appreciable enhancement. These circumscribed benign neoplasms are not to be confused with the similar, but distinct, appearance of lipomatous hypertrophy of the interatrial septum [68]. Malignant tumors account for 25% of primary cardiac masses, distinguishable from their benign counterparts by infiltrative behavior, irregular ill-defined margins, and vascular narrowing from neoplastic encasement or invasion [68].

Valves

Echocardiography remains the preferred modality for assessment of native and postoperative valvular disease due to the lack of ionizing radiation compared to CT and improved availability and relative speed of acquisition when compared to MRI. However, limitations of sonographic evaluation can result in suboptimal evaluation, particularly due to acoustic shadowing in the setting of prosthetic valves. Additionally, a number of conditions provide an unfavorable acoustic window, namely obesity and obstructive lung disease [69]. In addition to providing rapid acquisition and avoiding potential implantable device-related complications of MRI, CT provides for a 3D volumetric acquisition with high-resolution visualization of leaflet morphology and mobility, with the benefit of multiplanar evaluation from a single rapidly acquired axial dataset (Fig. 23.16).

Because valvular evaluation requires "cine" reconstructions to view valve leaflet mobility,

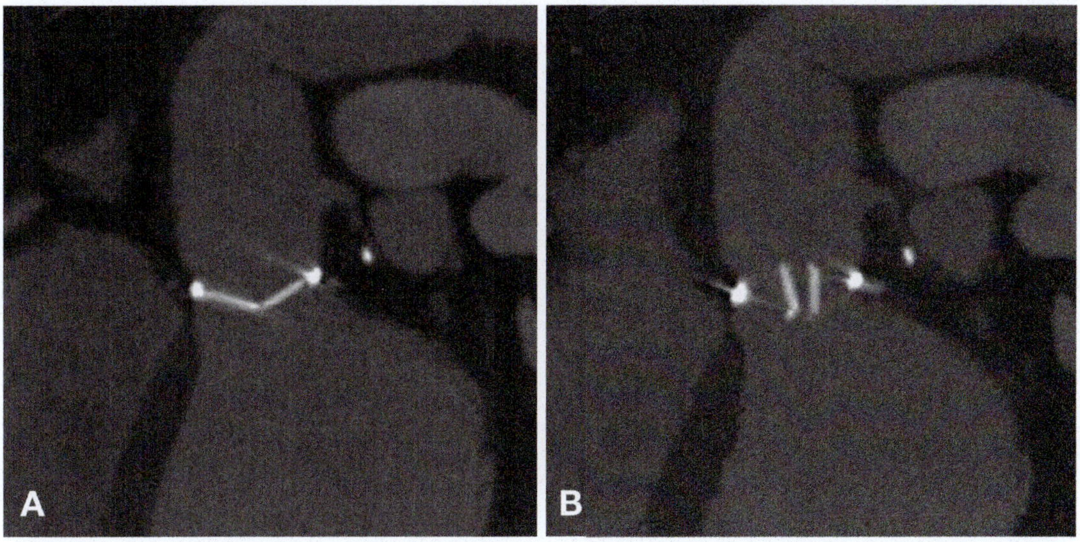

Fig. 23.16 Two of ten reconstructions from a retrospectively gated CT through a mechanical aortic valve prosthesis demonstrate normal function with the valve closed in diastole (**a**) and open in systole (**b**)

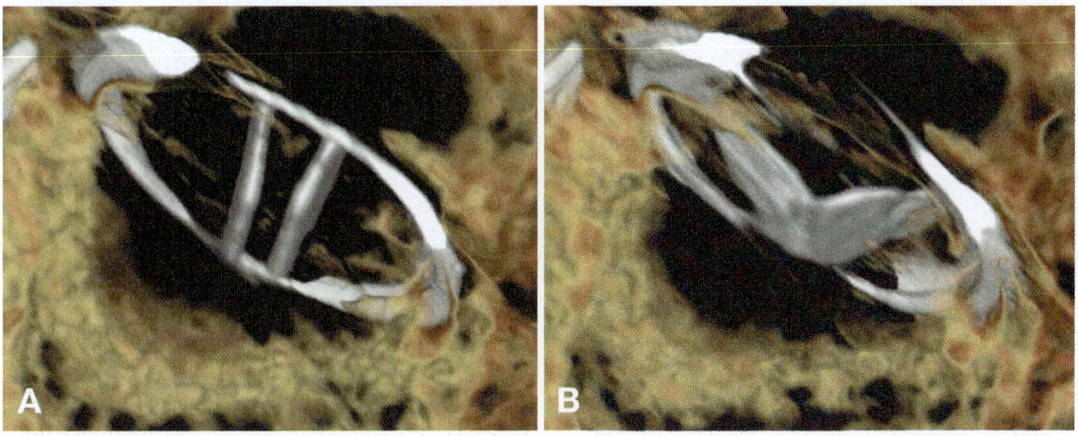

Fig. 23.17 Retrospectively gated CT from a patient with severe aortic vascular regurgitation following valve replacement surgery. A mechanical aortic valve opens fully in systole (**a**), but fails to close completely in diastole (**b**). Reoperation revealed panes growing into the valve opening, preventing closure of the left hemidisc

data must be acquired throughout the cardiac cycle using retrospective gating. The presence of streak/beam hardening artifact may be diminished through the use of specialized reconstruction kernels, dual-energy imaging, or thicker reconstructions [69].

Complications following valve replacement include regurgitation, pseudoaneurysm, dehiscence, infection, vascular injury, and functional obstruction caused by valvular thrombus/pannus [69]. MDCT may be utilized either as a primary means of evaluation, or to further evaluate abnormalities detected on echocardiography due to the superior spatial resolution of CT.

Regurgitation following valve replacement can occur due to impeded valvular closure (Fig. 23.17), or within abnormal channels allowing flow around the prosthetic annulus [69]. Such complications may occur following both conventional open and minimally invasive transcatheter techniques, with potentially significant morbidity and mortality if not appropriately recognized and managed [70].

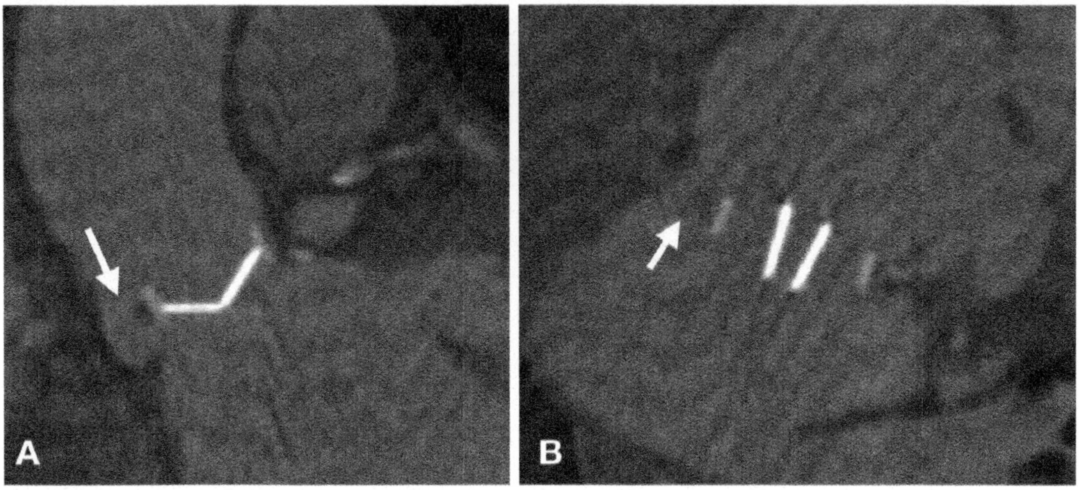

Fig. 23.18 Dehiscence of both a mechanical aortic valve prosthesis (**a**) and a mitral valve prosthesis (**b**) represents severe complications due to an extensive postoperative infection of the heart. Points of detachment of the valve rings are indicated by arrows with contrast opacification outside of the ring representing sources of regurgitation during diastole

Defects are appreciated as curvilinear regions of contrast opacification adjacent to the prosthetic valve ring which proximally communicate with the left ventricular outflow tract and distally with the supravalvular aorta (Fig. 23.18). Similarly, pseudoaneurysm, visualized as saccular dilation of the aorta, may occur as a result of dehiscence at anastomotic sites. In the setting of valvular obstruction, CT may assist in differentiating between thrombus (clot), pannus (fibrous tissue growth typically extending from the ventricular wall), and infective vegetation (small bacterial laden masses on the valvular surface) based on appearance, location, and attenuation.

Emerging and Future Applications

Having demonstrated unparalleled clinical value in noninvasive rapid angiographic evaluation of the coronary arteries, cardiac imagers quickly began to explore the potential application of cardiac CT in a variety of non-coronary applications, many of which have been established in routine clinical cardiac MRI (cMRI). Cardiac MRI has essentially become the "gold standard" with respect to detailed characterization of the myocardium and its function, largely owing to its inherent ability to provide soft tissue contrast resolution far beyond that of other modalities, including CT. However, despite increasing availability of cMRI, the essentially ubiquitous presence of CT with associated scan times now on the order of seconds (compared to 45–90 min for cMRI) as well as the absence of potential contraindications related to implanted devices complicating cMRI evaluation, has fueled research into a variety of new clinical applications of cardiac CT.

Infarction and Viability

An evaluation of myocardial "viability" is performed in patients with known coronary disease and severely reduced left ventricular systolic function in an effort to determine if revascularization may lead to recovery of some degree of myocardial function. Fundamentally, an imaging modality is required which allows for accurate determination of the extent of irreversibly scarred/infarcted myocardium, ideally also having the capability of acquiring simultaneous functional gated imaging to assess for regional wall motion abnormality. The latter requirement of wall motion abnormality allows for assessment of "hibernating" myocardium. Hibernating myocardium represents the sequelae of chronic ischemia, where diminished cellular metabolism prevents cellular death, but manifests clini-

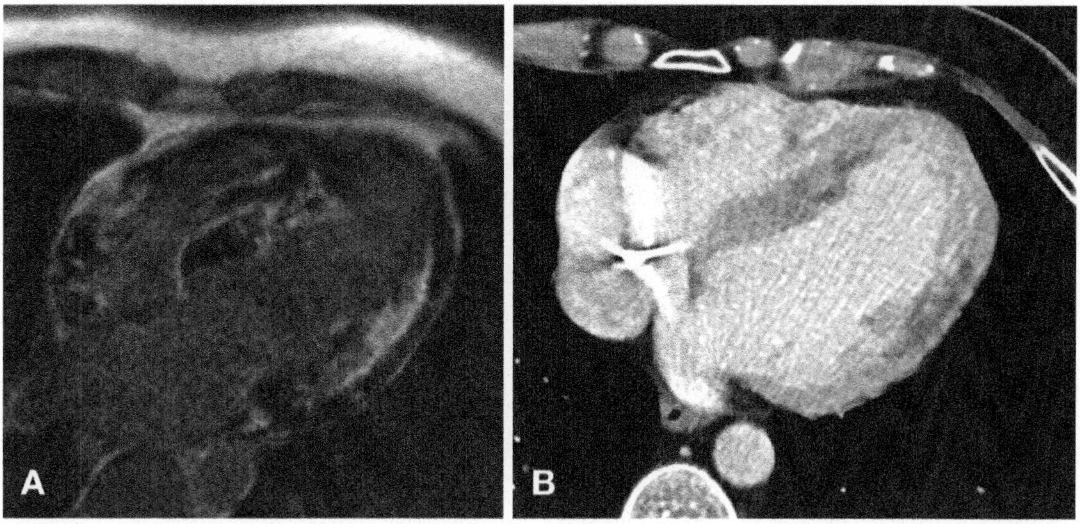

Fig. 23.19 (**a**) Delayed enhancement in a patient with nonischemic cardiomyopathy. Four-chamber MRI delayed enhancement post-contrast sequence demonstrates increased signal from gadolinium contrast deposition into scarred myocardium. This particular sequence suppresses (nulls) the signal of normal myocardium, which appears near black. This patchy distribution not following coronary artery vascular territories suggests an infectious or inflammatory etiology rather than sequela of infarcts from coronary atherosclerotic disease. (**b**) Contrast enhancement in a patient with nonischemic cardiomyopathy. Axial CT on the same patient with pattern of contrast enhancement similar to that of the MRI in (**a**). However, note that on this CT, regions correlating with scar on the MRI demonstrate impaired enhancement; whereas the intervening normal regions of myocardium demonstrate relatively homogenous enhancement. The appearance suggests that enhancement reflects perfusion – acquired in an earlier phase than the MRI in (**a**)

cally as significantly myocardial contractility in the setting of reduced myocardial perfusion.

"Delayed enhancement imaging" with cardiac MRI correlates with histologic infarction and serves as the reference standard for noninvasive determination of infarcted, non-recoverable myocardium [71]. The delayed enhancement sequences utilized in cMRI revolutionized the assessment for cardiac viability. By imaging after 5–10 min, when administered contrast has largely cleared from normal myocardium, preferential accumulation of contrast media in the expanded extracellular spaces of infarcted myocardium may be appreciated, allowing for accurate determination of myocardial scar [72]. Similar techniques are now being evaluated with cardiac CT using iodinated contrast and multispectral techniques to accentuate the subtle myocardial enhancement resulting from delayed myocardial accumulation of iodine (Fig. 23.19). Early work comparing established cMRI delayed gadolinium enhancement sequences with dual-energy spectral CT with late iodine enhancement mapping and iodine quantification has shown promising results [73] with significant potential for clinical use as techniques mature.

Myocardial Perfusion Imaging

Imaging of myocardial perfusion using either single emission photon topography or positron emission tomography is an important means of assessing the myocardium and an emerging application for CT scanning. This topic is addressed in a chapter specifically dedicated to the topic.

Summary

Imaging the heart with CT presents unique challenges often extending CT capabilities to their limits in order to achieve diagnostic studies across a range of patients. Nevertheless, the technical developments that support cardiac scanning have been astounding, and cardiac CT techniques continue to improve resulting in a more reliable and safer diagnostic test for an ever-expanding range of clinical applications.

References

1. Blanke P, Schoepf UJ, Leipsic JA. CT in transcatheter aortic valve replacement. Radiology. 2013;269(3):650–69.
2. O'Brien JP, Srichai MB, Hecht EM, Kim DC, Jacobs JE. Anatomy of the heart at multidetector CT: what the radiologist needs to know. Radiographics. 2007;27(6):1569–82.
3. Villa AD, Sammut E, Nair A, Rajani R, Bonamini R, Chiribiri A. Coronary artery anomalies overview: the normal and the abnormal. World J Radiol. 2016;8(6):537–55.
4. Hood WB Jr. Regional venous drainage of the human heart. Br Heart J. BMJ Publishing Group. 1968;30(1):105.
5. Kligerman S. Imaging of pericardial disease. Radiol Clin N Am. 2019;57(1):179–99.
6. Mahesh M, Cody DD. Physics of cardiac imaging with multiple-row detector CT. pubsrsnaorg. 2007.
7. Boudoulas H, Geleris P, Lewis RP, Chest SR. Linear relationship between electrical systole, mechanical systole, and heart rate. CHEST. 1981;80:613–7.
8. Chung CS, Karamanoglu M, Kovács SJ. Duration of diastole and its phases as a function of heart rate during supine bicycle exercise. Am J Phys Heart Circ Phys. 2004;287(5):H2003–8.
9. Garner KK, Pomeroy W, Arnold JJ. Exercise stress testing: indications and common questions. Am Fam Physician. 2017;96(5):293–9.
10. Achenbach S. Cardiac CT: state of the art for the detection of coronary arterial stenosis. J Cardiovasc Comput Tomogr. 2007;1(1):3–20.
11. Rubin GD. Emerging and evolving roles for CT in screening for coronary heart disease. J Am Coll Radiol. 10(12):943–8.
12. Saini S, Rubin GD, Kalra MK. MDCT: a practical approach. New York: Springer Science & Business Media; 2007.
13. Rubin GD, Leipsic J, Joseph Schoepf U, Fleischmann D, Napel S. CT angiography after 20 years: a transformation in cardiovascular disease characterization continues to advance. Radiology. 2014;271(3):633–52.
14. Janowitz WR. Current status of mechanical computed tomography in cardiac imaging. Am J Cardiol. 2001;88(2A):35E–8E.
15. Funabashi N, Kobayashi Y, Perlroth M, Rubin GD. Coronary artery: quantitative evaluation of normal diameter determined with electron-beam CT compared with cine coronary angiography initial experience. Radiology. 2003;226(1):263–71.
16. Moshage WE, Achenbach S, Seese B, Bachmann K, Kirchgeorg M. Coronary artery stenoses: three-dimensional imaging with electrocardiographically triggered, contrast agent-enhanced, electron-beam CT. Radiology. 1995;196:707–14.
17. Stehli J, Fuchs TA, Bull S, Clerc OF, Possner M, Buechel RR, et al. Accuracy of coronary CT angiography using a submillisievert fraction of radiation exposure: comparison with invasive coronary angiography. J Am Coll Cardiol. 2014;64(8):772–80.
18. Bischoff B, Hein F, Meyer T, Hadamitzky M, Martinoff S, Schömig A, et al. Impact of a reduced tube voltage on CT angiography and radiation dose: results of the PROTECTION I study. JACC: Cardiovasc Imaging. 2009;2(8):940–6.
19. Rybicki FJ, Otero HJ, Steigner ML, Vorobiof G, Nallamshetty L, Mitsouras D, et al. Initial evaluation of coronary images from 320-detector row computed tomography. Int J Cardiovasc Imaging. 2008;24(5):535–46.
20. Flohr TG, McCollough CH, Bruder H, Petersilka M, Gruber K, Süβ C, et al. First performance evaluation of a dual-source CT (DSCT) system. Eur Radiol. 2005;16(2):256–68.
21. Gassenmaier T, Petri N, Allmendinger T, Flohr T, Weng AM, Kunz AS, et al. In vitro comparison of second- and third-generation dual-source CT for coronary stent visualization at different tube potentials. Acad Radiol. 2016;23(8):961–8.
22. Goldman LW. Principles of CT: multislice CT. J Nucl Med Technol. Society of Nuclear Medicine. 2008;36(2):57–68.
23. Lin E, Alessio A. What are the basic concepts of temporal, contrast, and spatial resolution in cardiac CT? J Cardiovasc Comput Tomogr. 2009;3(6):403–8.
24. Ghekiere O, Salgado R, Buls N, Leiner T, Mancini I, Vanhoenacker P, et al. Image quality in coronary CT angiography: challenges and technical solutions. Br J Radiol. 2nd ed. Br Inst Radiol. 2017;90(1072):20160567.
25. Kitagawa K, George RT, Arbab-Zadeh A, Lima JAC, Lardo AC. Characterization and correction of beam-hardening artifacts during dynamic volume CT assessment of myocardial perfusion1. Radiology. Radiological Society of North America, Inc. 2010.
26. Kalisz K, Buethe J, Saboo SS, Abbara S, Halliburton S, Rajiah P. Artifacts at cardiac CT: physics and solutions. Radiographics. 2016;36(7):2064–83.
27. Pannu HK, Alvarez W Jr, Fishman EK. β-Blockers for cardiac CT: a primer for the radiologist. Am J Roentgenol. 2006;186(6_supplement_2):S341–5.
28. Sabarudin A, Sun Z. Beta-blocker administration protocol for prospectively ECG triggered coronary CT angiography. WJC. 2013;5(12):453–7.
29. Sato K, Isobe S, Sugiura K, Mimura T, Yotsudake Y, Meno C, et al. Optimal starting time of acquisition and feasibility of complementary administration of nitroglycerin with intravenous β-blocker in multislice computed tomography. J Comput Assist Tomogr. 2009;33(2):193–8.
30. Earls JP. How to use a prospective gated technique for cardiac CT. J Cardiovasc Comput Tomogr.. Elsevier. 2009;3(1):45–51.
31. Hausleiter J, Meyer T, Hermann F, Hadamitzky M, Krebs M, Gerber TC, et al. Estimated radiation dose associated with cardiac CT angiography. JAMA. American Medical Association. 2009;301(5):500–7.

32. Petersilka M, Bruder H, Krauss B, Stierstorfer K, Flohr TG. Technical principles of dual source CT. Eur J Radiol. 2008;68(3):362–8.
33. Fan L, Zhang J, Xu D, Dong Z, Li X, Zhang L. CTCA image quality improvement by using snapshot freeze technique under prospective and retrospective electrocardiographic gating. J Comput Assist Tomogr. 2015;39(2):202–6.
34. Liang J, Wang H, Xu L, Dong L, Fan Z, Wang R, et al. Impact of SSF on diagnostic performance of coronary computed tomography angiography within 1 heart beat in patients with high heart rate using a 256-row detector computed tomography. J Comput Assist Tomogr. 2018;42(1):54–61.
35. Einstein AJ, Henzlova MJ, Rajagopalan S. Estimating risk of cancer associated with radiation exposure from 64-slice computed tomography coronary angiography. JAMA.. American Medical Association. 2007;298(3):317–23.
36. Brenner DJ, Hall EJ. Computed tomography – an increasing source of radiation exposure. N Engl J Med. 2007;357(22):2277–84.
37. Hirshfeld JW, Ferrari VA, Bengel FM, Bergersen L, Chambers CE, Einstein AJ, et al. 2018 ACC/HRS/NASCI/SCAI/SCCT expert consensus document on optimal use of ionizing radiation in cardiovascular imaging-best practices for safety and effectiveness, part 1: radiation physics and radiation biology: a report of the American College of Cardiology Task Force on expert consensus decision pathways developed in collaboration with mended hearts. Catheter Cardiovasc Interv. 2018;92(2):203–21.
38. Stocker TJ, Deseive S, Leipsic J, Chen MY, Rubinshtein R, Heckner M, et al. Reduction in radiation exposure in cardiovascular computed tomography imaging: results from the PROspective multicenter registry on radiaTion dose estimates of cardiac CT angIOgraphy iN daily practice in 2017 (PROTECTION VI). Eur Heart J. 2018;39(41):3715–23.
39. Huda W, Magill D, He W. CT effective dose per dose length product using ICRP 103 weighting factors. Med Phys. John Wiley & Sons, Ltd. 2011;38(3):1261–5.
40. Lira D, Padole A, Kalra MK, Singh S. Tube potential and CT radiation dose optimization. Am J Roentgenol. 2015;204(1):W4–W10.
41. Hausleiter J, Meyer TS, Martuscelli E, Spagnolo P, Yamamoto H, Carrascosa P, et al. Image quality and radiation exposure with prospectively ECG-triggered axial scanning for coronary CT angiography: the multicenter, multivendor, randomized PROTECTION-III study. JACC Cardiovasc Imaging. 2012;5(5):484–93.
42. Matsubara K, Kawashima H, Chusin T, Okubo R. How to optimize radiation dose in computed tomography examinations: available methods and techniques. Med Phys Int. 2017;5(2):498.
43. Deseive S, Pugliese F, Meave A, Alexanderson E, Martinoff S, Hadamitzky M, et al. Image quality and radiation dose of a prospectively electrocardiography-triggered high-pitch data acquisition strategy for coronary CT angiography: the multicenter, randomized PROTECTION IV study. J Cardiovasc Comput Tomogr. 2015;9(4):278–85.
44. Seppelt D, Kolb C, Kühn JP, Speiser U, Radosa CG, Hoberück S, et al. Comparison of sequential and high-pitch-spiral coronary CT-angiography: image quality and radiation exposure. Int J Cardiovasc Imaging. Springer Netherlands. 2019;132:1–8.
45. Schoepf UJ, editor. CT of the heart. Totowa: Humana Press; 2019.
46. Detrano R, Guerci AD, Carr JJ, Bild DE, Burke G, Folsom AR, et al. Coronary calcium as a predictor of coronary events in four racial or ethnic groups. N Engl J Med. 2008;358(13):1336–45.
47. McCollough CH, Ulzheimer S, Halliburton SS, Shanneik K, White RD, Kalender WA. Coronary artery calcium: a multi-institutional, multimanufacturer international standard for quantification at cardiac CT1. Radiology. Radiological Society of North America. 2007.
48. Raggi P. Coronary calcium is all we need for risk assessment, yet we do not use it often enough. Atherosclerosis. 2019;282:167–8.
49. Takx RAP, Suchá D, Park J, Leiner T, Hoffmann U. Sublingual nitroglycerin Administration in Coronary Computed Tomography Angiography: a systematic review. Eur Radiol. Springer Berlin Heidelberg. 2015;25(12):3536–42.
50. Cury RC, Abbara S, Achenbach S, Agatston A, Berman DS, Budoff MJ, et al. CAD-RADS™: coronary artery disease – reporting and data system: an expert consensus document of the Society of Cardiovascular Computed Tomography (SCCT), the American College of Radiology (ACR) and the North American Society for Cardiovascular Imaging (NASCI). Endorsed by the American College of Cardiology. JACR. Elsevier. 2016;13(12):1458–9.
51. Budoff MJ, Dowe D, Jollis JG, Gitter M, Sutherland J, Halamert E, et al. Diagnostic performance of 64-multidetector row coronary computed tomographic angiography for evaluation of coronary artery stenosis in individuals without known coronary artery disease: results from the prospective multicenter ACCURACY (assessment by coronary computed tomographic angiography of individuals undergoing invasive coronary angiography) trial. JAC J Am Coll Cardiol. 2008;52(21):1724–32.
52. Tonino PAL, De Bruyne B, Pijls NHJ, Siebert U, Ikeno F, vant Veer M, et al. Fractional flow reserve versus angiography for guiding percutaneous coronary intervention. N Engl J Med. 2009;360(3):213–24.
53. Xaplanteris P, Fournier S, Pijls NHJ, Fearon WF, Barbato E, Tonino PAL, et al. Five-year outcomes with PCI guided by fractional flow reserve. N Engl J Med. 2018;379(3):250–9.
54. Ko BS, Cameron JD, Munnur RK, Wong DTL, Fujisawa Y, Sakaguchi T, et al. Noninvasive CT-derived FFR based on structural and fluid analysis: a comparison with invasive FFR for detection of

functionally significant stenosis. JACC Cardiovasc Imaging. 2017;10(6):663–73.

55. Koo B-K, Erglis A, Doh J-H, Daniels DV, Jegere S, Kim H-S, et al. Diagnosis of ischemia-causing coronary stenoses by noninvasive fractional flow reserve computed from coronary computed tomographic angiograms: results from the prospective multicenter DISCOVER-FLOW (diagnosis of ischemia-causing stenoses obtained via noninvasive fractional flow reserve) study. JAC J Am Coll Cardiol. 2011;58(19):1989–97.
56. Fairbairn TA, Nieman K, Akasaka T, Nørgaard BL, Berman DS, Raff G, et al. Real-world clinical utility and impact on clinical decision-making of coronary computed tomography angiography-derived fractional flow reserve: lessons from the ADVANCE Registry. Eur Heart J. 2018;39(41):3701–11.
57. Nørgaard BL, Terkelsen CJ, Mathiassen ON, Grove EL, Bøtker HE, Parner E, et al. Coronary CT angiographic and flow reserve-guided management of patients with stable ischemic heart disease. JAC. Elsevier. 2018;72(18):2123–34.
58. Kitabata H, Leipsic J, Patel MR, Nieman K, De Bruyne B, Rogers C, et al. Incidence and predictors of lesion-specific ischemia by FFRCT: learnings from the international ADVANCE registry. J Cardiovasc Comput Tomogr. Elsevier. 2018;12(2):95–100.
59. Meijboom WB, Van Mieghem CAG, van Pelt N, Weustink A, Pugliese F, Mollet NR, et al. Comprehensive assessment of coronary artery stenoses: computed tomography coronary angiography versus conventional coronary angiography and correlation with fractional flow reserve in patients with stable angina. JAC. Elsevier. 2008;52(8):636–43.
60. Kim SY, Seo JB, Do K-H, Heo J-N, Lee JS, Song J-W, et al. Coronary artery anomalies: classification and ECG-gated multi–detector row CT findings with angiographic correlation. Radiographics. 2006;26(2):317–33.
61. Lee BY. Anomalous right coronary artery from the left coronary sinus with an interarterial course: is it really dangerous? Korean Circ J. 2009;39(5):175–9.
62. Cronin P, Sneider MB, Kazerooni EA, Kelly AM, Scharf C, Oral H, et al. MDCT of the left atrium and pulmonary veins in planning radiofrequency ablation for atrial fibrillation: a how-to guide. Am J Roentgenol. 2004;183(3):767–78.
63. Jarcho JA. Biventricular pacing. N Engl J Med. 2006;355(3):288–94.
64. León AR, Abraham WT, Curtis AB, Daubert JP, Fisher WG, Gurley J, et al. Safety of transvenous cardiac resynchronization system implantation in patients with chronic heart failure: combined results of over 2,000 patients from a multicenter study program. J Am Coll Cardiol. 2005;46(12):2348–56.
65. Smith CR, Leon MB, Mack MJ, Miller DC, Moses JW, Svensson LG, et al. Transcatheter versus surgical aortic-valve replacement in high-risk patients. N Engl J Med. 2011;364(23):2187–98.
66. Kamdar AR, Meadows TA, Roselli EE, Gorodeski EZ, Curtin RJ, Sabik JF, et al. Multidetector computed tomographic angiography in planning of reoperative cardiothoracic surgery. Ann Thorac Surg. 2008;85(4):1239–45.
67. Steinberg DH, Staubach S, Franke J, Sievert H. Defining structural heart disease in the adult patient: current scope, inherent challenges and future directions. Eur Heart J Suppl. 2010;12(Suppl E):E2–9.
68. Chu LC, Johnson PT, Fishman EK. Cardiac CT angiography beyond the coronary arteries: what radiologists need to know and why they need to know it. Am J Roentgenol. American Roentgen Ray Society. 2014.
69. Pham N, Zaitoun H, Mohammed TL, DeLaPena-Almaguer E, Martinez F, Novaro GM, et al. Complications of aortic valve surgery: manifestations at CT and MR imaging. Radiographics. 2012;32(7):1873–92.
70. Wells JA, Condado JF, Kamioka N, Dong A, Ritter A, Lerakis S, et al. Outcomes after paravalvular leak closure: transcatheter versus surgical approaches. JACC Cardiovasc Interv. 2017;10(5):500–7.
71. Wagner A, Mahrholdt H, Holly TA, Elliott MD, Regenfus M, Parker M, et al. Contrast-enhanced MRI and routine single photon emission computed tomography (SPECT) perfusion imaging for detection of subendocardial myocardial infarcts: an imaging study. Lancet. 2003;361(9355):374–9.
72. Kim RJ, Wu E, Rafael A, Chen EL, Parker MA, Simonetti O, et al. The use of contrast-enhanced magnetic resonance imaging to identify reversible myocardial dysfunction. N Engl J Med. 2000;343(20):1445–53.
73. Bouleti C, Baudry G, Lung B, Arangalage D, Abtan J, Ducrocq G, et al. Usefulness of late iodine enhancement on spectral CT in acute myocarditis. JACC Cardiovasc Imaging. American College of Cardiology Foundation. 2017;10(7):826–7.
74. Bazan O, Ortiz JP. Duration of systole and diastole for hydrodynamic testing of prosthetic heart valves: comparison between ISO 5840 standards and in vivo studies. Braz J Cardiovasc Surg. 2016;31(2):171–3. https://doi.org/10.5935/1678-9741.20160036.

Index

© Springer Nature Switzerland AG 2020
E. Samei, N. J. Pelc (eds.), *Computed Tomography*, https://doi.org/10.1007/978-3-030-26957-9

The manufacturer's authorised representative in the EU is Springer
Nature Customer Service Centre GmbH, Europaplatz 3, 69115 Heidelberg,
Germany. If you have any concerns regarding our products, please
contact ProductSafety@springernature.com

Printed and bound by CPI Group (UK) Ltd, Croydon, CR0 4YY
12/08/2026
02194530-0001